DEVELOPMENTAL ENDOCRINOLOGY

CONTEMPORARY ENDOCRINOLOGY

P. Michael Conn, *SERIES EDITOR*

DEVELOPMENTAL ENDOCRINOLOGY

FROM RESEARCH TO CLINICAL PRACTICE

Edited by

ERICA A. EUGSTER, MD

Riley Hospital for Children,
Indiana University School of Medicine,
Indianapolis, IN

ORA HIRSCH PESCOVITZ, MD

Riley Hospital for Children,
Indiana University School of Medicine,
Indianapolis, IN

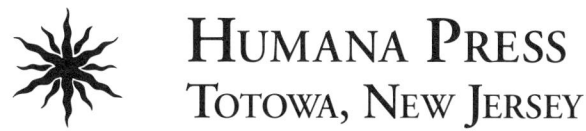

HUMANA PRESS
TOTOWA, NEW JERSEY

© 2002 Humana Press Inc.
999 Riverview Drive, Suite 208
Totowa, New Jersey 07512

www.humanapress.com

For additional copies, pricing for bulk purchases, and/or information about other Humana titles, contact Humana at the above address or at any of the following numbers: Tel: 973-256-1699; Fax: 973-256-8341; E-mail: humana@humanapr.com or visit our website at http://humanapress.com

This publication is printed on acid-free paper. ∞
ANSI Z39.48-1984 (American National Standards Institute)
Permanence of Paper for Printed Library Materials.

Production Editor: Mark J. Breaugh.

Cover Design by Patricia F. Cleary.

Printed in the United States of America. 10 9 8 7 6 5 4 3 2 1
Library of Congress Cataloging-in-Publication Data

Developmental Endocrinology : from research to clinical practice / edited by Erica A. Eugster, Ora Hirsch Pescovitz.
    p. cm. -- (Contemporary endocrinology)
  Includes bibliographical references and index.
  ISBN 0-89603-860-2 (alk. paper)
  1. Endocrinology, Developmental. I. Eugster, Erica A. II. Pescovitz, Ora Hirsch. III. Contemporary endocrinology (Totowa, N.J.)

QP187.6 .D484 2002
612'4--dc 21

2001051948

Preface

From the complex molecular control of endocrine cell differentiation to the amazing physiology of normal growth and puberty, developmental processes represent an integral and recurrent theme within the field of Endocrinology. Our goal in the creation of this book was to incorporate the latest scientific information regarding the development of endocrine systems into a larger context in which molecular genetics is combined with state-of-the-art understanding of endocrine physiology and optimal management of endocrine diseases. Each section is organized according to the chronologic development of the human organism, from the fetal/prenatal period through childhood, adolescence, and in some cases, into adulthood. In parallel with this sequence is a consistent progression of topics, which begins with a focus on molecular genetic aspects of endocrine development and concludes with chapters devoted to the diagnosis and treatment of endocrine disorders. Our hope is that the material contained herein will provide critical information for basic researchers regarding clinical applications of laboratory investigation, and will likewise benefit practitioners by elucidating the underlying pathophysiology of the many endocrinopathies encountered in the clinical setting. Ultimately, we aim to promote the collaborative translational efforts that are essential to the dual objectives of advancing knowledge of human biology and improving our ability to care for our patients. We wish to thank our authors for their invaluable contributions to this project. Lastly, this book is dedicated with utmost love and gratitude to our husbands and to our children, Aliza, Alex, Ari, Ariana, Naomi, Sophia, and Lydia: May you always follow your dreams!

Erica A. Eugster, MD
Ora Hirsch Pescovitz, MD

CONTENTS

CONTRIBUTORS

SHERI A. BERENBAUM, PhD, *Department of Psychology, Pennsylvania State University, University Park, PA*

GEORGE P. CHROUSOS, MD, *Pediatric and Reproductive Endocrinology Branch, National Institute of Child Health and Human Development, National Institutes of Health, Bethesda, MD*

JOAN DiMARTINO-NARDI, MD, *Division of Pediatric Endocrinology, Montefiore Medical Center, Bronx, NY*

LINDA ANNE DiMEGLIO, MD, *Section of Pediatric Endocrinology and Diabetology, James Whitcomb Riley Hospital for Children, Indiana University School of Medicine, Indianapolis, IN*

JAMES W. EDMONDSON, MD, *Section of Endocrinology, Indiana University, Indianapolis, IN*

ERICA A. EUGSTER, MD, *Section of Pediatric Endocrinology and Diabetology, James Whitcomb Riley Hospital for Children, Indiana University School of Medicine, Indianapolis, IN*

DELBERT A. FISHER, MD, *Quest Diagnostic Nichols Institute, San Juan Capistrano, CA*

LORRAINE A. FITZPATRICK, MD, *Division of Endocrinology, Metabolism and Nutrition, Mayo Clinic and Mayo Foundation, Rochester, MN*

JOHN S. FUQUA, MD, *Section of Pediatric Endocrinology and Diabetology, James Whitcomb Riley Hospital for Children, Indiana University School of Medicine, Indianapolis, IN*

ZEHRA HAIDER, MD, *Section of Endocrinology, Indiana University, Indianapolis, IN*

TAMARA S. HANNON, MD, *Section of Pediatric Endocrinology and Diabetology, James Whitcomb Riley Hospital for Children, Indiana University School of Medicine, Indianapolis, IN*

HELEN H. KIM, MD, *Department of Obstetrics and Gynecology and Section of Pediatric Endocrinology, The University of Chicago Children's Hospital, Chicago, IL*

ZVI LARON, MD, *Endocrinology and Diabetes Research Unit, Schneider Children's Medical Center, Tel Aviv University, Tel Aviv, Israel*

MICHAEL A. LEVINE, MD, *Division of Pediatric Endocrinology, Johns Hopkins School of Medicine, Baltimore, MD*

ANDREW N. MARGIORIS, MD, *Department of Clinical Chemistry, University of Crete School of Medicine, Crete, Greece*

SALVATORE MINISOLA, MD, *Dipartimento di Scienze Cliniche, Università degli Studi di Roma "La Sapienza", Rome, Italy*

GRETCHEN E. PARKER, PhD, *Department of Biology, Indiana University-Purdue University, Indianapolis, IN*

ORA HIRSCH PESCOVITZ, MD, *Section of Pediatric Endocrinology and Diabetology, James Whitcomb Riley Hospital for Children, Indiana University School of Medicine, Indianapolis, IN*

SALLY RADOVICK, MD, *Section of Pediatric Endocrinology, The University of Chicago Children's Hospital, Chicago, IL*

SIMON J. RHODES, PhD, *Department of Biology, Indiana University-Purdue University, Indianapolis, IN*

SCOTT A. RIVKEES, MD, *Section of Pediatric Endocrinology, Yale University, New Haven, CT*

KYLE W. SLOOP, PhD, *Department of Biology, Indiana University-Purdue University, Indianapolis, IN*

DIANE E. J. STAFFORD, MD, *Department of Obstetrics and Gynecology and Section of Pediatric Endocrinology, The University of Chicago Children's Hospital, Chicago, IL*

SOPHIA P. TSAKIRI, MD, *Department of Pediatrics, Venizelion Hospital, Heraklien, Crete, Greece*

GUY VAN VLIET, MD, *Endocrinology Service, Sainte-Justine Hospital; Department of Pediatrics, University of Montreal, Montréal, Quebec, Canada*

STEVEN G. WAGUESPACK, MD, *Sections of Pediatric Endocrinology and Diabetology and Endocrinology, Indiana University School of Medicine, Indianapolis, IN*

EMILY C. WALVOORD, MD, *Section of Pediatric Endocrinology and Diabetology, James Whitcomb Riley Hospital for Children, Indiana University School of Medicine, Indianapolis, IN*

PERRIN C. WHITE, MD, *Division of Pediatric Endocrinology, University of Texas Southwestern Medical Center, Dallas, TX*

ANDREW WOLFE, PhD, *Department of Obstetrics and Gynecology and Section of Pediatric Endocrinology, The University of Chicago Children's Hospital, Chicago, IL*

MARJORIE ZAKARIA, MD, *Department of Obstetrics and Gynecology and Section of Pediatric Endocrinology, The University of Chicago Children's Hospital, Chicago, IL*

I HYPOTHALAMUS/PITUITARY

1

Transcriptional Control of the Development and Function of the Hypothalamic-Pituitary Axis

Gretchen E. Parker, PhD, Kyle W. Sloop, PhD, and Simon J. Rhodes, PhD

CONTENTS

INTRODUCTION

Function of the Hypothalamic-Pituitary Axes and Their Hormone Products

The hypothalamic-pituitary (H-P) axis regulates many aspects of mammalian endocrine physiology by the controlled secretion of hormones. The hypothalamus is part of the diencephalon at the base of the brain beneath the third ventricle (*1*). It is physically located posterior to the optic chiasm and rostral to the mammillary bodies. The pituitary gland (or hypophysis) is a small organ located beneath the hypothalamus that weighs about 0.5 g in humans (*2*). The posterior pituitary lobe (or neurohypophysis or pars nervosa) develops directly from the brain (*see* below) and is connected to the hypothalamus by the infundibulum (or pituitary stalk). The anterior lobe (or adenohypophysis or

From: *Contemporary Endocrinology: Developmental Endocrinology: From Research to Clinical Practice*
Edited by: E. A. Eugster and O. H. Pescovitz © Humana Press Inc., Totowa, NJ

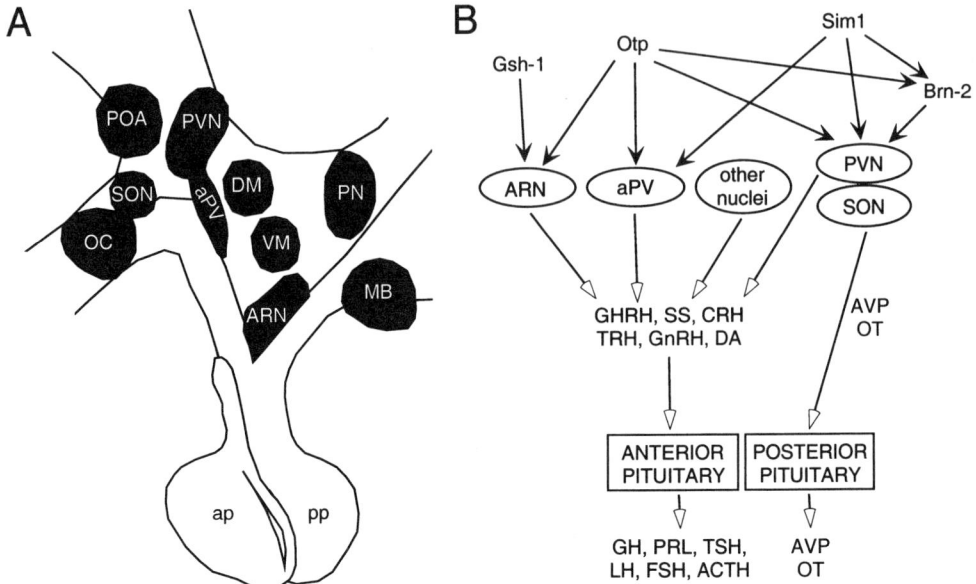

Fig. 1. Development of the hormone-secreting cell types of the hypothalamus. (**A**) Schematic diagram of a sagittal section of the ventral diencephalon region of the brain. Hypothalamic nuclei are shaded in black. POA, preoptic area; SON, supraoptic nucleus; OC, optic chiasm; PVN, paraventricular nucleus; aPV, anterior periventrucular nucleus; DM, dorsomedial nucleus; VM, ventromedial nucleus; ARN, arcuate nucleus; PN, posterior nucleus; MB, mammillary body; ap, anterior pituitary; pp, posterior pituitary. (**B**) The development of hypothalamic nuclei is dependent on the actions of the indicated transcription factors. Neurons in the differentiated nuclei then secrete the indicated hormones.

pars distalis) and intermediate lobe (or pars intermedia) of the pituitary have distinct embryological origins. In the mature gland, these structures are fused to the posterior pituitary, and some cells of the anterior pituitary proliferate up and around the pituitary stalk to form the pars tuberalis. The intermediate lobe is a poorly developed structure in adult humans and is absent in birds *(2)*. A vascular link called the portal system arises from the median eminence at the base of the hypothalamus and provides a connection for the passage of neurosecretory hormones from the hypothalamus to the anterior pituitary gland.

THE HYPOTHALAMUS

The hypothalamus can be subdivided into three groups of nuclei of neural cells: the supraoptic group, the tuberal (or middle) group, and the mammillary (or posterior) group of nuclei. Within the supraoptic group, the paraventricular (PVN) and supraoptic (SON) nuclei project their axons to the posterior lobe of the pituitary as the hypothalamic-hypophyseal tract (Fig. 1). Together, the large, highly vascularized cells of the PVN and SON are termed the magnocellular secretory system. These cells produce arginine vasopressin (AVP, also called antidiuretic hormone), and oxytocin (OT). OT and AVP are peptide hormones that are packaged in vesicles and then transported to the posterior pituitary for release. In the kidney, AVP promotes water retention; within the vasculature and heart, it activates blood pressure-sensitive receptors; and in the liver, it has glycogenolytic effects. Other actions of AVP include regulation of the secretion of pituitary hormones such as adrenocorticotropin (ACTH). OT induces uterine contraction during the later stages of pregnancy and promotes milk ejection during suckling. OT also has been proposed to have roles in mating and maternal behavior. Within the PVN, smaller cells form the parvocellular neurosecretory system. This system delivers neurohormones via the hypophyseal-portal system to control anterior pituitary function. Parvocellular neurons positioned in the PVN secrete corticotropin-releasing hormone (CRH), gonadotropin-releasing hormone (GnRH or LHRH), and thyrotropin-releasing hormone (TRH), which regulate pituitary corticotropes, gonadotropes, and thyrotropes, respectively. Other signaling molecules released by the parvocellular system into the median eminence include dopamine (DA), which acts at the pituitary as a prolactin (PRL) inhibitory factor.

The tuberal group of hypothalamic nuclei includes the ventromedial (VM), dorsomedial (DM), and arcuate (ARN) nuclei (Fig. 1). These nuclei also are important in pituitary regulation. Somatostatin (SS, or growth hormone-inhibiting hormone) and growth hormone-releasing hormone (GHRH, or growth hormone-releasing factor) are synthesized and released from the ARN. The ARN also is an autonomous generator of reproductive timing and rhythms.

The mammillary group of nuclei is less well-defined in their nuclear structure. Neurons in this region produce neurotransmitters such as gamma-aminobutyric acid, histamine, and also neuropeptides such as galanin, which has many roles within the body, including modulation of pituitary lactotrope function *(3)*.

THE PITUITARY GLAND

The pituitary gland secretes polypeptide hormones that regulate physiological functions including growth, the stress response, reproductive activity, metabolism, and lactation. The anterior pituitary hormones are released from five distinct cell types, and these peptide or protein hormones serve as characteristic, defining markers for each cell type (Fig. 2). The five cell types (and their respective hormone products) are corticotropes (producing ACTH by proteolytic processing of the product of the *proopiomelanocortin* [*POMC*] gene); gonadotropes (follicle-stimulating hormone [FSH] and luteinizing hormone [LH]); thyrotropes (thyroid-stimulating hormone [TSH]); somatotropes (growth hormone [GH]); and lactotropes (PRL). FSH, LH, and TSH are polypeptide heterodimers consisting of a common subunit, alpha glycoprotein (αGSU), and a distinct β subunit (FSHβ, LHβ, TSHβ). The anterior/intermediate pituitary also contains nonhormone-secreting cells known as folliculo-stellate cells that have glial-like properties *(4)*. The function and developmental origin of these cells is unclear, but some studies suggest that they arise in the region of Rathke's pouch (the primordial structure of the anterior/intermediate pituitary) closest to the posterior lobe *(5)*. In the intermediate pituitary, melanotrope cells secrete alpha-melanocyte stimulating hormone (α-MSH). As described earlier, the posterior lobe of the pituitary receives the peptide hormones AVP and OT directly from hypothalamic nuclei of the axons of the hypothalamic-hypophyseal tract. In addition, the posterior lobe contains modified glial cells known as pituicytes (reviewed in ref. *6*).

Embryology of the Hypothalamus-Pituitary Axis

The developmental programs that guide organogenesis of the hypothalamus and pituitary are highly interdependent processes. Inductive signals pass between the two developing structures, and these signals prime the transcriptional cascades that subsequently

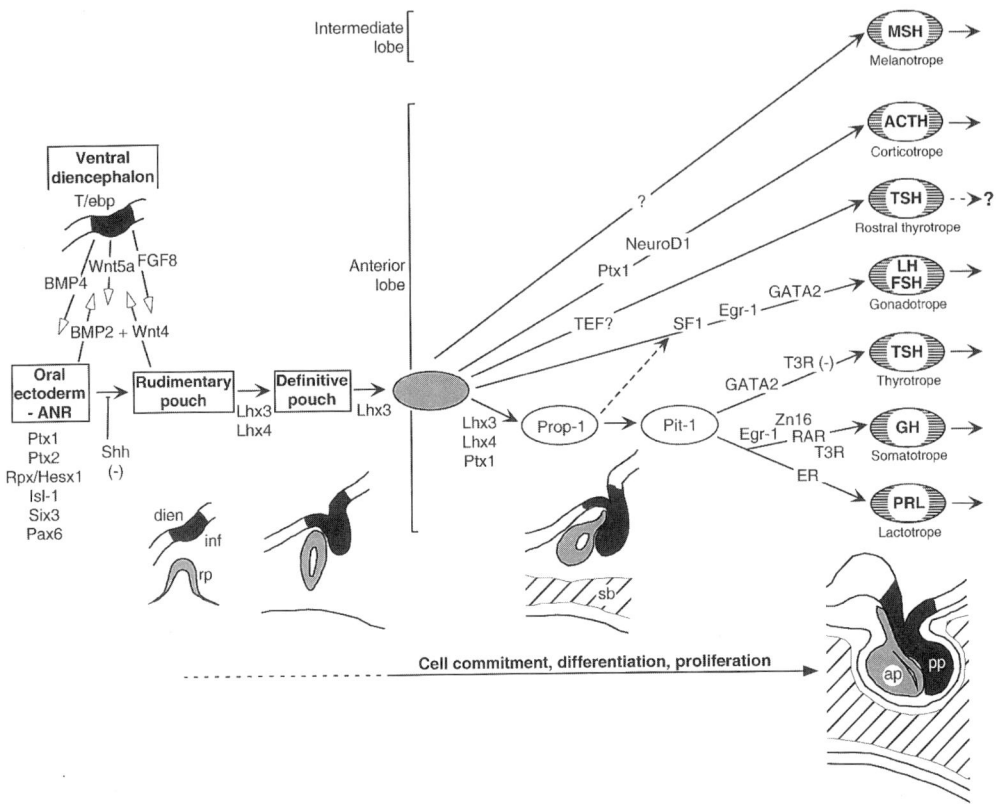

Fig. 2. Development of the hormone-secreting cell types of the mammalian pituitary gland. The pituitary arises as a result of interactions between the infundibulum (inf), a process of the ventral diencephalon (dien), and Rathke's pouch (rp). Rathke's pouch arises from the oral ectoderm at the most anterior end of the anterior neural ridge (ANR) and eventually is separated from the oral cavity by the developing sphenoid bone (sb). Pouch development occurs in distinct steps: first a rudimentary pouch is formed, followed by the establishment of the definitive pouch. Transcription factors and secreted protein signaling molecules that are important in development of the differentiated cell types of the anterior (ap) and intermediate lobes of the pituitary (the derivatives of Rathke's pouch) are shown. In the anatomical drawings Rathke's pouch and its derivatives are lightly shaded. The infundibulum and the resulting posterior pituitary (pp) are darkly shaded.

control specification of cell types within the two organs (*see Transcriptional Regulation of Endocrine Hypothalamus Development*). In humans, the hypothalamus is the first region of the brain to differentiate *(7)*. The hypothalamus is neuroectodermal in origin and develops from the floor of the diencephalon. By the 6th wk of human development, characteristic nuclei of the hypothalamus and the mammillary bodies can be discerned *(7)*.

In contrast to the hypothalamus, the mature pituitary gland is a composite organ. Like other endocrine glands, such as the adrenals and the thyroid, the tissues of the anterior/intermediate and posterior lobes have distinct embryological origins. The posterior pituitary lobe is neuroectodermal in origin and originates from the base of the diencephalon as an extension of the infundibulum (Fig. 2). The anterior and intermediate lobes arise from a pocket known as Rathke's pouch that develops in the roof of the stomodeum, the primitive oral cavity *(8)*. Rathke's pouch is conventionally described as being derived from the oral ectoderm *(8)*. Some studies, however, indicate that the endocrine cells of the eventual anterior/intermediate pituitary are committed very early during embryogenesis as part of the anterior neural ridge (ANR) of the neural plate *(7,9–17)*. Rathke's pouch can be clearly observed by the 4th wk of human gestation (corresponding to approx embryonic days 2, 9, and 11 of chick, mouse, and rat development, respectively [*7,17 18*]). The diverticulum of the diencephalon that becomes the infundibulum becomes distinct at about the 6th wk of human development *(18)*. After contacting the diencephalon, the pouch gradually moves in a caudal direction *(18)*. The pouch then is surrounded by proliferating mesodermal tissue and pinches off from the oral cavity after the 7th wk and associates with the developing posterior lobe *(18)*. The pituitary is morphologically developed by about the 13th wk of human development *(18)*. The order of the appearance of the hormone-secreting cell types of the anterior pituitary is similar in most mammals, including humans, rodents (reviewed in refs. *19,20*), and swine (*see* ref. *21*, and references therein). In humans, ACTH- and TSHβ-secreting cells can be detected by the 9th wk of gestation, followed by the appearance of GH- and FSHβ-positive cells by 13 wk, and the observation of LHβ- and PRL-containing cells by the 21st wk of pregnancy *(7,18)*.

Experiments using amphibian, chick, and rodent tissues indicate that the cell-cell contact relationship between the infundibulum (ventral diencephalon) and the developing Rathke's pouch is critical to correct pituitary-cell differentiation *(22–26)*. Similar inductive processes are found in the development of other embryonic structures such as during lens formation in the developing eye (reviewed in ref. *27*). Recent studies have begun to delineate the extrinsic and intrinsic signaling events that coordinate the earliest stages of pituitary organogenesis *(28–32)*. Protein signaling molecules such as bone morphogenetic protein 4 (BMP4), Wnt5a, and fibroblast growth factor 8 (FGF8) are expressed in the ventral diencephalon and exert important effects on the ectodermal tissue of Rathke's pouch (Fig. 2 and *see* p. 25). Sonic hedgehog (Shh) appears to be a boundary signal: it is expressed in the oral ectoderm but is excluded from the region from which Rathke's pouch originates *(29)*. Within the developing pouch, BMP2 and Wnt4 are crucial intrinsic signals that guide the ordered, positional development of pituitary cell types *(29,31,32)*. Studies of anencephalic human fetuses (which lack the hypothalamus) demonstrate the importance of brain-derived signals for the development of corticotropes, gonadotropes, and somatotropes, but also suggest that some of the other pituitary cell types can differentiate in the absence of the brain *(33–35)*.

During rodent embryogenesis, protein signaling pathways promote the development of Rathke's pouch-derived pituitary cell types in a distinct stratified pattern *(31,32)*. The dorsal side of Rathke's pouch becomes the intermediate pituitary lobe that contains the melanotropes. The anterior lobe develops by the proliferation and differentiation of the cells of the most ventral side of the pouch. In the developing anterior lobe, the gonadotropes form closest to the ventral BMP2 signal; thyrotropes arise in the central part of the lobe; and somatotropes and lactotropes (which have a common precursor; *see* Fig. 2) emerge in the most dorsal side of the anterior lobe *(31,32)*. The corticotropes also are located on the dorsal side of the anterior lobe portion of the developing gland but are concentrated towards the rostral tip *(31,32)*. A transient population of thyrotropes, known as the rostral thyrotropes, is found in the rostral region of the developing anterior lobe (*36*; Fig. 2; and *see* p. 17). It is interesting to note that the stratification of the secretory cells of the embryonic anterior lobe does not persist in most adult mammalian pituitaries: in the mature gland the cells are mostly homogeneously mixed *(2)*. By contrast, individual cell types are located in distinct zones in the pituitary glands of amphibians, birds, reptiles, and in many teleost fish *(2)*.

Over the past 12 yr, many gene regulatory proteins (transcription factors) that are important in the development of H-P endocrine tissues have been identified. The role of gene regulation in the development of the anterior pituitary has been intensively studied. The development of the five physiologically important anterior cell types in a precise order from a common origin (Fig. 2) make the anterior pituitary an excellent model system for the analysis of the transcriptional mechanisms that regulate the commitment and subsequent differentiation of specific phenotypes during mammalian organogenesis. Recently, however, transcription factors with roles in hypothalamic development have been identified and studied. This article is intended to provide an introduction to the H-P developmental transcription factors and to discuss their functions, control mechanisms, and involvement in human endocrine diseases.

TRANSCRIPTIONAL REGULATION
OF ENDOCRINE HYPOTHALAMUS DEVELOPMENT

Table 1 lists the properties of transcription factors that have been demonstrated to play roles in hypothalamic development. Some of these factors also are discussed in more detail below.

Thyroid-Specific Enhancer-Binding Protein

Thyroid-specific enhancer-binding protein (T/ebp, also known as TTF-1/Titf1/Nkx2.1) is a Nk-2 class homeodomain transcription factor that originally was identified as a regulator of thyroid gland development and later demonstrated to be an important transcription factor in the lung (*see* ref. *55*, and references therein). Recent analyses of mice with disrupted *T/ebp* genes have demonstrated the importance of this factor in hypothalamic development and have revealed signaling relationships between the hypothalamus and the primordial pituitary gland. Whereas *T/ebp* heterozygous mice develop normally, mice with ablated *T/ebp* genes are stillborn, lack lung parenchyma, and have no thyroid gland *(55)*. In addition, these mice lack the ARN, and the mammillary body and supramammillary nucleus of the posterior hypothalamus. Further, the entire pituitary gland is missing *(55)*. This result was unanticipated because T/ebp is not expressed in the developing anterior pituitary *(55)*. However, the diencephalon, which expresses T/ebp during development, is misformed in these animals, and recent experiments have demonstrated that expression of T/ebp is required for the hypothalamic production of FGF8, an essential early signal in pituitary-gland induction *(28)*. These studies illustrate the importance of T/ebp and the diencephalon in the development of Rathke's pouch. The related *Nkx2.2* and *Dlx* genes also are expressed in the developing hypothalamus, suggesting that this class of homeodomain genes is important in the differentiation of cells within this tissue *(56)*.

POU Domain Transcription Factors

The POU domain class of transcriptional regulatory proteins was named for its original members: Pit-1, Oct-1/2, and the *C. elegans* factor unc-86 (reviewed in ref. *57*). POU proteins are a subfamily of the homeodomain superfamily of transcription factors and contain a structurally related DNA binding domain, known as the POU domain. The POU

Table 1

Transcription Factors Important in Development of the Mammalian Hypothalamus

Factor	Class	Mutant phenotype/Expression pattern	References
Brn-2	POU-HD	Lethal; PVN, SON affected–loss of AVP, OT, CRH	37,38
c-Ets-1	Ets	Expressed during angiogenesis in H-P development	39
DAX-1	Nuclear receptor-like	Sex-reversal; congenital adrenal hypoplasia and hypogonadotropic hypogonadism. Expressed in developing hypothalamus.	40–43
Gsh-1	HD	Dwarfed, sexually infantile, absence of GHRH in arcuate nucleus	44
Mf3 (Fkh5/Hfh-e5.1)	Winged helix/forkhead	Variable phenotype–some lethality. Growth defects, unable to eject milk.	45
Nhlh2 (NSCL2)	bHLH	Hypogonadal, progressive obesity; male infertility	46
Otp	Paired-like HD	PVN, SON, aPV, ARN affected–loss of TRH, CRH, SS, OT, AVP	47
SF-1 (Ad4BP/*FtzF1*)	Nuclear receptor	Lethal; lack adrenals and gonads. Hypothalamus and pituitary defects. Sex reversal in humans.	48–51
Sim1	bHLH PAS	Lethal; PVN, SON, aPV affected–loss of AVP, OT, TRH, SS, CRH Loss of Brn-2	52
Six3	HD	Human patients with mutations have holoprosencephaly Expressed in anterior neural plate	53,54
T/ebp (Ttf-1/Titf1/Nkx2.1)	NK-2 HD	Lethal; lack lung parenchyma, thyroid, pituitary. Lack premammillary, ARN, mammillary body, supramammillary nuclei of hypothalamus	55

HD, homeodomain; bHLH, basic helix-loop-helix.

9

domain is a bipartite DNA-interacting structure consisting of the POU-specific domain joined by a linker region to a homeodomain, the POU homeodomain. The POU-specific domain adopts a helical structure reminiscent of the lambda and 434 bacteriophage repressor molecules, and the POU homeodomain is configured in a helix-turn-helix structure that is similar to classical homeodomains such as those within the *Drosophila* engrailed and antennapedia proteins *(58)*. The POU proteins form a large family of conserved factors that have been demonstrated to play critical roles in the development of many tissues. They are classified into subgroups based on their structural properties *(59)*.

BRN-2

Brn-2 is a class III POU domain transcription factor. This class of POU proteins is expressed predominantly in the central nervous system (CNS). *Brn-2* gene knockout mice die within 10 d of birth and lack expression of AVP, OT, and CRH in the PVN and SON of the hypothalamus *(37,38)*. These data imply that Brn-2 is necessary for the terminal differentiation and/or survival of magnocellar neurosecretory and parvocellar neurons of the PVN and SON. In the absence of *Brn-2* gene function, the posterior pituitary develops normally at first, but later, the pituicytes disappear, and there is a complete loss of the posterior lobe, suggesting that magnocellar axons produce trophic factors needed for pituicyte development *(37,38)*. The anterior and intermediate pituitary lobes of the *Brn-2* null mouse form normally, implying that the signals required for the proper development of these structures arise from the undifferentiated diencephalon and not the terminally differentiated cells of the hypothalamus. *Brn-2* heterozygotes are anatomically normal but express half of the normal levels of AVP, OT, and CRH, suggesting that Brn-2 may regulate expression of these genes *(37,38*; Fig. 1).

OTHER POU PROTEINS

Oct-2, a POU protein first described in the hematopoietic system, may be important in the hypothalamic neuroendocrine tissues as a regulator of puberty through activation of the *transforming growth factor-alpha* (*TGF-α*) gene *(60)*. Another POU factor, Tst-1/ Oct-6/SCIP, which is known to be required for peripheral nerve-cell differentiation myelination, recently has been shown to be a repressor of the *GnRH* gene promoter *(61)*. Tst-1, therefore, may play a role in the control of GnRH neuron activity.

Single-Minded

Several orthologs of the *Drosophila single-minded* gene have been described in mammals. These include *Sim1,* a gene that encodes Sim1, a basic helix-loop-helix (bHLH)-PAS transcription factor expressed during development in the PVN, SON, and anterior periventricular (aPV) nuclei of the hypothalamus *(52)*. Mice with deleted *Sim1* genes die shortly after birth and lack OT, AVP, TRH, CRH, and SS production in the developing PVN, SON, and aPV nuclei *(52)*. Further, these nuclei gradually lose expression of *Brn-2*, implying that *Sim1* functions upstream of *Brn-2*, which subsequently directs the terminal differentiation of neuroendocrine lineages within the hypothalamus (*52*; Fig. 1).

Orthopedia

Orthopedia (Otp), a homeodomain transcription factor, is expressed in neurons that give rise to the PVN, SON, aPV, and ARN hypothalamic nuclei *(47)*. Except in the ARN, *Otp* is temporally and spatially co-expressed with *Sim1*. Mice lacking the *Otp* gene die soon after birth and have reduced neuroendocrine cell proliferation and migration *(47)*. In these mutants, the parvocellular and magnocellular neurons of the PVN, SON, aPV, and ARN fail to terminally differentiate: axonal outgrowth is absent, and *TRH, CRH, SS, OT,* and *AVP* transcription does not occur *(47)*. As in the *Sim1* mutant, the Otp mutant animals gradually lose expression of Brn-2, which implies that both genes are important in control of the *Brn-2* gene (Fig. 1). These data, together with the studies described earlier, suggest that the aPV, PVN, and SON cell types are controlled developmentally by Otp, Brn-2, and Sim1. In addition, Otp also regulates development of the ARN.

Gsh-1

Gsh-1 is a homeobox gene that is expressed in the neural tube, hindbrain, telencephalon, mesencephalon, and diencephalon of the embryonic CNS *(62)*. Homozygous *Gsh-1* mutant mice display hypothalamic defects that cause secondary pituitary disease *(44)*. The mutants have hypoplastic pituitaries and are dwarfed, sexually infantile, and short-lived. Pituitary GH, PRL, and LH levels are reduced. Gsh-1 appears to be essential for *GHRH* gene expression in the ARN of the hypothalamus and binds to elements within the *GHRH* promoter (*44*; Fig. 1). Cell lines derived from *Gsh-1 -/-* hypothalamus tissue have been used as tools to probe DNA arrays and identify potential target genes of Gsh-1 *(63)*.

Nhlh2

Nhlh2 (NSCL2) is a bHLH transcription factor expressed in the developing hypothalamus and in the embryonic and adult pituitary gland *(46)*. *Nhlh2* knockout male mice are hypogonadal, infertile, have decreased levels of FSH and testosterone, have defects in spermatogenesis, and feature loss of sexual behavior *(46)*. Mutant females also are hypogonadal, but their reproductive systems do develop, and the mice are fertile after exposure to males. Both sexes of *Nhlh2* mutant mice have progressive adult obesity. Therefore, *Nhlh2* expression appears to be required at multiple levels of the H-P axes with important roles in the onset of puberty and the regulation of body-weight metabolism. Transgenic mouse experiments involving misexpression of the closely related bHLH factor, NSCL1, result in abnormal brain development *(64)*, suggesting that other members of this class of proteins also are important in brain embryogenesis.

Steroidogenic Factor-1

Steroidogenic factor-1 (SF-1, also known as Adrenal 4-binding protein) is encoded by the *Ftz-F1* gene *(65)*. SF-1 is an orphan nuclear receptor transcription factor that is expressed during development in the ventral diencephalon and in adrenal and gonadal tissues. *Ftz-F1* null mice die by postnatal day 8 and lack adrenals and gonads *(48)*. The mutant mice also exhibit altered structure of the VM nucleus of the hypothalamus *(66)*. In addition, SF-1 mutants lack pituitary gonadotropins *(49)*, and SF-1 has been demonstrated to be an activator of the αGSU gene promoter *(49,67)*. SF-1, therefore, is required for the development of steroidogenic organs and for all levels of the reproductive axis formation. A recent report has described a mutation of the human *FTZ-F1* gene that causes XY sex reversal and adrenal failure *(51)*. The actions of SF-1 and of other transcription factors important in sex determination, such as Dax-1 (*see* below) and Wilm's tumor 1 (WT1), appear to be functionally interdependent *(68,69)*.

DAX-1

The *DAX-1* gene encodes a nuclear receptor-related protein and is located in the dosage sensitive sex reversal (DSS) region of the X chromosome (*see* ref. *43*, and references therein). *DAX-1* may serve as an "antitestis" gene because XY patients with DSS region duplications exhibit male-to-female sex reversal *(43)*. Human patients with *DAX-1* gene mutations also may develop X-linked congenital adrenal hypoplasia and hypogonado-tropic hypogonadism *(40,41,70)*. In mice, *Dax-1* is expressed during adrenal and gonadal differentiation and in the developing hypothalamus, suggesting a regulatory role in these tissues *(42)*.

Mf3

The *Mf3* gene, which encodes a winged helix/forkhead transcription factor also known as Fkh5/HFH-e5.1, is expressed in the developing hypothalamus. Mice lacking the *Mf3* gene have variable phenotypes, suggesting that the gene may be necessary at several stages of embryonic and postnatal development *(45)*. Some mutant embryos have an open neural tube in the diencephalon and midbrain region and die *in utero*; others display a severe reduction of the posterior body axis and also die *in utero*. Surviving mutants have a normal phenotype at birth but postnatally exhibit growth retardation, and one-third die before weaning. In these animals, GH and TSH levels are normal *(45)*. Surviving knock-out animals are fertile, but the females cannot eject milk during suckling. This defect can be corrected by injections of OT. These studies suggest that Mf3 is necessary for hypothal-amic development and may play a role in postnatal growth and lactation.

Other Transcription Factors in the Developing Hypothalamus

SINE OCULIS-3

Sine oculis-3 (Six3) is a homeobox gene related to the *Drosophila sine oculis* gene. In the mouse, the *Six3* gene is expressed at the most anterior border of the neural plate and later in the developing retina, lens, hypothalamus, and in Rathke's pouch *(53,71,72)*. Mutations in the homeodomain of human SIX3 cause holoprosencephaly, demonstrating that SIX3 is involved in the development of head midline structures by regulating gene expression in the developing anterior neural plate *(54)*.

C-ETS1

The *c-ets1* proto-oncogene encodes an Ets domain transcription factor that is expressed in the H-P system and has been proposed to play a role in angiogenesis in the hypothala-mus, pituitary, and placenta *(39)*.

TRANSCRIPTIONAL REGULATION OF PITUITARY DEVELOPMENT

Table 2 lists the properties of transcription factors that have been demonstrated to play roles in mammalian pituitary development. Some of these factors also are important in hypothalamic development and have been discussed earlier; others are discussed in more detail below.

The Ptx Family

Three members of the Ptx family of bicoid-related homeodomain transcription factors have been described in mammals to date (reviewed in refs. *103,104*). These factors play

Table 2

Transcription Factors Important in Pituitary Gland Development

Factor	Class	Mutant phenotype/Expression pattern/Role	References
Brm–4	POU-HD	Ventrally induced factor during pituitary development	31
DAX-1	Nuclear receptor-like	Sex-reversal; congenital adrenal hypoplasia and hypogonadotropic hypogonadism. Expressed in developing hypothalamus	40–43
Egr-1 (Krox24/NGFIA/Zif268)	Zinc finger	Reduced growth, female infertility, LHβ deficiency	73,74
ER alpha	Nuclear receptor	*PRL* and gonadotropin gene expression affected. Lactotrope growth reduced	75
GATA2	Zinc finger	Regulation of gonadotrope and thyrotrope cell differentiation	31,76
Isl-1	LIM-HD	Expressed in Rathke's Pouch	77
Isl-2	LIM-HD	Expressed in Rathke's Pouch	78
Lhx3 (P-Lim/LIM3)	LIM-HD	Hypoplastic anterior pituitary; no differentiation Loss of GH, PRL, TSH, LH, FSH	79–81
Lhx4 (Gsh4)	LIM-HD	Hypoplastic anterior pituitary: some differentiation	80
Msx1	HD	Expressed in thyrotropes; can activate the αGSU gene	82
NeuroD1 (Beta2)	bHLH	Important in *POMC* gene regulation	83
Nhlh2 (NSCL2)	bHLH	Hypogonadal, progressive obesity; male infertility	46
Nzf-1 (MyT1)	Zinc finger	Expressed in the pituitary: can regulate the *Pit-1* gene	84
Otx1	Bicoid-related HD	Transient dwarfism, hypogonadism. Can activate the *GH, αGSU, LHβ, FSHβ* genes	85
Pax6	HD	Establishes early boundary between dorsal and ventral pituitary cell types	32
P-Frk1	Winged-helix	Expressed in early pituitary	29,31
Pit-1 (GHF-1/*POU1F1*)	POU-HD	Dwarfism, hypothyroidism, hypoplastic anterior pituitary Loss of GH, PRL, and TSH	86
Prop-1	Paired-like HD	Dwarfism, hypoplastic anterior pituitary Loss of GH, PRL, and TSH	87
Ptx1 (P-Otx/Pitx1/Otlx1)	Bicoid-related HD	Lethal, pituitary and limb defects	88,89
Ptx2 (RIEG/Pitx2/Otlx2)	Bicoid-related HD	Lethal; regulates lung asymmetry, cardiac positioning, and pituitary and tooth morphogenesis	90–95
RAR	Nuclear receptor	Involved in *Pit-1* and *GH* gene regulation	20,96
Rpx (Hesx1)	Paired-like HD	Anterior defects; septooptic dysplasia	97,98
SF-1 (Ad4BP/*FtzF1*)	Nuclear receptor	Lethal; lack adrenals and gonads. Hypothalamus and pituitary defects Sex reversal in humans.	49–51
Six3	Sine oculis HD	Expressed in the developing pituitary	53
T3R	Nuclear receptor	Affects pituitary-thyroid axis, growth, and bone maturation	99
TEF	PAR bZIP	Can activate the *TSHβ* gene	100
Zn16 (Zn15/Zfp15)	Zinc finger	Can activate the *GH* gene	101,102

HD, homeodomain; T3R, thyroid hormone receptor; RAR, retinoic acid receptor.

13

critical roles in many aspects of mammalian development, including pituitary organo-genesis. Ptx1 (also known as P-OTX/Pitx1/Otlx1) was identified as an activator of the *POMC* gene *(105)* and as an interaction partner of Pit-1 *(106)*. *Ptx1* is expressed early in pituitary development *(107,108)* and appears to play a broad role in the transcriptional activation of many pituitary hormone genes *(105,106,109–111)*. Ptx1 also is proposed to be an upstream regulator of the *Lhx3* LIM homeodomain gene *(109)*, a critical pituitary transcription factor (*see* p. 14,15). Mice with ablated *Ptx1* genes exhibit defects in both hindlimb and pituitary development *(88,89)*.

The *Ptx2* gene also is expressed early in pituitary development *(112)*. Targeted disrup-tion of the *Ptx2* gene (the Ptx2 protein also is known as Pitx2/RIEG/Otlx2/solurshin) demonstrated that it is essential for proper left-right asymmetry, cardiac positioning, and pituitary, tooth, and craniofacial development *(90–95)*.

Egr-1

Egr-1 is a zinc finger-transcription factor that also is known as Krox24/NGFIA/Zif268. An analysis of *Egr-1* gene mutant mice demonstrated that the males were fertile, but females were infertile due to reduced levels of LHβ *(73)*. This study also demonstrated the abilities of Egr-1 and SF-1 to activate the *LHβ* gene *(73)*. An independent study of mice homozygous for an *Egr-1* gene mutation described mutant animals with reduced body size and sterility in both males and females *(74)*. This phenotype was related to defects in the anterior pituitary of both sexes and in the ovary *(74)*. In the pituitary, two cell lineages expressing *Egr-1* are affected differentially by the mutation: somatotropes display abnormal cytological features and are decreased in number, consistent with the reduced GH content observed in *Egr-1* null animals *(74)*. By contrast, gonadotropes are normal in number but fail to synthesize LHβ *(74)*.

Egr-1 also may play a role in hypothalamic signaling to the pituitary. For example, the effects of GnRH-induced signals from the hypothalamus on transcription of gonadotro-pin genes are not well-understood. GnRH is a stimulator of *Egr-1* but not *Ptx1* or *SF-1* expression *(113)*. Egr-1 interacts directly with Ptx1 and with SF-1, leading to an augmen-tation of Ptx1/SF-1-induced *LHβ* gene transcription *(113)*. Egr-1, therefore, may be a central mediator of GnRH-induced signals for transcriptional activation of the *LHβ* gene.

LIM Homeodomain Transcription Factors

Many LIM homeodomain transcription factors, including Lhx2 (also known as LH-2), Lhx3 (P-Lim/LIM3), Lhx4 (Gsh4), Isl-1, and Isl-2, are expressed during pituitary develop-ment. The LIM homeodomain proteins regulate many aspects of mammalian organogene-sis and development (reviewed in ref. *114*). Several of these factors have been demonstrated to be essential for the establishment of Rathke's pouch and the subsequent differentiation of the specialized trophic hormone-secreting cell types of the pituitary. These transcrip-tion factors contain two cysteine-rich, zinc finger-like LIM motifs that mediate protein-protein interactions with other transcription factors and regulatory proteins. In addition, proteins in this class possess a characteristic DNA-binding homeodomain.

Lhx3 is transiently expressed in the embryonic neural cord and brainstem and then is detected during pituitary organogenesis, first appearing in the forming Rathke's pouch and persisting in the pituitary throughout adulthood *(79,80,115–119)*. Cross-species com-parisons of Lhx3 protein sequences reveals conservation of the LIM and homeodomain regions and of a motif in the carboxyl-termini of these orthologs known as the Lhx3/LIM3-specific domain *(118–121)*. Lhx3 can activate pituitary trophic hormone genes, including the *PRL, TSHβ, αGSU,* and *Pit-1* genes *(117–119,122–124)*. Another LIM homeodomain factor, Lhx2, also can induce transcription from the αGSU gene *(125)*. Both Lhx2 and Lhx3 specifically bind to the pituitary glycoprotein basal element within the proximal region of the αGSU promoter. In transgenic mice, this element is required to correctly restrict expression of the αGSU gene to pituitary gonadotropes and thyrotropes *(126)*. In activation of other promoters, such as the *PRL* and *Pit-1* gene promoters, Lhx3 has been shown to transcriptionally synergize with pituitary transcription factors such as Pit-1 and Ptx1 *(117–119,122–124;* Fig. 3).

Mice with disrupted *Lhx3* genes are stillborn or die soon after birth and lack the anterior and intermediate lobes of the pituitary gland *(79)*. In these animals, pituitary development is arrested after the initial formation of Rathke's pouch, and most of the differentiated hormone-secreting cells are missing; a few corticotrope cells can be detected *(79,80)*. Lhx3, therefore, is critical for both early structural events and for the specification and proliferation of the lactotrope, somatotrope, gonadotrope, and thyrotrope pituitary-cell lineages *(79,80)*. The structurally-related Lhx4 LIM homeodomain factor also is required for complete development of Rathke's pouch; but unlike Lhx3, this factor is not essential for the determination and specification of differentiated pituitary cell types *(80)*. Studies of mice lacking both *Lhx3* and *Lhx4* genes have revealed that the formation of Rathke's pouch is a multistep process requiring LIM homeodomain gene function. *Lhx3/Lhx4* null mice do not develop a definitive Rathke's pouch but rather form a rudimentary pouch structure *(80)*. For this early step, there is redundancy of genetic control: either Lhx3 or Lhx4 is required during this early stage of pituitary development *(80)*.

Pit-1

Biochemical analyses of the *GH* and *PRL* gene promoters suggested that a common pituitary-specific *trans*-acting factor bound to important A/T-rich elements within the promoters and was critical for activation of these genes (reviewed in ref. *20*). The subsequent cloning of this transcription factor (known as Pit-1/ or GHF-1; the human gene locus is classified as *POU1F1*) revealed that the protein contained a DNA-binding homeodomain. Several studies have reported expression of the *Pit-1* RNA in all five anterior pituitary-cell types *(127,128)*, but the Pit-1 protein appears to be restricted to the thyrotrope, somatotrope, and lactotrope lineages. Consistent with this, the functions ascribed to Pit-1 involve genes expressed in these three cell types. Pit-1 has been shown to activate anterior pituitary genes, including those encoding GH, PRL, TSHβ, the GHRH receptor, and the thyroid hormone receptor beta type 2 promoter (reviewed in ref. *20*). In addition, Pit-1 positively autoregulates the *Pit-1* gene (reviewed in refs. *19,20*), providing a mechanism for the maintenance and stability of committed Pit-1-dependent anterior pituitary-cell lineages. Pit-1 target genes possess clusters of characteristic Pit-1 binding sites that tend to conform to an A/T-rich consensus sequence (reviewed in ref. *20*).

Pit-1 is a founder member of the POU domain family of developmental regulatory transcription factors. Both the POU-specific and POU homeodomain subdomains of Pit-1 are required for high-affinity binding of Pit-1 dimers to DNA sites. The amino terminus of Pit-1 contains the major *trans*-activation domain, but the POU-specific domain also appears to contribute to Pit-1 *trans*-activation function (reviewed in ref. *20*). High-resolution

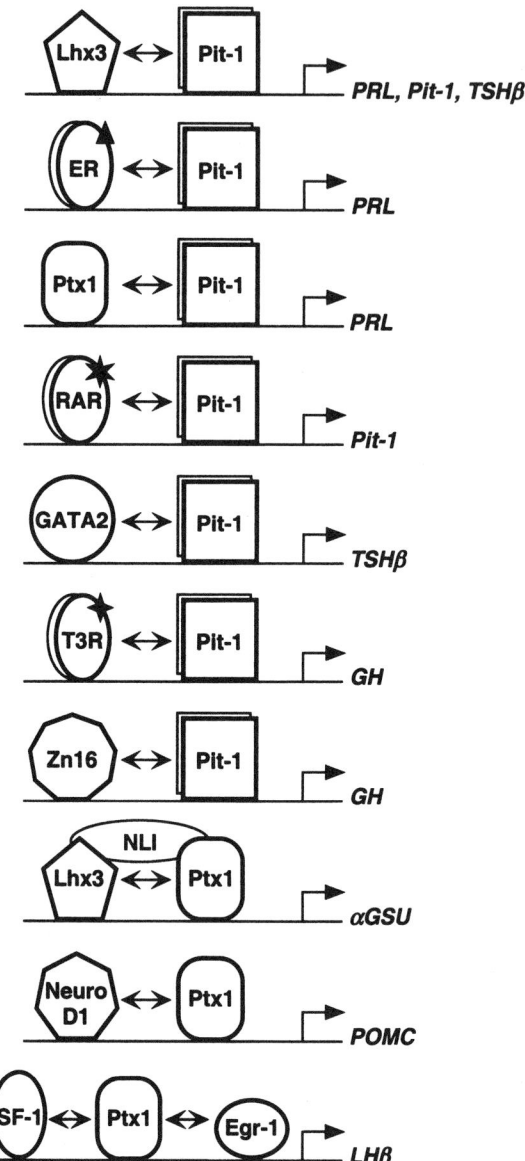

Fig. 3. Synergistic actions of pituitary transcription factors and their cofactors. The diagram depicts examples of reported cooperative effects of various transcription factors in activation of anterior pituitary target genes. Symbols denote ligands for nuclear receptors.

X-ray analysis of the Pit-1 POU domain bound to a DNA element revealed that the molecule binds as a homodimer in an unusual conformation *(58)*. These data provide structural explanations for the molecular basis of disease-causing mutations in PIT-1 *(see* p. 22) and also provide insights into the mechanism by which Pit-1 can synergistically induce transcription from pituitary genes in cooperation with a variety of other types of transcription factors, including nuclear receptors, homeodomain factors, and LIM homeodomain proteins (Fig. 3).

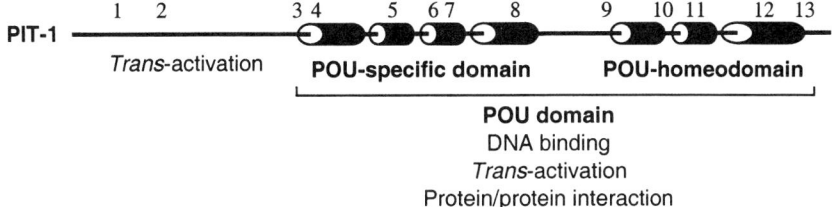

	Mutation	Effect on protein	Inheritance	Reference
1	CCT→CTT	Pro14Leu	Dominant	129
2	CCT→CTT	Pro24Leu	Dominant	130
3	TTT→TGT	Phe135Cys	Recessive	131
4	CGA→CAA	Arg143Gln	Recessive	130
5	GCA→CCA	Ala158Pro	Recessive	132
6	CGA→TGA	Arg172Ter	Recessive	133
7	GAA→GGA	Glu174Gly	Recessive	134
8	TGG→CGG	Trp193Arg	Recessive	135
9	AAA→GAA	Lys216Glu	Dominant	136
10	CCT→CCC	Pro239Ser	Recessive	137
11	GAA→TAA	Glu250Ter	Recessive	138
12	TGG→TGT	Trp261Cys	Recessive	86 (Snell mouse)
13	CGG→TGG	Arg271Trp	Dominant	139-145

Fig. 4. Mutations of the PIT-1 anterior pituitary transcription factor associated with compound pituitary diseases in humans and animal models. A schematic representation of the domains of the PIT-1 protein is shown. The functions of domains are indicated. Numbers denote the locations of mutations, and the nature of each mutation is described in the table below the protein diagram.

The importance of Pit-1 in the development of the thyrotrope, somatotrope, and lactotrope pituitary lineages was confirmed by the molecular analysis of naturally-occurring strains of dwarf mice (reviewed in refs. *19,20*). The Snell (*dw*) and Jackson (*dw^J*) dwarf mice carry recessive genetic defects that segregate with chromosome 16 and lack the thyrotrope, somatotrope, and lactotrope cell types and their respective hormone products. Li and colleagues *(86)* mapped the *Pit-1* gene to mouse chromosome 16 and then demonstrated that the Snell mouse *Pit-1* gene contains a single point mutation that disables the POU DNA binding domain (Fig. 4) and that the Jackson *Pit-1* gene is rearranged and does not produce a functional protein.

The demonstration that the Pit-1-defective Snell dwarf mouse lacked thyrotrope cells suggested that functional Pit-1 was required for the proliferation and/or maintenance of this cell type *(86)*. In support of this hypothesis, Pit-1 has been shown to transcriptionally activate the *TSHβ* gene, and modulators of *TSHβ* gene activity have been demonstrated to act through Pit-1-binding sites within the gene (reviewed in ref. 20). However, the detection of *TSHβ* transcripts in the developing pituitary before *Pit-1* gene activation indicated that Pit-1 was not required for the appearance of differentiated thyrotrope cells *(127)*. This puzzle was solved by an analysis of *TSHβ* gene expression during pituitary development in wild-type and Snell mice that revealed that there are two spatially and temporally distinct populations of thyrotrope cells (*36*; Fig. 2). The first population is found in the rostral tip of the developing pituitary (a region that eventually contributes to the pars tuberalis) and is independent of Pit-1 activity. The rostral thyrotropes are detected in both normal and Pit-1-defective animals during the early stages of pituitary development and have been reported to disappear at around the time of birth *(36)*. The second thyrotrope population appears at the time of *Pit-1* gene activation and co-localizes with Pit-1-positive cells. These caudomedial thyrotropes are absent in the Pit-1-defective Snell dwarf mouse, demonstrating their dependence on Pit-1. The Pit-1-dependent thyrotropes form the thyrotropes of the adult animal. More recent experiments have described a population of Pit-1-independent thyrotropes that is associated with the pars tuberalis and that persists in the adult gland *(146)*. The mechanism that controls the initial appearance of the Pit-1-independent population(s) of cells is unclear. Thyrotrope embryonic factor (TEF; ref. 100), a PAR leucine zipper transcription factor that is expressed in the developing pituitary and that can potently activate *TSHβ* promoter reporter genes, is a possible candidate for involvement in the initial activation of these thyrotropes (Fig. 2).

Prophet of Pit-1

Prophet of Pit-1 (Prop-1) is a paired class homeodomain transcription factor that is specifically expressed in the pituitary gland *(87)*. In the adult, expression continues at low levels *(21)*. Mutations in the *Prop-1* gene cause compound pituitary diseases in human patients (*see* below). This factor was identified by the positional cloning of the gene that is defective in the Ames dwarf mouse (*87*; Fig. 5). Similar to the Pit-1-defective Snell and Jackson mice, in Ames mice the lactotrope, thyrotrope, and somatotrope cell types are absent or occur in low numbers. Ames mice also exhibit reduced secretion of the gonadotropin pituitary hormones *(164)*. Analyses of these animal models during development demonstrated that *Prop-1* is genetically epistatic to *Pit-1*. For example, the size of the nascent Ames pituitary is reduced earlier during development compared to the Snell; *Pit-1* expression is deficient in the Ames dwarf; and the three Pit-1-dependent cell lineages fail to proliferate and differentiate in the Ames pituitary *(87,165–167)*. In addition, Prop-1 appears to be required for the repression of early pituitary transcription-factor genes, including the gene encoding Rpx/Hesx1 *(168)*. Little is known about the direct transcriptional targets of Prop-1, although there are potential sites within *Pit-1* gene regulatory regions that may mediate Prop-1 activities *(87)*.

Rpx/Hesx1

Rpx/Hesx1 is a paired-like homeobox transcription factor *(169,170)*. *Rpx* is expressed in the early developing mouse embryo, being later expressed in the neural plate, and finally is restricted to Rathke's pouch *(170)*. The *Rpx* gene is down regulated when the mature hormone-secreting cells of the pituitary begin to differentiate *(170)*. Rpx, therefore, is an early marker of pituitary organogenesis and may be important for the determination of the pouch where it is controlled by other pituitary regulatory genes. For example, whereas Lhx3 is necessary for maintaining the expression of *Rpx* in the first stages of pituitary formation *(80)*, Prop-1 is required to repress *Rpx* gene prior to pituitary-cell differentiation *(168)*. Mice lacking Rpx exhibit variable anterior CNS defects and pituitary dysplasia *(97)*. Human patients with mutations in RPX display septo-optic dysplasia (*see* p. 20). Therefore, Rpx/RPX plays a role in forebrain, midline, and pituitary development in mouse and human.

Pax6

Pax6 is an evolutionarily conserved paired-class homeodomain transcription factor that is expressed in the developing CNS (reviewed in ref. *171*). During human embryo-

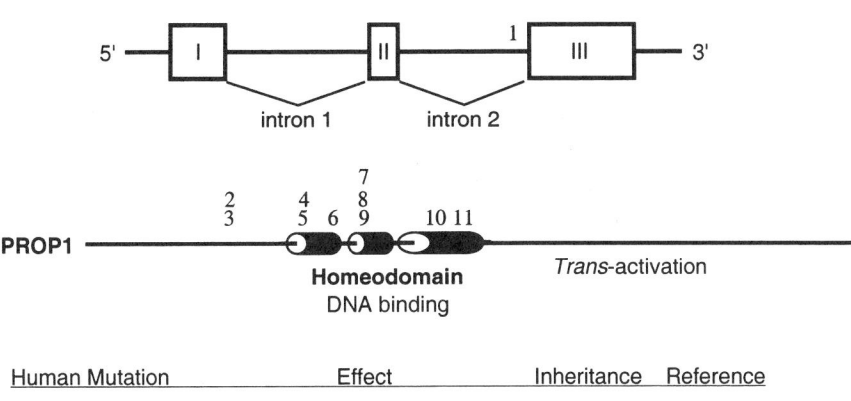

Fig. 5. Mutations of the PROP-1 anterior pituitary transcription factor identified as causing combined pituitary hormone deficiency in human patients and in rodent models. A schematic representation of the domains of the *PROP-1* gene and protein are shown. Exons are labeled in Roman numerals. The functions of protein domains are indicated. Numbers denote the locations of mutations, and the nature of each mutation is described in the table below the protein diagram.

genesis, PAX6 is expressed in the ventricular zone of telencephalon and diencephalon, in the ventricular and ventral intermediate zones of the medulla oblongata, in the spinal cord, in the optic cup, in the optic stalk, and in the prospective corneal epithelium *(172)*. Expression also is detected in the human infundibulum and Rathke's pouch *(172)*. The role of Pax6 in eye development is well-established: this function is strikingly conserved from flies to humans (reviewed in ref. *171*). Analyses of mice carrying *Pax6* mutations also indicate important roles for this gene in ocular, neural, pancreatic, and pituitary development *(32,173,174)*. In the developing pituitary, the transient dorsal expression of *Pax6* is essential for establishing a boundary between the dorsal and ventral cell types, perhaps by confining the ventral actions of BMP2 *(32)*.

NeuroD1

NeuroD1 (also known as Beta2) is a bHLH transcription factor. Mice homozygous for a deletion at the *NeuroD1* locus fail to develop a granule-cell layer within the dentate gyrus, one of the principal structures of the hippocampal formation, and exhibit spontaneous seizures *(175)*. It has been reported that transcription of the *POMC* gene in pituitary corticotrope cells depends on the synergistic actions of Ptx1 and bHLH heterodimers containing NeuroD1 *(83)*. Direct interactions occur between the bHLH of NeuroD1 and the homeodomain of Ptx1 *(110)*.

Estrogen Receptor

The actions of estrogen are critical to hypothalamic and pituitary function at many times. Estrogen regulates the synthesis and secretion of several pituitary hormones during the reproductive cycle. Of the two estrogen receptors, ER alpha and ER beta, the alpha receptor appears to be the predominant receptor expressed in the pituitary gland *(176)*. A recent analysis of mice lacking the *ER alpha* gene indicated that ER alpha is involved in *PRL* and gonadotropin gene transcription and plays an important role in lactotrope cell growth but is not necessary for specification of lactotrope cell phenotype *(75)*.

PITUITARY TRANSCRIPTION FACTORS IN HUMAN DISEASE

PTX2/RIEG

The human *PTX2/RIEG* gene contains 4 exons and maps to chromosome 4 at position 4q24-q25 *(177)*. Rieger syndrome is an autosomal dominant disorder that often features eye, dental, craniofacial, umbilical, limb, and pituitary developmental defects (*see* ref. *177*, and references therein). Six mutations have been identified in the *PITX2/RIEG* gene in patients with Rieger syndrome (*177*; Fig. 6). These include two splicing mutations, three homeodomain mutations, and one mutation that introduces a premature stop codon in the carboxyl terminus of the molecule. However, these particular patients did not display abnormal pituitary function *(177)*. Mutations in *PTX2/RIEG* also have been found in patients with iridogoniodysgenesis syndrome *(179)*, autosomal dominant iris hypoplasia type 2 *(180)*, and Peter's anomaly (*178*; Fig. 6). Molecular characterization of some of these mutations indicates that the Thr68Pro and Leu54Gln defects reduce the ability of *PTX2/RIEG* to induce transcription. These mutations appear to impair the protein-protein interaction and protein stability characteristics of the molecule, respectively *(181)*.

RPX/HESX1

RPX/HESX1 is one of the earliest factors expressed in the embryonic pituitary gland *(169,170)*. Interestingly, *Hesx1* knockout mice possess developmental abnormalities of the corpus callosum, the anterior and hippocampal commissures, and the septum pellucidum *(97)*. This phenotype is similar to that seen in humans with septo-optic dysplasia. The human *HESX1* gene contains 4 exons and maps to chromosome 3p21.2-p21.1 *(97)*. A brother and sister with septo-optic dysplasia have been shown to be homozygous for an Arg160Cys missense mutation in homeodomain of RPX/HESX (*97*; Fig. 7). Septo-optic dysplasia in these patients is characterized by agenesis of the corpus callosum and panhypopituitarism and is inherited in an autosomal recessive fashion *(97)*, although patients with dominant mutations may exist *(98)*. Molecular characterization of the

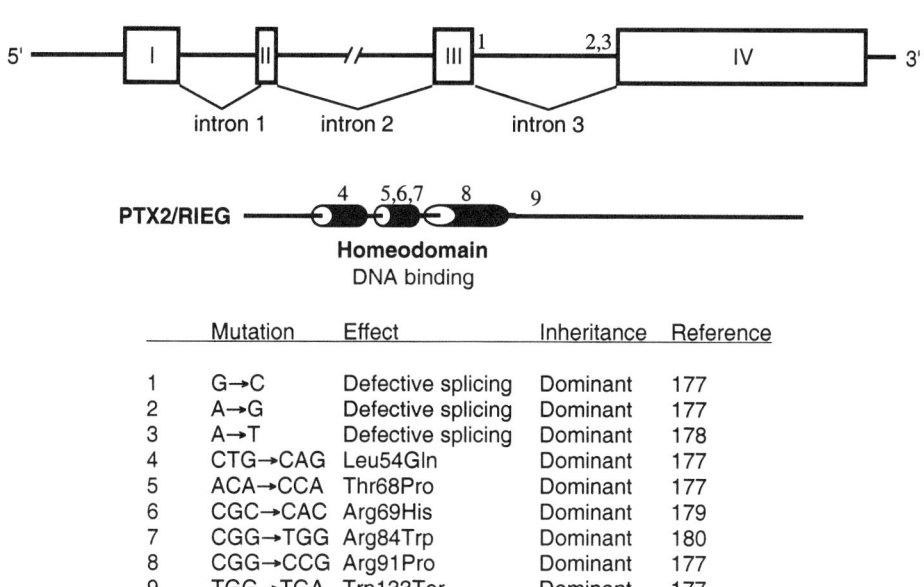

	Mutation	Effect	Inheritance	Reference
1	G→C	Defective splicing	Dominant	177
2	A→G	Defective splicing	Dominant	177
3	A→T	Defective splicing	Dominant	178
4	CTG→CAG	Leu54Gln	Dominant	177
5	ACA→CCA	Thr68Pro	Dominant	177
6	CGC→CAC	Arg69His	Dominant	179
7	CGG→TGG	Arg84Trp	Dominant	180
8	CGG→CCG	Arg91Pro	Dominant	177
9	TGG→TGA	Trp133Ter	Dominant	177

Fig. 6. Mutations of the PTX2/RIEG transcription factor associated with Rieger's syndrome. A schematic representation of the domains of the *PTX2/RIEG* gene and protein are shown. Exons are labeled in Roman numerals. Numbers denote the locations of mutations, and the nature of each mutation is described in the table below the protein diagram.

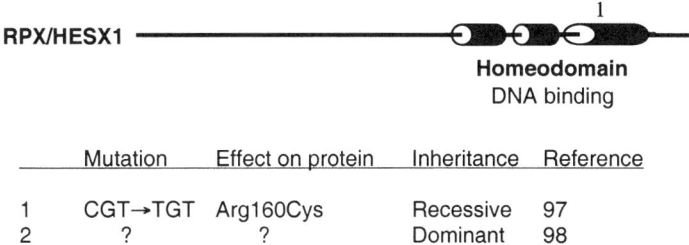

	Mutation	Effect on protein	Inheritance	Reference
1	CGT→TGT	Arg160Cys	Recessive	97
2	?	?	Dominant	98

Fig. 7. Mutations of the RPX/HESX1 transcription factor associated with septo-optic dysplasia and pituitary diseases. A schematic representation of the domains of the protein is shown. The functions of domains are indicated. Numbers denote the locations of mutations, and the nature of each mutation is described in the table below the protein diagram.

mutant protein indicates that the mutation inhibits the ability of RPX/HESX1 to bind DNA *(97)*.

LHX3

Two human LHX3 isoforms exist, and these factors may regulate transcription of different target genes *(119)*. The human *LHX3* gene contains 7 exons and maps to chromosome 9q34.3 *(81,182)*. Humans with mutations in *LHX3* are growth retarded and have combined pituitary hormone deficiency (CPHD), featuring deficiencies of the anterior pituitary hormones with the exception of ACTH *(81)*. Interestingly, they also have elevated and anteverted shoulders that appear as a stubby neck associated with severe restriction of rotation of the cervical spine *(81)*. Patients with a Tyr116Cys mutation have severe pituitary hypoplasia *(81;* Fig. 8). However, one patient with an intragenic deletion in

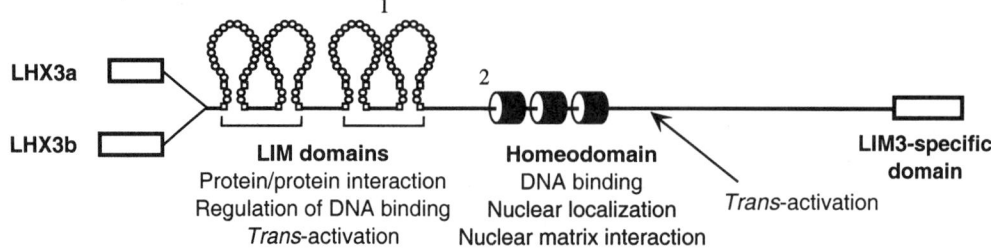

	Mutation	Effect on protein	Inheritance	Reference
1	TAC→TGC	Tyr116Cys	Recessive	81
2	23 nt deletion	Truncation - no homeodomain	Recessive	81

Fig. 8. Mutations of the LHX3 transcription factor associated with compound pituitary disease. A schematic representation of the domains of the two LHX3 protein isoforms is shown. The functions of domains of the LHX3 molecule are indicated. Numbers denote the locations of mutations, and the nature of each mutation is described in the table below the protein diagram.

LHX3 that results in a truncated protein lacking the DNA-binding homeodomain possesses an enlarged anterior pituitary gland *(81)*, a structure similar to that found in some patients with PROP-1 mutations *(162)*. To date, only patients with homozygous mutations in *LHX3* have been identified. CPHD associated with posterior pituitary ectopia does not appear to be caused by mutations in *LHX3 (183)*.

PIT-1

As described earlier, Pit-1 is necessary for the specification of the anterior pituitary-cell types that produce GH, PRL, and TSH, and gene defects in *Pit-1* have been shown to cause hypopituitarism in the Jackson and Snell dwarf mice. The human *PIT-1 (POU1F1)* gene contains 6 exons and is located on chromosome 3 at position 3p11 *(184)*. Mutations in the *PIT-1* gene in humans lead to the development of a hypoplastic anterior pituitary gland and CPHD with postnatal growth failure. Patients with *PIT-1* mutations commonly exhibit loss of circulating GH and PRL and low or absent TSH levels that lead to the development of central hypothyroidism. Similar to the phenotype of the Jackson and Snell mice, these patients possess normal gonadotrope and corticotrope function. Mutations have been identified in each of the regions of the *PIT-1* gene that encode the functional domains of the factor. Homozygous (recessive mutation), compound heterozygous (recessive), and heterozygous (dominant) patients have been described (Fig. 4). Two autosomal dominant mutations have been found in the amino terminal transcriptional activation domain, several autosomal recessive mutations have been identified in the POU specific domain, and both dominant and recessive mutations have been characterized in the POU homeodomain (Fig. 4).

Mutations in PIT-1 impair its ability to induce transcription by several mechanisms. For example, the Ala158Pro *(132)* and Pro239Ser *(137)* mutations reduce the ability of the molecule to induce transcription of pituitary target genes. Nonsense mutations such as Arg172Ter *(133)* and Glu250Ter *(138)* result in shortened proteins that do not contain the DNA-binding POU homeodomain. Interestingly, the common Arg271Trp mutation may exert a dominant negative effect by enabling PIT-1 to bind certain DNA elements better than the wild-type protein *(130,139,140,185)*. In addition, the Arg271Trp mutation may affect dimerization of the molecule in a site-specific DNA-binding manner *(58)*. CPHD also occurs in heterozygous patients carrying the Pro14Leu *(129)* or Pro24Leu *(130)* mutations, but it is as yet unclear how these mutations impair PIT-1 and cause pituitary disease. Recently, the Lys216Glu mutation has been shown to be defective in cooperating with the retinoic acid receptor in induction of the *Pit-1* gene via the distal enhancer *(186)*.

PROP-1

Prop-1 is necessary for the initial determination of the Pit-1-dependent pituitary-cell types *(87)*. The finding that a mutation in Prop-1 (Ser83Pro) is the genetic defect responsible for hypopituitarism and pituitary hypoplasia in the Ames dwarf mouse (*87*; Fig. 5) enabled further molecular analyses of human pituitary disease. The human *PROP-1* gene contains 3 exons and maps to the distal end of chromosome 5q *(147,156,161,187)*. Mutations in *PROP-1* also cause CPHD. Similar to CPHD patients with *PIT-1* mutations, these patients typically have hypoplastic anterior pituitary glands and deficiencies of GH, PRL, and TSH, however, they also may display low or absent levels of the circulating gonadotropins, LH and FSH, and many patients do not spontaneously enter puberty or experience pubertal delay *(147,156,157)*. CPHD in patients with *PROP-1* gene defects appears to be more variable compared to the phenotype of patients with *PIT-1* mutations. This variability may be a function of the severity of the specific type of *PROP-1* mutation, but phenotypic differences in the timing of hormone loss in individuals with the same mutation also have been described *(163)*. In addition, a few *PROP-1* mutant patients have normal-sized or enlarged pituitaries rather than hypoplastic glands *(151,160,162)*. Interestingly, some older individuals with *PROP-1* mutations develop adrenal insufficiency later in life as a result of ACTH deficiency *(175,162,163)*, while others do not *(152)*.

Several different *PROP-1* mutations cause CPHD, and most of these affect the homeodomain of the molecule (Fig. 5). Homozygous and compound heterozygous patients with *PROP-1* mutations have been identified *(156)*. To date, dominant-negative *PROP-1* mutations have not been described. Nucleotide deletions at three different positions that disrupt the reading frame and lead to a premature stop codon resulting in a truncated protein without a complete DNA-binding homeodomain have been described (Fig. 5). One of these deletions, the 301-302delAG, is found in what appears to be a mutational "hot spot" region and is the most common *PROP-1* genetic defect yet identified (Fig. 5). Similar to the Ser83Pro Prop-1 mutation in the Ames mouse, the Phe88Ser, Phe117Ile, and Arg120Cys mutations in human PROP-1 decrease its ability to bind DNA *(154,156)*.

ALTERNATE FORMS OF HYPOTHALAMUS-PITUITARY TRANSCRIPTION FACTORS

The production of more than one protein isoform from a single gene provides an increased capacity for regulatory transcription factors and may allow higher levels of control in complex regulatory mechanisms. Recent studies have demonstrated that many H-P transcription factor genes encode more than one protein isoform. The structural differences between the various isoforms vary, ranging from isoforms with amino acid sequences missing to isoforms with distinct domain structures. The focus of most investigations of the variant forms of H-P transcription factors has been to determine whether the alternate proteins possess distinct transcriptional properties from the "wild-type" form. Indeed, functional differences in activation of trophic hormone target genes, for example, have been noted (*see* below). The biological relevance of such observations is, however, only likely to be significant if the variant isoforms are expressed at levels high enough to exert their unique effects, or if they are expressed in distinct locations or at discrete times from the "common" or "wild-type" form. Of course, if the variant isoform exhibits entirely separate activities from the wild-type form, then such corollaries may not apply.

Variant forms of the Rpx/Hesx1, Ptx1, and Ptx2 early pituitary transcription factors have been reported (*97,103,111,112*), and the Ptx2 isoforms appear to have different activities in assays using amphibian model systems (*188*). By contrast, experiments using pituitary-hormone promoter-reporter genes have suggested similar activities for Ptx1 and Ptx2 isoforms (*111*). Although isoforms of the Prop-1 pituitary transcription factor protein have not been described, the human and porcine *PROP-1* genes produce alternate messenger RNAs that are found in the adult pituitary at similar levels to the wild-type RNA (*21*; Sloop and Rhodes, unpublished observations). To date, however, the characterized variant RNAs do not appear to encode functional proteins, and their role therefore is unclear.

The *Pit-1* gene produces multiple alternate protein isoforms (reviewed in refs. *19,20*). These forms, which were originally characterized in rodents, may be expressed at much lower levels than the wild-type form (which is sometimes called Pit-1/Pit-1α/GHF-1). One variant, Pit-1β/GHF-2/Pit-1a, contains an insertion of 26 amino acids in the amino terminal *trans*-activation domain of the protein. A second Pit-1 splice product (Pit-1T) results from the insertion of 14 amino acids at the same position as the Pit-1β insertion. Pit-1T has been speculated to have a role in transcription of the *TSHβ* promoter. A third class of Pit-1 isoform results from a splice choice that excludes exon 4 coding information, removing most of the POU-specific domain. Variant forms of Pit-1 also are detected in primates such as humans and rhesus monkeys (*189*). Interestingly, multiple forms of Pit-1 also are found in nonmammalian species, such as birds and fish, suggesting that the alternate forms may have been adapted to specialized roles during evolution (*190,191*). In addition, the mammalian and nonmammalian Pit-1 molecules have provided valuable models for analysis of the functions of Pit-1 protein domains: using "natural mutagenesis" to test the roles of specific amino acid sequences (*191,192*). In addition to alternate Pit-1 forms that are generated from differently spliced RNAs, alternative translation initiation-site usage results in two forms of the major Pit-1/Pit-1α molecule (*193*).

As described earlier, the *Lhx3* LIM homeodomain transcription factor gene is critical to both the early development of Rathke's pouch and for the later commitment and differentiation events that mediate the establishment of the hormone-secreting cell types of the anterior and intermediate lobes of the pituitary gland. The mouse *Lhx3* gene has been demonstrated to produce two isoforms, Lhx3a and Lhx3b (*117,194*). These isoforms share common LIM domains and homeodomain sequences but possess alternate amino terminal sequences that are encoded by alternate exons (*182,194*; Fig. 8). In contrast to Pit-1, the *Lhx3* genes of nonmammalian species (often known as LIM3 class genes) do not appear to encode multiple protein isoforms. The *Lhx3* gene may use distinct promoters to generate RNAs encoding the two isoforms (*182,194*). Analysis of the human LHX3 isoforms has revealed that LHX3a is a more potent activator of pituitary-gene promoters such as those from the αGSU and TSHβ genes (*119*). The different *trans*-activation abilities of LHX3a and LHX3b correlate with observed differences in DNA binding affinities for binding sites within these genes, consistent with the b-specific domain serving a repressive function on this type of DNA-recognition element *(119)*. These experiments suggest that the two isoforms may serve distinct roles during pituitary development. In accord with this hypothesis, the two forms display distinct expression patterns, both in the timing of their appearance and in their levels of expression in various pituitary cell types *(119,194*; Sloop and Rhodes, unpublished observations).

REGULATION OF HYPOTHALAMUS-PITUITARY TRANSCRIPTION FACTOR FUNCTION

Inductive Events and Extracellular Signals

As described earlier, recent studies have begun to delineate the signaling events between the infundibulum (ventral diencephalon) and Rathke's pouch that coordinate the earliest stages of pituitary organogenesis. Protein-signaling molecules such as BMP4, BMP2, FGF8, and Shh appear to be critical to the activation of the transcription factors that regulate H-P development *(28–30)*. For example, BMP4 appears to be required for the early expression of the *Isl-1* LIM homeodomain gene in the primordial Rathke's pouch. Later, FGF8 signals cause repression of *Isl-1* expression and activation of the *Lhx3* gene. Expression of the T/ebp homeodomain transcription factor in the ventral diencephalon is a critical step in these early events. In mice lacking the *T/ebp* gene, pituitary development is arrested *(28,55)*. It is clear that the further elucidation of the extracellular-signaling pathways that activate H-P transcription-factor programs will be an important focus of future research in this field.

Post-Translational Modification

Control of protein activity by post-translational modification is a common regulatory mechanism in eukaryotic cells. Modifications include the removal or addition of phosphate groups; the addition of carbohydrate moieties; the addition of lipid, methyl, acetyl, sulfate, or isoprenoid groups; and proteolytic processing. Little is known about the possible involvement of post-translational modification in the regulation of most H-P transcription factors. However, the role of phosphorylation in the activities of Pit-1 has been extensively studied. Signaling pathways have been demonstrated to exert their actions on pituitary hormone genes through Pit-1 DNA recognition elements (reviewed in ref. *20*). Pit-1 is phosphorylated at three positions by enzymes including protein kinase A (PKA) and protein kinase C (PKC). Phosphorylation can modulate binding to specific pituitary hormone target-gene sequences *(195)*. However, other studies have suggested that the basal *trans*-activation function of Pit-1 may be independent of the phosphorylation status of the protein *(196,197)*. Phosphorylation may serve to repress Pit-1 function by lowering its DNA binding affinity or by reducing stability of the protein. For example, activin, an endocrine growth factor, represses pituitary somatotrope proliferation and GH biosynthesis and secretion by increasing Pit-1 phosphorylation and decreasing its stability *(198)*. In another study, a cell cycle-regulated kinase was observed to inhibit Pit-1 DNA binding *(199)*. A mutation near one of the defined Pit-1 phosphorylation sites may interfere with human PIT-1 phosphorylation causing altered PIT-1 function and pituitary disease *(200)*. In summary, the precise role of Pit-1 phosphorylation is unclear. Pit-1 certainly is a key mediator of hormone gene responses to cyclic AMP and growth factors; however, these effects may be mediated by regulation of Pit-1 interaction with cofactor proteins that serve coregulatory functions for these pathways *(186,201*, and *see* p. 26).

Transcription Factor Cofactors: Regulation and Execution of Activity

It is evident that most transcription factors (even those that are expressed in tissue- or cell-specific fashion) do not function in isolation; rather, they work in combination with other transcription factors and cofactor/corepressor proteins to regulate the rate of RNA polymerase activity at a particular target-gene promoter. Over the past five years, critical aspects of the biochemical mechanisms by which transcription factors activate and repress target genes have been determined. These studies, which primarily began with studies of nuclear receptors, have now demonstrated that many types of transcription factors recruit coactivator and corepressor proteins to their transcriptional complexes (reviewed in refs. *202–204*; Fig. 9). The coactivators acetylate chromatin histone proteins, either directly or by the recruitment of additional factors with histone acetyltransferase (HAT) enzyme activities. By contrast, corepressor factors cause histone deacetylation by the recruitment of deacetylase (HDAC) enzymes. HATs acetylate lysine residues of chromatin histone proteins resulting in greater accessibility of chromatin regions containing transcription factor binding sites, thereby promoting gene activation. Histone deactylases catalyze the removal of acetyl groups from the lysine residues, promoting tighter assembly of chromatin complexes and therefore reduced levels of transcription.

Some coregulatory proteins, such as the GRIP1 and SRC-1 nuclear receptor coactivators, appear to serve as ligand-dependent coactivators for specific types of transcription factors such as the nuclear receptors *(205,206)*. As described earlier, nuclear receptors, especially those with hormone ligands such as the estrogen receptors, appear to play critical roles in the establishment and control of H-P cell types. Other transcription factor cofactors, such as the CREB-binding protein and p300 "cointegrator" proteins, the p/CAF and p/CIP coactivator proteins, and the N-CoR/SMRT and mSIN3 corepressor proteins, interact with many types of transcription factors *(201,207–213)*. The co-integrator factors may serve multiple roles, acting as bridging molecules in transcriptional complexes and also directly providing histone-modifying activities *(214–216)*. Co-integrator, coactivator, and corepressor factors have been demonstrated to interact with important H-P developmental transcription factors, including Pit-1 and Rpx/Hesx1 *(186,201,217)*. These studies also provide important insights into the mechanism of how H-P transcription factors mediate intracellular responses to hormone and growth-factor signals resulting in altered expression of tissue-specific genes, such as the *GH* and *TSHβ* genes. Intriguingly, some nuclear-receptor coactivators may even act as RNAs, rather than as proteins *(218)*. It will be interesting to see if any coactivators of non-nuclear receptor H-P transcription factors function by similar biochemical mechanisms. Such discoveries might allow the design of nucleic acid-based therapies for diseases of the H-P axis.

LIM homeodomain class transcription factors, including the Lhx3, Lhx4, and Isl-1 proteins, appear to interact with multiple regulatory cofactor proteins. The LIM domains of the molecules mediate the cofactor interactions. One extensively studied class of LIM protein cofactors is the nuclear LIM interactor proteins (NLI, also known as Ldb/CLIM/CHIP). The NLI proteins are broadly expressed nuclear factors that can mediate higher order complexes involving one or more type of LIM homeodomain proteins and can modulate LIM protein activity and cellular location (reviewed in refs. *114,219*). Interestingly, a recent report has demonstrated that the NLI class of factors may regulate a broader range of target molecules, including homeodomain proteins *(220)*. This finding has important implications for H-P development where many of the key regulatory transcrip-

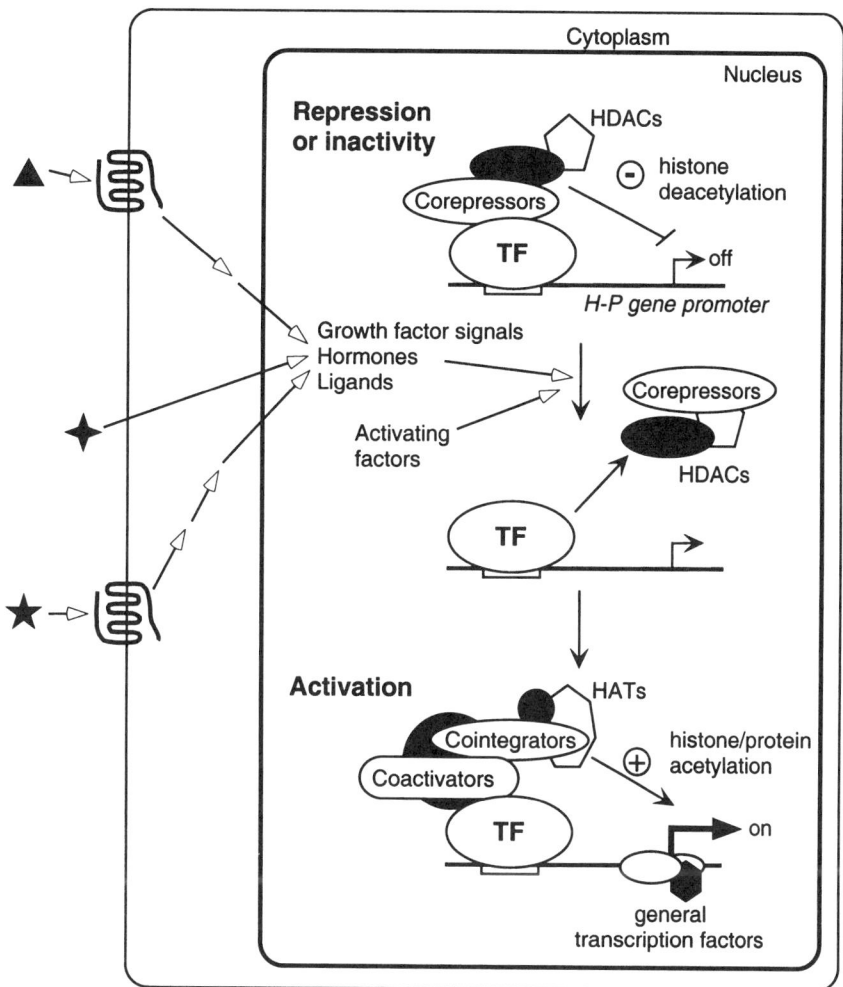

Fig. 9. Chromatin-modifying cofactor proteins may mediate the actions of many H-P transcription factors. In the absence of ligands or positive influences, H-P transcription factors (TF, including both nuclear receptor and non-nuclear receptor factors) may interact with DNA binding elements of repressed or silent target genes as complexes with corepressor and histone deacetylase (HDAC) proteins. In the presence of ligands, hormones, signals (represented by the symbols on the left of the figure), or positive regulatory factors, the corepressor and HDAC molecules are released and replaced by coactivators, cointegrators, and histone acetylases (HATs) leading to gene activation.

tion factors are homeodomain class DNA binding proteins (reviewed in refs. *221,222*). Some cofactor proteins may be more selective in their interactions. For example, the SLB molecule appears to interact with specific LIM homeodomain transcription factors, including Lhx3 and Lhx4, and may serve a repressive function for *PRL* gene expression *(123)*. The mechanism of action of many cofactors is unknown. However, recent experiments have demonstrated that factors such as RLIM, an inhibitory protein that interacts with Lhx3, may recruit HDAC-associated protein complexes, thereby creating the chromatin environment that does not support transcription as described above *(223)*. Further, another LIM-interacting cofactor, MRG1, is a positive regulator of α*GSU* promoter reporter genes and has been demonstrated by Glenn and Maurer *(124)* to interact with the p300 cointegrator molecule and with the TATA element-binding protein, TBP.

Regulation of Intranuclear Location

A further level of regulation of H-P transcription factor function may be achieved by the functional partitioning of these factors within the nucleus. The nucleus is a complex structure that includes components such as the nucleoplasm, chromatin, and the nuclear matrix. After entering the nucleus, transcription factors may undergo additional trafficking, including targeting to the nuclear matrix. The nuclear matrix is a proteinaceous substructure that resists nuclease digestion and high salt extraction *(224)*. The nuclear matrix is composed of proteins such as the nuclear mitotic apparatus protein, NuMA *(225)*. It has been proposed that transcriptionally active genes are associated with the nuclear matrix, and multiple proteins involved in gene regulation (including HATs) have been demonstrated to be associated with the matrix. The nuclear matrix may provide a functional scaffold for chromatin and has been proposed to mediate the actions of both extranuclear and extracellular regulatory signals that result in altered gene expression (reviewed in ref. *226*). Recent studies have demonstrated that the pituitary transcription factors Pit-1 and Lhx3 are associated with the nuclear matrix *(227,228)*. Intriguingly, these two transcription factors cooperate in synergistic activation of the *PRL*, *TSHβ*, and *Pit-1* pituitary-specific genes *(117–119)*, and it has been speculated that the interaction of these two factors with the nuclear matrix may contribute to the transcriptional activation of pituitary target genes *(228)*. Consistent with this hypothesis, another homeodomain protein, Oct-1, also is present within the nuclear-matrix fraction, and this interaction has been proposed to play a role in regulation of the *TSHβ* gene *(229)*.

COMBINATIONS OF HYPOTHALAMUS-PITUITARY TRANSCRIPTION FACTORS IN THE SPECIFICATION OF CELL TYPES

Although some H-P-specific transcription factors have been identified, it is clear that the commitment and differentiation pathways that regulate terminal H-P cell type specification involve interactions of both tissue-specific and ubiquitous or widespread transcription factors of many kinds (Figs. 1 and 2). For example, in considering the determination of the Pit-1-dependent anterior pituitary-cell lineages, the transcription factor "equations" that specificy the thyrotrope, somatotrope, and lactotrope phenotypes must include Pit-1 plus other factors, such as nuclear receptors. Such combinatorial codes mediate the activation of the trophic hormone genes and the other cell-specific gene products that characterize these cells, such as receptors for hypothalamic peptides. Consistent with this model, synergy between H-P transcription factors has been observed in studies of many H-P genes (Fig. 3). For example, Pit-1 has been observed to synergize with the retinoic acid receptor (RAR) in autoregulation of its own gene *(96)*; synergism has been reported between the thyroid hormone receptor (T_3R) and the zinc-finger protein Zn15/Zn16 and Pit-1 in the rat *GH* gene promoter (reviewed in ref. *20*); and between the estrogen receptor and Pit-1 in regulation of the rat *PRL* gene distal enhancer (reviewed in refs. *20,230*). The Lhx3 LIM-homeodomain factor also appears to be important in the development of these cells, and synergy has been demonstrated between Lhx3 and Pit-1 in induction of the *Pit-1*, *PRL,* and *TSHβ* genes *(117–119,123,228)*. The outcome of interactions between transcription factors may be dependent on (or may determine) the differentiated phenotype of particular H-P cell types. For example, recent studies have demonstrated that Pit-1 can synergize with the GATA2 zinc-finger protein in activation of the *TSHβ* gene in thyrotropes *(31,76)*. Within this cell type, Pit-1 also may repress gonadotrope-specific genes in a DNA-independent fashion *(31)*. Further, in the gonadotrope, GATA2 may repress the *Pit-1* gene and participate in the induction of gonadotrope-specific genes *(31)*. The restriction of terminal H-P differentiated cell types, therefore, likely requires both inductive and repressive activities of transcription factors and may involve complex protein/ protein interactions, some of which may not be DNA-dependent.

The biochemical mechanism underlying H-P transcription factor synergy is not clear, although direct protein-protein interaction between partners often has been observed *(31, 76,106,110,117,118,122,230)*. Further, these transcription factor combinations may promote the recruitment of coregulatory proteins to transcriptional complexes, as described earlier. An increased comprehension of the mechanisms that drive such transcriptional synergy will be vital to understanding the processes that regulate the establishment of the specialized endocrine cells of the hypothalamus and pituitary.

CONCLUSIONS

Following the pivotal identification and cloning of Pit-1 in the late 1980s, substantial progress has been made in our understanding of the tissue-specific transcriptional mechanisms that regulate the development and function of the hypothalamus and pituitary. As summarized in this article, many transcription factors that are expressed in developing H-P tissues have been cloned. The roles of some of these factors have been elucidated by experiments with transgenic and knockout mice; by the analysis of the naturally occurring mutant animals; and by the molecular diagnosis of patients with H-P diseases. In addition, elegant transgenic experiments have provided insights into the developmental lineages of specific terminal, differentiated cell types. Together, these investigations have allowed us to generate a preliminary "road map" that outlines some of the molecular and cellular decisions that occur during H-P organ development. This map will provide a foundation for the significant questions that must next be answered. These include: 1) What are the precise transcriptional codes that program the establishment of each of the specialized cell types of the mature hypothalamus and pituitary (including determination of the functions of alternate and modified forms of H-P transcription factors)? 2) What are the extracellular signaling events that activate and repress H-P transcription factors? 3) What are the intracellular pathways that modulate H-P transcription factor function? and 4) How do H-P transcription factors exert their effects at the chromatin level? Solutions to these questions will provide tools that will permit future gene or small molecule therapies that specifically target transcriptional regulatory pathways in the treatment of H-P diseases. Further, the central role of the H-P axes in controlling growth, reproduction, and metabolism will make similar protocols useful in the animal agriculture and aquaculture industries.

ACKNOWLEDGMENTS

The authors apologize to colleagues whose work was not cited due to space constraints. Research in the laboratory of SJR is supported by grants from the National Science Foundation and the U.S. Department of Agriculture National Research Initiative Competitive Grants Program.

REFERENCES

1. Romer AS. The Vertebrate Body. 4th ed. (Shorter version) WB Saunders, Philadelphia, PA, 1971, pp. 554–559.
2. Mikimi SI. Hypophysis. In: Matsumoto A, Ishi S, eds. Atlas of Endocrine Organs: Vertebrates and Invertebrates. Springer-Verlag, New York, 1992, pp. 39–62.
3. Wynick D, Small CJ, Bacon A, Holmes FE, Norman M, Ormandy CJ, et al. Galanin regulates prolactin release and lactotroph proliferation. Proc Natl Acad Sci USA 1998;95:12,671–12,676.
4. Rinehart JF, Farquhar MG. The fine vascular organization of the pituitary gland. An electron microscopic study with histochemical correlations. Anat Rec 1955;121:207–240.
5. Coates P, Doniach I. Development of folliculo-stellate cells in the human pituitary. Acta Endocrinologica 1988;119:16–20.
6. Hatton GI. Pituicytes, glia and control of terminal secretion. J Exp Biol 1988;139:67–79.
7. Dubois P, ElAmraoui A, Heritier A. Development and differentiation of pituitary cells. Microsc Res Tech 1997;38:98–113.
8. Schwind J. The development of the hypophysis cerebri of the albino rat. Am J Anat 1928;41:295–319.
9. Jacobson A, Miyamoto D, Mai S. Rathke's pouch morphogenesis in the chick embryo. J Exp Zool 1979;207:351–366.
10. Couly G, Le Douarin N. Mapping of the early neural primordium in quail-chick chimeras. I. Developmental relationships between placodes, facial ectoderm, and prosencephalon. Dev Biol 1985;110:422–439.
11. Couly G, Le Douarin N. Mapping of the early neural primordium in quail-chick chimeras. II. The prosencephalic neural plate and neural folds: implications for the genesis of cephalic human congenital abnormalities. Dev Biol 1987;120:198–214.
12. Couly G, Le Douarin N. The fate map of the neural primordium at the presomitic to the 3-somite stage in the avian embryo. Development 1988;103:101–113.
13. Eagleson G, Harris W. Mapping of the presumptive brain regions in the neural plate of Xenopus laevis. J Neurobiol 1990;21:427–440.
14. Dubois P, Hemming F. Fetal development and regulation of pituitary cell types. J Electron Microsc Tech 1991;19:2–20.
15. Couly G, Coltey P, Le Douarin N. The developmental fate of the cephalic mesoderm in quail-chick chimeras. Development 1992;114:1–15.
16. Osumi-Yamashita N, Ninomiya Y, Doi H, Eto K. The contribution of both forebrain and midbrain crest cells to the mesenchyme in the frontonasal mass of mouse embryos. Dev Biol 1994;164:409–419.
17. Dubois P, ElAmraoui A. Embryology of the pituitary gland. Trends Endo Metab 1995;6:1–7.
18. Ikeda H, Suzuki J, Sasano N, Niizuma H. The development and morphogenesis of the human pituitary gland. Anat Embryol 1988;178:327–336.
19. Rhodes SJ, DiMattia GE, Rosenfeld MG. Transcriptional mechanisms in anterior pituitary cell differentiation. Curr Opin Genet Dev 1994;4:709–717.
20. Rhodes SJ, Rosenfeld MG. Molecular involvement of the pit-1 gene in pituitary cell commitment. J Animal Sci 1996;74/2:94–106.
21. Sloop KW, McCutchan Schiller A, Blanton JR Jr, Meier BC, Rohrer G, Smith TPL, Rhodes SJ. Biochemical and genetic characterization of the porcine Prophet of Pit-1 pituitary transcription factor. Mol Cell Endocrinol 2000;168:77–87.
22. Watanabe YG. Effects of brain and mesenchyme upon the cytogenesis of rat adenohypophysis in vitro. Cell Tissue Res 1982;227:257–266.
23. Watanabe YG. An organ culture study of the site of determination of ACTH and LH cells in the rat adenohypophysis. Cell Tissue Res 1982;227:267–275.
24. Daikoku S, Chikamori M, Adachi T, Maki Y. Effect of the basal diencephalon on the development of Rathke's pouch in rats: a study in combined organ cultures. Dev Biol 1982;90:198–202.
25. Daikoku S, Chikamori M, Adachi T, Okamura Y, Nishiyama T, Tsuruo Y. Ontogenesis of hypothalamic immunoreactive ACTH cells in vivo and in vitro: role of Rathke's pouch. Dev Biol 1983;97:81–88.
26. Gleiberman A, Fedtsova N, Rosenfeld MG. Tissue interactions in the induction of anterior pituitary: role of the ventral diencephalon, mesenchyme, and notochord. Dev Biol 1999;213:340–353.
27. Grainger R, Henry J, Saha M, Servetnick M. Recent progress on the mechanisms of embryonic lens formation. Eye 1992;6:117–122.
28. Takuma N, Sheng H, Furuta Y, Ward J, Sharma K, Hogan B, et al. Formation of Rathke's pouch requires dual induction from the diencephalon. Development 1998;125:4835–4840.

29. Treier M, Gleiberman A, O'Connell S, Szeto D, McMahon J, McMahon A, Rosenfeld MG. Multistep signaling requirements for pituitary organogenesis in vivo. Genes Dev 1998;12:1691–1704.

30. Ericson J, Norlin S, Jessell T, Edlund T. Integrated FGF and BMP signaling controls the progression of progenitor cell differentiation and the emergence of pattern in the embryonic anterior pituitary. Development 1998;125:1005–1015.

31. Dasen J, O'Connell SM, Flynn S, Treier M, Gleiberman A, Szeto D, et al. Reciprocal interactions of Pit1 and GATA2 mediate signaling gradient-induced determination of pituitary cell types. Cell 1999;97: 587–598.

32. Kioussi C, O'Connell S, St-Onge L, Treier M, Gleiberman AS, Gruss P, Rosenfeld MG. Pax6 is essential for establishing ventral-dorsal cell boundaries in pituitary gland development. Proc Natl Acad Sci USA 1999;96:14,378–14,382.

33. Begeot M, Dubois M, Dubois P. Growth hormone and ACTH in the pituitary of normal and anencephalic human fetuses: immunocytochemical evidence for hypothalamic influences during development. Neuroendocrinology 1977;24:208–220.

34. Osamura R. Functional prenatal development of anencephalic and normal anterior pituitary glands. Acta Path Jap 1977;27:495–509.

35. Pilavdzic D, Kovacs K, Asa S. Pituitary morphology in anencephalic human fetuses. Neuroendocrinology 1997;65:164–172.

36. Lin SC, Li S, Drolet DW, Rosenfeld MG. Pituitary ontogeny of the Snell dwarf mouse reveals Pit-1-independent and Pit-1-dependent origins of the thyrotrope. Development 1994;120:515–522.

37. Nakai S, Kawano H, Yudate T, Nishi M, Kuno J, Nagata A, et al. The POU domain transcription factor Brn-2 is required for the determination of specific neuronal lineages in the hypothalamus of the mouse. Genes Dev 1995;9:3109–3121.

38. Schonemann MD, Ryan AK, McEvilly RJ, O'Connell SM, Arias CA, Kalla KA, et al. Development and survival of the endocrine hypothalamus and posterior pituitary gland requires the neuronal POU domain factor Brn-2. Genes Dev 1995;9:3122–3135.

39. Laurent-Huck FM, Egles C, Kienlen P, Stoeckel ME, Felix JM. Expression of the c-ets1 gene in the hypothalamus and pituitary during rat development. Brain Res Dev Brain Res 1996;97:107–117.

40. Zanaria E, Muscatelli F, Bardoni B, Strom TM, Guioli S, Guo W, et al. An unusual member of the nuclear hormone receptor superfamily responsible for X-linked adrenal hypoplasia congenita. Nature 1994;372:635–641.

41. Muscatelli F, Strom TM, Walker AP, Zanaria E, Recan D, Meindl A, et al. Mutations in the DAX-1 gene give rise to both X-linked adrenal hypoplasia congenita and hypogonadotropic hypogonadism. Nature 1994;372:672–676.

42. Swain A, Zanaria E, Hacker A, Lovell-Badge R, Camerino G. Mouse Dax1 expression is consistent with a role in sex determination as well as in adrenal and hypothalamus function. Nat Genet 1996;12: 404–409.

43. Goodfellow PN, Camerino G. DAX-1, an 'antitestis' gene. Cell Mol Life Sci 1999;55:857–863.

44. Li H, Zeitler P, Valerius M, Smal, K, Potter S. Gsh-1, an orphan Hox gene, is required for normal pituitary development. EMBO J 1996;15:714–724.

45. Labosky PA, Winnier GE, Jetton TL, Hargett L, Ryan AK, Rosenfeld MG, et al. The winged helix gene, Mf3, is required for normal development of the diencephalon and midbrain, postnatal growth and the milk-ejection reflex. Development 1997;124:1263–1274.

46. Good DJ, Porter FD, Mahon KA, Parlow AF, Westphal H, Kirsch IR. Hypogonadism and obesity in mice with a targeted deletion of the Nhlh2 gene. Nat Genet 1997;15:397–401.

47. Acampora D, Postiglione MP, Avantaggiato V, Di Bonito M, Vaccarino FM, Michaud J, Simeone A. Progressive impairment of developing neuroendocrine cell lineages in the hypothalamus of mice lacking the Orthopedia gene. Genes Dev 1999;13:2787–2800.

48. Luo X, Ikeda Y, Parker K. A cell specific nuclear receptor is essential for adrenal and gonadal development and sexual differentiation. Cell 1994;77:481–490.

49. Ingraham HA, Lala D, Ikeda Y, Luo X, Shen W, Nachtigal M, et al. The nuclear receptor steroidogenic factor 1 acts as multiple levels of the reproductive axis. Genes Dev 1994;8:2302–2312.

50. Nomura M, Bartsch S, Nawata H, Omura T, Morohashi K. An E box element is required for the expression of the ad4bp gene, a mammalian homologue of ftz-f1 gene, which is essential for adrenal and gonadal development. J Biol Chem 1995;270:7453–7461.

51. Achermann JC, Ito M, Ito M, Hindmarsh PC, Jameson JL. A mutation in the gene encoding steroidogenic factor-1 causes XY sex reversal and adrenal failure in humans. Nat Genet 1999;22:125–126.

52. Michaud JL, Rosenquist T, May NR, Fan CM. Development of neuroendocrine lineages requires the bHLH-PAS transcription factor SIM 1. Genes Dev 1998;12:3264–3275.

53. Oliver G, Mailhos A, Wehr R, Copeland NG, Jenkins NA, Gruss P. Six3, a murine homologue of the sine oculis gene, demarcates the most anterior border of the developing neural plate and is expressed during eye development. Development 1995;121:4045–4055.

54. Wallis DE, Roessler E, Hehr U, Nanni L, Wiltshire T, Richieri-Costa A, et al. Mutations in the homeodomain of the human SIX3 gene cause holoprosencephaly. Nat Genet 1999;22:196–198.

55. Kimura S, Hara Y, Pineau T, Fernandez-Salguero P, Fox C, Ward J, Gonzalez F. The T/ebp null mouse: thyroid-specific enhancer binding protein is essential for the organogenesis of the thyroid, lung, ventral forebrain and pituitary. Genes Dev 1996;10:60–69.

56. Price M, Lazzaro D, Pohl T, Matte MG, Ruther U, Olivo JC, et al. Regional expression of the homeobox gene Nkx-2.2 in the developing mammalian forebrain. Neuron 1992;8:241–255.

57. Schonemann MD, Ryan AK, Erkman L, McEvilly RJ, Bermingham J, Rosenfeld MG. POU domain factors in neural development. Adv Exp Med Biol 1998;449:39–53.

58. Jacobson EM, Li P, Leon-del-Rio A, Rosenfeld MG, Aggarwal AK. Structure of Pit-1 POU domain bound to DNA as a dimer: unexpected arrangement and flexibility. Genes Dev 1997;11:198–212.

59. Wegner M, Drolet DW, Rosenfeld MG. POU-Domain proteins: structure and function of developmental regulators. Curr Op Cell Biol 1993;5:488.

60. Ojeda SR, Hill J, Hill DF, Costa ME, Tapia V, Cornea A, Ma YJ. The Oct-2 POU domain gene in the neuroendocrine brain: A transcriptional regulator of mammalian puberty. Endocrinology 1999;140: 3774–3789.

61. Wierman ME, Xiong X, Kepa JK, Spaulding AJ, Jacobsen BM, Fang Z, et al. Repression of gonadotropin-releasing hormone promoter activity by the POU homeodomain transcription factor SCIP/Oct-6/ Tst-1: a regulatory mechanism of phenotype expression? Mol Cell Biol 1997;17:1652–1665.

62. Valerius MT, Li H, Stock JL, Weinstein M, Kaur S, Singh G, Potter SS. Gsh-1: a novel murine homeobox gene expressed in the central nervous system. Dev Dyn 1995;203:337–351.

63. Li H, Schrick JJ, Fewell GD, MacFarland KL, Witte DP, Bodenmiller DM, et al. Novel strategy yields candidate Gsh-1 homeobox gene targets using hypothalamus progenitor cell lines. Dev Bio 1999;211: 64–76.

64. Li CM, Yan RT, Wang SZ. Misexpression of a bHLH gene, cNSCL1, results in abnormal brain development. Dev Dyn 1999;215:238–247.

65. Lala DS, Ikeda Y, Luo X, Baity LA, Meade JC, Parker KL. A cell-specific nuclear receptor regulates the steroid hydroxylases. Steroids 1995;60:10–14.

66. Ikeda Y, Luo X, Abbud R, Nilson JH, Parker KL. The nuclear receptor steroidogenic factor 1 is essential for the formation of the ventromedial hypothalamic nucleus. Mol Endocrinol 1995;9:478–486.

67. Barnhart KM, Mellon PL. The orphan nuclear receptor, steroidogenic factor-1, regulates the glycoprotein hormone alpha-subunit gene in pituitary gonadotropes. Mol Endocrinol 1994;8:878–885.

68. Ikeda Y, Swain A, Weber TJ, Hentges KE, Zanaria E, Lalli E, et al. Steroidogenic factor 1 and Dax-1 colocalize in multiple cell lineages: potential links in endocrine development. Mol Endocrinol 1996; 10:1261–1272.

69. Nachtigal MW, Hirokawa Y, Enyeart-VanHouten DL, Flanagan JN, Hammer GD, Ingraham HA. Wilm's tumor 1 and Dax-1 modulate the orphan nuclear receptor SF-1 in sex specific gene expression. Cell 1998;93:445–454.

70. Merke DP, Tajima T, Baron J, Cutler GB Jr. Hypogonadotropic hypogonadism in a female caused by an X-linked recessive mutation in the DAX1 gene. N Engl J Med 1999;340:1248–1252.

71. Bovolenta P, Mallamaci A, Puelles L, Boncinelli E. Expression pattern of cSix3, a member of the Six/ sine oculis family of transcription factors. Mech Dev 1998;70:201–203.

72. Leppert GS, Yang JM, Sundin OH. Sequence and location of SIX3, a homeobox gene expressed in the human eye. Ophthalmic Genet 1999;20:7–21.

73. Lee SL, Sadovsky Y, Swirnoff AH, Polish JA, Goda P, Gavrilina G, Milbrandt J. Luteinizing hormone deficiency and female infertility in mice lacking the transcription factor NGFI-A (Egr-1). Science 1996;273:1219–1221.

74. Topilko P, Schneider-Maunoury S, Levi G, Trembleau A, Gourdji D, Driancourt MA, et al. Multiple pituitary and ovarian defects in Krox-24 (NGFI-A, Egr-1)-targeted mice. Mol Endocrinol 1998;12: 107–122.

75. Scully KM, Gleiberman AS, Lindzey J, Lubahn DB, Korach KS, Rosenfeld MG. Role of estrogen receptor-alpha in the anterior pituitary gland. Mol Endocrinol 1997;11:674–681.

76. Gordon DF, Lewis SR, Haugen BR, James RA, McDermott MT, Wood WM, Ridgway EC. Pit-1 and GATA-2 interact and functionally cooperate to activate the thyrotropin beta-subunit promoter. J Biol Chem 1997;272:24,339–24,347.

77. Thor S, Ericson J, Brannstrom T, Edlund T. The homeodomain LIM protein Isl-1 is expressed in subsets of neurons and endocrine cells in the adult rat. Neuron 1991;7:881–889.

78. Varela-Echavarria A, Pfaff SL, Guthrie S. Differential expression of LIM homeobox genes among motor neuron subpopulations in the developing chick brain stem. Mol Cell Neurosci 1996;8:242–257.

79. Sheng HZ, Zhadanov AB, Mosinger B Jr, Fujii T, Bertuzzi S, Grinberg A, et al. Specification of pituitary cell lineages by the LIM homeobox gene Lhx3. Science 1996;272:1004–1007.

80. Sheng HZ, Moriyama K, Yamashita T, Li H, Potter SS, Mahon KA, Westphal H. Multistep control of pituitary organogenesis. Science 1997;278:1809–1812.

81. Netchine I, Sobrier ML, Krude H, Schnabel D, Maghnie M, Marcos E, et al. Mutations in LHX3 result in a new syndrome revealed by combined pituitary hormone deficiency. Nat Genet 2000;25:182–186.

82. Sarapura VD, Strouth HL, Gordon DF, Wood WM, Ridgway EC. Msx1 is present in thyrotropic cells and binds to a consensus site on the glycoprotein hormone alpha-subunit promoter. Mol Endocrinol 1997;11:1782–1794.

83. Poulin G, Turgeon B, Drouin J. NeuroD1/beta2 contributes to cell-specific transcription of the pro-opiomelanocortin gene. Mol Cell Biol 1997;17:6673–6682.

84. Jiang Y, Yu VC, Buchholz F, O'Connell S, Rhodes SJ, Candeloro C, et al. A novel family of Cys-Cys, His-Cys zinc finger transcription factors expressed in developing nervous system and pituitary gland. J Biol Chem 1996;271:10,723–10,730.

85. Acampora D, Mazan S, Tuorto F, Avantaggiato V, Tremblay JJ, Lazzaro D, et al. Transient dwarfism and hypogonadism in mice lacking Otx1 reveal prepubescent stage-specific control of pituitary levels of GH, FSH and LH. Development 1998;125:1229–1239.

86. Li S, Crenshaw EB III, Rawson EJ, Simmons DM, Swanson LW, Rosenfeld MG. Dwarf locus mutants lacking three pituitary cell types result from mutations in the POU-domain gene pit-1. Nature 1990; 347:528–533.

87. Sornson MW, Wu W, Dasen JS, Flynn SE, Norman DJ, O'Connell SM, et al. Pituitary lineage determination by the Prophet of Pit-1 homeodomain factor defective in Ames dwarfism. Nature 1996;384: 327–333.

88. Lanctot C, Moreau A, Chamberland M, Tremblay ML, Drouin J. Hindlimb patterning and mandible development require the Ptx1 gene. Development 1999;126:1805–1810.

89. Szeto DP, Rodriguez-Esteban C, Ryan AK, O'Connell SM, Liu F, Kioussi C, et al. Role of the Bicoid-related homeodomain factor Pitx1 in specifying hindlimb morphogenesis and pituitary development. Genes Dev 1999;13:484–494.

90. Ryan AK, Blumberg B, Rodriguez-Esteban C, Yonei-Tamura S, Tamura K, Tsukui T, et al. Pitx2 determines left-right asymmetry of internal organs in vertebrates. Nature 1998;394:545–551.

91. Logan M, Pagan-Westphal SM, Smith DM, Paganessi L, Tabin CJ. The transcription factor Pitx2 mediates situs-specific morphogenesis in response to left-right asymmetric signals. Cell 1998;94:307–317.

92. Piedra ME, Icardo JM, Albajar M, Rodriguez-Rey JC, Ros MA. Pitx2 participates in the late phase of the pathway controlling left-right asymmetry. Cell 1998;94:319–324.

93. Yoshioka H, Meno C, Koshiba K, Sugihara M, Itoh H, Ishimaru Y, et al. Pitx2, a bicoid-type homeobox gene, is involved in a lefty-signaling pathway in determination of left-right asymmetry. Cell 1998;94: 299–305.

94. Lu MF, Pressman C, Dyer R, Johnson RL, Martin JF. Function of Rieger syndrome gene in left-right asymmetry and craniofacial development. Nature 1999;401:276–278.

95. Lin CR, Kioussi C, O'Connell S, Briata P, Szeto D, Liu F, et al. Pitx2 regulates lung asymmetry, cardiac positioning and pituitary and tooth morphogenesis. Nature 1999;401:279–282.

96. Rhodes SJ, Chen R, DiMattia GE, Scully KM, Kalla KA, Lin SC, et al. A tissue-specific enhancer confers Pit-1-dependent morphogen inducibility and autoregulation on the pit-1 gene. Genes Dev 1993; 7:913–932.

97. Dattani MT, Martinez-Barbera JP, Thomas PQ, Brickman JM, Gupta R, Martensson IL, et al. Mutations in the homeobox gene HESX1/Hesx1 associated with septo-optic dysplasia in human and mouse. Nat Genet 1998;19:125–133.

98. Dattani MT, Martinez-Barbera JP, Thomas PQ, Brickman JM, Gupta R, Wales JK, et al. HESX1: a novel gene implicated in a familial form of septo-optic dysplasia. Acta Paediatr Suppl 1999;88:49–54.

99. Gothe S, Wang Z, Ng L, Kindblom JM, Barros AC, Ohlsson C, et al. Mice devoid of all known thyroid hormone receptors are viable but exhibit disorders of the pituitary-thyroid axis, growth, and bone maturation. Genes Dev 1999;13:1329–1341.

100. Drolet DW, Scully KM, Simmons DM, Wegner M, Chu KT, Swanson LW, Rosenfeld MG. TEF, a transcription factor expressed specifically in the anterior pituitary during embryogenesis, defines a new class of leucine zipper proteins. Genes Dev 1991;5:1739–1753.

101. Lipkin SM, Naar AM, Kalla KA, Sack RA, Rosenfeld MG. Identification of a novel zinc finger protein binding a conserved element critical for Pit-1-dependent growth hormone gene expression. Genes Dev 1993;7:1674–1687.

102. VanderHeyden TC, Wojtkiewicz PW, Voss TC, Mangin TM, Harrelson Z, Ahlers KM, et al. Mouse growth hormone transcription factor Zn-16: unique bipartite structure containing tandemly repeated zinc finger domains not reported in rat Zn-15. Mol Cell Endocrinol 2000;159:89–98.

103. Gage PJ, Suh H, Camper SA. The bicoid-related Pitx gene family in development. Mamm Genome 1999;10:197–200.

104. Drouin J, Lamolet B, Lamonerie T, Lanctot C, Tremblay JJ. The PTX family of homeodomain transcription factors during pituitary development. Mol Cell Endocrinol 1998;140:31–36.

105. Lamonerie T, Tremblay JJ, Lanctot C, Therrien M, Gauthier Y, Drouin J. Ptx1, a bicoid-related homeo box transcription factor involved in transcription of the pro-opiomelanocortin gene. Genes Dev 1996; 10:1284–1295.

106. Szeto DP, Ryan AK, O'Connell SM, Rosenfeld MG. P-OTX: a PIT-1-interacting homeodomain factor expressed during anterior pituitary gland development. Proc Natl Acad Sci USA 1996;93:7706–7710.

107. Lanctot C, Lamolet B, Drouin J. The bicoid-related homeoprotein Ptx1 defines the most anterior domain of the embryo and differentiates posterior from anterior lateral mesoderm. Development 1997; 124:2807–2817.

108. Lanctot C, Gauthier Y, Drouin J. Pituitary homeobox 1 (Ptx1) is differentially expressed during pituitary development. Endocrinology 1999;140:1416–1422.

109. Tremblay JJ, Lanctot C, Drouin J. The pan-pituitary activator of transcription, Ptx1 (pituitary homeobox 1), acts in synergy with SF-1 and Pit1 and is an upstream regulator of the Lim-homeodomain gene Lim3/Lhx3. Mol Endocrinol 1998;12:428–441.

110. Poulin G, Lebel M, Chamberland M, Paradis FW, Drouin J. Specific protein-protein interaction between basic helix-loop-helix transcription factors and homeoproteins of the Pitx family. Mol Cell Biol 2000; 20:4826–4837.

111. Tremblay JJ, Goodyer CG, Drouin J. Transcriptional properties of ptx1 and ptx2 isoforms. Neuroendocrinology 2000;71:277–286.

112. Gage P, Camper S. Pituitary homeobox 2, a novel member of the bicoid-related family of homeobox genes, is a potential regulator of anterior structure formation. Hum Mol Genet 1991;6:457–464.

113. Tremblay JJ, Drouin J. Egr-1 is a downstream effector of GnRH and synergizes by direct interaction with Ptx1 and SF-1 to enhance luteinizing hormone beta gene transcription. Mol Cell Biol 1999;19: 2567–2576.

114. Hobert O, Westphal H. Functions of LIM-homeobox genes. Trends Genet 2000;16:75–83.

115. Seidah NG, Barale JC, Marcinkiewicz M, Mattei MG, Day R, Chretien M. The mouse homeoprotein mLIM-3 is expressed early in cells derived from the neuroepithelium and persists in adult pituitary. DNA Cell Biol 1994;13:1163–1180.

116. Zhadanov AB, Bertuzzi S, Taira M, Dawid IB, Westphal H. Expression pattern of the murine LIM class homeobox gene Lhx3 in subsets of neural and neuroendocrine tissues. Dev Dyn 1995;202: 354–364.

117. Bach I, Rhodes SJ, Pearse RV II, Heinzel T, Gloss B, Scully KM, et al. P-Lim, a LIM homeodomain factor, is expressed during pituitary organ and cell commitment and synergizes with Pit-1. Proc Natl Acad Sci USA 1995;92:2720–2724.

118. Meier BC, Price JR, Parker GE, Bridwell JL, Rhodes SJ. Characterization of the porcine Lhx3/LIM-3/P-Lim LIM homeodomain transcription factor. Mol Cell Endocrinol 1999;147:65–74.

119. Sloop KW, Meier BC, Bridwell JL, Parker GE, Schiller AM, Rhodes SJ. Differential activation of pituitary hormone genes by human Lhx3 isoforms with distinct DNA binding properties. Mol Endocrinol 1999;13:2212–2225.

120. Glasgow E, Karavanov AA, Dawid IB. Neuronal and neuroendocrine expression of lim3, a LIM class homeobox gene, is altered in mutant zebrafish with axial signaling defects. Dev Biol 1997;192:405–419.

121. Thor S, Andersson SGE, Tomlinson A, Thomas JB. A LIM-homeodomain combinatorial code for motor neuron pathway selection. Nature 1999;397:76–80.

122. Bach I, Carrière C, Ostendorff HP, Anderson B, Rosenfeld MG. A family of LIM domain-associated cofactors confer transcriptional synergism between LIM and Otx homeodomain proteins. Genes Dev 1997;11:1370–1380.

123. Howard PW, Maurer RA. Identification of a conserved protein that interacts with specific LIM homeodomain transcription factors. J Biol Chem 2000;275:13,336–13,342.

124. Glenn DJ, Maurer RA. MRG1 binds to the LIM domain of Lhx2 and may function as a coactivator to stimulate glycoprotein hormone alpha-subunit gene expression. J Biol Chem 1999;274:36,159–36,167.

125. Roberson MS, Schoderbek WE, Tremml G, Maurer RA. Activation of the glycoprotein hormone α-subunit promoter by a LIM-homeodomain transcription factor. Mol Cell Biol 1994;14:2985–2993.

126. Brinkmeier ML, Gordon DF, Dowding JM, Saunders TL, Kendall SK, Sarapura VD, et al. Cell-specific expression of the mouse glycoprotein hormone-alpha subunit gene requires multiple interacting DNA elements in transgenic mice and cultured cells. Mol Endocrinol 1998;12:622–633.

127. Simmons DM, Voss JW, Ingraham HA, Holloway JM, Broide RS, Rosenfeld MG, Swanson LW. Pituitary cell phenotypes involve cell-specific Pit-1 mRNA translation and synergistic interactions with other transcription factors. Genes Dev 1990;4:695–711.

128. Malagon MM, Garrido JC, Dieulois C, Hera C, Castrillo JL, Dobado-Berrios PM, Gracia-Navarro F. Expression of the pituitary transcription factor GHF-1/PIT-1 in cell types of the adult porcine adenohypophysis. J Histochem Cytochem 1996;44:621–627.

129. Fofanova O, Takamura N, Kinoshita E, Yoshimoto M, Tsuji Y, Peterkova V, et al. Rarity of Pit-1 involvement in children from Russia with combined hormone deficiency. Am J Med Genet 1998;77: 360–365.

130. Ohta K, Nobukuni Y, Mitsubuchi H, Fujimoto S, Matsuo N, Inagaki H, et al. Mutations in the Pit-1 gene in children with combined pituitary hormone deficiency. Biochem Biophys Res Commun 1992;189: 851–855.

131. Pellegrini-Bouiller I, Belicar P, Barlier A, Gunz G, Charvet J, Jaquet P, et al. A new mutation of the gene encoding the transcription factor Pit-1 is responsible for combined pituitary hormone deficiency. J Clin Endocrinol Metab 1996;81:2790–2796.

132. Pfäffle R, DiMattia G, Parks J, Brown M, Wit J, Jansen M, et al. Mutation of the POU-specific domain of Pit-1 and hypopituitarism without pituitary hypoplasia. Science 1992;257:1118–1121.

133. Tatsumi K, Miyai K, Notomi T, Kaibe K, Amino N, et al. Cretinism with combined hormone deficiency caused by a mutation in the Pit-1 gene. Nat Genet 1992;1:56–58.

134. Brown M, Parks J, Adess M, Rich B, Rosenthal I, Voss T, et al. Central hypothyroidism reveals compound heterozygous mutations in the Pit-1 gene. Horm Res 1998;49:98–102.

135. Bakker B, Jansen M, Hendriks-Stegeman B. A new mutation in the *Pit-1* gene, discovered by the neonatal congenital hypothyroidism (CH) screening program. Horm Res 1997;201:161.

136. Botero D, Brue T, Cohen L, Hashimoto Y, Zanger K, Radovick S. Defective interaction of a mutant Pit-1, K216E, with CBP inhibits human prolactin gene expression. Abstracts of 2000 Endocrine Society Meeting, p. 168, The Endocrine Society Press, Bethesda, MD.

137. Pernasetti F, Milner R, Al Ashwal A, Zegher F, Chavez V, Muller M, Martial J. Pro239Ser: a novel recessive mutation of the Pit-1 gene in seven middle eastern children with growth hormone, prolactin, and thyrotropin deficiency. J Clin Endocrinol Metab 1998;83:2079–2083.

138. Irie Y, Tatsumi K, Ogawa M, Kamijo T, Preeyasombat C, Suprasongsin C, Amino N. A novel E250X mutation of the Pit-1 gene in a patient with combined pituitary hormone deficiency. Endocr J 1995; 42:351–354.

139. Radovick S, Nations M, Du Y, Berg L, Weintraub B, Wondisford F. A mutation in the POU-homeodomain of Pit-1 responsible for combined pituitary hormone deficiency. Science 1992;257:1115–1118.

140. Aarskog D, Eiken H, Bjerknes R, Myking O. Pituitary dwarfism in the R271W Pit-1 gene mutation. Eur J Pediatr 1997;156:829–834.

141. Ward L, Chavez M, Huot C, Lecocq P, Collu R, Decarie J, et al. Severe congenital hypopituitarism with low prolactin levels and age-dependent anterior pituitary hypoplasia: a clue to a Pit-1 mutation. J Pediatr 1998;132:1036–1038.

142. Arnhold I, Nery M, Brown M, Voss T, VanderHeyden T, Adess M, et al. Clinical and molecular characterization of a Brazilian patient with Pit-1 deficiency. J Pediatr Endocrinol Metab 1998;11:623–630.

143. Martineli A, Braga M, De Lacerda L, Raskin S, Graf H. Description of a Brazilian patient bearing the R271W Pit-1 gene mutation. Thyroid 1998;8:299–304.

144. Holl R, Pfäffle R, Kim C, Sorgo W, Teller W, Heimann G. Combined pituitary deficiencies of growth hormone, thyroid stimulating hormone and prolactin due to Pit-1 gene mutation: a case report. Eur J Pediatr 1997;156:835–837.

145. Okamoto N, Wada Y, Ida S, Koga R, Ozono K, Chiyo H, et al. Monoallelic expression of normal mRNA in the Pit-1 mutation heterozygotes with normal phenotype and biallelic expression in the abnormal phenotype. Hum Mol Genet 1994;3:1565–1568.

146. Sakamoto S, Kitagawa Y, Muraki T, Inoue K, Sakai T. Immunohistochemical Evidence of Two Independent Thyrotrope Cell Lineages. Abstracts of 2000 Endocrine Society Meeting, p. 385.

147. Duquesnoy P, Roy A, Dastot F, Ghali I, Teinturier C, Netchine I, et al. Human Prop-1: cloning, mapping, genomic structure. Mutations in familial combined pituitary hormone deficiency. FEBS Lett 1998;437:216–220.

148. Deladoëy J, Flück C, Büyükgebiz A, Kuhlmann BV, Eblé A, Hindmarsh PC, et al. "Hot spot" in the PROP1 gene responsible for combined pituitary hormone deficiency. J Clin Endocrinol Metab 1999;84: 1645–1650.

149. Fofanova O, Takamura N, Kinoshita E, Parks JS, Brown M, Peterkova V, et al. A mutational hot spot in the PROP-1 gene in Russian children with combined pituitary hormone deficiency. Pituitary 1998; 1:45–49.

150. Fofanova O, Takamura N, Kinoshita E, Parks JS, Brown M, Peterkova V, et al. Compound heterozygous deletion of the PROP-1 gene in children with combined pituitary hormone deficiency. J Clin Endocrinol Metab 1998;83:2601–2604.

151. Fofanova O, Takamura N, Kinoshita E, Vorontsov A, Vladimirova V, Dedov I, et al. MR imaging of the pituitary gland in children and young adults with congenital combined pituitary hormone deficiency associated with PROP1 mutations. AJR Am J Roentgenol 2000;174:555–559.

152. Krzisnik C, Kolacio Z, Battelino T, Brown M, Parks JS, Laron Z. The "little people" of the island of Krk-revisited. Etiology of hypopituitarism revealed. J Endo Genet 1999;1:9–19.

153. Vallette-Kasic S, Barlier A, Manavela M, Teinturier C, Brue T. Two hot spots in the PROP1 gene of patients with multiple pituitary hormone deficiency. Abstracts of 2000 Endocrine Society Meeting, p. 448, The Endocrine Society Press, Bethesda, MD.

154. Osorio M, Kopp P, Marui S, Latronico A, Mendonca B, Arnhold I. A novel mutation of a highly conserved residue (F88S) in the homeodomain of Prop1 impairs DNA-binding and causes combined pituitary hormone deficiency. Abstracts of 2000 Endocrine Society Meeting, p. 510, The Endocrine Society Press, Bethesda, MD.

155. Vieira TC, Silva M, Cerutti J, Borges M, Brunner E, Abucham J. A novel mutation Arg99Gln in the hot spot region of Prop-1 gene causing familial combined pituitary hormone deficiency. Abstracts of 2000 Endocrine Society Meeting, p. 538, The Endocrine Society Press, Bethesda, MD.

156. Wu W, Cogan J, Pfäffle R, Dasen J, Frisch H, O'Connell S, et al. Mutations in PROP1 cause familial combined pituitary hormone deficiency. Nat Genet 1998;18:147–149.

157. Pernasetti F, Toledo S, Vasilyev V, Hayashida C, Cogan J, Ferrari C, et al. Impaired adrenocorticotropin-adrenal axis in combined pituitary hormone deficiency caused by a two-base pair deletion (301-302delAG) in the prophet of Pit-1 gene. J Clin Endocrinol Metab 2000;85:390–397.

158. Takamura N, Fofanova O, Kinoshita E, Yamashita S. Gene analysis of PROP1 in dwarfism with combined pituitary hormone deficiency. Growth Horm IGF Res 1999;9:12–17.

159. Nogueira C, Sabacan L, Jameson J, Medeiros-Neto G, Kopp P. Combined pituitary hormone deficiency in an inbred Brazilian kindred associated with a mutation in the PROP-1 gene. Mol Genet Metab 1999;67:58–61.

160. Rosenbloom AL, Almonte AS, Brown MR, Fisher DA, Baumbach L, Parks JS. Clinical and biochemical phenotype of familial anterior hypopituitarism from mutation of the PROP1 gene. J Clin Endocrinol Metab 1999;84:50–57.

161. Cogan J, Wu W, Phillips J III, Arnhold I, Agapito A, Fofanova O, et al. The PROP1 2-base pair deletion is a common cause of combined pituitary hormone deficiency. J Clin Endocrinol Metab 1998;83: 3346–3349.

162. Mendonca BB, Osorio MG, Latronico AC, Estefan V, Lo LS, Arnhold IJ. Longitudinal hormonal and pituitary imaging changes in two females with combined pituitary hormone deficiency due to deletion of A301,G302 in the PROP1 gene. J Clin Endocrinol Metab 1999;84:942–945.

163. Flück C, Deladoëy J, Rutishauser K, Eble A, Marti U, Wu W, Mullis P. Phenotypic variability in familial combined pituitary hormone deficiency caused by a PROP1 gene mutation resulting in the substitution of Arg—>Cys at codon 120(R120C). J Clin Endocrinol Metab 1998;83:3727–3734.

164. Tang K, Bartke A, Gardiner CS, Wagner TE, Yun JS. Gonadotropin secretion, synthesis, and gene expression in human growth hormone transgenic mice and in Ames dwarf mice. Endocrinology 1993; 132:2518–2524.

165. Andersen B, Pearse II RV, Jenne K, Sornson M, Lin SC, Bartke A, Rosenfeld MG. The Ames dwarf gene is required for Pit-1 gene activation. Dev Biol 1995;172:495–503.

166. Gage PJ, Lossie AC, Scarlett LM, Lloyd RV, Camper SA. Ames dwarf mice exhibit somatotrope commitment but lack growth hormone-releasing factor response. Endocrinology 1995;136:1161–1167.

167. Gage PJ, Roller ML, Saunders TL, Scarlett LM, Camper SA. Anterior pituitary cells defective in the cell-autonomous factor, df, undergo cell lineage specification but not expansion. Development 1996; 122:151–160.

168. Gage PJ, Brinkmeier ML, Scarlett LM, Knapp LT, Camper SA, Mahon KA. The Ames dwarf gene, df, is required early in pituitary ontogeny for the extinction of Rpx transcription and initiation of lineage-specific cell proliferation. Mol Endocrinol 1996;10:1570–1581.

169. Thomas PQ, Johnson BV, Rathjen J, Rathjen PD. Sequence, genomic organization, and expression of the novel homeobox gene Hesx1. J Biol Chem 1995;270:3869–3875.

170. Hermesz E, Mackem S, Mahon KA. Rpx: a novel anterior-restricted homeobox gene progressively activated in the prechordal plate, anterior neural plate and Rathke's pouch of the mouse embryo. Development 1996;122:41–52.

171. Gehring WJ, Ikeo K. Pax 6: mastering eye morphogenesis and eye evolution. Trends Genet 1999;15: 371–377.

172. Terzic J, Saraga-Babic M. Expression pattern of PAX3 and PAX6 genes during human embryogenesis. Int J Dev Biol 1999;43:501–508.

173. Bentley CA, Zidehsarai MP, Grindley JC, Parlow AF, Barth-Hall S, Roberts VJ. Pax6 is implicated in murine pituitary endocrine function. Endocrine 1999;10:171–177.

174. Dohrmann C, Gruss P, Lemaire L. Pax genes and the differentiation of hormone-producing endocrine cells in the pancreas. Mech Dev 2000;92:47–54.

175. Liu M, Pleasure SJ, Collins AE, Noebels JL, Naya FJ, Tsai MJ, Lowenstein DH. Loss of BETA2/ NeuroD leads to malformation of the dentate gyrus and epilepsy. Proc Natl Acad Sci USA 2000;97:865–870.

176. Pelletier G, Labrie C, Labrie F. Localization of oestrogen receptor alpha, oestrogen receptor beta and androgen receptors in the rat reproductive organs. J Endocrinol 2000;165:359–370.

177. Semina E, Reiter R, Leysens N, Lee W, Alward M, Small K, et al. Cloning and characterization of a novel bicoid-related homeobox transcription factor gene, RIEG, involved in Rieger syndrome. Nat Genet 1996;14:392–399.

178. Doward W, Perveen R, Lloyd IC, Ridgway AE, Wilson L, Black GC. A mutation in the RIEG1 gene associated with Peters' anomaly. J Med Genet 1999;36:152–155.

179. Kulak SC, Kozlowski K, Semina EV, Pearce WG, Walter MA. Mutation in the RIEG1 gene in patients with iridogoniodysgenesis syndrome. Hum Mol Genet 1998;7:1113–1117.

180. Alward WL, Semina EV, Kalenak JW, Heon E, Sheth BP, Stone EM, Murray JC. Autosomal dominant iris hypoplasia is caused by a mutation in the Rieger syndrome (RIEG/PITX2) gene. Am J Ophthalmol 1998;125:98–100.

181. Amendt B, Sutherland L, Semina E, Russo A. The molecular basis of Rieger syndrome. J Biol Chem 1998;273:20,066–20,072.

182. Sloop KW, Showalter AD, Von Kap-Herr C, Pettenati MJ, Rhodes SJ. Analysis of the human LHX3 neuroendocrine transcription factor gene and mapping to the subtelomeric region of chromosome 9. Gene 2000;245:237–243.

183. Sloop KW, Walvoord EC, Showalter AD, Pescovitz OH, Rhodes SJ. Molecular analysis of LHX3 and PROP-1 in pituitary hormone deficiency patients with posterior pituitary ectopia. J Clin Endo Metab 2000;85:2701-2708.

184. Ohta K, Nobukuni Y, Mitsubuchi H, Ohta T, Tohma T, Jinno Y, et al. Characterization of the gene encoding human pituitary-specific transcription factor, Pit-1. Gene 1992;122:387–388.

185. Cohen LE, Wondisford FE, Salvatoni A, Maghnie M, Brucker-Davis F, Weintraub BD, Radovick S. A "hot spot" in the Pit-1 gene responsible for combined pituitary hormone deficiency: clinical and molecular correlates. J Clin Endocrinol Metab 1995;80:679–684.

186. Cohen LE, Hashimoto Y, Zanger K, Wondisford F, Radovick S. CREB-independent regulation by CBP is a novel mechanism of human growth hormone gene expression. J Clin Invest 1999;104:1123–1130.

187. Nakamura Y, Usui T, Mizuta H, Murabe H, Muro S, Suda M, et al. Characterization of Prophet of Pit-1 gene expression in normal pituitary and pituitary adenomas in humans. J Clin Endocrinol Metab 1999;84:1414–1419.

188. Essner J, Branford W, Zhang J, Yost H. Mesendoderm and left-right brain and gut development are differentially regulated by pitx2 isoforms. Development 2000;127:1081–1093.

189. Schanke JT, Conwell CM, Durning M, Fisher JM, Golos TG. Pit-1/growth hormone factor 1 splice variant expression in the rhesus monkey pituitary gland and the rhesus and human placenta. J Clin Endocrinol Metab 1997;82:800–807.

190. Kurima K, Weatherly KL, Sharova L, Wong EA. Synthesis of turkey Pit-1 mRNA variants by alternative splicing and transcription initiation. DNA Cell Biol 1998;17:93–103.

191. Majumdar S, Irwin DM, Elsholtz HP. Selective constraints on the activation domain of transcription factor Pit-1. Proc Natl Acad Sci USA 1996;93:10,256–10,261.

192. Voss JV, Wilson L, Rhodes SJ, Rosenfeld MG. An alternative RNA splicing product reveals modular binding and non-modular transcriptional activities of the Pit-1 POU-specific domain. Mol Endocrinol 1993;7:1551–1560.

193. Voss JW, Yao TP, Rosenfeld MG. Alternative translation initiation site usage results in two structurally distinct forms of Pit-1. J Biol Chem 1991;266:12,832–12,835.

194. Zhadanov AB, Copeland NG, Gilbert DJ, Jenkins NA, Westphal H. Genomic structure and chromosomal localization of the mouse LIM/homeobox gene Lhx3. Genomics 1995;27:27–32.

195. Kapiloff MS, Farkash Y, Wegner M, Rosenfeld MG. Variable effects of phosphorylation of Pit-1 dictated by the DNA response elements. Science 1991;253:786–789.

196. Fischberg DJ, Chen XH, Bancroft C. A Pit-1 phosphorylation mutant can mediate both basal and induced prolactin and growth hormone promoter activity. Mol Endocrinol 1994;8:1566–1573.

197. Okimura Y, Howard PW, Maurer RA. Pit-1 binding sites mediate transcriptional responses to cyclic adenosine 3',5'-monophosphate through a mechanism that does not require inducible phosphorylation of Pit-1. Mol Endocrinol 1994;8:1559–1565.

198. Gaddy-Kurten D, Vale WW. Activin increases phosphorylation and decreases stability of the transcription factor Pit-1 in MtTW15 somatotrope cells. J Biol Chem 1995;270:28,733–28,739.

199. Caelles C, Hennemann H, Karin M. M-phase-specific phosphorylation of the POU transcription factor GHF-1 by a cell cycle-regulated protein kinase inhibits DNA binding. Mol Cell Biol 1995;15:6694–6701.

200. Cohen LE, Zanger K, Brue T, Wondisford FE, Radovick S. Defective retinoic acid regulation of the Pit-1 gene enhancer: a novel mechanism of combined pituitary hormone deficiency. Mol Endocrinol 1999;13:476–484.

201. Xu L, Lavinsky RM, Dasen JS, Flynn SE, McInerney EM, Mullen TM, et al. Signal-specific co-activator domain requirements for Pit-1 activation. Nature 1998;395:301–306.

202. Wolffe AP, Hayes JJ. Chromatin disruption and modification. Nucleic Acids Res 1999;27:711–720.

203. Lemon BD, Freedman LP. Nuclear receptor cofactors as chromatin remodelers. Curr Opin Genet Dev 1999;9:499–504.

204. Glass CK, Rosenfeld MG. The coregulator exchange in transcriptional functions of nuclear receptors. Genes Dev 2000;14:121–141.

205. Spencer TE, Jenster G, Burcin MM, Allis CD, Zhou J, Mizzen CA, et al. Steroid receptor coactivator-1 is a histone acetyltransferase. Nature 1997;389:194–198.

206. Xu J, Qui Y, DeMayo FJ, Tsai SY, Tsai MJ, O'Malley BW. Partial hormone resistance in mice with disruption of the steroid receptor coactivator-1 (SRC-1) gene. Science 1998;279:1922–1925.

207. Kamei Y, Xu L, Heinzel T, Torchia J, Kurokawa R, Gloss B, et al. A CBP integrator complex mediates transcriptional activation and AP-1 inhibition by nuclear receptors. Cell 1996;85:403–414.

208. Korzus E, Torchia J, Rose DW, Xu L, Kurokawa R, McInerney EM, et al. Transcription factor-specific requirements for coactivators and their acetyltransferase functions. Science 1998;279:703–707.

209. Chen H, Lin RJ, Schiltz RL, Chakravarti D, Nash A, Nagy L, et al. Nuclear receptor coactivator ACTR is a novel histone acetyltransferase and forms a multimeric activation complex with P/CAF and CBP/p300. Cell 1997;90:569–580.

210. Heinzel T, Lavinsky RM, Mullen TM, Soderstrom M, Laherty CD, Torchia J, et al. A complex containing N-CoR, mSin3 and histone deacetylase mediates transcriptional repression. Nature 1997;387:43–48.

211. Torchia J, Rose DW, Inostroza J, Kamei Y, Westin S, Glass CK, Rosenfeld MG. The transcriptional co-activator p/CIP binds CBP and mediates nuclear-receptor function. Nature 1997;387:677–684.

212. Utley RT, Ikeda K, Grant PA, Cote J, Steger DJ, Eberharter A, et al. Transcriptional activators direct histone acetyltransferase complexes to nucleosomes. Nature 1998;394:498–502.

213. Lavinsky RM, Jepsen K, Heinzel T, Torchia J, Mullen TM, Schiff R, et al. Diverse signaling pathways modulate nuclear receptor recruitment of N-CoR and SMRT complexes. Proc Natl Acad Sci USA 1998;95:2920–2925.

214. Smith CL, Onate SA, Tsai MJ, O'Malley BW. CREB binding protein acts synergistically with steroid receptor coactivator-1 to enhance steroid receptor-dependent transcription. Proc Natl Acad Sci USA 1996;93:8884–8888.

215. Kawasaki H, Eckner R, Yao TP, Taira K, Chiu R, Livingston DM, Yokoyama KK. Distinct roles of the co-activators p300 and CBP in retinoic-acid-induced F9-cell differentiation. Nature 1998;393:284–289.

216. Perissi V, Dasen JS, Kurokawa R, Wang Z, Korzus E, Rose DW, et al. Factor-specific modulation of CREB-binding protein acetyltransferase activity. Proc Natl Acad Sci USA 1999;96:3652–3657.

217. Zanger K, Cohen LE, Hashimoto K, Radovick S, Wondisford FE. A novel mechanism for cyclic adenosine 3',5'-monophosphate regulation of gene expression by CREB-binding protein. Mol Endocrinol 1999;13:268–275.

218. Lanz RB, McKenna NJ, Onate SA, Albrecht U, Wong J, Tsai SY, et al. A steroid receptor coactivator, SRA, functions as an RNA and is present in an SRC-1 complex. Cell 1999;97:17–27.

219. Bach I. The LIM domain: regulation by association. Mech Dev 2000;91:5–17.

220. Torigoi E, Bennani-Baiti IM, Rosen C, Gonzalez K, Morcillo P, Ptashne M, Dorsett D. Chip interacts with diverse homeodomain proteins and potentiates bicoid activity in vivo. Proc Natl Acad Sci USA 2000;97:2686–2691.

221. Watkins-Chow DE, Camper SA. How many homeobox genes does it take to make a pituitary gland? Trends Genet 1998;14:284–290.

222. Burrows HL, Douglas KR, Seasholtz AF, Camper SA. Genealogy of the anterior pituitary gland: tracing a family tree. Trends Endocrinol Metab 2000;10:343–352.

223. Bach I, Rodriguez-Esteban C, Carriere C, Bhushan A, Krones A, Rose DW, et al. RLIM inhibits functional activity of LIM homeodomain transcription factors via recruitment of the histone deacetylase complex. Nat Genet 1999;22:394–399.

224. Fey EG, Wan J, Penman S. Epithelial cytoskeletal framework and nuclear matrix-intermediate filament scaffold: three-dimensional organization and protein composition. J Cell Biol 1984;19:1973–1984.

225. Merdes A, Cleveland DW. The role of NuMA in the interphase nucleus. J Cell Sci 1998;111:71–79.

226. Bidwell JP, Alvarez M, Feister H, Onyia J, Hock J. Nuclear matrix proteins and osteoblast gene expression. J Bone Min Res 1998;13:155–167.

227. Mancini MG, Liu B, Sharp ZD, Mancini MA. Subnuclear partitioning and functional regulation of the Pit-1 transcription factor. J Cell Biochem 1999;72:322–338.

228. Parker GE, Sandoval RM, Feister HA, Bidwell JP, Rhodes SJ. The homeodomain coordinates nuclear entry of the Lhx3 neuroendocrine transcription factor and association with the nuclear matrix. J Biol Chem 2000;275:23,891–23,898.

229. Kim MK, Lesoon-Wood LA, Weintraub BD, Chung JH. A soluble transcription factor, Oct-1, is also found in the insoluble nuclear matrix and possesses silencing activity in its alanine-rich domain. Mol Cell Biol 1996;16:4366–4377.

230. Holloway JM, Szeto DP, Scully KM, Glass CK, Rosenfeld MG. Pit-1 binding to specific DNA sites as a monomer or dimer determines gene-specific use of a tyrosine-dependent synergy domain. Genes Dev 1995;9:1992–2006.

II GROWTH

2

Molecular Mutations
in the Human Growth Hormone Axis

Zvi Laron, MD

CONTENTS

INTRODUCTION

Human growth hormone (hGH) is secreted from somatomammotrophic cells in the anterior pituitary in a pulsatile pattern that results from a diurnal rhythmically changing disequilibrium between two hypothalamic hormones: GHRH (GH-releasing hormone) and SMS (somatostatin = GH secretion inhibiting hormone) *(1)*. GHRH induces hGH synthesis and secretion whenever the somatostatinergic tone is low *(2)*. It is thus evident that SMS plays a central role in the regulation of GH secretion. The actions of SMS are not restricted to GH alone, but also affect other hormones, as seen in Fig. 1, which illustrates the GH cascade. Not illustrated is the inhibitory effect of somatostatin on TSH,

From: *Contemporary Endocrinology: Developmental Endocrinology: From Research to Clinical Practice*
Edited by: E. A. Eugster and O. H. Pescovitz © Humana Press Inc., Totowa, NJ

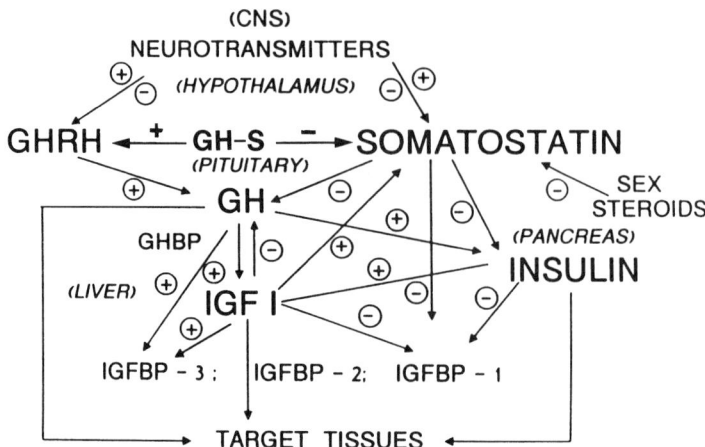

Fig. 1. The growth hormone axis. GH, growth hormone; GH-S, GH secretagog; GHRH, GH-releasing hormone; IGF-1, insulin-like growth factor-1; GHBP, GH binding protein; IGFBP, insulin-like growth factor; binding proteins; +, stimulates; −, inhibits.

and glucagon secretion *(3)*. The regulation of somatostatin secretion is not yet completely elucidated, but there is evidence that insulin-like growth factor-1 (IGF-1) stimulates SMS *(4)*, and that GH-S (GH secretagogs) inhibit SMS secretion *(5)*. Growth hormone secretagogs are small peptides, or nonpeptide substances synthesized in recent years, that act in synergism with GHRH to stimulate GH secretion *(6)*. Several analogs of these substances have been found active in vitro and in vivo; however, whether they are natural products or man-invented pharmacological substances related to natural products remains to be elucidated. The finding of a GH-S receptor *(7)* indicated that such a hormone exists in reality.

Indeed recently Kojima et al. *(8)* described a 28 amino acid peptide extracted from the stomach that specifically binds to this receptor. It is called GHRELIN and releases GH both in vitro and in vivo. Its human gene has been encoded *(8)* and is located on chromosome 3p26-25 *(9)*. It has 4 exons spanning 4.1 Kb of genomic DNA. The 117 amino acids have a 82% homology with the rat gene. It is also expressed in the arcuate nucleus of the hypothalamus *(8)*.

Recent studies have shown a close relationship between Ghrelin and Motilin, another hormone synthesized in the stomach *(10)*. Thus, the amino acid sequence of human prepro-motilin-related peptide (Prepro-MTLRP) is identical with human prepro-ghrelin, except Serine 26, which is not octanoylated in Prepro-MTLRP *(11)*. Also the gastrointestinal motilin receptor (MTL-R) and the GHS-R are both G-protein-coupled receptors that show a high degree of homology *(12)*. Motilin has also been found in the central nervous system (CNS) *(13)*. Interactivity between these two hormones is not yet clear, but Ghrelin in addition to stimulating GH release in humans *(14)* releases appetite-stimulatory signals from the stomach *(15)*, and induces adiposity in rodents *(16)*. The orexigenic effect of Ghrelin does not seem to be GH-dependent, but acts by increasing hypothalamic neuropeptide y (NPY) *(17)*. Standard meal intake after an overnight fast in 10 healthy young adults resulted in a significant decrease in plasma Ghrelin (120 min after the meal) correlating with the gastric emptying time *(18)*. Thus Ghrelin seems to regulate between nutrient intake, gastric motility, and the CNS.

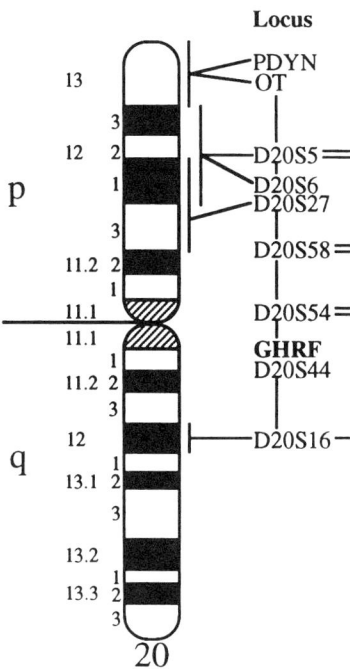

Fig. 2. Representation of chromosome 20 and location of the GHRH gene. Adapted with permission from ref. (*26*).

Ghrelin has also been identified in the placenta (*19*). Whether it plays a role in the secretion of placental lactogen remains to be established, as is the possibility that mutations in Ghrelin or its receptor may be involved in overeating and obesity.

The cloning of the genes of the hormones of the GH axis and their receptors in recent years and the advancement in molecular biology techniques have enabled the elucidation of the etiology of many conditions of abnormal growth. This chapter is a review of what is known at present on molecular defects in man related to the GHRH, GH, and IGF-1 molecules and their receptors, as well as a summary of the resulting clinical sequelae.

GROWTH HORMONE RELEASING HORMONE (GHRH)

Historical Perspective

In 1961, Reichlin demonstrated that lesions of the ventromedial nucleus of the rat hypothalamus resulted in cessation of growth as a result of GH deficiency (*20*). The isolation and characterization of human GHRH was made possible by the extraction of pancreatic tumors causing acromegaly (*21,22*).

The GHRH Gene

The GHRH gene is a member of a large family of hormones and factors, which includes glucagon, secretin, vasoactive intestinal polypeptide (VIP), and others (*23,24*). Humans have a single copy of the GHRH gene (*25*). It is localized on chromosome 20q12 and p11.23 (*26*) (Fig. 2) and has 5 exons spanning over 10 kilobase pairs (Fig. 3). GHRH is localized in the arcuate and ventromedial nuclei of the hypothalamus, but also in the

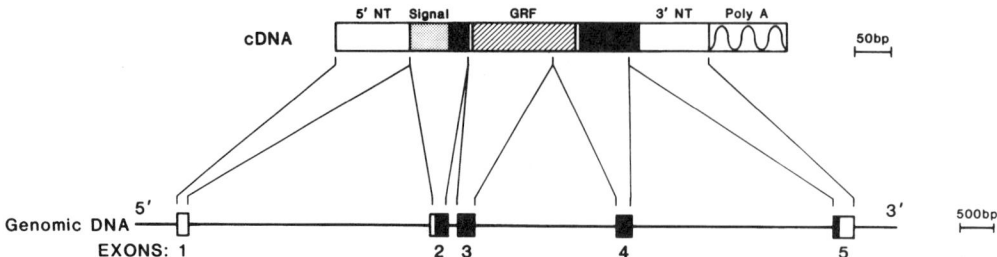

Fig. 3. Structure of the human GHRH cDNA and gene. GRF, GHRH. Adapted with permission from ref. (*25*).

gastrointestinal tract including pancreas *(27)*, the testis and placenta *(28)*, and other tissues as well as tumors *(29,30)*.

Chemical Structure

GHRH is secreted in three molecular forms GHRH 1-44NH2, GHRH 1-40-OH, and GHRH 1-37-OH *(31)*. All three forms are biologically active, even a 1-29 fragment *(32)*.

GHRH Gene Defects

Although isolated GH deficiency (IGHD) owing to complete or partial absence of GHRH has been diagnosed by indirect methods *(33–35)*, no patients with a GHRH gene deletion or mutation in the GHRH gene have been described so far.

Clinical Aspects

The patients suspected or proved to have GHRH deficiency present the clinical and biochemical changes typical of IGHD (*see* later). The diagnosis is made by finding a GH response to GHRH and a negative one to insulin hypoglycemia and/or clonidine, or arginine.

THE GHRH-RECEPTOR (GHRH-R)

Historical Perspective

GHRH stimulates the transcription of the GH gene *(36)* and induces proliferation of the somatotroph cell *(37)* acting as a hypophyseotropic hormone. Successful cloning of the GHRH-R was achieved in 1992 by Mayo *(38)*. This enabled a better insight into the mechanism of action of GHRH on the GH synthesis and secretion *(39)*. The first abnormalities in the GHRH-R gene were detected in the little (lit) mouse *(40)*, which paved the way to findings in man.

The Human GHRH Receptor Gene

The GHRH-R gene is located in the anterior hypophysis. GHRH stimulates adenylate cyclase resulting in increased cyclic adenosine monophosphate (cAMP) production indicating the intermediary action of a G-protein *(41)*. The GHRH-R is homologous to a subfamily of G-protein-coupled receptors, which include VIP, GLP-1, secretin, glucagon, GIP, PACAP, calcitonin, PTH, and CRH *(42)*. The human GHRH-R gene is located on chromosome 7p 13-p21 *(43)* (Fig. 4) and probably at p15 *(44)*. It contains a frame of 1269

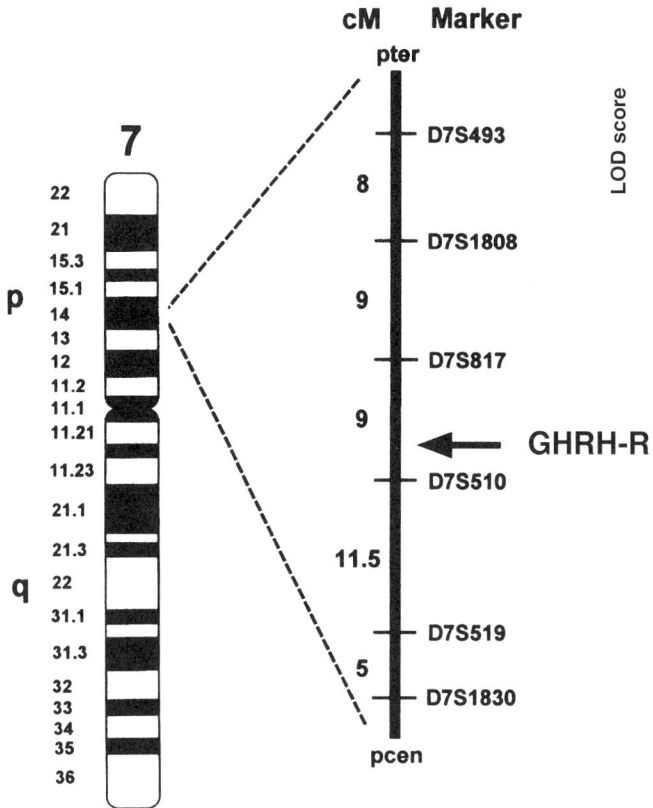

Fig. 4. Representation of chromosome 7 with location of the GHRH receptor gene. Adapted with permission from ref. (*46*).

bp coding for 432 amino-acids and 7 transmembrane-spanning helices *(38)* (Fig. 5). The mature GHRH-R is a 401 amino acid residue peptide with a large extracellular domain of 108 amino acids.

GHRH-Receptor Gene Mutations in Man

The finding of an inactivating mutation in the GHRH-R in the little (lit) mouse *(40)* suggested that similar defects may occur in man. So far four kindreds have been described, three originating from the Indian peninsula and one from Northeast Brazil *(45–48)*. The first described patients by Wajnrajch et al. *(45)* are Indian Moslems and originate from Bombay. They belong to a very consanguineous kindred of which two cousins, a boy (age 16 yr) and a girl (3.5 yr) were investigated. Both were very short (–4.2 and –7.4 height SDS), and had frontal bossing and truncal obesity, the typical phenotype of severe isolated GH deficiency (IGHD) *(49)* or GH resistance (Laron syndrome; LS) *(50)*. They had IGHD as demonstrated by no rise in serum GH upon oral clonidine, insulin hypoglycemia, and intravenous GHRH after sex-hormone priming. All other pituitary hormones were normal. DNA analysis revealed a nonsense mutation in the extracellular domain of the GHRH receptor, namely a G→T transversion at position 265 resulting in a Glu 72 stop (calculated with the signal protein). Treatment by hGH resulted in a growth spurt of 13 and 17 cm, respectively, in the first year of treatment.

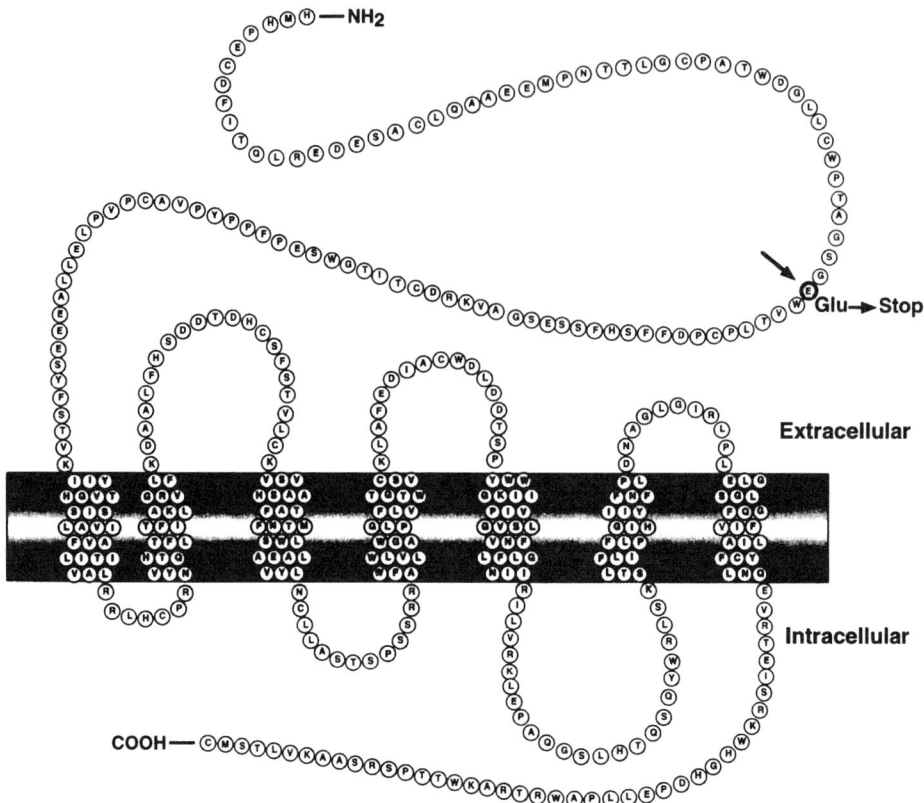

Fig. 5. The GHRH receptor gene and the GHRH-R mutation in the Brazilian kindred *(48)*. Adapted with permission from ref. *(46)*.

The second consanguineous kindred originated in Sindh/Pakistan. Mahashwari et al. *(46)* examined 18 affected subjects, all very short (−7.2 to −8.3 height SDS), with a small head circumference (−4.3 SDS), possible facial hypoplasia, and some increase in adiposity. Puberty was delayed and the patients had high-pitched voices. Four patients had endocrine evaluations and no response of serum hGH was found to various stimuli, including GHRH. As expected, serum IGF-1 and IGFBP-3 were very low: 5.2 ± 2 ng/mL and 420 ± 130 ng/mL, respectively. Serum GHRH was found within the normal range and not elevated *(46)*. DNA analysis revealed the same mutation as in the patients reported by Wajnrajch et al. *(45)*.

Two additional brothers reported by Netchine et al. *(47)* were of Tamilian origin from Delf, an island between India and Srilanka. They were very short (−4 and −5 height SDS) and not responsive to GHRH stimulation. Despite having the same GHRH-R defect causing a truncated nonactive receptor as the patients previously reported, they had no frontal bossing, nor a small penis. MRI of the skull revealed a hypoplastic anterior pituitary. They too responded well to hGH therapy.

A fourth report coming from Itabaininha in Northeastern Brazil, a region with a population with a high degree of consanguinity, described 22 very short patients (−4.5 to −6 height SDS) belonging to a kindred of at least 105 affected families *(48)*. Adult statures ranged from 105–135 cm; they were obese, had delayed puberty but normal

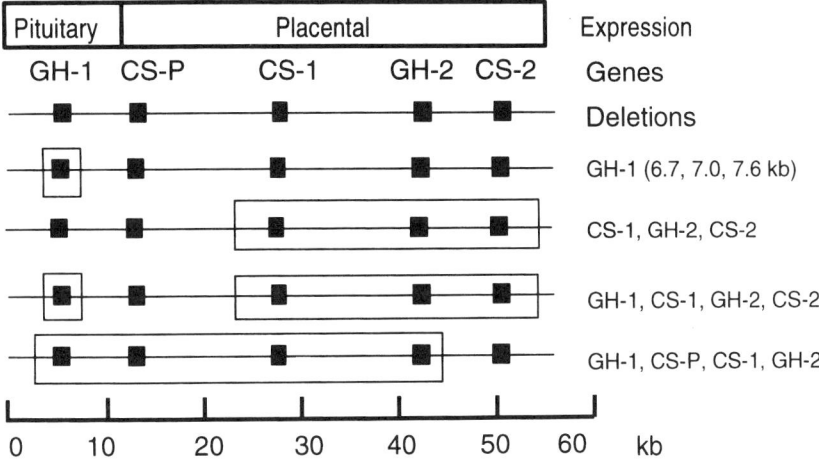

Fig. 6. The growth hormone and chorionic somatotropin gene cluster. Adapted with permission from ref. (*84*).

reproduction, and high-pitched voices. All 22 patients investigated had no response of hGH to stimuli including GHRH, and IGF-1 and IGFBP-3 were very low. DNA analysis revealed a novel mutation affecting the junction of exon 1 with intron 1 IVS1+1 G→A) (Fig. 5). Thirty of the affected subjects were homozygous for this mutation. The heterozygote subjects had a normal phenotype.

CONCLUSIONS

The patients with GHRH-R defects identified so far stem from inbred populations and all have been described to have various degrees of the typical phenotype of IGHD *(49)* or GH insensitivity (LS) *(50)*. Of interest is the finding of a hypoplastic anterior pituitary in one report *(47)*.

Diagnostic Hint

Patients with severe IGHD that show no rise of serum GH upon intravenous administration of GHRH should be screened for a defect in the GHRH-R.

HUMAN PITUITARY GROWTH HORMONE (hGH)

Historical Perspective

Human GH was isolated in 1956 *(51)* and its gene cloned in 1979 *(52)*. The diagnosis of IGHD was made possible only after the introduction of specific radioimmunoassays *(53)* and immunocytochemistry *(54)*.

The hGH Gene Family

Human GH consists of a cluster of five similar genes in the following order: 5 hGH-1, (or−N), CSHP (chorionic somatomammotropin pseudo gene, CSH-1 (chorionic somato-mammotropin); hGH-2 (or V) or placental GH, which differs from the primary sequence of hGH-N by 13 amino acids *(55)* and replaces pituitary GH in the maternal circulation during the second half of pregnancy (Fig. 6). The hGH genes are located on a 78kb section of the long arm of chromosome 17q22-24 *(56)*.

CSH-1 and CSH-2 encode chorionic somatomammotropin, and CSH-P gives rise to low levels of alternatively spliced mRNAs and does not encode a known hormone *(57)*. Only hGH-1 has anabolic growth promoting actions. The genes for GH and chorionic somatomammotropins have 5 exons separated by 4 introns. The human CSH genes have no anabolic or growth activity *(58)*.

hGH Chemical Structure

Human GH is produced as a single chain, 191 amino acid 22-Kd protein *(59)*. It contains two disulfide bonds and shares homology with GH-2. Under normal conditions 75% of pituitary hGH is of the mature 22Kd form. Alternate splicing of the second codon resulting in deletion of amino acids 31–46 yields a 20 Kd form (about 5–10% of pituitary hGH) *(60)*. A small amount of 17 Kd hGH is formed as well *(61)*. The spectrum of biological activity of the 20 Kd hGH form is very similar to that of the 22 Kd hGH *(62)* although a lesser insulinotropic effect has been occasionally found.

The relationship between the integrity of the GH molecule and its biological activities has been a topic of great interest since the isolation of hGH. In contradistinction to ACTH and GHRH in which shortened molecules are fully active; with respect to hGH this seems to be true only for the 20 and 22 Kd variants. Nevertheless, it is of interest that hGH fragments 1-43 and 44-191 have been found to have potent in vivo effects on glucose homeostasis in rodents, and the 44-191 fragment has low-affinity binding to recombinant hGHBP *(63)*.

MOLECULAR DEFECTS
IN THE HUMAN GH GENE AND HORMONE

Abnormalities in the structure of the hGH molecule or GH gene deletion have been suspected to occur in humans for some time, but could not be proven until adequate laboratory methods were developed and the right patients found.

A seemingly innocuous defect is the omission of exon 3, which causes the production of 17 Kd hGH *(64)*. hGH-N gene deletions are being diagnosed more and more frequently in patients with hereditary IGHD from consanguineous families. A classification attempt has been made *(65)* (Table 1). Three or possibly four forms of IGHD due to defects in the hGH-1 gene are now recognized. In some forms of familial IGHD the exact molecular defect has not yet been found.

IGHD Type IA

Type IA was first described by Illig et al. *(66)* in a Swiss inbred family. Phillips et al. *(67)* found that the etiology was the lack of the hGH-1 gene. There followed descriptions from other countries *(68–81)*. The sizes of the deletions are heterogenous. DNA analysis revealed that most (70–80%) patients with IGHD Type I have a 6.7 kb deletion in the GH gene, the remainder (20–30%) have a 7.6 or 7.0 kb deletion *(81)*.

The frequency of GH-1 deletions as a cause of IGHD varies among populations. Analyzing patients with severe IGHD (height SDS below 4) the prevalences cited by Mullis et al. *(82)* are 9.4% (Northern Europe), 13.6% (Mediterranean), 16.6% (Turkey), 38% (Oriental Jews), and 12% Chinese. Parks et al. *(83)* suggest that GH gene deletion is the most common cause of severe GHD among Oriental Jewish children. This seems to be true also for the Israeli Arab including Bedouin population (Laron, unpublished observation).

Table 1
Isolated Growth Hormone Deficiencies (IGHD)

Category	Inheritance	GH-RIA	Candidate Gene	Status
IGHD IA	Autosomal recessive	Absent	hGH-1	Deletions
				Mutations (signal peptide)
IGHD IB	Autosomal recessive	Absent/low	hGH-1	Frameshifts
				Stop codon
				Splice site mutations
			GHRH	Unlikely
			GHRH-receptor	Mutations
			Trans-*acting* factors	Mutations/deletions
			Cis-*acting* elements	Mutations/deletions
IGHD II	Autosomal dominant	Low	hGH-1	Splice site mutations
IGHD III	X-linked	Low	Unknown	

Adapted with permission from ref. *(65)*.

Dependent on the size of the deletion also the CSH cluster or hGH-2 genes can also be deleted *(79)*, although the clinical implications of such deletions is unknown. Institution of hGH replacement therapy induces in most patients the formation of high titers of hGH antibodies leading to growth arrest *(69)*. It is not yet understood why some patients do not develop antibodies *(70,78)*. It seems that patients with a 7.6 kb gene deletion respond well to hGH treatment without antibody formation in contradistinction to patients with a 6.7 kb gene deletion. Gene deletion could result from incorrect alignment of chromosomes during meiosis.

Missense and nonsense mutations as well as small deletions of the GH-1 gene also cause familial IGHD *(84)*. Thus a homozygous nonsense mutation in codon 20 of the signal peptide was reported in two patients of a Turkish family *(85)*. Igarashi et al. *(86)* reported a Japanese compound heterozygote patient with a 6.7kb deletion and a 2bp deletion in exon 3 of the GH-1 gene, which produced a frameshift and generated a stop codon at amino acid residue 131 in exon 4. Nishi et al. *(87)* reported an affected child with a compound heterozygous deletion of 6.7 kb inherited from the mother and point mutations (at positions 123 and 250) inherited from the father. Phenotypically the patients are very short (> −4 SDS), with protruding forehead, acromicria, and obesity.

Treatment

The patients with hGH-1 gene deletions who do not develop antibodies against hGH or only low titers, can be treated by hGH *(70,88)*. The patients who develop blocking antibodies to hGH need to be treated by IGF-1 *(89)*.

Isolated GH Deficiency Type IB

IGHD Type IB is a not very clearly defined entity *(65,90)*. It also has an autosomal recessive mode of inheritance and is characterized by low but detectable levels of serum hGH after stimulation (partial GHD). This is in contradistinction to Type IA IGHD where no circulating hGH is detectable. Cogan et al. *(85)* reported two patients from a Saudi Arabian family in which a first-base transition of the intron 4 (+1G→C) causes an activation of a cryptic splice in exon 4, thereby deleting aminoacids 103 to 126 (in exon 4) and the frameshift in exon 5.

Recently, Abdul-Latif et al. *(91)* described several patients with IGHD belonging to a large consanguineous Bedouin kindred in Israel. They were short (height SDS between −3.6 to −5.2) and revealed no or very low-serum GH response to pharmacological stimuli. This family presented a novel mutation: a G→C transversion at the fifth base of intron 4, but it resulted in the same cryptic splice site as the patients from Saudi Arabia *(85,90)*. The excess of patients with IGHD among Arab families may reflect the high incidence of consanguinity rather than spontaneous mutations *(92)*.

Isolated GH Deficiency Type II

In contrast to IGHD Type I, IGHD Type II has an autosomal dominant mode of inheritance *(65,84)*. The diagnostic criteria resemble IGHD Type IB. The patients are short but less than type IA and respond to hGH treatment. In a Turkish family a T→C transition of base 6 of the donor splice site of intron 3 caused the splicing out or skipping of exon 3 and the loss of amino acids 32–71 of the hGH molecule *(81)*, so that the truncated molecule corresponds to the 17.5 Kd isoform of hGH. Saitoh et al. *(93)* reported a 1-yr-old Japanese boy and his father with IGHD. Both were found to have a G→C transition of the first base of the donor splice site of intron 3 of the hGH-1 gene.

Subsequently, a G→A transition at the first base of intron 3 has been identified in several families of different ethnic backgrounds *(94–96)*. Recently Hayashi et al. *(97)* described a de novo mutation in a Japanese boy. He had a G→C transversion at the fifth nucleotide of intron 3, causing the skipping of exon 3.

Isolated GH Deficiency Type III

This type of IGHD has an X-linked recessive mode of inheritance. Some patients have hypo- or agammaglobulinemia (deficiency of IgG, IgA, IgM, and IgE) *(98,99)*. As the hGH-1 gene is normal, this disease is considered to affect steps proximal to the hGH-1 gene *(100)* or a combination between X-linked agammaglobulinemia and hGH gene deletions *(101)*. Some patients with IGHD have been found to have interstitial deletion at chromosome X p22.3 *(102)* or duplication of X q13.3- q21.2 *(103)*. Recently four patients with 22q 11.2 deletion, short stature and GH deficiency were reported *(104)*. Two of them had a hypoplastic anterior pituitary gland and one of them also had an abnormal insertion of the infundibular stalk.

CONCLUSION

IGHD can be caused by various defects of the hGH-1 gene, from deletions to single mutations *(105)*. Whereas IGHD Type IA and Type II seem clearly defined, the etiologies and definitions of Type IB and Type III remain to be improved.

Diagnostic Hint

Patients with severe IGHD, who show no rise of serum GH upon intravenous administration of GHRH should also be screened for a defect in the hGH-1 gene; patients with a family history of short stature and partial GHD on repeated tests, should also be investigated, as well as short children with immunoglobulin deficiencies.

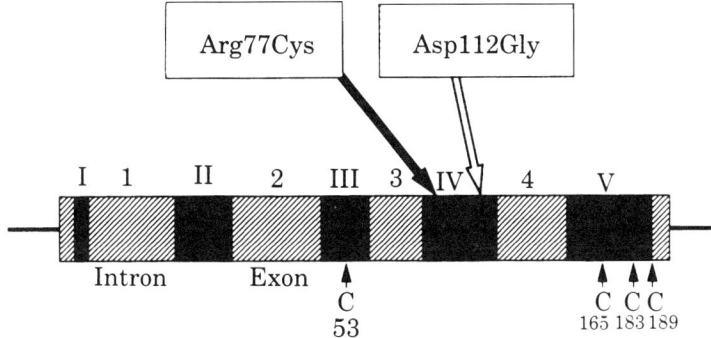

Fig. 7. The localizations of the mutations of the hGH-1 gene leading to bio-inactive growth hormone. Adapted with permission from ref. *(108)*.

Growth Hormone Deficiency Owing to Mutant Human Growth Hormone

Although the existence of short stature due to biologically inactive growth hormone had been postulated, the case was only proven recently. Takahashi et al. *(106,107)* reported the first documented patients. Both are products of nonrelated parents. The first patient *(106)* had a birth length of 39 cm and measured 81.7 cm at age 4.9 yr (−6.1 height SDS). He had a prominent forehead, serum hGH levels ranged from 7–14 μg/mL, and rose upon pharmacological stimulation to 35 μg/mL. Serum GHBP was low 70 pmol/L (normal: 107–337 pmol/L). Linear growth responded only temporarily to hGH. The molecular analysis of the hGH gene revealed a heterozygous missense mutation, which converted codon 77 in exon 4 from Arg→Cys (Fig. 7) *(108)*. The second patient *(107)*, a girl, was born with a normal length but slowed her growth so that at the age 3 she measured 79.4 cm (−3.6 height SDS). Her mother was also short (147 cm). She had a prom-inent forehead. Serum hGH rose from 11 to 26 μg/mL upon hypoglycemia stimulation and up to 51 μg/mL after intravenous GHRH. The low IGF-1 rose from 0.28 U/mL to 1.21 U/mL after 3 daily hGH injections and further after successful treatment (11cm/yr) of 1 yr hGH treatment. DNA analysis revealed a heterozygous missense mutation which converted codon 112 in exon 4 from Asp→Gly. The presence of mutant hGH was further confirmed in both patients by isoelectric focusing. In addition, the functional properties of the mutant hGHs were determined by the investigation. The 112 G mutant tended to form a 1:1 GH-GHBP complex instead of a 1:2 complex as produced by the wild-type hGH, a crucial step for GH signal transmission. Thus the mutant was less potent in the phosphorylation of JAK 2 and activation of STAT 5 in IM-9 cells (*see* later). In the case of the other patient, the affinity of the mutant hGH to GHBP was six times higher than the wild-type hGH, and act-ing as an antagonist failed to stimulate tyrosine phosphorylation and inhibited the activity of wild-type hGH upon simultaneous addition in vitro.

Diagnostic Hint

Whenever there is severe short stature (−3.5 height SDS or more) and the pheno-type resembles IGHD, the serum hGH is measurable and responsive to stimuli, but serum IGF-1 is low and only partially responsive to exogenous hGH, the presence of a mutant, biologically inactive hGH molecule should be considered.

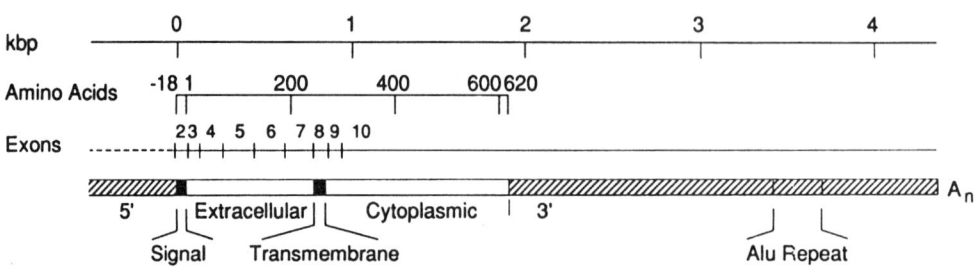

Fig. 8. The hGH receptor gene. Adapted with permission from ref. *(111).*

THE GROWTH HORMONE RECEPTOR

The growth hormone receptor (GH-R) belongs to the family of cytokine receptors which includes receptors for prolactin, erythropoietin, and interleukins *(109)*. The human GH-R gene was cloned in 1987 by Leung et al. *(110)*. It is a protein of 620 aminoacids and consists of 10 exons and spans 87 Kb *(111)*. Exons 2 through 7 encode the extracellular domain (246 residues), exon 8 the single membrane-spanning domain (23 residues), and exons 9 and 10 the intracellular (cytoplasmatic) domain (351 residues) (Fig. 8) *(111)*. The extracellular domain is identical in structure to the GH binding protein (GHBP) *(110)*. The human GH-R gene is located on the short arm of chromosome 5p 13.1 *(112)*.

GH-R form homodimers in the course of binding a single GH molecule *(113,114)*. First the hGH molecule binds at binding site A and then at site B on the second receptor molecule. Sites A and B of binding on hGH are distinct but those on the GHBP overlap *(115)*. The species specificity in the recognition of hGH by the human GH-R is claimed to reside in the interaction between an aspartic acid residue at position 171 of hGH with an arginine residue 43 of the GH-R *(116)*. The binding sites of hGH to the GH-R are located in the cysteine-rich domain of the extracellular domain *(115)*. Receptor occupancy leads to auto-phosphorylation of the Janus 2 (JAK 2) kinase *(117)* and subsequent phosphorylation of the receptor itself. The intracellular signalling cascade includes activation of mitogen-activated protein kinase (MAPK) and of transcription factors known as STATS (signal transducers and activation of transcription) *(118)*.

GROWTH HORMONE BINDING PROTEIN (GHBP)

Herington et al. *(119)* and Baumann et al. *(120)* independently described a serum protein capable of binding GH with high affinity. This GH binding protein (GHBP) was shown to be identical in structure with the extracellular hormone-binding domain of the GH-R *(110)*. Its quantitative measurements revealed that its serum concentrations change with age, being low in neonates and reaching maximal values in young adulthood *(121)*. Whether GHBP can be synthesized de novo, in addition to being formed by the splicing of the extracellular domain of the GH-R *(122)* with which it shares structural identity *(110)* is not known. The presence of mutated GHBP in the circulation has not yet been described. Between 30–50% of the circulating GH is bound to this protein.

Determination of serum GHBP can be used as a simple quantitative estimation of the extracellular domain of the GH-R; its absence indicating a defect in this domain of the receptor and resulting in classical Laron syndrome *(50,123,124)*. A low-serum GHBP concentration in relatives of patients with LS helps identify heterozygous carriers *(125)* of mutations in the extracellular domain of the receptor.

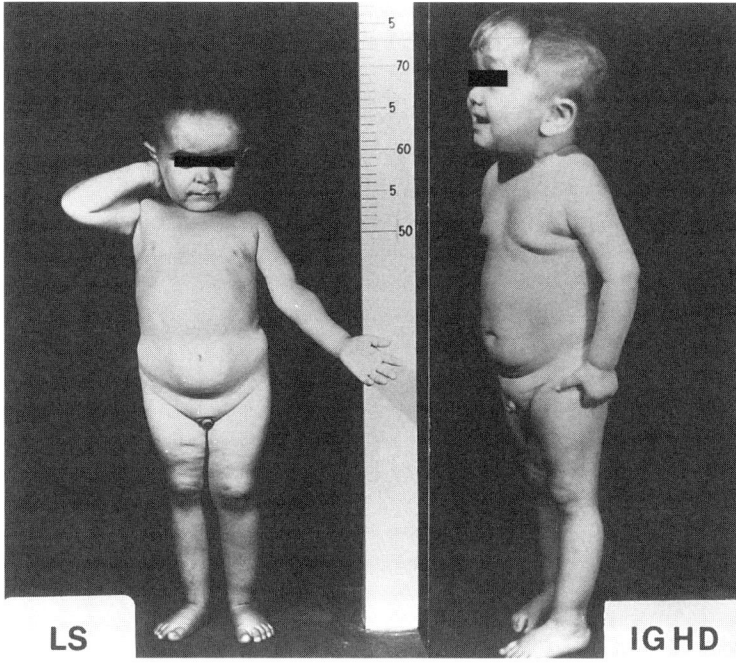

Fig. 9. Similarity between a boy with Laron syndrome (LS) and one with isolated GH deficiency (IGHD) due to GH-1 gene deletion.

Normal or elevated serum GHBP in typical LS patients denotes a defect in the transmembrane, intracellular or downstream of the GH-R.

MOLECULAR DEFECTS OF THE HUMAN GH RECEPTOR (LARON SYNDROME)

Historical Perspective

The first description of patients with this syndrome was made by Laron et al. in 1966 *(126)* who reported 22 patients in 1968 *(127)*. The patients resembled phenotypically those with IGHD (Fig. 9) but had excessively high circulating GH levels, and very low serum IGF-1 (sulfation factor) generation *(128)*, which did not respond to administration of exogenous GH *(129)*. The first assumption that the GH molecule is abnormal was excluded by findings between 1973 and 1985 that their high circulating hGH was normal both by immunologic *(130,131)* and radioreceptor testing *(132,133)*. The proof that the GH resistance, the characteristic of these patients, is the result of a defect in the GH-R was provided by Eshet et al. in 1984 *(134)* by demonstrating that liver membranes of two patients prepared from open biopsies do not bind human GH. The cloning of the GH-receptor in 1986 *(111)* enabled the study of molecular defects.

Geographical Distribution

Following the early descriptions, patient reports from many continents followed, a majority originating from the Mediterranean, Mid-Eastern, or South Asian regions, known to have a high incidence of consanguineous marriages.

Today several hundreds of patients are known; the majority, though, are probably still undiagnosed. The largest cohorts known so far are in Ecuador: 79 patients *(135)*, consisting of subjects originating in Spain, possibly of Jewish origin, and the Israeli cohort consisting of 51 Jews originating from Yemen, Iran, Afghanistan, Middle East, North Africa, and Israeli Arabs *(136)*, with smaller cohorts in Turkey *(137)*, Iran *(138)*, India *(123)*, and Bahamas *(140)*. Patients in families or isolated patients have been reported from Italy, France, Spain, Denmark, Germany, Slovakia, Slovenia, Russia, Poland, North Africa, Japan, Vietnam, Cambodia, Mexico, and South and North America. They are listed in review papers *(141–143)*. Recently an additional 14-yr-old girl of Slavic origin from Russia was reported *(144)*.

Analysis of the Israeli cohort led to the conclusion that LS is caused by an autosomal fully penetrant recessive mechanism *(145)* with one exception of a father and two of his children in whom a dominant transmission is assumed *(146)*.

DEFECTS OF THE GH-RECEPTOR (GH-R)

In 1989 Godowski et al. *(111)* characterized the genomic organization of the GH-R gene and reported two patients from the Israeli cohort who were homozygous for the deletion of exons 3, 5 and 6. In the same year Amselem et al. *(147)* using the newly developed polymerase chain reaction (PCR) methodology described several point mutations in patients with Laron syndrome. Since then a series of patients have been investigated and the findings are listed in Table 2 *(148–163)*. As seen, the molecular defects range from deletions, nonsense-frameshift, splice to missense mutations. The majority of defects reported today are located in the extracellular domain of the human GH-R gene. In almost all instances the patients were found to be homozygous for the same mutant allele, as expected in recessive hereditary transmission. However, occasionally there were patients who were compound heterozygotes for mutations *(160,161)*.

As the GHBP is identical in structure to the extracellular domain *(110)*, mutations in this part of the receptor usually result in undetectable or very low serum GHBP. This measurement represents a simple and fast screening for the ascertainment of a molecular defect in the extracellular domain of the GH-R, and identification of heterozygotes for defects in this domain *(125)*.

So far only two mutations in the transmembrane region (exon 8) *(156,157)* and three instances of mutations in the intracellular domain (exons 9 or 10) *(159–161)* have been reported. In all these patients the serum levels of GHBP are normal or high. The patients described by Ayling et al. *(160)* had a dominant transmitted single heterozygous mutation: from mother to daughter, a G→C transversion at 876-1 affecting the 3' splice receptor site preceding exon 9, causing the deletion. The patients of Iida et al. *(161)* also had a G→A transversion at 876, and also revealed a dominant negative transmission from mother to two children.

Post GH-R Defects

Until now only two reports on downstream defects in Laron syndrome have been described. Laron et al. *(163)* described three siblings of Palestinian Arab origin, with high serum hGH, normal GHBP, and a normal GH-R structure. Exogenous administration of hGH for 7 d did not raise the undetectable or very low-serum IGF-1, but caused a rise in serum IGFBP-3, indicating a functioning GH-R. The exact defect is under study. Freeth et al. *(164)* described four girls with LS of two unrelated Asian families with normal GHBP in whom no mutations of the GH-R were detected. Further studies of the GH signaling pathway performed in skin fibroblasts of these patients *(165)* revealed that GH failed to activate the STAT pathway in fibroblasts of one family, being normal in the second family denoting different signalling defects in the two families.

Clinical Features

The clinical and biochemical characteristics of patients with primary IGF-1 deficiency (GH insensitivity = Laron syndrome) in childhood and adulthood are summarized in Table 3. Despite a wide spectrum of variability *(141,143,146,166)*, the characteristic clinical features resemble IGHD (Fig. 9), i.e., severe growth failure (−4 to −10 height SDS), small cranium, underdevelopment of the facial bones resulting in protruding forehead *(141)*, sparse hair *(167)*, crowded and defective teeth *(127)*, acromicria, and small genitalia and gonads *(168)*. Most patients have a high-pitched voice *(127,146)*. Body proportions show a high upper/lower ratio; skeletal maturation is markedly retarded *(169)*, with osteopenia and osteoporosis developing in young adulthood *(170)*. There is delayed motor development *(50,127)* and intellectual impairments of variable degrees *(171)*. Puberty is delayed *(172)* but reproductive potential is preserved *(50)*, the heterozygote children having a normal phenotype. Obesity is evident in young age and progresses markedly in adulthood *(173)*, the patients also developing hyperlipidemia and insulin resistance despite a tendency for hypoglycemia *(174)*. Final height ranges from 108–136 cm in females and 119–142 cm in males *(50)*. Some of the patients with positive serum GHBP, i.e., those with a molecular defect in the transmembane, intracellular, or postreceptor pathways, seem to be slightly less short *(166,175)*. The few patients with a postreceptor defect seem to be less obese *(163,164)*, possibly due to a preserved direct GH effect.

Nomenclature

The nomenclature used for this syndrome is confusing. A consensus nomenclature has been published, proposing that primary GH resistance or insensitivity (GHIS) be synonymous with Laron syndrome (LS), differentiating it from secondary GH resistance *(176)*. Some authors use only GHIS, without differentiation; others use GH receptor deficiency (GHRD) *(135,177)*.

Diagnostic Hint

The findings of abnormally high serum GH levels in patients with the clinical characteristics of IGHD should serve as an alert to the diagnosis of LS. The confirmation is low-serum IGF-1, which does not rise upon the daily administration of exogenous hGH for 4–7 d *(129,146)*. Location of a defect in the extracellular domain of the GH-R is evidenced by a low or undetectable serum GHBP *(119,120)*. The finding of a normal or high serum GHBP denotes a defect in the transmembrane or intracellular domain.

Treatment

The only possible therapy is administration of IGF-1, which has been practiced by us since 1988 *(178)* and subsequently by three other groups in the US, Ecuador, and Europe *(179–181)*. IGF-1 stimulates linear growth *(179–183)*, but is less efficient than hGH in the treatment of IGHD *(184)*. IGF-1 treatment improves also biochemical abnormalities

Table 2
Growth Hormone Receptor Mutations Reported in Patients with Laron Syndrome[a]

Mutations	Molecular defect	Nucleotide change	Exon involved	Domain[b]	GHBP[c]	Authors	Reference
Deletion	Exons 3-5-6		Exons 3-5-6			Godowski et al. (1989)	(111)
Nonsense	C38X	C→A at 168	4	EC	–	Amselem et al. (1991)	(148)
	R43X	C→T at 181	4	EC	–	Amselem et al. (1991)	(148)
	Q65X	C→T at 197	4	EC	–	Sobrier et al. (1997)	(150)
	W80X	C→A at 293	5	EC	–	Sobrier et al. (1997)	(150)
	W157X	C→A at 525	6	EC	?	Sobrier et al. (1997)	(150)
	E183X	C→T at 601	6	EC	?	Berg et al. (1994)	(151)
	R217X	C→T at 703	7	EC	–	Amselem et al. (1993)	(152)
	Z224X	G→T at 724	7	EC	–	Kaji et al. (1997)	(242)
Frameshift	21delTT	delTT at 118	4	EC	–	Counts and Cutler (1995)	(153)
	36delC	delC at 162	4	EC	–	Sobrier et al. (1997)	(150)
	46delTT	delTTat192-193	4	EC	–	Berg et al. (1993)	(154)
	230delT	delT at 744	7	EC	–	Sobrier et al. (1997)	(150)
	230delAT	delATat 743-744	7	EC	–	Berg et al. (1993)	(154)
	309delC	delC at 981	10	IC	–	Kaji et al. (1997)	(242)
Splice	Intron 2	G→A at 70+1		EC	?	Sobrier et al. (1997)	(150)
	Intron 4	G→A at 266+1		EC	–	Amselem et al. (1993)	(152)
	Intron 5	G→A at 71+1		EC		Berg et al. (1993)	(154)
	Intron 5	G→C at130-1		EC		Berg et al. (1994)	(151)
	Intron 6	G→T at 189-1		EC		Berg et al. (1993)	(154)
	Intron 5	G→C at 440-1		EC	–	Amselem et al. (1993)	(152)
	Intron 6	G→T at 619-1		EC	–	Berg et al. (1993)	(154)
	E180splice	A→G at 594	6	EC	+	Berg et al. (1992)	(155)
	Gly236GLY	C→T at 766		EC	–	Baumbach et al. (1997)	(140)
	G223G	C→T at 723	7	EC	–	Sobrier et al. (1997)	(150)
	Intron 7	G→C at 785-1	7/8	EC/TM	+++	Silbergeld et al. (1997)	(156)

R274T	G→C at 874	8	TM	++	Woods et al. (1996)	(157)
GHR(1-277)[d]	G→A at 876+1	9	TM/IC	++	Iida et al. (1998)	(161)
GHR(1-277)[e]	G→C at 876-1	9	TM/IC	+	Ayling et al. (1997)	(160)
Missense						
C38S	T→A at 166	4	EC	?	Sobrier et al. (1997)	(150)
S40L	C→T at 173	4	EC	?	Sobrier et al. (1997)	(150)
W50R	T→C at 202	4	EC	–	Sobrier et al. (1997)	(150)
R71K	G→A at 266	4	EC	–	Amselem et al. (1993)	(152)
F96S	T→C at 341	5	EC	–	Amselem et al. (1989)	(147)
V125A	T→C at 428	5	EC	–	Amselem et al. (1993)	(152)
P131Q	C→A at 446	6	EC	?	Walker et al. (1998)	(162)
V144D	T→A at 485	6	EC	–	Amselem et al. (1993)	(152)
D152H	G→C at508	6	EC	+	Duquesnoy et al. (1994)	(158)
R161C	C→T at 535	6	EC	–	Amselem et al. (1993)	(152)
R211G	C→G at 685	7	EC	–	Amselem et al. (1993)	(152)
C422F[f]	C→T at 1362	10	IC	–	Kou et al. (1993)	(159)
P561T[f]	C→T at 1778	10	IC	–	Kou et al. (1993)	(159)

[a]Primary growth hormone insensitivity = resistance.

[b]EC, extracellular; TM, transmembrane; IC, intracellular.

[c]?, not available; +, detectable; ++, high levels; +++, very high levels.

[d]at the +1 position of the 5'-donor splice site of intron 9.

[e]at the 3'-splice acceptor site preceding exon 9.

[f]These two mutations were identified on the same GHR allele.

Table 3
Early and Late Consequences of Primary IGF-1 Deficiency[a]

Perinatal and during childhood
Subnormal birth length (−10–30%)
Disproportional growth
Acromicria including facial bones
Defective and crowded teeth
Sparse hair growth
Small gonads and genitalia
Obesity
Retarded skeletal maturation
Retarded brain growth (head circumference)
Delayed motor development
Narrow larynx (high-pitched voice)
Delayed puberty
Hypoglycemia
High-serum GH

Adulthood
Very short stature (final height: 108–142 cm, i.e., −4 to −10 height SDS)
Marked progressive obesity
Osteoporosis
Muscle underdevelopment and weakness
Cardiomicria
Varying intellectual deficits (from retardation to normal)
Hyperinsulinemia
Hypercholesterolemia
Glucose intolerance and diabetes

[a]GH insensitivity = Laron Syndrome.

such as hyperlipidemia, insulin resistance, glucose utilization, and renal function in children as well as adults *(170,173,174)*.

It is regrettable that IGF-1 is available to only a very few of the many patients in need of replacement therapy *(185)*.

PARTIAL GROWTH HORMONE INSENSITIVITY (GHI)

In recent years the possible existence of partial GH insensitivity as one of the causes of so-called idiopathic short stature (ISS) has been raised *(186)* as children with ISS do not respond to exogenous hGH as well as children with GHD. Goddard et al. *(187)* found in 14 out of a series of children with ISS, selected because of low GHBP in the presence of normal GH levels, 5 GH receptor mutations. in four patients. One patient was a double heterozygote with a missense mutation in exon 4 (GLU44→Lys) and a missense mutation in exon 6 (Arg161→Cys). The exon 4 mutation was inherited from the father and the exon 6 mutation from the mother. It is of interest that this patient did not have severe growth failure. Three other patients were heterozygotes for a nonsense mutation in exon 5 introducing a premature stop codon (Cys 122 stop) and two other patients were heterozygotes for missense mutations in exon 7 (Arg211→His or GLU 224→ASP), without defects in the other allele.

There is no strong evidence that heterozygous mutations of only one allele cause GH resistance as most children studied by Goddard et al. *(187)* showed a response to GH therapy. In our cohort of patients with classical LS *(50)*, 1/15 heterozygote males and 10/16 heterozygote females were below the 3rd centile of height (Tanner charts). However, because most belonged to a generation of new immigrants from underprivileged countries, it is possible that the growth failure resulted from environmental circumstances. Some of the short and normal-sized heterozygous of classical LS patients had below normal GHBP values *(125)*.

In conclusion, the clinical and biochemical features of partial GHI have not yet been clearly elucidated *(186)* and this entity appears to be very rare. Some double heterozygotes for a GH-R mutation have severe GH resistance and the complete LS phenotype *(161)*, although some do not *(187)*. Most heterozygous family members described so far were of normal height.

The Pygmies

The African Pygmies resemble patients with LS (primary GH insensitivity) in several aspects *(188)*. They are short, both at birth and at final height (males: 145–150 cm; females: 130–145 cm) *(189)*. They have full sexual development and normal reproduction. Their serum GH levels are normal and upon stimulation by hypoglycemia or arginine reach levels up to 30 ng/mL and they are hypoglycemia-unresponsive *(190)*. Serum IGF-1 is low *(191,192)* and does not rise upon short-term hGH administration *(192,193)*, denoting GH resistance. The molecular cause of the GH receptor abnormality in pygmies is still unknown, however, like patients with LS, it was found that they have reduced GHBP *(194)*. Furthermore, it has been shown that both GH and IGF-1 fail to augment colony formation of T-lymphocytes from Efe pygmies *(195)*, denoting hormone resistance in vitro.

The absence of high levels of serum GH in the pygmies may disprove classical GH resistance, as do the low IGF-1 levels preclude IGF-1 resistance. Studies are needed to determine the molecular etiology of these short people.

INSULIN-LIKE GROWTH FACTOR-1 (IGF-1)

Historical Perspective

The IGFs (1 and 2) were identified in 1957 by Salmon and Daughaday *(196)* and designated sulfation factor by their ability to stimulate ^{35}sulfate incorporation into rat cartilage. Froesch et al. *(197)* described the nonsuppressible insulin-like activity (NSILA) of two soluble serum components (NSILA I and II). In 1972 the labels "sulfation factor" and "NSILA" were replaced by the term "somatomedin," denoting a substance under control and mediating the effects of GH *(198)*. In 1976 Rinderknecht and Humbel *(199)* isolated two active substances from human serum and due to this structural resemblance to proinsulin were renamed "insulin-like growth factor I and II" (IGF-1 and 2). IGF-1 is the mediator of the anabolic and mitogenic activity of GH *(200)*.

Chemical Structure

The IGFs are members of a family of insulin-related peptides, which include relaxin and several peptides isolated from lower invertebrates *(201)*. IGF-1 is a small peptide consisting of 70 amino acids with a molecular weight of 7649 Da *(202)*. Like insulin, IGF-1 has

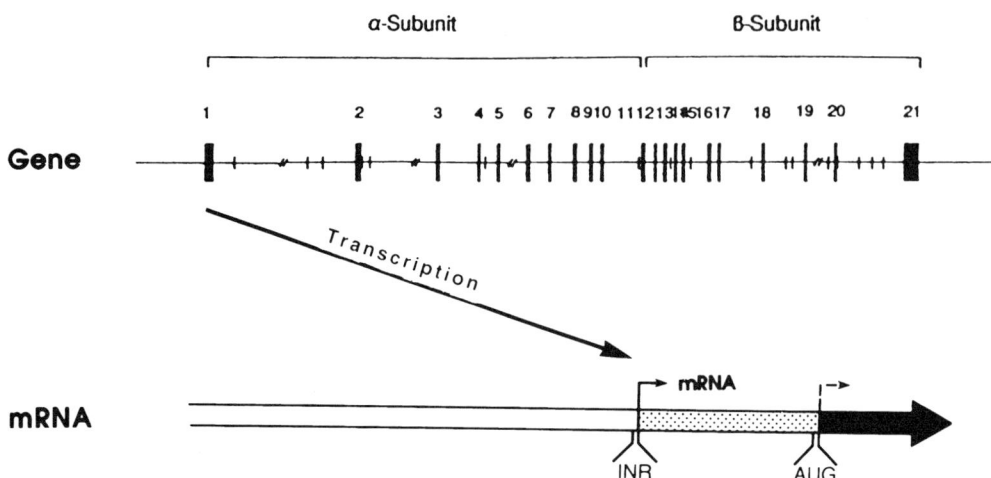

Fig. 10. The Type 1 IGF receptor gene and mRNA. Adapted with permission from ref. (*206*).

an A and B chain connected by disulfide bonds. The C-peptide region has 12 amino acids. The structural similarity to insulin explains the ability of IGF-1 to bind (with low affinity) to the insulin receptor.

The IGF-1 Gene

The IGF-1 gene is encoded on the long arm of chromosome 12q23-23 *(203,204)*. The human IGF-1 gene consists of 6 exons including two leader exons and has two promoters *(205)* (Fig. 10).

INSULIN-LIKE GROWTH FACTOR BINDING PROTEINS (IGFBPs)

The IGFs circulate in plasma 99% complexed to a family of binding proteins that modulate the availability of free IGF-1 to various tissues. There are 6 binding proteins *(207)*, and possibly more *(208)*. In humans almost 80% of circulating IGF-1 is carried by IGFBP-3 a ternary complex consisting of one molecule of IGF-1, one molecule of IGFBP-3, plus a molecule of an 88 Kd protein named acid-labile subunit (ALS) *(209)*. IGFBP-1 is regulated by insulin and IGF-1 *(210)*. IGFBP-3 is controlled mainly by GH but also to some degree by IGF-1 *(211)* In states of GHD, serum IGFBP-3 is low *(212)* but IGFBP-1 is elevated *(210)* due to a negative insulin and IGF-1 feedback mechanism.

The IGF-1 Receptor

The human IGF-1 receptor (Type 1 receptor) is the product of a single-copy gene spanning over 100 Kb of genomic DNA at the end of the long arm of chromosome 15q 25-26 *(213)*. The gene contains 21 exons (Fig. 10) and its organization resembles that of the structurally related insulin receptor *(214)*. The Type-1 IGF-receptor gene is expressed in virtually every tissue and cell type even during embryogenesis *(215)*.

It is of interest that the liver, the organ with the highest levels of IGF-1 ligand expression, exhibits almost undetectable levels of IGF-1 receptor mRNA, possibly due to the downregulation of the receptor by the local production of IGF-1. Like the insulin recep-

Insulin Receptor   IGF-I-Receptor

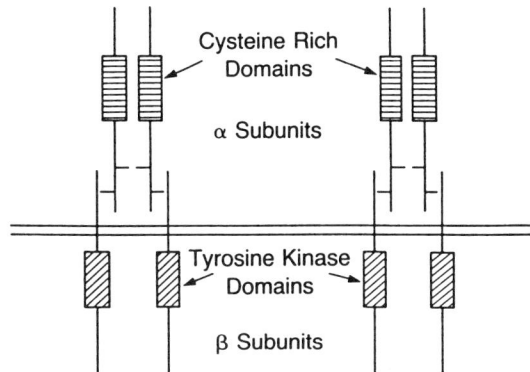

Fig. 11. Resemblance between the IGF-1 and insulin receptors.

tor, the Type-1 IGF receptor is a heterotetramer composed of two extracellular-spanning α subunits and transmembrane β subunits. The α subunits have the binding sites for IGF-1 and are linked by disulfide bonds (Fig. 11). The β subunit has a short extracellular domain, a transmembrane, and an intracellular domain. The intracellular part contains a tyrosine kinase domain, which constitutes the signal-transduction mechanism. Similar to the insulin receptor, the IGF-1 receptor undergoes ligand-induced autophosphorylation, mainly on tyrosines 1131, 1135, and 1136 *(216)*. The activated IGF-1 receptor is capable of phosphorylating other tyrosine-containing substrates, such as IRS-1 (insulin receptor substrate 1) and continue a cascade of enzyme activations via PI3-kinase (phosphatidylinositol-3 kinase), Grb2 (growth factor receptor-bound protein 2), Syp (a phosphotyrosine phosphatase), and Nck (an oncogenic protein) *(217–219)*. Another pathway of the activated IGF-1 receptor is phosphorylation of Shc (src homology domain-protein), which associates with Grb2, and activates Raf leading to a cascade of protein kinases including Raf, MAP kinase, 5 G kinase, and others *(220)*.

Physiological Aspects

IGF-1 is secreted by many tissues and the secretory site seems to determine its actions. The majority of IGF-1 is secreted by the liver and by its transport to other tissues, it acts as an endocrine hormone *(221)*. IGF-1 secreted by other tissues *(222)*, such as cartilagenous cells, acts locally in a paracrine fashion *(223)*. It is also assumed that IGF-1 can act in an autocrine manner as an oncogene *(224,225)*.

The role of IGF-1 in the metabolism of many tissues has recently been reviewed *(211, 226)*. Its effect on pre- and postnatal growth of the skeleton, organs, and tissues including the nervous system have been clearly established in man *(227)* and experimentally in animals, including knockout of the IGF-1 gene *(228)*.

DEFECTS OF THE IGF-1 GENE AND RECEPTOR

Only one patient with a defective IGF-1 gene has been described so far. In 1996 Woods et al. *(229)* described a very short 15.8-yr-old boy (height 119 cm = −6.9 height SDS). He had a small head circumference, small jaw, hypogonadism, and mental retardation, and severe bilateral sensorineural deafness. He had high-serum hGH (stimulated peaks up to 175 μg/mL; normal IGFBP-3 levels, but undetectable serum IGF-1). DNA analysis revealed deletion of exons 4 and 5 of the IGF-1 gene. One year of treatment with hGH resulted in poor growth, indicating that he was GH-resistant.

IGF-1 Resistance

Very few reports of short children fit this category, and so far no convincing evidence of a true homozygous IGF-1 receptor defect has been reported. Two heterozygous deletions of the distal arms of chromosome 15, the site of the IGF-1 receptor gene in man, have been reported.

Bierich et al. *(230)* described a very short girl with typical features of LS. Her birth length was 48 cm, she had hypoglycemic episodes, and both her basal GH and IGF-1 were high. In addition there was a 50% reduction of the specific binding of IGF-1 by the patient's fibroblasts. Momoi et al. *(231)* reported a 14-yr-old dwarfed girl born after 40 wk gestation with a birth length of 43 cm. There is no mention of her appearance but on several occasions her serum GH and IGF-1 were high, the latter reaching values of 4860 U/L. Not consistent with resistance to IGF-1 was the finding that the patient's cultured fibroblast-bound IGF-1 similarly to control cells. A possible etiology of IGF-1 resistance may be the deletion of one copy of the gene encoding the IGF-1 receptor on the long arm of chromosome 15 *(232,233)*.

Diagnostic Hints

Children born very short (≥-4 SDS height) with decreased postnatal growth who may not present with all the signs of congenital IGF-1 deficiency but who have elevated serum GH levels should be investigated for a possible abnormality in the IGF-1 gene (low to undetectable serum IGF-1) or IGF-1 receptor gene (high serum IGF-1 levels), once a defect in the GH-R has been excluded.

Comment

Experimental animal models such as the IGF-1 gene knockout *(228)* are helpful in the study of the basic physiological role of IGF-1. A recent report on the selective knockout of the hepatic IGF-1 gene challenges the concept that circulating IGF-1 (originating from the liver) can replace GH for normal postnatal growth *(234)*. However, IGF-1 plays an essential role in GH-induced postnatal growth *(235)*. IGF-1 receptor knockout mice do not survive after birth *(228)*.

Treatment

Patients with IGF-1 gene deletion or gene mutations should be treated by exogenous IGF-1 administration. For potential patients with IGF-1 receptor defects, there are no available treatments.

Table 4
Similarities and Differences Between Patients
with Molecular Defects in the hGH or IGF-1 Genes or Their Receptors (R)

Characteristics	GHRH-R gene mutation	hGH-1 gene deletion	hGH-1 deletion or mutation		Post-hGH-R mutation GHBP+	IGF-1 gene deletion	IGF-1-R mutation
			GHBP−	GHBP+			
Dwarfism	+	+	+	+	+	+	+
Short at birth	+	+	+	+	+	+	+
Small cranium	+	+	+	+	+	+	+
Acromicria	+	+	+	+	+	+	?
Obesity	±	+	+	+	−	−	+
Small genitalia and testes	+	+	+	+	+	+	?
Serum hGH	↓	↓	↑	↑	↑	↑	↑
Serum IGF-1	↓	v↓	v↓	v↓	v↓	v↓	↑
Serum insulin	↓	↓	↑	↑	N	?	↓

v, very.

GENOTYPE-PHENOTYPE RELATIONSHIP

Patients with genetic abnormalities along the GH axis present a wide spectrum of phenotypic expression (236,237) (Table 4); however, they have in common severe short stature from −3.5 to −10 height SDS below the mean normal (Tanner growth charts). Typical features of the classical LS (50,183) have been described in patients ranging from receptor defects (45,48) to IGF-1 resistance (230). These patients have a small head circumference, a protruding forehead, acromicria, hypogenitalism, and hypogonadism.

Insufficient data is available to explain the variations of expression in the nervous tissue, including psychological maturation (171,238–240), glucose and adipose tissue metabolism, and so forth (113,114). Some differences in the latter may be explained by the absence or presence of GH signal transmission in instances of mutations downstream of the GH-R, thus permitting some non-IGF-1-dependent actions. It was observed that there are slight differences between the height of GHBP- positive and GHBP-negative patients with LS, the former being slightly less short (175,241,242). As more molecular data becomes available both from patients and their family members, a better understanding of variations in the phenotypic expression of molecular defects along the GH axis will become available.

ACKNOWLEDGMENT

Thanks are due to Mrs. Gila Waichman for her invaluable technical assistance in the preparation of this chapter.

REFERENCES

1. Tannenbaum GS, Ling N. The interrelationship of growth hormone (GH)-releasing factor and somatostatin in generation of the ultradian rhythm of GH secretion. Endocrinology 1984;115:1952–1957.
2. Devesa J, Lima L, Tresquerres AF. Neuroendocrine control of growth hormone secretion in humans. Trends Endocrinol Metab 1992;3:175–183.
3. Reichlin, S. Somatostatin. N Engl J Med 1983;309:1495–1501.

4. Gil-Ad I, Koch Y, Silbergeld A, Dickerman Z, Kaplan B, Weizman A, Laron Z. Differential effect of insulin-like growth factor I (IGF-1) and growth hormone (GH) on hypothalamic regulation of GH secretion in the rat. J Endocrinol Invest 1996;19:542–547.

5. Jaffe CA, Ho, PJ, Demott-Friberg R, Bowers CY, Barkan AL. Effects of a prolonged growth hormone (GH)-releasing peptide infusion on pulsatile GH secretion in normal men. J Clin Endocrinol Metab 1993;77:1641–1647.

6. Ghigo E, Boghen M, Casanneva FF, Dieguez C, eds. Growth Hormone Secretagogues. Basic Findings and Clinical Implications. Elsevier, Amsterdam, 1994, pp. 325.

7. Howard AD, Feighner SD, Cully DF, Arena JP, Liberator PA, Rosenblum CI, et al. A receptor in pituitary and hypothalamus that functions in growth hormone release. Science 1996;273:974–977.

8. Kojima M, Hosoda H, Date Y, Nakazato M, Matsuo H, Kangawa K. Ghrelin is a growth-hormone-releasing acylated peptide from stomach. Nature 1999;402:656–660.

9. Wajnrajch MP, Ten IS, Gertner JM, Leibel RL. Genomic organization of the human GHRELIN gene. J Endocrine Genet 2000;1:231–233.

10. Folowaczny C, Chang JK, Tschoep M. Ghrelin and motilin: two sides of one coin? Eur J Endocrinol 2001;144:R1–R3.

11. Tomasseto C, Karam S, Riberias S, Masson R, Lefebvre O, Staub A, et al. Identification and characterization of a novel gastric peptide hormone: the motilin-related peptide. Gastroenterology 2000;119: 395–405.

12. Feighner SD, Tan SP, McKee KK, Palyha OC, Hreniuk DL, Pong SS, et al. Receptor for motilin identified in the human gastrointestinal system. Science 1999;284:2184–2188.

13. Itoh Z. Motilin and clinical application. Peptides 1997;18:693–698.

14. Peino R, Baldelli R, Rodriguez-Garcia J, Rodriguez-Segade S, Kojima M, Kangawa K, et al. Ghrelin-induced growth hormone secretion in humans. Eur J Endocrinol 2000;143:R11–R14.

15. Asakawa A, Inui A, Kaga T, Yuzuriha H, Nagata T, Ueno N, et al. Ghrelin is an appetite-stimulatory signal from stomach with structural resemblance to motilin. Gastroenterology 2001;120:337–345.

16. Tschoep M, Smiley DL, Heiman ML. Ghrelin induces adiposity in rodents. Nature 2000;407:908–913.

17. Shintani M, Ogawa Y, Ebihara K, Aizawa-Abe M, Miyanaga F, Takaya K, et al. Ghrelin, an endogenou growth hormone secretagogue, is a novel orexigenic peptide that antagonizes leptin action through the activation of hypothalamic neuropeptide Y/Y1 receptor pathway. Diabetes 2001;50:227–232.

18. Tschoep M, Wawarta RL, Friedrich S, Bidlingmaier M, Landrag R, Folwaczny C. Post-prandial decrease of circulating human Ghrelin levels. J Endocrinol Invest 2001;24:RC19–RC21.

19. Gualillo O, Caminos JE, Blanco M, Garcia-Caballero T, Kojima M, Kangawa K, et al. Ghrelin, a novel placental-derived hormone. Endocrinology 2001;142:788–794.

20. Reichlin S. Growth hormone content of pituitaries in rats with hypothalamic lesions. Endocrinology 1961;69:225–230.

21. Guillemin R, Brazeau P, Bohlen P, Esch F, Ling N, Wehrenberg WB. Growth hormone-releasing factor from a human pancreatic tumor that caused acromegaly. Science 1981;218:585–587.

22. Spiess J, Rivier J, Thorner M, Vale W. Sequence analysis of a growth hormone releasing factor from a human pancreatic islet tumor. Biochemistry 1982;21:6037–6040.

23. Campbell RM, Scanes CG. Evolution of the growth hormone-releasing factor (GRF) family of peptides. Growth Regul 1992;2:175–191.

24. Hofman PL, Pescovitz OH. Growth hormone releasing hormone: biological and molecular aspects. In: Handwerger S, ed. Molecular and Cellular Pediatric Endocrinology. Humana Press, Totowa, NJ, 1999, pp. 85–112.

25. Mayo KE, Cerelli GM, Lebo RV, Bruce BD, Rosenfeld MG, Evans RM. Gene encoding human growth hormone-releasing factor precursor: structure, sequence, and chromosomal assignment. Proc Natl Acad Sci USA 1985;82:63–67.

26. Perez Jurado, LA, Phillips JA III, Summar ML, Mao J, Weber JL, Schaefer FV, et al. Genetic mapping of the human growth hormone-releasing factor gene (GHRF) using two intragenic polymorphism detected by PCR amplification. Genomics 1994;20:132–134.

27. Bosman FT, Van Assche C, Nieuwenhuyzen Kruseman AC, Jackson S, Lowry PJ. Growth hormone releasing factor (GRF) immunoreactivity in human and rat gastrointestinal tract and pancreas. J Histochem Cytochem 1984;32:1139–1144.

28. Berry SA, Srivastava CH, Rubin LR, Phipps WR, Pescovitz OH. Growth hormone-releasing hormone-like messenger ribonucleic acid and immunoreactive peptide are present in human testis and placenta. J Clin Endocrinol Metab 1992;75:281–284.

29. Rivier J, Spiess J, Thorner M, Vale W. Characterization of a growth hormone-releasing factor from a human pancreatic islet tumour. Nature 1982;300:276–278.

30. Asa SL, Kovacs J, Thorner MO, Leong DA, Rivier J, Vale W. Immunohistological localization of growth hormone-releasing hormone in human tumors. J Clin Endocrinol Metab 1985;60:423–427.

31. Guillemin R, Zeytin F, Ling N, Bohlen P, Esch F, Brazeau P, et al. Growth hormone-releasing factor: chemistry and physiology (41813). Proc Soc Exp Biol Med 1984;175:407–413.

32. Laron Z. Usefulness of the growth hormone-releasing hormone test regardless of which fragment is used (GHRH 1-44, 1-40 or 1-29). Isr J Med Sci 1991;27:343–345.

33. Schriock EA, Lustig RH, Rosenthal SM, Kaplan SL, Grumbach MM. Effect of growth hormone (GH)-releasing hormone (GRH) on plasma GH in relation to magnitude and duration of GH deficiency in 26 children and adults with isolated GH deficiency or multiple pituitary hormone deficiencies: evidence for hypothalamic GRH deficiency. J Clin Endocrinol Metab 1984;58:1043–1049.

34. Pertzelan A, Keret R, Bauman B, Ben-Zeev Z, Olsen DB, Comaru-Schally AM, et al. Plasma GH response to synthetic GH-RH 1-44 in 52 children and adults with GH deficiency of various etiologies. Horm Res 1985;22:24–31.

35. Keret R, Josefsberg Z, Kinarti H, Silbergeld A, Szoke B, Schally AV, Laron Z. Discrimination between growth hormone (GH) deficiency of hypothalamic or pituitary origin: an aid in selecting patients for GH-releasing hormone (RH) prolonged therapy. Isr J Med Sci 1988;24:207–211.

36. Barinaga M, Yamamoto G, Rivier C, Vale W, Evans R, Rosenfeld MG. Transcriptional regulation of growth hormone gene expression by growth hormone-releasing factor. Nature 1983;306:84–85.

37. Billestrup N, Swanson LW, Vale W. Growth hormone-releasing hormone stimulates proliferation of somatotrophs *in vitro*. Proc Natl Acad Sci USA 1986;83:6854–6857.

38. Mayo KE. Molecular cloning and expression of a pituitary-specific receptor for growth hormone-releasing hormone. Mol Endocrinol 1992;6:1734–1744.

39. Gaylinn BD, Harrison JK, Zysk JR, Lyons CE, Lynch KR, Thorner MO. Molecular cloning and expression of a human anterior pituitary receptor for growth hormone-releasing hormone. Mol Endocrinol 1993;7:77–84.

40. Godfrey P, Rahal JO, Beamer WC, Copeland NH, Jenkins NA, Mayo KE. GHRH receptor of *little* mice contains a missense mutation in the extracellular domain that disrupts receptor function. Nat Genet 1993;4:227–232.

41. Labrie F, Gagne B, Lefevre G. Growth hormone-releasing factor stimulates adenylate cyclase activity in the anterior pituitary gland. Life Sci 1983;33:2229–2233.

42. Mayo KE. Molecular cloning and expression of a pituitary-specific receptor for growth hormone-releasing hormone. Mol Endocrinol 1992;6:1734–1744.

43. Vamvakopoulos NC, Kunz J, Olberding U, Scherer SW, Sioutopoulou TO, Schneider V, et al. Mapping the human growth hormone-releasing hormone receptor (GHRHR) gene to the short arm of chromosome 7 (7p13-p21) near the epidermal growth factor receptor (EGFR) gene. Genomics 1994;20:338–340.

44. Wajnrajch MP, Chua SC, Green ED, Leibel RL. Human growth hormone-releasing hormone receptor (GHRHR) maps to a YAC at chromosome 7p15. Mamm Genet 1994;5:595.

45. Wajnrajch MP, Gertner JM, Harbison MD, Chua SC Jr, Leiberl RL. Nonsense mutation in the human growth hormone-releasing hormone receptor causes growth failure analogous to the little (*lit*) mouse. Nature Genet 1996;12:88–90.

46. Maheshwari HG, Silverman BL, Dupuis J, Baumann G. Phenotype and genetic analysis of a syndrome caused by an inactivating mutation in the growth hormone releasing hormone receptor. Dwarfism of Sindh. J Clin Endocrinol Metab 1998;83:4065–4074.

47. Netchine I, Talon P, Dastot F, Vitaux F, Goossens M, Amselem S. Extensive phenotypic analysis of a family with growth hormone (GH) deficiency caused by a mutation in the GH-releasing hormone receptor gene. J Clin Endocrinol Metab 1998;83:432–436.

48. Salvatori R, Hayashida CY, Aguilar-Oliveira MH, Phillips JA III, Souza AHO, Gondo RG, et al. Familial dwarfism due to a novel mutation in the growth hormone-releasing hormone receptor gene. J Clin Endocrinol Metab 1999;84:914–923.

49. Laron Z. Deficiencies of growth hormone and somatomedins in man. In: Cohen MP, Foa PP, eds. Special Topics in Endocrinology and Metabolism, vol. 5. Alan R. Liss, Inc., New York, 1983, pp. 149–199.

50. Laron Z. Natural history of the classical form of primary growth hormone (GH) resistance (Laron syndrome). J Pediatr Endocrinol Metab 1999;12:231–249.

51. Li CH, Papapkoff H, Preparation and properties of growth hormone from human and monkey pituitary glands. Science 1956;124:1293–1294.

52. Miller WL, Eberhart NL. Structure and evaluation of the growth hormone gene family. Endocr Rev 1983;4:97–130.
53. Laron Z, Mannheimer S. Measurement of human growth hormone. Description of the method and its clinical applications. Isr J Med Sci 1966;2:115–119.
54. Schechter J, Kovacs K, Rimoin D. Isolated growth hormone deficiency: immunocytochemistry. J Clin Endocrinol Metab 1984;59:798–800.
55. Frankenne F, Closset J, Gomez F, Scippo ML, Smal J. Hennen G. The physiology of growth hormones (GHs) in pregnant women and partial characterization of the placental GH variant. J Clin Endocrinol Metab 1988;66:1171–1180.
56. George DL, Phillips JA III, Francke U, Seeburg PH. The genes for growth hormone and chorionic somatomammotropin are on the long arm of human chromosome 17 in region q21-qter. Hum Genet 1981;57:138–141.
57. MacLeod JN, Lee AK, Liebhaber SA, Cooke NE. Developmental control and alternative splicing of the placentally expressed transcripts from the human growth hormone gene cluster. J Biol Chem 1992; 267:14,219–14,226.
58. Parks JS, Nielsen PV, Sexton LA, Jorgensen EH. An effect of gene dosage on production of human chorionic somatomammotropin. J Clin Endocrinol Metab 1985;50:994–997.
59. Lewis U J, Singh RNP, Tutwiler GH, Siegel MB, Van der Laan EF, Van der Laan WP. Human growth hormone: a complex of proteins. Rec Progr Horm Res 1980;36:477–508.
60. Lewis UJ, Bonewald LF Lewis LJ. The 20,000 dalton variant of human growth hormone: location of the amino acid deletions. Biochem Biophys Res Comm 1980;92:511–516.
61. Cooke NE, Ray J. Watson MA, Ester PA, Kuo BA, Liebhaber SA. Human growth hormone gene and the highly homologous growth hormone variant gene display different splicing patterns. J. Clin Invest 1988;82:270–275.
62. Culler FL, Kaufman S, Frigeri LG, Jones KL. Comparison of the acute metabolic effects of 22,000-dalton and 20,000-dalton growth hormone in human subjects. Horm Metab Res 1988;20:107–109.
63. Rowlinson SW, Waters MJ, Lewis UJ, Barnard R. Human growth hormone fragments 1-43 and 44-191: *in vitro* somatogenic activity and receptor binding characteristics in human and nonprimate systems. Endocrinology 1996;137:90–95.
64. Ray J, Jones BK, Liebhaber SA, Cooke NE. Glycosylated human growth hormone variant. Endocrinology 1989;125:566–568.
65. Kuhlmann BV, Mullis PE. Genetics of the growth hormone axis. J Pediatr Endocrinol Metab 1997;10: 161–174.
66. Illig R, Prader A, Ferrandez M, Zachman M. Hereditary prenatal growth hormone deficiency with increased tendency to growth hormone antibody formation. A type of isolated growth hormone deficiency. Acta Paediat Scand 1971;60(Suppl):607.
67. Phillips JA III, Hjelle B, Seeburg PH, Zachmann M. Molecular basis for familial isolated growth hormone deficiency. Proc Natl Acad Sci USA 1981;78:6372–6375.
68. Nishi Y, Aihara K, Usui T, Phillips JA III, Mallonee RL, Migeon CJ. Isolated growth hormone deficiency type IA in a Japanese family. J Pediatr 1984;104:885–889.
69. Rivarola MA, Phillips JA III, Migeon CJ, Heinrich JJ, Hjelle BL. Phenotypic heterogeneity in familial isolated growth hormone deficiency type I-A. J Clin Endocrinol Metab 1984;59:34–40.
70. Laron Z, Kelijman M, Pertzelan A, Keret R, Shoffner JM, Parks JS. Human growth hormone gene deletion without antibody formation or growth arrest during treatment: a new disease entity. Isr J Med Sci 1985;21:999–1006.
71. Braga S, Phillips JA III, Joss E, Schwarz H, Zuppinger K. Familial growth hormone deficiency resulting from a 7.6 kb deletion within the growth hormone gene cluster. Am J Med Genet 1986;25:443–452.
72. Frisch H, Phillips JA III. Growth hormone deficiency due to GH-N gene deletion in an Austrian family. Acta Endocrinol (Copenh) 1986;27(Suppl):107–112.
73. Goossens M, Brauner R, Czernichow P, Duquesnoy P, Rappaport R. Isolated growth hormone (GH) deficiency type IA associated with a double deletion in the human GH gene cluster. J Clin Endocrinol Metab 1986;62:712–716.
74. Matsuda I, Hata A, Jinno Y, Endo F, Akaboshi I, Nishi Y, et al. Heterogeneous phenotypes of Japanese cases with a growth hormone gene deletion. Jpn J Human Genet 1987;32:227–235.
75. Vnencak-Jones CL, Phillips JA III, Chen EY, Seeburg PH. Molecular basis of human growth hormone gene deletion. Proc Natl Acad Sci USA 1988;85:5615–5619.

76. He YA, Chen SS, Wang YX, Lin XY, Wang DF. A Chinese familial growth hormone deficiency with a deletion of 7.1 kb of DNA. J Med Genet 1990;27:151–154.

77. Duquesnoy P, Amselem S, Gourmelen M, Le Bouc Y, Goossens M. A frame shift mutation causing isolated growth hormone deficiency type IA. Am J Hum Genet 1990;47:A110.

78. Nishi Y, Masuda H, Nishimura S, Kihara M, Suwa S, Tachibana K, et al. Isolated human deficiency due to the hGH-I gene deletion with (type IA) and without (the I Israeli-type) hGH antibody formation during hGH therapy. Acta Endocrinol (Copenh) 1990;122:267–271.

79. Akinci A, Kanaka C, Eble A, Akar N, Vidialisan S, Mullis PE. Isolated growth hormone (GH) deficiency type IA associated with a 45-kilobase gene deletion within the human GH gene cluster. J Clin Endocrinol Metab 1992;75:437–441.

80. Kamijo T, Phillips JA III. Detection of molecular heterogeneity in GH-I gene deletions by analysis of polymerase chain reaction amplification products. J Clin Endocrinol Metab 1992;75:786–789.

81. Cogan JD, Phillips JA III, Sakati N, Frisch H, Schober E, Milner RDG. Heterogenous growth hormone (GH) gene mutations in familial GH deficiency. J Clin Endocrinol Metab 1993;76:1124–1128.

82. Mullis PE, Akinci A, Kanaka Ch, Eble A, Brook CGD. Prevalence of human growth hormone-I gene deletions among patients with isolated growth hormone deficiency from different populations. Pediatr Res 1992;31:532–534.

83. Parks JS, Meacham LR, McKean MC, Keret R, Josefsberg Z, Laron Z. Growth hormone (GH) gene deletion is the most common cause of severe GH deficiency among oriental Jewish children. Pediatr Res 1989;25:90A.

84. Parks JS, Faase E. GH and GH-receptor genes. In: Merimee TJ, Laron Z, eds. Growth Hormone, IGF-1 and Growth: New Views of Old Concepts. Modern Endocrinology and Diabetes, vol. 4. Freund Publishing House Ltd., London, Tel Aviv, 1996, pp. 23–43.

85. Cogan JD, Phillips JA III, Schenkman SS, Milner RDG, Sakati N. Familial growth hormone deficiency: a model of dominant and recessive mutations affecting a monometric protein. J Clin Endocrinol Metab 1994;79:1261–1265.

86. Igarashi Y, Ogawa M, Kamijo T, Iwatani N, Nishi Y, Kohno H, et al. A new mutation causing inherited growth hormone deficiency: a compound heterozygote of a 6.7 kb deletion and a two base deletion in the third exon of the GH-I gene. Hum Mol Genet 1993;2:1073–1074.

87. Nishi Y, Ogawa M, Kamijo T, Igarashi Y, Iwatani N, Kohno H, et al. A case of isolated growth hormone (GH) deficiency with compound heterozygous abnormality at the GH-1 gene locus. J Pediatric Endocrinol Metab 1997;10:73–76.

88. De Luca F, Duquesnoy P, Arrigo T, Lombardo F, Goossens M. Long-lasting catch-up growth under bio-methionyl growth hormone treatment in an infant with isolated growth hormone deficiency Type 1A. Acta Paediatr Scand 1991;80:1235–1240.

89. Arnhold IJP, Oliveira SB, Osorio MGF, Mendonca BB. Insulin-like growth factor-1 treatment in two children with growth hormone gene deletions. J Pediatr Endocrinol Metab 1999;12:499–506.

90. Phillips JA III, Cogan JD. Genetic basis of endocrine disease. Molecular basis of familial human growth hormone deficiency. J Clin Endocrinol Metab 1994;78:11–16.

91. Abdul-Latif H, Leiberman E, Brown MR, Carmi R, Parks JS. Growth hormone deficiency type IB caused by cryptic splicing of the GH-1 gene. J Pediatr Endocrinol Metab 2000;13:21–38.

92. Jaber L, Bailey-Wilson JE, Haj-Yehia M, Hernandez J, Shohat M. Consanguineous matings in an Israeli-Arab community. Arch Pediatr Adolesc Med 1994;148:412–415.

93. Saitoh H, Fukushima T, Kamoda T, Tanae A, Kamijo T, Yamamoto M, et al. A Japanese family with autosomal dominant growth hormone deficiency. Eur J Pediatr 1999;158:624–627.

94. Missarelli C, Herrera L, Mericq V, Carvallo P. Two different 5' splice site mutations in the growth hormone gene causing autosomal dominant growth hormone deficiency. Hum Genet 1997;101:113–117.

95. Kamijo T, Hayashi Y, Shimatsu S, Kinoshita E, Yoshimoto M, Ogawa M, Seo H. Mutations in intron 3 of GH-I gene associated with isolated GH deficiency type II in three Japanese families. Clin Endocrinol (Oxford) 1999;51:355–360.

96. Hayashi Y, Yamamoto M, Ohmori S, Kamijo T, Ogawa M, Seo H. Inhibition of growth hormone secretion by a mutant *GH-I* gene product in neuroendocrine cells containing secretory granules: an implication for isolated growth hormone deficiency. J Clin Endocrinol Metab 1999;84:2134–2139.

97. Hayashi Y, Kamijo T, Yamamoto M, Ohmori S, Phillips JA III, Ogawa M, et al. A novel mutation at the donor splice site of intron 3 of the *GH-I* gene in a patient with isolated growth hormone deficiency. GH IGF Res 1999;9:434–437.

98. Fleisher TA, White RM, Broder S. X-linked hypogammaglobulinemia and isolated growth hormone deficiency. N Engl J Med 1980;302:1429–1434.

99. Tang MLK, Kemp AS. Growth hormone deficiency and combined immunodeficiency. Arch Dis Child 1993;68:231–232.

100. Phillips JA III. Regulation and defects in expression of growth hormone genes. In: Isaksoon O, Binder C, Hall K, Hokfelt B, eds. Growth Hormone. Basic and Clinical Aspects. International Congress Series. Excerpta Medica, Amsterdam, 1987, pp. 11–27.

101. Conley ME, Burks AW, Herrod HG, Puck JM. Molecular analysis of X-linked aggammaglobulinemia with growth hormone deficiency. J Pediatr 1991;119:392–397.

102. Ogata T, Petit C, Rappold G, Matsuo N, Matsumoto T, Goodfellow P. Chromosomal localization of a pseudoautosomal growth gene(s). J Med Genet 1992;29:624–628.

103. Yokoyawa Y, Narahara K, Tsuji K, Moriwake T, Kanzaki S, Murakami M, et al. Growth hormone deficiency and empty sella syndrome in a boy with dup(X)-q13.3 → q21.2). Am J Med Genet 1992;42:660–664.

104. Weinzimer SA, McDonald-McGinn DM, Driscoll DA, Emanual BS, Zackai EH, Moshang T Jr. Growth hormone deficiency in patients with a 22q11.2 deletion: expanding the phenotype. Pediatrics 1998;101:929–932.

105. Wagner JK, Eble A, Hindmarsh PC, Mullis PE. Prevalence of human *GH-I* gene alterations in patients with isolated growth hormone deficiency. Pediatr Res 1998;43:105–110.

106. Takahashi Y, Kaji H, Okimura Y, Goji K, Abe H, Chihara K. Brief report: short stature caused by a mutant growth hormone. N Engl J Med 1996;334:432–436.

107. Takahashi Y, Shirono H, Arisaka O, Takahashi K, Yagi T, Koga J, et al. Biologically inactive growth hormone caused by an amino acid sub-situation. J Clin Invest 1997;100:1159–1165.

108. Takahashi Y, Chihara K. Short stature by mutant growth hormones. GH IGF Res 1999;9(Suppl B):37–41.

109. Kelly PA, Goujon L, Sotiropoulos A, Dinerstein H, Esposito N, Edery M, et al. The GH receptor and signal transduction. Horm Res 1994;42:133–139.

110. Leung DW, Spencer SA, Cachianes G, Hammonds RG, Collins C, Henzel WJ, et al. Growth hormone receptor and serum binding protein: purification, cloning and expression. Nature 1987;330:537–543.

111. Godowski PJ, Leung DW, Meacham LR, Galgagni JP, Hellmiss R, Keret R, et al. Characterization of the human growth hormone receptor gene and demonstration of a partial gene deletion in two patients with Laron type dwarfism. Proc Natl Acad Sci USA 1989;86:8083–8088.

112. Barton DE, Foellmer BE, Wopod WI, Francke U. Chromosome mapping of the growth hormone receptor gene in man and mouse. Cytogenet Cell Genet 1989;50:137–141.

113. Cunningham BC, Ultsch M, de Vos AM, Mulkerrin MG, Clauser KR, Wells JA. Dimerization of the extracellular domain of the human growth hormone receptor by a single hormone molecule. Science 1991;254:821–825.

114. De Vos AM, Ultsch M, Kossiakioff AA. Human growth hormone and extracellular domain of its receptor: crystal structure of the complex. Science 1992;255:306–312.

115. Bass SH, Mulkerrin MG, Wells JA. A systematic mutational analysis of hormone-binding determinants in the human growth hormone receptor. Proc Natl Acad Sci USA 1991;88:4498–4502.

116. Souza SC, Frick GP, Wang X, Kopchick JJ, Lobo RB, Goodman HM. A single arginine residue determines species specificity of the human growth hormone receptor. Proc Natl Acad Sci USA 1995;92:959–963.

117. Argetsinger LS, Campbell GS, Yang X, Witthuhn BA, Silvennoinen O, Ihle JN, Carter-Su C. Identification of JAK2 as a growth hormone receptor-associated tyrosine kinase. Cell 1993;74:237–244.

118. Smit LS, Myer DJ, Billestrup N, Norstedt G, Schwartz J, Carter-Su C. The role of the growth hormone (GH) receptor and JAK1 and JAK2 kinases in the activation of Stats 1, 3, and 5 by GH. Mol Endocrinol 1996;10:519–533.

119. Herington AC, Ymer S, Stevenson J. Identification and characterization of specific binding proteins for growth hormone in normal human sera. J Clin Invest 1986;77:1817–1823.

120. Baumann G, Stolar MN, Amburn K, Barsano CP, DeVries BC. A specific GH-binding protein in human plasma: initial characterization. J Clin Endocrinol Metab 1986;62:134–141.

121. Silbergeld A, Lazar L, Erster B, Keret R, Tepper R, Laron Z. Serum growth hormone binding protein activity in healthy neonates, children and young adults correlation with age, height and weight. Clin Endocrinol 1989;31:295–303.

122. Sotiropoulos A, Goujon L, Simonin G, Kelly PA, Postel-Vinay MC, Finidori J. Evidence for genetation of the growth hormone-binding protein through proteolysis of the growth hormone membrane receptor. Endocrinology 1993;132:1863–1865.

123. Silbergeld A, Keret R, Selman-Almonte A, Klinger B, Laron Z. Serum growth hormone binding protein in Laron syndrome patients and their relatives. In: Laron Z, Parks JS, eds. Lessons from Laron Syndrome (LS) 1966–1992. Pediatric and Adolescent Endocrinology, vol. 24. Karger, Basel, New York, 1993, pp. 153–159.

124. Laron Z. Prismatic cases: Laron Syndrome (primary growth hormone resistance). From patient to laboratory to patient. J Clin Endocrinol Metab 1995;80:1526–1573.

125. Laron Z, Klinger B, Erster B, Silbergeld A. Serum GH binding protein activity identifies the heterozygous carriers for Laron type dwarfism. Acta Endocrinol 1989;121:603–608.

126. Laron Z, Pertzelan A, Mannheimer S. Genetic pituitary dwarfism with high serum concentration of growth hormone. A new inborn error of metabolism? Isr J Med Sci 1966;2:152–155.

127. Laron Z, Pertzelan A, Karp M. Pituitary dwarfism with high serum levels of growth hormone. Isr J Med Sci 1968;4:883–894.

128. Daughaday WH, Laron Z, Pertzelan A, Heins JN. Defective sulfation factor generation: a possible etiological link in dwarfism. Trans Assoc Am Phys 1969;82:129–138.

129. Laron Z, Pertzelan A, Karp M, Kowadlo-Silbergeld A, Daughaday WH. Administration of growth hormone to patients with familial dwarfism with high plasma immunoreactive growth hormone. Measurement of sulfation factor, metabolic, and linear growth responses. J Clin Endocrinol Metab 1971;33: 332–342.

130. Eshet R, Laron Z, Brown M, Arnon R. Immunoreactive properties of the plasma hGH from patients with the syndrome of familial dwarfism and high plasma IR-hGH. J Clin Endocrinol Metab 1973;37:819–821.

131. Eshet R, Laron Z, Brown M, Arnon R. Immunological behaviour of hGH from plasma of patients with familial dwarfism and high IR-hGH in a radioimmunoassay system using the cross-reaction between hGH and HCS. Horm Metab Res 1974;6:79–81.

132. Jacobs LS, Sneid DS, Garland JT, Laron Z, Daughaday WH. Receptor-active growth hormone in Laron dwarfism. J Clin Endocrinol Metab 1976;43:403–407.

133. Eshet R, Peleg S, Josefsberg Z, Laron Z. Characterization of hGH from patients with LTD by a human liver radioreceptor assay (RRA) (abstract). Pediatr Res 1981;15:89.

134. Eshet R, Laron Z, Pertzelan A, Dintzman M. Defect of human growth hormone in the liver of two patients with Laron type dwarfism. Isr J Med Sci 1984;20:8–11.

135. Rosenbloom AL, Guevarra-Aguire J, Rosenfeld RG, Francke U. Growth hormone receptor deficiency in Ecuador. J Clin Endocrinol Metab 1999;84:4436–4443.

136. Laron Z. Laron Syndrome: from description to therapy. Endocrinologist 1993;3:21–28.

137. Yordam N, Kandemir N, Erkul I, Kurdoglu S, Hatun S. Review of Turkish patients with growth hormone insensitivity (Laron type). Eur J Endocrinol 1995;133:539–542.

138. Razzaghy-Azar M. Laron Syndrome: a review of 8 Iranian patients with Laron syndrome. In: Laron Z, Parks JS, eds. Lessons from Laron Syndrome (LS) 1966–1992. Pediatric and Adolescent Endocrinology, vol. 24. Karger, Basel-New York, 1993, pp. 93–100.

139. Desai MP, Colaco P, Choksi CS, Sanghavi KP, Ambedkar MC, Vaz FEE. Endogenous growth hormone nonresponsive dwarfism in Indian children. In: Laron Z, Parks JS, eds. Lessons from Laron Syndrome (LS) 1966–1992. Pediatric and Adolescent Endocrinology, vol. 24. Karger, Basel-New York, 1993, pp. 81–92.

140. Baumbach L, Schiavi A, Bartlett R, Perera E, Day J, Brown MR, et al. Clinical, biochemical and molecular investigations of a genetic isolate of growth hormone insensitivity (Laron's syndrome). J Clin Endocrinol Metab 1997;82:444–451.

141. Laron Z. Laron type dwarfism (hereditary somatomedin deficiency): a review. In: Frick P, Von Harnack GA, Kochsiek GA, Prader A, eds. Advances in Internal Medicine and Pediatrics. Springer-Verlag, Berlin, 1984, pp. 117–150.

142. Rosenbloom AL, Guevara-Aguirre J. Lessons from the genetics of Laron Syndrome. TEM 1998;9: 276–283.

143. Laron Z. Laron syndrome: primary growth hormone resistance. In: Jameson JL, ed. Hormone Resistance Syndromes. Contemporary Endocrinology, vol. 2. Humana Press, Totowa, NJ, 1999, pp. 17–37.

144. Tiulpakov AN, Orlovsky IV, Kalintchenko NU, Lonina DA, Kalesnikova GS, Peterkova VA, et al. Growth hormone insensitivity (Laron Syndrome) in a Russian girl of Slavic origin caused by a common mutation of the GH receptor gene. J Endocrine Genet 1999;1:95–100.

145. Pertzelan A, Adam A, Laron Z. Genetic aspects of pituitary dwarfism due to absence of biological activity of growth hormone. Isr J Med Sci 1968;4:895–900.

146. Laron Z, Pertzelan A, Karp M, Keret R, Eshet R, Silbergeld A. Laron syndrome: a unique model of IGF-1 deficiency. In: Laron Z, Parks JS, eds. Lessons from Laron Syndrome (LS) 1966–1992. Pediatric and Adolescent Endocrinology, vol. 24. Karger, Basel-New York, 1993, pp. 3–23.

147. Amselem S, Duquesnoy P, Attree O, Novelli G, Bousnina S, Postel-Vinay MC, Goosens M. Laron dwarfism and mutations of the growth hormone-receptor gene. N Engl J Med 1989;321:989–995.

148. Amselem S, Sobrier ML, Duquesnoy P, Rappaport R, Postel-Vinay MS, Gourmelen M, et al. Recurrent nonsense mutations in the growth hormone receptor from patients with Laron dwarfism. J Clin Invest 1991;87:1098–1102.

149. Meacham WR, Brown MR, Murphy TL, Keret R, Silbergeld A, Laron Z, Parks JS. Characterization of a noncontiguous gene deletion of the growth hormone receptor in Laron's syndrome. J Clin Endocrinol Metab 1993;77:1379–1383.

150. Sobrier ML, Dastot F, Duquesnoy P, Kandemir N, Yordam N, Goossens M, Amselem S. Nine novel growth hormone receptor gene mutations in patients with Laron syndrome. J Clin Endocrinol Metab 1997;82:435–437.

151. Berg MA, Peoples R, Perez-Jurado L, Guevara-Aguirre J, Rosenbloom AL, Laron Z, et al. Receptor mutations and haplotypes in growth hormone receptor deficiency: a global survey and identification of the Ecuadorean E180splice mutation in an oriental Jewish patient. Acta Paediatr 1994;399(Suppl): 112–114.

152. Amselem S, Duquesnoy P, Duriez B, Dastot F, Sobrier ML, Valleix, S. Spectrum of growth hormone receptor mutations and associated haplotypes in Laron syndrome. Hum Mol Genet 1993;2:355–359.

153. Counts DR, Cutler GB. Growth hormone insensitivity syndrome due to point deletion and frame shift in the growth hormone receptor. J Clin Endocrinol Metab 1995;80:1978–1981.

154. Berg MA, Argente J, Chernausek S, Gracia R, Guevara-Aguirre J, Hopp M, et al. Diverse growth hormone receptor gene mutations in Laron syndrome. Am J Hum Genet 1993;52:998–1005.

155. Berg MA, Guevara-Aguirre J, Rosenbloom AL, Rosenfeld RG, Francke U. Mutation creating a new splice site in the growth hormone receptor genes of 37 Ecuadorean patients with Laron syndrome. Hum Mutation 1992;1:124–134.

156. Silbergeld A, Dastot F, Klinger B, Kanety H, Eshet R, Amselem S, Laron Z. Intronic mutation in the growth hormone (GH) receptor gene from a girl with Laron Syndrome and extremely high serum GH binding protein: extended phenotypic study in a very large pedigree. J Pediatr Endocrinol Metab 1997; 10:265–274.

157. Woods KA, Fraser NC, Postel-Vinay MC, Dusquenoy P, Savage MO, Clark AJL. A homozygous splice site mutation affecting the intracellular domain of the growth hormone (GH) receptor resulting in Laron syndrome with elevated GH-binding protein. J Clin Endocrinol Metab 1996;81:1686–1690.

158. Duquesnoy P, Sobrier ML, Duriez B, Dastot F, Buchanan CR, Savage MO, et al. A single amino acid substitution in the exoplasmic domain of the human growth hormone (GH) receptor confers familial GH resistance (Laron syndrome) with positive GH-binding activity by abolishing receptor homodimerization. EMBO J 1994;13:1386–1395.

159. Kou K, Lajara R, Rotwein P. Amino acid substitutions in the intracellular part of the growth hormone receptor in a patient with the Laron syndrome. J Clin Endocrinol Metab 1993;76:54–59.

160. Ayling RM, Ross R, Towner P, Von Laue S, Finidori J, Moutoussamy S, et al. A dominant-negative mutation of the growth hormone receptor causes familial short stature. Nature Genet 1997;16:13–14.

161. Iida K, Takahashi Y, Kaji H, Nose O, Okimura Y, Hiromi A, Chihara K. Growth hormone (GH) insensitivity syndrome with high serum GH-binding protein levels caused by a heterozygous splice site mutation of the GH receptor gene producing a lack of intracellular domain. J Clin Endocrinol Metab 1998;83:531–537.

162. Walker JL, Crock PA, Behncken SN, Rowlinson SW, Nicholson LM, Boulton TJC, Waters MJ. A novel mutation affecting the interdomain link region of the growth hormone receptor in a Vietnamese girl, and response to long-term treatment with recombinant human insulin-like growth factor-1 and luteinizing hormone-releasing hormone analogue. J Clin Endocrinol Metab 1998;83:2554–2561.

163. Laron Z, Klinger B, Eshet R, Kanety H, Karasik A, Silbergeld A. Laron Syndrome due to a post-receptor defect: response to IGF-1 treatment. Isr J Med Sci 1993;29:757–763.

164. Freeth JS, Ayling RM, Whatmore AJ, Towner P, Price DA, Norman MR, Clayton PE. Human skin fibroblasts as a model of growth hormone action in growth hormone receptor-positive Laron's Syndrome. Endocrinology 1997;138:55–61.

165. Freeth JS, Silva CM, Whatmore AJ, Clayton PE. Activation of the signal transducers and activators of transcription signaling pathway by growth hormone (GH) in skin fibroblasts from normal and GH binding protein-positive Laron Syndrome children. Endocrinology 1998;139:20–28.

166. Woods KA, Savage MO. Laron syndrome: typical and atypical forms. Bailliere's Clin Endocrinol Metab 1996;10:371–387.

167. Laron Z, Klinger B, Grunebaum M. Laron type dwarfism. Special feature: picture of the month. Am J Dis Child 1991;145:473–474.

168. Laron Z, Sarel R. Penis and testicular size in patients with growth hormone insufficiency. Acta Endocrinol 1970;63:625–633.

169. Arad I, Laron Z. Standards for upper/lower body segment ratio/sitting height: subischial leg length from birth to 18 years in girls and boys. In: Proceedings 1st International Congress of Auxology, Rome, 1977 Milan, Centro Auxologia Italiano di Piancavallo, 1979, pp. 159–164.

170. Laron Z, Klinger B. IGF-1 treatment of adult patients with Laron syndrome. Clin Endocrinol 1994;41:631–638.

171. Galatzer A, Aran O, Nagelberg N, Rubitzek J, Laron Z. Cognitive and psychosocial functioning of young adults with Laron syndrome. In: Laron Z, Parks JS, eds. Lessons from Laron Syndrome (LS) 1966–1992. Pediatric and Adolescent Endocrinology, vol. 24. Karger, Basel-New York, 1993, pp. 53–60.

172. Laron Z, Sarel R, Pertzelan A. Puberty in Laron type dwarfism. Eur J Pediatr 1980;134:79–83.

173. Laron Z, Klinger B. Body fat in Laron syndrome patients: effect of insulin-like growth factor I treatment. Horm Res 1993;40:16–22.

174. Laron Z, Avitzur Y, Klinger B. Insulin resistance in Laron Syndrome (primary insulin-like growth factor-1 [IGF-1] deficiency) and effect of IGF-1 replacement therapy. J Pediat Endocrinol Metab 1997;10(Suppl 1):105–115.

175. Laron Z, Desai M, Silbergeld A. Girls with Laron syndrome having positive growth hormone binding protein (GHBP) are less retarded in height than those lacking GHBP. J Pediatr Endocrinol Metab 1997;10:305–307.

176. Laron Z, Blum W, Chatelain P, Ranke M, Rosenfeld R, Savage M, Underwood L. Classification of growth hormone insensitivity syndrome. J Pediatr 1993;122:241.

177. Rosenbloom AL, Martinez V, Kranzier JH, Bachrach LK, Rosenfeld RG, Guevarra-Aguire J. Natural history of growth hormone receptor deficiency. Acta Paediatr 1999;428(Suppl):153–156.

178. Laron Z, Klinger B, Erster B, Anin S. Effect of acute administration of insulin-like growth factor in patients with Laron-type dwarfism. Lancet 1988;ii:1170–1172.

179. Azcona C, Preece MA, Rose SJ, Fraser N, Rappaport R, Ranke MB, Savage MO. Growth response to rhIGF-1 80 µg/kg twice daily in children with growth hormone insensitivity syndrome: relationship to severity of clinical phenotype. Clin Endocrinol 1999;51:787–792.

180. Backeljauw PF, Underwood LE and the GHIS Collaborative Group. Prolonged treatment with recombinant insulin-like growth factor-1 in children with growth hormone insensitivity syndrome: a Clinical Research Center study. J Clin Endocrinol Metab 1996;81:3312–3317.

181. Guevara-Aguirre J, Rosenbloom AL, Vasconez O, Martinez V, Gargosky SE, Allen L, Rosenfeld RG. Two-year treatment of growth hormone (GH) receptor deficiency with recombinant insulin-like growth factor-1 in 22 children: comparison of two dosage levels and to GH-treated GH deficiency. J Clin Endocrinol Metab 1997;82:629–633.

182. Klinger B, Laron Z. Three year IGF-1 treatment of children with Laron Syndrome. J Pediatr Endocrinol Metab 1995;8:149–158.

183. Laron Z. The essential role of IGF-1. Lessons from the long-term study and treatment of children and adults with Laron syndrome. J Clin Endocrinol Metab 1999;84:4397–4404.

184. Laron Z, Klinger B. Comparison of the growth-promoting effects of insulin-like growth factor I and growth hormone in the early years of life. Acta Paediatr 2000;88:38–41.

185. Laron Z. Clinical use of insulin-like growth factor-1—Yes or no? (Leading Article). Paediatr Drugs 1999;1:155–159.

186. Johnston LB, Savage MO. Partial growth hormone insensitivity. J Pediatr Endocrinol Metab 1999;12(Suppl 1):251–257.

187. Goddard AD, Covello R, Luoh S-M, Clackson T, Attie KM, Gesundheit N, et al. Growth hormone receptor mutations in idiopathic short stature. N Engl J Med 1995;333:1093–1098.

188. Merimee TJ, Laron Z. The Pygmy. In: Growth Hormone, IGF-1 and Growth: New Views of Old Concepts. Freund Publishing House Ltd., London, 1996, pp. 217–240.

189. Cavalli-Sforza LL. Ed. Anthropometric Data in African Pygmies. Academic Press, New York, 1986, pp. 81–94.
190. Merimee TJ, Rimoin DL, Cavalli-Sforza LL. Metabolic studies in the African pygmy. J Clin Invest 1972;51:395–401.
191. Merimee TJ. Growth hormone and IGF abnormalities of the African pygmy. In: LeRoith D, Raizada M, eds. Molecular and Cellular Biology of Insulin Like Growth Factors and Their Receptors. Plenum Press, New York, 1989, pp. 73–81.
192. Merimee TJ, Zapf J, Froesch ER. Insulin like growth factors in pygmies and subjects with the pygmy trait. J Clin Endocrinol Metab 1982;55:1081–1088.
193. Rimoin DL, Merimee TJ, Rabinowitz D, Cavalli-Sforza LL, McKusick VA. Peripheral subresponsiveness to human growth hormone in the African pygmies. N Engl J Med 1969;281:1383–1388.
194. Merimee TJ, Baumann G, Daughaday W. Growth hormone binding protein II. Studies in pygmies and normal statured subjects. J Clin Endocrinol Metab 1990;71:1183–1188.
195. Geffner ME, Bailey RC, Bersch N, Vera JC, Golde DW. Insulin-like growth factor I unresponsiveness in a Efe pygmy. Biochem Biophys Res Comm 1993;193:1216–1220.
196. Salmon WD Jr, Daughaday W. A hormonally controlled serum factor which stimulates sulfate incorporation by cartilage in vitro. J Lab Clin Med 1957;49:825–836.
197. Froesch ER, Burgi H, Ramseier EB, Bally P, Labhart A. Antibody-suppressible and nonsuppressible insulin-like activities in human serum and their physiologic significance. An insulin assay with adipose tissue of increased precision and specificity. J Clin Invest 1963;42:1816–1834.
198. Daughaday WH, Hall K, Raben MS, Salmon WD Jr, Van den Brande JL, Van Wyk JJ. Somatomedin: a proposed designation for the sulfation factor. Nature 1972;235:107.
199. Rinderknecht E, Humbel RE. Polypeptides with non-suppressible insulin-like and cell-growth promoting activities in human serum: isolation, chemical characterization, and some biological properties of forms I and II. Proc Natl Acad Sci USA 1976;73:2365–2369.
200. Laron Z. Somatomedin-1 (recombinant insulin-like growth factor-1). Clinical pharmacology and potential treatment of endocrine and metabolic disorders. BioDrugs 1999;11:55–70.
201. Blundell TL, Humbel RE. Hormone families: pancreatic hormones and homologous growth factors. Nature 1980;287;781–787.
202. Rinderknecht E, Humbel RE. The amino acid sequence of human insulin like growth factor I and its structural homology, with proinsulin. J Biol Chem 1978;253:2769–2776.
203. Brissenden JE, Ullrich A, Francke U. Human chromosomal mapping of genes for insulin-like growth factors I and II and epidermal growth factor. Nature 1984;310:781–784.
204. Mullis PE, Patel MS, Brickell PM, Hindmarsh PC, Brook CD. Growth characteristics and response to growth hormone therapy in patients with hypochondroplasia: genetic linkage of the insulin-like growth factor I gene at chromosome 12q23 to the disease in a subgroup of these patients. Clin Endocrinol 1991; 34:265–274.
205. Rotwein P. Structure, evolution, expression and regulation of insulin-like growth factors I and II. Growth Factors 1991;5:3–18.
206. Werner H. Molecular biology of the Type I IGF receptor. In: Rosenfeld RG, Roberts CT Jr, eds. The IGF System: Molecular Biology, Physiology and Clinical Applications. Humana Press, Totowa, NJ, 1999, pp. 63–88.
207. Hwa V, Oh Y, Rosenfeld RG. The insulin-like growth factor binding protein (IGFBP) superfamily. Endocr Rev 1999;20:761–787.
208. Collet C, Candy J. At the cutting edge: how many insulin-like growth factor binding proteins? Mol Cell Endocrinol 1998;139:1–6.
209. Lewitt MS, Saunders H, Phuyal JL, Baxter RC. Complex formation by human insulin-like growth factor-binding protein-3 and human acid-labile subunit in growth hormone-deficient rats. Endocriology 1994;134:2402–2409.
210. Laron Z, Suikkairi, AM, Klinger B, Silbergeld A, Pertzelan A, Seppala M, Koivisto VA. Growth hormone and insulin-like growth factor regulate insulin-like growth factor-binding protein-1 in Laron type dwarfism, growth hormone deficiency and constitutional short stature. Acta Endocrinol 1992;127: 351–358.
211. Kanety H, Karasik A, Klinger B, Silbergeld A, Laron Z. Long-term treatment of Laron type dwarfs with insulin-like growth factor I increases serum insulin-like growth factor-binding protein 3 in the absence of growth hormone activity. Acta Endocrinol 1993;128:144–149.

212. Laron Z, Klinger B, Blum WF, Silbergeld A, Ranke MB. IGF binding protein-3 in patients with Laron-type dwarfism: effect of exogenous rIGF-1. Clin Endocrinol 1992;36:301–304.

213. Abbott AM, Bueno R, Pedrini MT, Murray JM, Smith RJ. Insulin-like growth factor I receptor gene structure. J Biol Chem 1992;267:10,759–10,763.

214. Seino S, Seino M, Nishi S, Bell GI. Structure of the human insulin receptor gene and characterization of its promoter. Proc Natl Acad Sci USA 1989;86:114–118.

215. Bondy CA, Werner H, Roberts CT Jr, LeRoith D. Cellular pattern of insulin-like growth factor I (IGF-1) and type I IGF receptor gene expression in early organogenesis: comparison with IGF-2 gene expression. Mol Endocrinol 1990;4:1386–1398.

216. Kato H, Faria TN, Stannard B, Roberts CT Jr, LeRoith D. Essential role of tyrosine residues 1131, 1135, and 1136 of the insulin-like growth factor-1 (IGF-1) receptor in IGF-1 action. Mol Endocrinol 1994;8: 40–50.

217. Shemer J, Adamo M, Wilson GI, Heffez D, Zick Y, LeRoith D. Insulin and insulin-like growth factor-1 stimulate a common endogenous phosphoprotein substrate (pp185) in intact neuroblastoma cells. J Biol Chem 1987;262:15,476–15,482.

218. Kuhne MR, Pawson T, Lienhard GE, Feng GS. The insulin receptor substrate-I associate with the SH2-containing phosphotyrosine phosphatase Syp. J Biol Chem 1993;268:11,479–11,481.

219. Skolnik EY, Batzer A, Li N, Lee CH, Lowenstein E, Mohammadi M, et al. The function of GRB2 in linking the insulin receptor to ras signaling pathways. Science 1993;260;1953–1955.

220. LeRoith D, Werner H, Beitner-Johnson D, Roberts CT Jr. Molecular and cellular aspects of the insulin-like growth factor I receptor. Endocr Rev 1995;16:143–163.

221. Merimee TJ, Laron Z, eds. Growth Hormone, IGF-1 and Growth: New Views of Old Concepts. Freund Publishing House Ltd., London, 1996.

222. D'Ercole AJ, Applewhite GT, Underwood LE. Evidence that somatomedin is synthesized by multiple tissues in the fetus. Dev Biol 1980;75:315–328.

223. Nilsson A, Isgaard J, Lindhahl A, Dahlstrom A, Skottner A, Isaksson OGP. Regulation by growth hormone of number of chondrocytes containing IGF-1 in rat growth plate. Science 1986;233:571–574.

224. Baserga R. The IGF-1 receptor in cancer research. Exp Cell Res 1999;253:1–6.

225. Kaleko M, Rutter WJ, Miller AD. Overexpression of the human insulin-like growth factor I receptor promotes ligand-dependent neoplastic transformation. Mol Cell Biol 1990;10:464–473.

226. Rosenfeld RG, Roberts CT Jr (eds). The IGF System: Molecular Biology, Physiology and Clinical Applications. Humana Press, Totowa, NJ, 1999, pp. 787.

227. Zapf J, Froesch ER. Insulin-like growth factor I actions on somatic growth. In: Kostyo J, ed. Handbook of Physiology, vol. V. American Physiol. Society, Washington DC, 1999, pp. 663–699.

228. Liu J-P, Baker J, Perkins AS, Robertson EJ, Efstratiadis A. Mice carrying null mutations of the genes encoding insulin-like growth factor I (IGF-1) and type 1 IGF receptor (IGF1r). Cell 1993;75: 59–72.

229. Woods KA, Camacho-Hubner C, Savage MO, Clark AJ. Intrauterine growth retardation and postnatal growth failure associated with deletion of the insulin-like growth factor I gene. N Engl J Med 1996;335: 1363–1367.

230. Bierich JR, Moeller H, Ranke MB, Rosenfeld RG. Pseudopituitary dwarfism due to resistance to somatomedin: a new syndrome. Eur J Pediatr 1984;142:186–188.

231. Momoi T, Yamanaka C, Kobayashi M, Haruta T, Sasaki H, Yorifuji T, et al. Short stature with normal growth hormone and elevated IGF-1. Eur J Pediatr 1992;152:321–325.

232. Siebler T, Lopaczynski W, Terry CL, Casella SJ, Munson P, De Leon DD, et al. Insulin-like growth factor I receptor expression and function in fibroblasts from two patients with deletion of the distal long arm of chromosome 15. J Clin Endocrinol Metab 1995;80:3447–3457.

233. Tamura T, Tohma T, Ohta T, Soejima H, Harada H, Abe K, Niikawa N. Ring chromosome 15 involving deletion of the insulin-like growth factor 1 receptor gene in a patient with features of Silver-Russell syndrome. Clin Dysmorphol 1997;2:106–113.

234. Yakar S, Liu S-L, Stannard B, Butler A, Accili D, Sauer B, LeRoith D. Normal growth and development in the absence of hepatic insulin-like growth factor I. Develop Biol 1999;96:7324–7329.

235. Liu JL, LeRoith D. Insulin-like growth factor I is essential for postnatal growth in response to growth hormone. Endocrinology 1999;140:5178–5184.

236. Laron Z. Short stature due to genetic defects affecting growth hormone activity. N Engl J Med 1996; 334:463–465.

237. Clayton PE, Freeth JS, Norman MR. Congenital growth hormone insensitivity syndromes and their relevance to idiopathic short stature. Clin Endocrinol 1999;50:275–283.
238. Frankel JJ, Laron Z. Psychological aspects of pituitary insufficiency in children and adolescents with special reference to growth hormone. Isr J Med Sci 1968;4:953–961.
239. Kranzler JH, Rosenbloom AL, Martinez V, Guevara-Aguirre J. Normal intelligence with severe insulin-like growth factor I deficiency due to growth hormone receptor deficiency: a controlled study in a genetically homogenous population. J Clin Endocrinol Metab 1998;83:1953–1958.
240. Laron Z, Galatzer A. A comment on normal intelligence in growth hormone receptor deficiency. (Letter to the Editor). J Clin Endocrinol Metab 1999;83:4528.
241. Woods KA, Clark AJL, Amselem S, Savage MO. Relationship between phenotype and genotype in growth hormone insensitivity syndrome. Acta Paediatr 1999;88(Suppl 428):158–162.
242. Kaji H, Nose O, Tajiri H, Takahashi Y, Iida K, Takahashi T, et al. Novel compound heterozygous mutations of growth hormone (GH) receptor gene in a patient with GH insensitivity syndrome. J Clin Endocrinol Metab 1997;82:3705–3709.

3   Normal and Abnormal Growth

Emily C. Walvoord, MD
and Erica A. Eugster, MD

CONTENTS

INTRODUCTION

Growth has been described as the work of childhood. Very few things are as important, or as good a barometer of a child's health, as his or her growth. Under normal circumstances, growth proceeds in a predictable fashion from conception to adulthood. Abnormal growth can be a harbinger of a pathologic condition of any organ system, as well as a psychosocial problem.

NORMAL GROWTH

Phases of Growth

INFANCY

Linear growth can be divided into three separate components: infancy, childhood, and puberty. The infancy component of growth begins immediately following birth and reflects a continuation of fetal influences. Growth continues to be very rapid, but the rate steadily decelerates until around 9 mo of age when the childhood stage of growth begins *(1)*.

CHILDHOOD

Most normal children shift centiles during the first 18–24 mo of life, but then grow along a genetically predicted growth channel during the remainder of childhood.

Growth during childhood is not a continuous, smooth, linear process. Seasonal variations appear, with the highest rate of growth occurring in the spring and summer *(2,3)*. Although poorly understood, studies of growth rates in blind children as compared to partially sighted and normal children reveal that blind children do not appear to have a seasonal variation in their growth pattern, suggesting that normal retinal exposure to light seems to influence and possibly synchronize growth patterns *(4)*. Normal growth can also

From: *Contemporary Endocrinology: Developmental Endocrinology: From Research to Clinical Practice*
Edited by: E. A. Eugster and O. H. Pescovitz © Humana Press Inc., Totowa, NJ

vary significantly over a short time period. Intervals of rapid growth spurts have been described to be manifest over a period of days *(5)* to weeks *(2,6)*, separated by periods of very slow or nonexistent growth. This nonlinear pattern is termed "saltatory growth" *(5)*, but the concept has not been universally accepted. Likewise, serum concentrations of growth hormone (GH) and insulin-like growth factor-1 (IGF-1) show considerable day-to-day variability *(7)*.

PUBERTY

Growth velocity greatly accelerates again during puberty until a peak height velocity is reached. This is followed by a decelerating growth rate until final height is attained. The average peak in height velocity occurs in girls at around age 11 yr, corresponding to Tanner stage 2–3, and at around age 13 yr in boys, Tanner stage 3–4. This corresponds to the timing of maximal GH secretion that shows parallel sex differences during puberty *(8)*. Interestingly, the duration of the growth spurt is inversely related to the age of onset of the growth spurt. Thus, normal children with a later onset of puberty do not necessarily attain greater adult heights than their counterparts with an earlier onset of puberty *(9,10)* as the duration of their puberty is shorter. The average total pubertal height gain is 25–29 cm in girls and 28–31 cm in boys *(11,12)*. Therefore, adult stature is a product of the prepubertal height, the average height velocity during puberty, and the duration of the pubertal growth spurt. Adult heights usually fall within 1 standard deviation (SD), or SCM, of genetic height potential.

Nutritional Control

Adequate caloric intake is obviously a necessity for normal growth. However, concerns about the effects of nontraditional diets on growth seem to be largely unfounded. Longitudinal studies comparing the growth of well-matched, prepubertal, school-aged children reveal that children who ate vegetarian diets obtained mean heights similar to or even slightly taller than omnivores, as long as eggs, milk, or fish were included in the diet *(13,14)*. The data are more controversial for infants and preschool children, but also seem to be reassuring *(15)*. Diets of reduced saturated fat and cholesterol, even in children less than 1 yr of age, are compatible with normal growth *(16,17)*. However, this is true only when the diet consists of roughly at least 25% fat and otherwise provides proper amounts of protein, calcium, zinc, and other essential nutrients *(18,19)*.

Hormonal Control

GROWTH HORMONE

Linear growth occurs at the epiphyseal plates of long bones primarily under the influence of GH. GH itself seems to have a direct effect by stimulating proliferation of prechondrocytes *(20)* as well as an indirect effect through the systemic and local production of IGF-1 *(21)*. Interestingly, the importance of circulating IGF-1 levels in the maintenance of normal growth has recently been called into question. Knockout mice unable to produce IGF-1 in the liver were found to have normal tissue concentrations of IGF-1 and had normal growth. This suggests an autocrine/paracrine action of IGF-1 on bone, even in the setting of extremely low circulating levels of IGF-1 *(22)*.

THYROID HORMONE

Thyroid hormone is essential for normal growth. At the level of the pituitary, normal GH secretion in response to growth hormone-releasing hormone (GHRH) stimulation requires the presence of normal levels of triiodothyronine *(23)*. In the periphery, GH-stimulated hepatic IGF-1 production seems to be augmented by the presence of T3 *(24–26)*, although an independent affect of T3 on IGF-1 production is unlikely. Finally, thyroid hormone increases bone turnover through a direct action on osteoblasts, which then signals osteoclast resorption of bone *(27)*.

Unlike GH, thyroid hormone is essential for normal linear growth during infancy and for a normal onset of the childhood component of growth *(28)*. Untreated congenital hypothyroidism results in profound short stature and mental retardation. If detected and treated early, final adult height does not appear to be compromised *(29)*.

SEX STEROIDS

Sex steroids are necessary for a normal pubertal growth spurt. Under their influence, both GH secretory rates and the amount of GH secreted per burst increase during puberty *(30)*. In the absence of sex steroids, continuous linear growth continues and normal or even supernormal height may be attained. However, a lack of sex steroids results in disproportionate growth of the limbs as compared to the trunk, resulting in a eunuchoid body habitus *(31)*.

Clinical trials and naturally occurring human genetic mutations have aided in determining the interplay between sex steroids and the growth axis. Studies of nonaromatizable androgens as compared to testosterone *(32)*, estrogen receptor blockade with tamoxifen *(33)*, and androgen receptor blockade with flutamide *(34)* strongly suggest that it is estrogen, not testosterone, that stimulates the increase in GH production seen in both males and females during puberty. Additional evidence regarding the importance of estrogen in normal bone maturation in both men and women has been seen in naturally occurring human examples. Prepubertal bone ages and osteopenia were seen in men with either estrogen receptor mutations or aromatase deficiency prior to the initiation of hormone replacement *(35–37)*.

Growth Without Growth Hormone

Numerous cases have been reported of children who experience normal growth despite biochemical evidence of growth hormone deficiency (GHD). Normal growth following the surgical resection of hypothalamic tumors, especially craniopharyngiomas, with complete absence of GH secretion is the most widely recognized situation. A similar phenomenon has been observed in rare children with idiopathic GHD who have maintained normal growth in the presence of extremely low GH levels *(38,39)*. The mechanism of growth in these cases is unknown, but may result from the presence of one or more serum factors with potent growth-stimulating activity. Alternatively, normal growth in the setting of hypothalamic obesity has been postulated to be due to hyperinsulinism with cross-reactivity at the level of IGF-1.

ABNORMAL GROWTH

Short Stature

Concern about poor growth and short stature is the leading reason for referral to a pediatric endocrinologist. However, short stature alone is usually not reason enough to initiate a work-up. A combination of height that is less than 2.5 SD below the mean and a growth rate of less than the 10th percentile for age increases the likelihood of pathology. Standardized curves of normal growth velocities at differing ages are available and the determination of an accurate growth velocity often provides the single most useful parameter in the assessment of short stature.

Although the concern of an undiagnosed disease process underlies much of the concern regarding growth retardation, the perceived psychosocial consequences of short stature are also of paramount importance to patients, parents, and physicians. However, well-performed studies of children with all causes of short stature reveal that girls with short stature do not have a higher incidence of behavior or social problems than their taller counterparts. Although the parents of short boys report more problems compared to normal controls (but less compared to a psychiatric referral sample), the boys themselves report only decrements in social activities without any decreases in feelings of self-worth *(40–42)*. In one study, IQ measurements were lower in short children than controls, but social class had a much more profound influence than did height *(42)*. Additionally, psychosocial outcomes in GHD adults are no different than same sex siblings and are not dependent on final adult heights *(43)*. Finally, a recent review of multiple public health studies suggests that shorter individuals may have an overall health advantage, as they have an increased life expectancy and a lower incidence of malignancy compared with the general population *(44)*.

Normal Variations

The two most common causes of short stature in childhood are genetic, or familial short stature, and constitutional delay of growth and/or puberty.

GENETIC SHORT STATURE

Approximately half of all children referred for evaluation of short stature are normal children with short parents and short predicted adult heights. Most of these children have normal GH responses to provocative testing as well as normal spontaneous GH secretion *(45)* and do not appear to have GH resistance or increased levels of bioactive GH *(46)*. However, short children do appear to have more prolonged periods of growth stasis and less frequent growth bursts as compared to children of normal stature *(5)*, possibly accounting for their short stature.

In following 236 short normal children to adult height, Ranke et al. *(46a)* found that the majority of patients reached adult heights above the third percentile, although still below their target heights. A final height of less than 2 SD seems to be associated with an earlier age at presentation for evaluation, a shorter predicted height and target height, and a reduced amount of bone age delay as compared to other short children who reach heights greater than the 3rd percentile. Interestingly, it has been observed that short children gain approx 0.5 SD in height during the pubertal growth spurt *(47)*, possibly contributing to a final height that is greater than initial predictions. The treatment of genetic short stature with exogenous GH is not Food and Drug Administration (FDA)-approved and remains controversial. A large study of a heterogeneous group of short, GH-sufficient children revealed that 2–10 yr of GH therapy resulted in final heights 5–6 cm above predicted adult heights *(48)*. Whether this same improvement in height would be seen in children with pure genetic short stature remains unknown.

CONSTITUTIONAL DELAY

Constitutional delay of growth and puberty (CDGP) is characterized by normal growth until around 6–18 mo of age followed by a slowing of the growth rate. Thereafter, children with CDGP frequently cross growth percentiles and usually end up growing at or below the 3rd percentile until puberty, which is typically delayed. Skeletal maturation is also delayed. Thus, this condition may be very difficult to distinguish from true GHD on the basis of clinical criteria. Often times there is a family history of this same type of growth pattern, especially in boys *(49)*. Mutations in the transcription factor gene *Otx-1* in mice results in a phenotype remarkably similar to CDGP in humans *(50)*. Human mutations in OTX-1 have yet to be reported.

Treatment with oxandrolone, a nonaromitazable androgen, has been shown to significantly increase the growth rate of prepubertal and pubertal boys with CDGP, possibly by a direct effect at the growth plate in the former and via increases in GH secretion in the later *(51–53)*. However, there is no evidence that oxandrolone improves final height. Although nearly 80% of patients with CDGP reach an adult height within 2 SD of the mean *(54)*, final heights are on average 5 cm less than calculated target heights *(49)*. The combination of genetic short stature and CDGP, as well as poor height gain during puberty, seem to be poor prognostic factors for final height *(54,55)*.

Endocrine Causes of Short Stature

GROWTH HORMONE DEFICIENCY (GHD)

GHD can be congenital or acquired. Classic features of congenital GHD include central adiposity, frontal bossing, hypoplasia of facial bones, and an overall physical appearance that is younger than the chronologic age (Fig. 1). However, GHD presents prior to 2 yr of age in less than 2% of all GH-deficient patients *(56)*. In fact, in very young children, GHD usually presents with hypoglycemia or generalized "failure to thrive," with poor weight gain as well as linear growth failure.

Diagnosing GHD based on spontaneous vs stimulated GH levels has been the subject of much debate. Normal children have highly variable GH secretion patterns during serial collections as well as after stimulation testing, making abnormal tests results difficult to interpret. Provocative testing for GHD through the use of levodopa, arginine, glucagon, clonidine, or insulin is less cumbersome than collecting serial GH measurements and is arguably more sensitive than mean overnight or 24 h GH levels *(57)*.

Currently, the widely accepted, yet arbitrary, cut-off to define GHD is a peak of less than 10 µg/L after two provocative stimuli. However, measurements of spontaneous secretion rates appear to be more specific for GHD *(58)*. Recently, the combination of GHRH and a somatostatin inhibitor, either arginine or pyridostigmine, has been shown to differentiate normal children from GHD children better than other currently available tests *(59)*. However, this is not currently in widespread clinical practice. Others have argued that GHD is best diagnosed based on auxologic data and low IGF-1 and IGFBP-3 levels alone, without formal GH testing *(60)*. Magnetic resonance imaging (MRI) of the pituitary region has revealed either a hypoplastic anterior pituitary or an interrupted pituitary stalk with an ectopic posterior pituitary (Fig. 2) in a large number of children with isolated GHD *(61)*.

Theoretically, defects anywhere along the growth axis can lead to functional GHD and resultant short stature. (An extensive discussion of these defects can be found in Chapter 4). Although no mutations have been identified to date in the GHRH gene, such mutations undoubtedly exist. GHRH receptor mutations have been identified as a rare cause of isolated short stature in highly consanguineous populations *(62)*. Complete deletions *(63)* and mutations *(64)* of the growth hormone gene (GH-N) have been identified that result in either absent or very low levels of circulating GH, respectively. Two biologi-

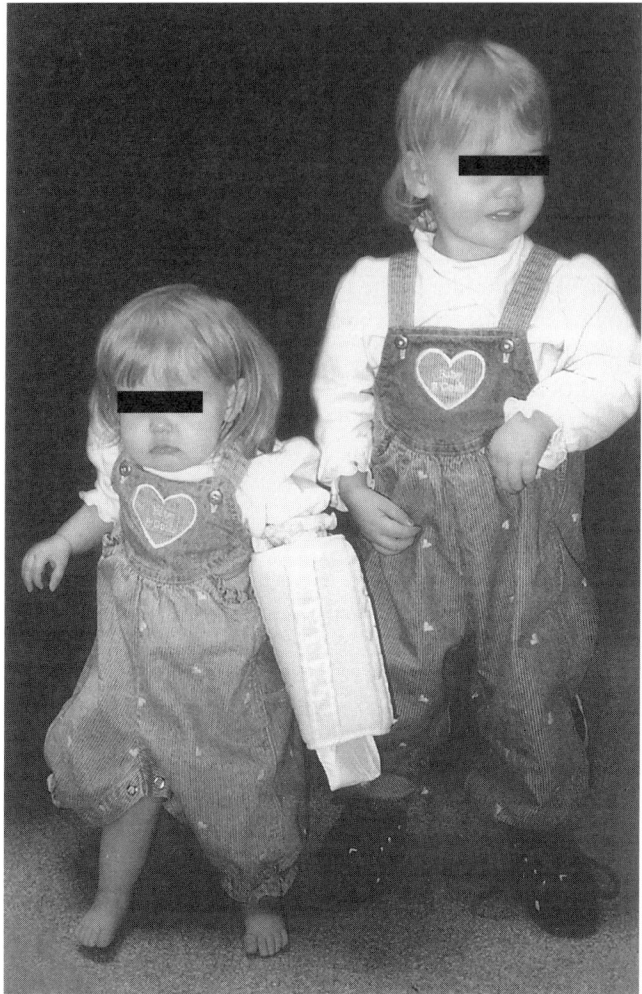

Fig. 1. The presence of her normal fraternal twin sister highlights the classic features of congenital growth hormone deficiency in this 3-yr-old girl. Note the profound short stature, cherubic appearance, and mid-face hypoplasia.

cally inactive forms of GH, resulting from point mutations of GH-N, have also been identified in two very short children with relatively high GH and low IGF-1 levels *(65)*. GH insensitivity as a result of a growth hormone receptor (GH-R) mutation is manifest in its complete form as Laron syndrome (LS) *(66)* (*see* Chapter 4). These patients have a classical phenotype of severe postnatal growth failure, acral hypoplasia, sparse hair, prominent forehead, hypoplastic nasal bridge, and a high-pitched voice *(67)*. Partial GH insensitivity due to heterozygous mutations in the GH-R has received much interest of late as it has been identified as the cause of 5–8% of cases of idiopathic short stature (ISS) *(68,69)*. Interestingly, obligate carriers of the mutation may have normal heights, thus it can be inferred that still unknown factors influence the expression of this phenotype.

The presence of the recently identified endogenous ligand of the GH secretagog receptor, ghrelin *(70)*, may also play an important physiologic role in GH output.

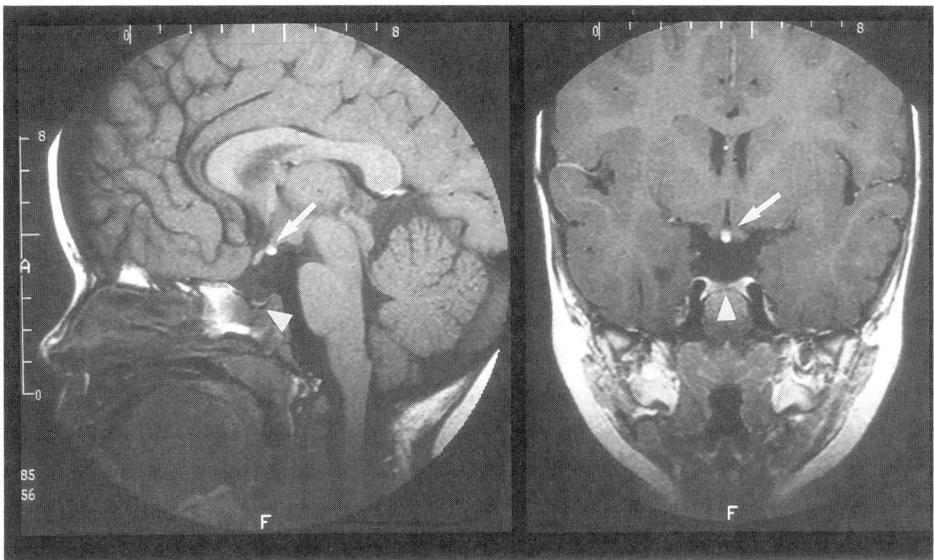

Fig. 2. Sagittal and coronal views of an MRI scan of a growth hormone-deficient patient with an ectopic posterior pituitary (arrow) and a hypoplastic anterior pituitary (arrowhead).

Defects in IGF-1 signaling may also result in short stature. Only one patient to date has been found to have an IGF-1 mutation *(71)*. This boy had prenatal and postnatal growth failure as well as mental retardation and dysmorphic facial features. Rare patients with isolated short stature have been suspected to posses tissue-specific IGF-1 receptor mutations *(72,73)*, based on elevated GH and IGF-1 levels in the face of poor growth, but no mutations have been identified to date.

Abnormal development of the pituitary gland due to a transcription-factor defect can also lead to GHD in combination with other pituitary abnormalities (*see* Chapter 1). Many of these transcription factors are also important for the maintenance of pituitary cells. Much is known about the role of many of the pituitary-transcription factors in the murine model, but to date, mutations in only 5 human pituitary transcription factors have been shown to result in hypopituitarism. HESX1, also known as Rpx1, is the earliest transcription factor expressed in the pituitary. Homozygous mutations in HESX1 have been found in two familial cases of septo-optic dysplasia (SOD) and hypopituitarism *(74)*. Sporade heterozygous mutations in HESX1 have also been recently described to result in phenotypes ranging from isolated GH deficiency with or without SOD to anhypopituitarism *(74a)*. Mutations in Ptx2, or Reig, result in Reiger syndrome that consists of pituitary, eye, and craniofacial abnormalities *(75)*. LHX3, another transcription factor expressed during early Rathke's pouch formation, when mutated has recently been shown to result in deficiencies of GH, thyroid-stimulating hormone (TSH), follicle-stimulating hormone (FSH), luteinizing hormone (LH), and prolactin but not ACTH. Interestingly, patients with this mutation also have cervical-spine abnormalities resulting in limitations of neck rotation *(76)*. The two most well-described factors important for pituitary development and function are Prop-1 and Pit-1. Prop-1, the prophet of Pit-1, is expressed only during pituitary development and specifies gonadotroph development in addition to somatotroph, lactotroph, and thyrotroph development. Interestingly, clinical phenotypes vary widely between different mutations in the PROP-1 gene and even among patients with the same mutation. Short stature is invariable. MRI findings vary as well, from a hyperplastic appearing pituitary gland to findings of an empty sella. Late onset adrenal insufficiency is often seen, but the cause of this is unclear, as Prop-1 is not known to directly effect corticotroph function *(76a)*. Finally, Pit-1 is expressed late in pituitary development and specifies somatotroph, lactotroph and thyrotroph development and function *(77)*. Familial cases of hypopituitarism should be considered to result from a transcription-factor defect and in many cases, a genetic diagnosis can now be identified.

Combined data from 11 studies of GHD children that received recombinant GH revealed that final adult heights are −1.4 SD from the mean, an improvement of 1.5 SD from the start of therapy. Outcome data are confounded by different doses of GH, variable ages at the start of GH therapy, and unstandardized criteria for the diagnosis of GHD. Most centers now use 0.3 mg/kg/wk given daily until epiphyseal fusion or until the family is satisfied with the current height. Improved outcomes are associated with a younger age at the start of therapy, delayed puberty, and a taller mid-parental height *(61,78)*. Height gained prior to the onset of puberty correlates well with adult height, as pubertal gains during GH therapy are similar to the height gains seen in normal children *(78,79)*.

Hypothyroidism

Acquired primary hypothyroidism is a leading cause of unexplained growth deceleration and growth arrest in children, even in the absence of a goiter or other recognizable symptoms of hypothyroidism. At the time of diagnosis, most children have significantly delayed skeletal maturation as well as abnormal growth (Fig. 3). Unfortunately, even with appropriate therapy, complete catch-up growth is usually not attained owing to the discordant, rapid advancement in skeletal maturation *(80,81)*. Final heights in patients with severe acquired primary hypothyroidism have been reported to be 2 SD below the mean as well as below mid-parental heights *(81)*. Interestingly, pubertal delay and the unusual finding of continued linear growth for more than 2 yr following menarche can be seen in girls treated for acquired hypothyroidism *(80)*.

Glucocorticoid Excess

Exposure to supraphysiologic levels of glucocorticoids, even at doses as low as 12–15 mg/M^2/d of hydrocortisone, is a well-known cause of growth suppression in children *(82)*. Glucocorticoids inhibit both osteoblast and chondrocyte function and disrupt normal pulsatile release of GH. They also suppress growth indirectly by altering calcium metabolism and sex-steroid secretion *(83)*.

Studies evaluating the growth of children with chronic inflammatory conditions requiring long-term glucocorticoid therapy have revealed that prednisone doses greater than 0.1 mg/kg/d result in impaired growth. Alternate-day administration schedules may improve growth as compared to every-day dosing, but still result in a slowing of the growth rate in some patients *(84,85)*. Catch-up growth does occur once therapy is stopped, but may be incomplete *(83)*. A large study of cystic fibrosis (CF) patients revealed that 2 yr after an alternate-day regimen of prednisone had been halted, girls exhibited adequate catch-up growth and had similar heights as compared to placebo-treated girls. However, the boys on alternate-day prednisone therapy did not exhibit this same catch-up growth, and at 18 yr were 4 cm shorter than placebo-treated boys *(86)*.

The use of exogenous GH to counteract the GH impairment and catabolic effects of pharmacologic doses of glucocorticoids has been proposed. Large studies are lacking,

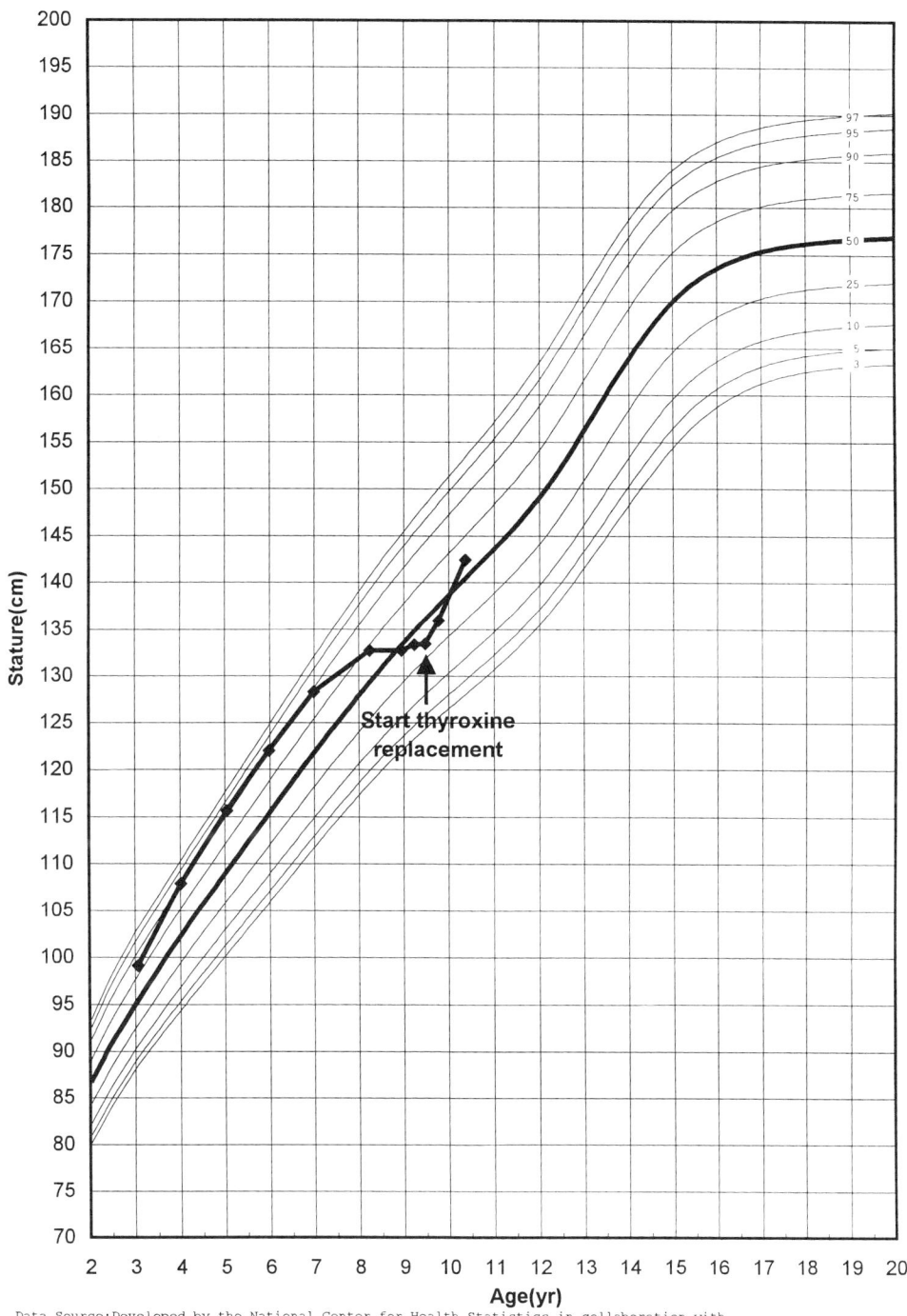

Data Source:Developed by the National Center for Health Statistics in collaboration with
the National Center for Chronic Disease Prevention and Health Promotion (2000).

Fig. 3. This boy's growth chart illustrates the growth arrest observed in untreated, acquired hypothyroidism with the subsequent rapid catch-up growth seen after therapy is instituted. Initial laboratory data revealed a TSH of 457 IU/mL and high titers of thyroperoxidase and antithyroglobulin antibodies. (Growth chart design graciously provided by Dr. Ernest M. Post.)

but it appears that GH is useful in improving the growth rates of children on small doses of prednisone, but is unable to overcome the growth-suppressing effects of prednisone at doses higher than 0.35 mg/kg/d *(87)*. It also remains controversial as to whether inhaled corticosteroids suppress growth in asthmatic children. A few controlled trials seem to indicate that regular beclomethasone use does result in mild, but measurable, growth suppression *(88,89)*. However, lower daily doses, once-daily dosing *(90)* and less potent formulations may not have the same effects *(91)*.

Nonendocrine Causes of Short Stature

INTRAUTERINE GROWTH RETARDATION

Causes of IUGR are multifactorial and in many cases, poorly understood. A single case of an IGF-1 mutation causing both prenatal and postnatal growth failure has been described and mutations in the IGF-1 receptor are hypothesized to result in IUGR although no cases have been identified to date. Multiple familial cases suggest a genetic influence of IUGR *(92)*, but a significant number of children have no known etiology.

Hormonal evaluation of children with IUGR reveals elevated GH levels and diminished IGF-1 levels as compared to controls *(47,93,94)*. These differences have been found to persist into the sixth year of life, particularly in children who fail to show expected catch up growth. It is unknown whether this pattern represents GH resistance or abnormalities in the growth axis secondary to fetal-growth restriction.

A number of metabolic derangements later in life have been shown to be associated with a history of IUGR, including hypertension, insulin resistance, elevated fibrinogen levels, and coronary artery disease *(95)*. Recently, it has been found that a subset of IUGR infants have elevated cortisol to cortisone ratios, suggesting a partial 11-B hydroxysteroid dehydrogenase type 2 defect *(96)*. Interestingly, as compared to other IUGR children with normal ratios, these children also exhibit significantly lower childhood heights and are at an increased risk for the subsequent development of additional medical problems such as hypertension, glucose intolerance, and lipid abnormalities.

Children with IUGR are 5–7 times more likely to be short as adults than are children born of appropriate size for gestational age *(47)*. Despite this, the majority of children with IUGR attain normal adult heights (<2 SD from the population mean). The vast majority of catch-up growth is seen in the first 2–5 mo of life *(47,97,98)*. However, 10–15% of children with a history of IUGR fail to experience catch-up growth, are still short at 2 yr of age, and frequently have adult heights >2 SD below the mean. A short birth length, as opposed to a low birth weight only, has been identified as a risk factor for poor postnatal catch-up growth *(97)*.

Recently, a large cohort of short children born with IUGR was treated for 5 yr with high-dose GH. By the end of the study, all of the children achieved heights within 2 SD from the mean for age, with many eventually growing along their target height percentile. Body mass index (BMI) also normalized *(99)*. The long-term safety of high dose GH in these patients, who, as previously mentioned, are already at risk for glucose intolerance, remains to be determined.

SKELETAL DYSPLASIAS

Osteochondrodysplasias are characterized by abnormal bone formation and abnormal body proportions. Achondroplasia is the most common osteochondrodysplasia that results in short stature. Clinically these patients display rhizomelic dwarfism (proximal shortening of the limbs), macrocephaly with frontal bossing, midface hypoplasia, and lumbar lordosis. Achondroplasia is inherited in an autosomal dominant pattern, but most cases are due to new mutations in the fibroblast growth factor receptor (FGFR) 3 gene *(100)*. Interestingly, 97% of all cases arise from the same point mutation causing constitutive activation of the receptor that disrupts normal osteogenesis, endochondral bone formation, and growth *(101)*. Hypochondroplasia and the more severe thanatophoric dysplasia are also due to mutations in the same gene, but in other distinct locations. Additionally, mutations in FGFR genes 1 and 2 also result in a variety of skeletal dysplasias including Apert, Pfeiffer, and Crouzon syndromes.

Numerous other skeletal dysplasias that are characterized by short stature have been described. A few may not be obvious at birth, including Albright hereditary osteodystrophy and spondyloepiphyseal dysplasia tarda, but may present in later childhood with short stature as one of the many phenotypic features.

Syndromes

Growth retardation is a feature of a countless number of syndromes. The cause of poor growth and short stature is often unknown, highlighting the multifactorial control of linear growth. Some of the more common syndromes associated with short stature include Down syndrome, Turner syndrome, Noonan syndrome, Russel-Silver syndrome, Seckel's syndrome, CHARGE association, and Prader Willi syndrome (PWS).

The etiology of the short stature associated with some syndromes has been at least partially elucidated. PWS patients are thought to suffer from a hypothalamic defect resulting in GHRH deficiency. GH replacement results not only in sustained catch-up growth, similar to that seen in classical GHD children, but also in a significant increase in muscle and fat-free mass in children with PWS *(102)*. The etiology of the short stature associated with Turner's syndrome is thought to be due, at least in part, to haploinsufficiency of the SHOX (short stature homeobox-containing gene) gene *(103)*. SHOX is found in the pseudoautosomal region on the short arm of both the X and the Y chromosome and has also been implicated as the cause of short stature in Leri-Weil syndrome, Langer dwarfism *(104)*, and a small proportion of ISS patients *(105)*. It does not appear that differing levels of mosaicism play a role in growth retardation seen in Turner's syndrome *(106)*, thus implying that the short stature seen in Turner syndrome is due only in part to haploinsufficiency of X chromosome genes.

Recent studies of girls with Turner syndrome using high-dose human growth hormone (hGH) therapy instituted at a relatively early age, indicate that final height may be improved by 10 cm or more with prolonged therapy *(107–109)*. However, a subset of patients respond poorly to hGH therapy for reasons that are unclear *(110)*. The doses of hGH required to improve growth rates in girls with Turner syndrome are higher than those used in patients with GHD. This is postulated to be due to subtle GH or IGF-1 resistance. An earlier age at the onset of therapy, a taller target height and a later onset of puberty all seem to confer the greatest benefit of GH therapy *(107,111)*. The optimal timing of estrogen replacement in girls without the spontaneous onset of puberty remains controversial.

PSYCHOSOCIAL DWARFISM

The concept of psychosocial dwarfism was first introduced in 1951 after studying the growth of children in orphanages *(112)*. Since that time, other reports consisting of small numbers of children report that stunted growth can be seen without any organic etiology

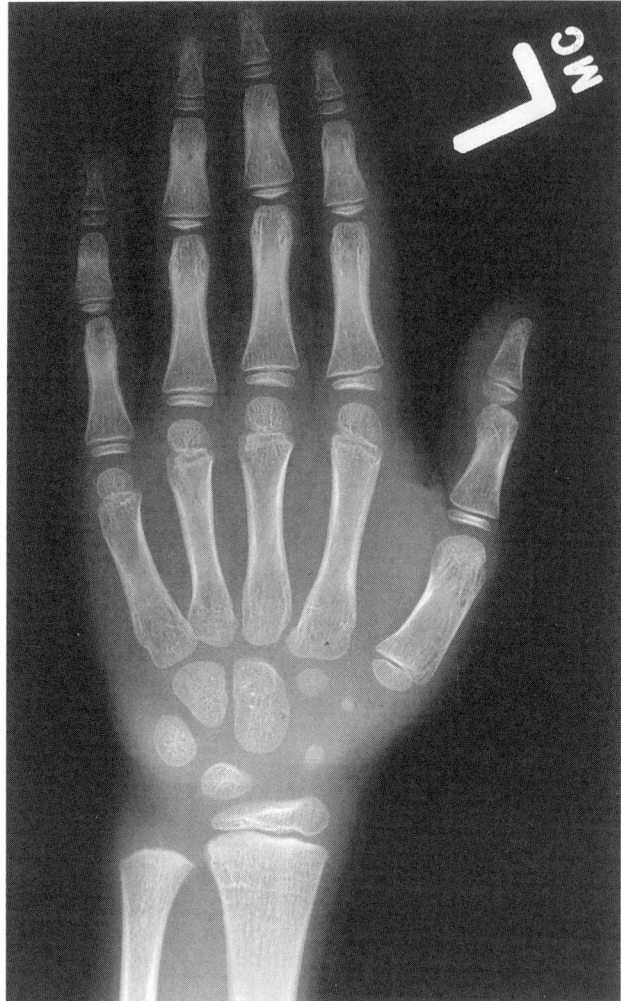

Fig. 4. Bone age X-ray of a 9-yr-old boy with a history of psychosocial dwarfism, who was eventually adopted from a Rumanian orphanage. The growth lines seen in the distal radius indicate periods of cessation of growth with subsequent recovery.

in the face of severe stress, emotional abuse, or psychological isolation *(113)*. These children present with growth failure as well as developmental and behavioral abnormalities and exhibit profound catch-up growth once they are removed from their family environment *(114)*. Long-bone radiographs often reveal periods of arrested growth with subsequent recovery. This abnormal growth pattern may occur even during periods while the child is in the troubled environment *(115)* (Fig. 4). Poor childhood socioeconomic conditions, without abuse or isolation, may also play a minor but significant role as an independent risk factor for a shorter adult height *(116)*.

CHRONIC DISEASE

Perturbations of any organ system leading to decreased caloric intake, malabsorption, or increased caloric demands can lead to growth failure. Chronic illnesses that may present as isolated short stature include inflammatory bowel disease, celiac disease, renal tubular acidosis, chronic infections, chronic anemia, and metabolic diseases. Unfortunately, correcting the underlying etiology does not always lead to full recovery of growth potential.

Tall Stature

Many fewer patients are evaluated for tall stature as compared to short stature. This reflects both the comparative rarities of pathologic tall stature as well as societies' heightism, or positive bias towards tall stature.

Normal Variant

Familial Tall Stature. Familial, constitutional, or genetic tall stature is the most common cause of tall stature. It is defined as a height more than 2 SD above the population means. This corresponds to an adult height greater than 5 feet 9 inches (175 cm) in American women or greater than 6 feet 3 inches (190 cm) in American men. The diagnosis is usually easily made in the presence of a normal history, a physical exam without signs of dysmorphic features, a normal timing of the onset of puberty, and a family history of tall stature. In fact, it is believed that 50–90% of height is controlled by genetic factors. Although it is known that GH and IGF-1 levels correlate with growth rate *(117)*, investigations of the GH-IGF-1 axis in tall children have not conclusively revealed any abnormalities. Children with constitutional tall stature usually exhibit very rapid growth in early childhood and are clearly taller than their peers by 3–4 years of age. Growth then slows to a normal rate and these children parallel the growth curve thereafter, albeit above the 97% *(118)*.

The usual reasons that children come to medical attention for tall stature are concerns of psychological adjustment, and, less frequently, the risk of scoliosis. Although no long-term prospective study of the psychological outcome after intervention for tall stature exists, retrospective data reveals that most tall adults are happy with their stature and most psychosocial problems exist only during adolescence, regardless of intervention *(119,120)*. Nonetheless, treatment options exist, with either ethinyl estradiol or conjugated estrogens being the mainstay for females and testosterone therapy for males. Final heights are, on average, 5 cm less than predicted at the start of therapy, with best results seen if therapy is initiated before a bone age of 13 yr *(120–122)*. Ethinyl estradiol (EE) at doses as low as 0.1 mg/d are effective *(123)*. Earlier regimens utilizing 11.25 mg/d of conjugated estrogens or 0.3 mg of EE resulted in significant weight gain, elevated triglycerides, increased platelet aggregation, and reports of thrombotic events *(124)*. Due to theoretical long-term risks of endometrial and breast carcinoma, it is not recommended to begin therapy until after the commencement of spontaneous puberty. Fertility does not appear to be affected *(125)*. Additional growth of approx 3 cm is often seen after the cessation of therapy, possibly due to incomplete fusion of epiphyses or late spinal growth *(122)*, thus continuation of treatment until near complete or complete epiphyseal fusion is recommended. Results of the treatment of males with constitutional tall stature with testosterone are even less impressive. Recent studies suggest no net benefit, as testosterone increases growth velocity initially, unless treatment is started before a bone age of 14 yr and continued to near complete fusion of epiphyses *(122,126)*. Octreotide, a long-acting somatostatin analog, has shown promising results in small studies in children with tall stature, with significant decreases in growth velocities and final heights *(127,128)*. However, it is currently not considered standard treatment.

ENDOCRINE ABNORMALITIES

True endocrinologic causes of tall stature are quite rare. Although hyperthyroidism and precocious puberty (either central or peripheral) can cause growth acceleration, it is at the cost of excessive skeletal maturation and eventually leads to a stunted adult height.

Growth Hormone Excess. GH excess causing gigantism in childhood is extremely rare. Sporadic cases are occasionally reported in the literature, but the incidence rate is unclear. Patients present as early as infancy with excessive growth rates, tall stature for age, large heads, large hands and feet, and thick fingers and toes. Laboratory evaluation reveals high IGF-1 and IGFBP-3 levels for age and frequently elevated prolactin levels. The gold standard for diagnosis has been considered to be the inability to suppress GH levels to less than 1 ng/mL following an oral glucose tolerance test (OGT). However, the specificity of this test is questionable, as 30% of tall children without gigantism fail to show suppression of GH after on OGT (129). TRH and CRF stimulation testing may also aid in the diagnosis with a paradoxical rise in GH reported in some cases of acromegaly, thought to be due to dedifferentiation of somatotroph receptors, but the utility of these tests in children with gigantism is unproven (130,131).

The etiology of GH excess in childhood is somewhat different than in adults. Pituitary adenomas in children are frequently mammosomatotrophs, resulting in elevated prolactin levels in addition to GH (132,133). This specific tumor type is rarely seen in adults, as mammosomatotrophs, found in fetal pituitaries, are thought to disappear by adult life (134). Both micro and macroadenomas occur, with childhood adenomas tending to be more invasive than those seen in adults (133).

Gigantism may also appear as part of an inherited syndrome. GH secreting pituitary adenomas arise in patients with multiple endocrine neoplasia type 1 (MEN 1), but occur primarily in adults, resulting in acromegaly. Ten to twenty percent of patients with Carney complex develop GH secreting pituitary adenomas resulting in either gigantism or acromegaly. This autosomal dominantly inherited disease also includes primary pigmented nodular adrenocortical disease, cardiac myxomas, spotty facial and labial pigmentation. The gene for Carney complex has yet to be identified, but has been mapped to chromosome 2p16 (135) as well as chromosome 17q2 (136). Interestingly, isolated familial somatotropinomas, a third form of inherited GH-secreting adenomas, have been reported to be linked to a locus on chromosome 11q13 (137), very near to, but not including the MEN 1 gene and to a second locus, chromosome 2p16-12, the same location also implicated in Carney complex (138), thus establishing a link between all three diseases.

Hypothalamic overproduction of GHRH leads to mammosomatotroph hyperplasia and GH excess. Infiltration of the somatostatin inhibitory inputs from the hypothalamus has been reported to cause gigantism in a patient with an optic glioma (139), and has been suggested to at least contribute to the GH excess seen in other patients with optic-pathway tumors associated with neurofibromatosis that extend into the hypothalamus (140,141) (Fig. 5). Patients with McCune Albright syndrome (MAS) may also develop gigantism due to somatotroph hyperplasia, a pituitary adenoma (142), or GH excess without signs of a pituitary abnormality, suggesting hypothalamic dysfunction (143). Interestingly, 35–40% of all GH secreting adenomas are due to activating mutations of the $Gs\alpha$ gene resulting in the oncogene gsp (144,145) not associated with the MAS. Finally, ectopic production of GHRH, most commonly from pancreatic, thymic, lung, adrenal, or bowel neoplasias, has also been reported to lead to acromegaly (146), but not gigantism.

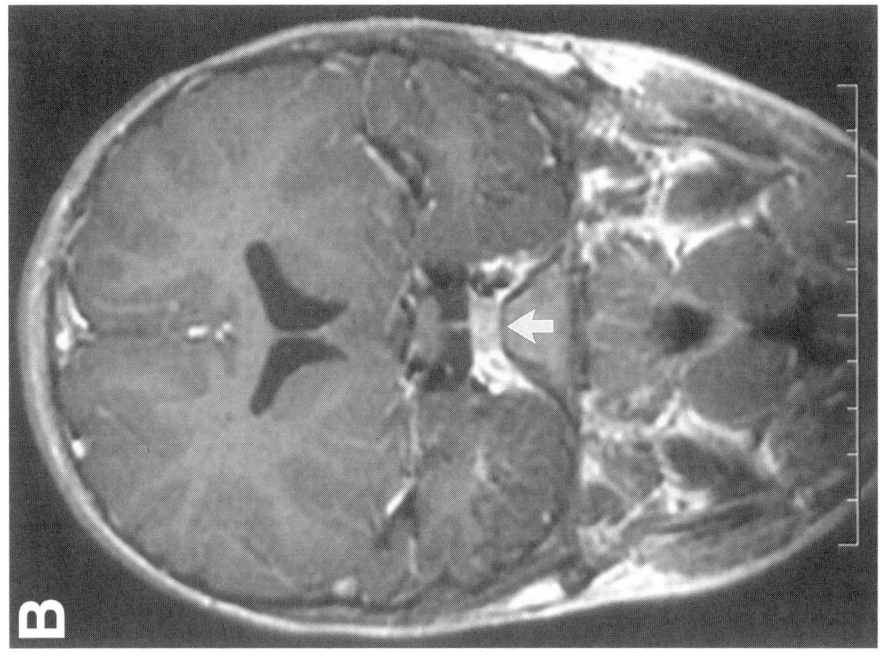

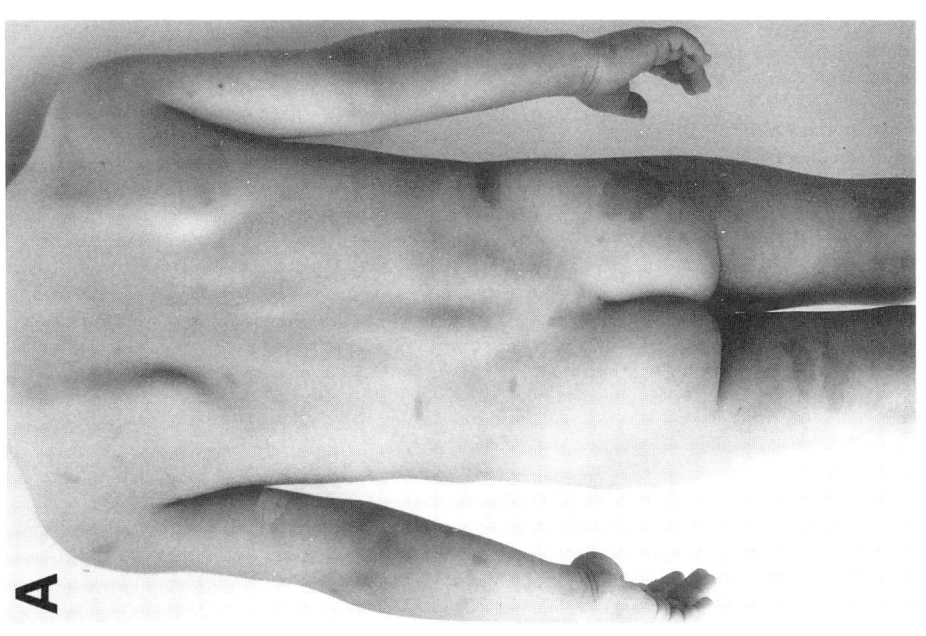

Fig. 5. (**A**) Multiple café-au-lait spots in a boy with Neurofibromatosis and gigantism. (**B**) The MRI of this boy revealing a large optic pathway glioma (arrow), presumably interfering with somatostatin inhibition of GH release.

Treatment includes medical, surgical, or radioablative options. Octreotide, a potent long-acting somatostatin analog, is often effective and may be combined with bromo-criptine if hyperprolactinemia is also present. Bromocriptine alone may even be effective in select cases *(141)*. Patients who have failed intermittent octreotide dosing schedules may be more effectively treated by continuous pump infusion of somatostatin *(147,148)*, or the new long-acting depot form of somatostatin. Another option, transfrontal or transphenoidal surgical removal of pituitary adenomas may be curative in up to 50% of children *(133)*. However, certain patients, for example those with MAS and significant cranial-bone involvement may not be good surgical candidates. Finally, radiotherapy may be effective as a primary or adjuvant therapy, but carries a high risk of permanent hypopituitarism *(149,150)*. Combination therapy may be needed for complete cure. Long-term sequelae of GH hypersecretion in children, besides tall stature, includes severe kyphosis, osteoarthritis, bitemporal hemianopia, depression, hypogonadism, and an increased risk of death due to cardiovascular, cerebrovascular, respiratory, and malig-nant disease *(151)*.

Estrogen Deficiency. Tall stature has also been associated with the extremely rare condition of functional estrogen deficiency due to either an estrogen-receptor mutation or aromatase deficiency. Untreated, these patients exhibit continued linear growth well into adulthood. The 1994 report of a man with osteoporosis, tall stature, and open epiphyses at age 28 yr and a mutation in the estrogen receptor gene resulting in a premature stop codon, definitively proved that estrogen is crucial for a normal epiphyseal fusion *(35)*. Severe aromatase deficiency also results in delayed skeletal maturation, tall stature with eunuchoid body proportions, and osteopenia with epiphyseal fusion only occurring after the administration of exogenous estrogens *(36,152)*. These patients also fail to exhibit a normal pubertal growth spurt.

ISOLATED PRENATAL GROWTH EXCESS

Full-term infants whose birth weights are above 2 SD or exceed 4000 grams are con-sidered large for gestational age (LGA). Pre-gestational or gestational diabetes is the most common cause of prenatal growth excess. Chronically high glucose levels with ensuing fetal hyperinsulinemia result in macrosomia. Other risk factors for fetal macrosomia with normal maternal glucose tolerance include maternal obesity, increased maternal age, and higher parity. However, even with normal glucose tolerance in the mother, one-third of these LGA infants have elevated cord-blood insulin levels *(153)* and some macrosomic infants of nondiabetic mothers even exhibit beta-cell hyperplasia *(154)*. Out-come studies of infants of diabetic mothers reveal that even though the overgrowth pres-ent at birth resolves by 1 yr, these children are at significant risk for obesity and impaired glucose tolerance, even as early as the teenage years *(155)*.

OVERGROWTH SYNDROMES

Beckwith-Wiedemann Syndrome. Beckwith-Wiedemann syndrome (BWS) is char-acterized by somatic overgrowth, with mean birth weights and lengths greater than the 90th percentiles, macroglossia, omphalocele, ear creases or pits, midface hypoplasia, and visceromegaly *(156)* (Fig. 6). Two imprinted loci on chromosome 11 have been strongly implicated in causing this disease. Overexpression of IGF-2, a paternally expressed growth factor, results in the Beckwith-Wiedemann phenotype. This may result from either loss of imprinting of the maternal IGF-2 gene, or paternal uniparental disomy. Mutations

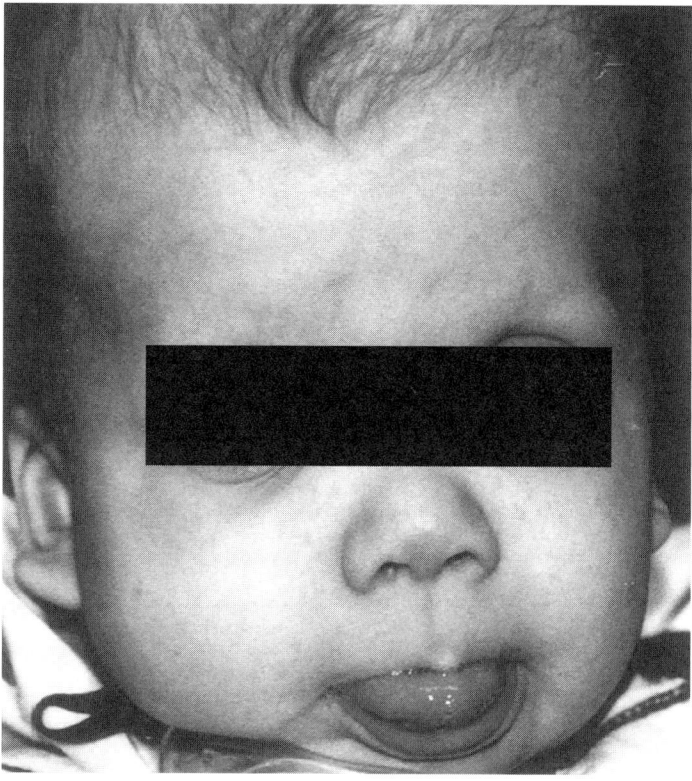

Fig. 6. An 11-mo-old boy with typical stigmata of Beckwith-Wiedemann syndrome, macrosomia, macroglossia, large eyes, and ear creases.

in p57 (KIP2), a maternally expressed cyclin-dependent kinase inhibitor, have also been found in BWS patients *(157)*. Interestingly, high IGF-2 levels downregulate p57 (KIP2) expression *(158)* implicating this cascade as critical to normal growth in numerous tissues.

Weaver Syndrome. Patients with Weaver syndrome are typically greater than the 95% for weight and length at birth and display advanced skeletal maturation, camptodactyly (permanent flexion of one or more of the interphalangeal joints), hypertonia, a hoarse cry, characteristic facies, and prolonged neonatal indirect hyperbilirubinemia *(159)*. An autosomal mode of inheritance has been suggested *(160)*, but as yet, the cause is unknown.

Simpson-Golabi-Behmel. A similar syndrome, Simpson-Golabi Behmel syndrome (SGBS) is an X-linked recessive condition resulting in overgrowth, coarse facial features, and finger anomalies. This syndrome shares common features with BWS as well, notably earlobe creases, visceromegaly, macroglossia, and neonatal hypoglycemia *(161)*. The link between the two syndromes seems to be mediated by IGF-2. SGBS results from mutations in glypican-3, a heparan-sulfated proteoglycan that complexes with IGF-2 *(162)*. Glypican-3 is thought to act locally under normal circumstances by inhibiting IGF-2 actions in the specific tissues known to exhibit overgrowth in this syndrome *(163)*.

Sotos Syndrome. Patients with Sotos syndrome, also known as cerebral gigantism, display prenatal and postnatal overgrowth with advanced skeletal maturation. Other characteristic features include megalencephaly, dolichocephaly, strabismus, hypertelorism, developmental delay *(164)*, and an increased risk of malignancy *(165)*. Significantly increased growth acceleration is seen in the first few years of life, but final heights are within the normal range, +1.5 SD for men and +1.8 SD for women, but still well above genetically predicted target heights *(166)*. The etiology of Sotos syndrome is still unknown. Multiple reports of familial cases suggest an autosomal dominant inheritance with variable penetrance *(167)*. However, numerous different chromosomal translocations in patients with Sotos syndrome have also been reported *(168–170)*, suggesting a multigenic phenomenon. Two children with Sotos syndrome have described who possess partial duplications of the short arm of chromosome 20. Included in this segment is the somatostatin receptor 4 gene, a logical candidate as the cause of growth excess in Sotos syndrome, as GH and IGF-1 secretion seems to be normal in these patients *(164,171)*.

Marfan Syndrome. The most common presentation of Marfan syndrome, a disorder of musculoskeletal, cardiovascular, and ocular abnormalities, is tall stature, usually noted by 2 yr of age *(172)*. Marfan syndrome is due to a mutation in the fibrillin 1 gene. Fibrillin 1 is a major component of microfibrils that play an important role in elastic tissue formation as well as extracellular matrix (ECM) organization. Mutations result in abnormal microfibrillar organization from a dominant-negative effect *(173)*. The disease is inherited in an autosomal dominant fashion, with 20–30% of cases resulting from new mutations. Interestingly, nearly every kindred has a unique mutation in this extremely large gene. The heights of most children with Marfan syndrome parallel the 97th percentile while their weights follow the 50th percentile *(172)*. Other musculoskeletal manifestations of the disease include arachnodactyly, an arm span at least 5 cm greater than height, scoliosis, chest-wall deformities, and a high, arched palate. Ectopia lentis, with an upward dislocation and aortic-root dilation are also commonly present *(174)*. Treatment involves careful monitoring of cardiac status, routine slit lamp exams, and consideration of sex steroid therapy to limit excessive linear growth.

Homocystinuria. Homocystinuria is an autosomal recessive condition usually due to cystathionine- B-synthase deficiency, resulting in the accumulation of methionine and homocystine in plasma and leading to excessive urinary excretion of homocystine. The clinical features are quite similar to Marfan syndrome, in that these patients also exhibit tall stature, scoliosis, a high arched palate, occasional arachnodactyly, and ectopia lentis, but in the downward direction. The phenotypic features result from interference with normal collagen cross-linking by excessive levels of homocystine *(175)*. Additional complications include mental retardation and life-threatening thromboembolic events *(176)*.

Many of the overgrowth syndromes share common features. Phenotype/genotype characteristics of the aforementioned syndromes are summarized in Table 1.

SEX CHROMOSOME ABNORMALITIES

A variety of sex-chromosome aneuploidies frequently result in tall stature. Men with Klinefelter syndrome, an XXY karyotype, exhibit an accelerated rate of growth as compared to age-matched controls throughout early childhood. The etiology of this supranormal growth velocity is unknown, as these boys have normal GH and IGF-1 levels *(177)*. Mean final heights are at the 75% and are, on average, 7 cm greater than their midparental heights *(177,178)*. These patients also classically suffer from primary hypogonadism, gynecomastia, learning and behavior problems, and eunuchoid body proportions. Interestingly, the disproportionate lower leg length is present prepubertally *(177)*, suggesting an etiology other than sex-steroid inadequacy.

Table 1
Overgrowth Syndrome

Syndrome	Phenotype	Genetic abnormality	Biochemical abnormality	Chromosomal location	Mode of inheritance
Beckwith Wiedemann	LGA, macroglossia, hypertelorism, hypoglycemia, omphalocele, organomegaly with malignant potential	1a. Loss of imprinting of normally silenced maternal IGF-2 gene 1b. Paternal Uniparental Disomy of IGF-2 gene 2. Loss of function mutation of maternal p57(KIP2) gene	IGF-2 overexpression	11p15 cluster of imprinted genes	Sporadic
Simpson Golabi Behmel Syndrome	LGA, macroglossia, coarse facial features, enlarged kidneys, hypoplastic nails, congenital midline anomalies	Mutation of GPC-3 gene	Abnormal function of glypican which normally limits IGF-2 actions	Xq26	X-linked recessive
Weaver Syndrome	LGA, hypertelorism, broad forehead, large ears, hoarse cry, camptodactyly	Unknown	Unknown	Unknown	Autosomal dominant; sporadic
Marfan Syndrome	Tall stature, long thin limbs (dolichostenomelia), long thin fingers (arachnodactyly), joint laxity, scoliosis, aortic dilation, upward subluxation of lens	Mutation of FBN-1 gene	Defective fibrillin protein resulting in abnormal microfibrils	15q21.1	Autosomal dominant; 15% new mutations
Homocystinuria	Tall stature, dolichostenomelia, arachnodactyly, scoliosis, mental retardation, thrombolembolic events, downward subluxation of lens	Most common: Cystathione-B-synthase deficiency	Acculmulation of homocysteine and methionine	21q22.3	Autosomal recessive
Sotos Syndrome	LGA, dolichocephaly, hypertelorism, prominent forehead, high arched palate, mental retardation, high risk of malignancy	Unknown	Unknown	Unknown	Autosomal dominant; sporadic

Males with XYY karyotypes also suffer from delayed development and behavior problems as well as excessive growth rates prepubertally. However, distinct from Klinefelter males, they have a mildly delayed puberty and a longer pubertal growth spurt as compared to normal boys, resulting in final heights that are between the 75th and 90th percentile *(179)* and, on average, 13 cm greater than paternal heights *(177)*. Additional phenotypic findings include nodular cystic acne and large teeth *(180)*.

47 XXX females have final heights that are often greater than the mean. However, conflicting reports exist, with some investigators reporting final heights of these girls to be near the 90th percentile *(178)*, while others report final heights that are no different than control girls *(177)*. Puberty is mildly delayed, resulting in a taller height at the take-off of the pubertal growth spurt. Interestingly, these girls also have disproportionately long legs pre- and postpubertally, similar to boys with Klinefelter syndrome *(178,181)*, suggesting a dosage effect of the additional X chromosome genes. Other similarities include behavior problems and reports of premature ovarian failure *(177,182)*.

REFERENCES

1. Karlberg J, Engstrom I, Karlberg P, Fryer JG. Analysis of linear growth using a mathematical model. Acta Paediatr Scand 1987;76:478–488.
2. Thalange NK, Foster PJ, Gill MS, Price DA, Clayton PE. Model of normal prepubertal growth. Arch Dis Child 1996;75:427–431.
3. Gelander L, Karlberg J, Albertsson-Wikland K. Seasonality in lower leg length velocity in prepubertal children. Acta Paediatr 1994;83:1249–1254.
4. Marshall WA, Swan AV. Seasonal variation in growth rates of normal and blind children. Hum Biol 1971;43:502–516.
5. Lampl M, Veldhuis JD, Johnson ML. Saltation and stasis: a model of human growth [see comments]. Science 1992;258:801–803.
6. Tillmann V, Thalange NK, Foster PJ, Gill MS, Price DA, Clayton PE. The relationship between stature, growth, and short-term changes in height and weight in normal prepubertal children. Pediatr Res 1998;44:882–886.
7. Gill MS, Thalange NK, Foster PJ, et al. Regular fluctuations in growth hormone (GH) release determine normal human growth. Growth Horm IGF Res 1999;9:114–122.
8. Albertsson-Wikland K, Rosberg S, Karlberg J, Groth T. Analysis of 24-hour growth hormone profiles in healthy boys and girls of normal stature: relation to puberty. J Clin Endocrinol Metab 1994;78:1195–1201.
9. Marti-Henneberg C, Vizmanos B. The duration of puberty in girls is related to the timing of onset. J Pediatr 1997;131:618–621.
10. Tanner JM, Davies PS. Clinical longitudinal standards for height and height velocity for North American children [see comments]. J Pediatr 1985;107:317–329.
11. Abbassi V. Growth and normal puberty. Pediatrics 1998:507–511.
12. Tanner JM, Whitehouse RH, Marubini E, Resele LF. The adolescent growth spurt of boys and girls of the Harpenden growth study. Ann Hum Biol 1976;3:109–126.
13. Nathan I, Hackett AF, Kirby S. A longitudinal study of the growth of matched pairs of vegetarian and omnivorous children, aged 7–11 years, in the north-west of England. Eur J Clin Nutr 1997;51:20–25.
14. Sabate J, Lindsted KD, Harris RD, Sanchez A. Attained height of lacto-ovo vegetarian children and adolescents. Eur J Clin Nutr 1991;45:51–58.
15. Herbert JR. Relationship of vegetarianism to child growth in South India. Am J Clin Nutr 1985;42:1246–1254.
16. Niinikoski H, Lapinleimu H, Viikari J, et al. Growth until 3 years of age in a prospective, randomized trial of a diet with reduced saturated fat and cholesterol. Pediatrics 1997;99:687–694.
17. Friedman G, Goldberg SJ. An evaluation of the safety of a low-saturated-fat, low-cholesterol diet beginning in infancy. Pediatrics 1976;58:655–657.
18. Boulton TJ, Magarey AM. Effects of differences in dietary fat on growth, energy and nutrient intake from infancy to eight years of age. Acta Paediatr 1995;84:146–150.

19. Lifshitz F, Moses N. Growth failure. A complication of dietary treatment of hypercholesterolemia. Am J Dis Childhood 1989;80:175–182.

20. Isaksson OG, Jansson JO, Gause IA. Growth hormone stimulates longitudinal bone growth directly. Science 1982;216:1237–1239.

21. Ohlsson C, Bengtsson B, Isaksson OGP, Andreassen TT, Slootweg MC. Growth hormone and bone. Endocr Rev 1998;19:55–79.

22. Yakar S, Liu JL, Stannard B, et al. Normal growth and development in the absence of hepatic insulin-like growth factor I. Proc Natl Acad Sci USA 1999;96:7324–7329.

23. Williams T, Maxon H, Thorner MO, Frohman LA. Blunted growth hormone (GH) response to GH-releasing hormone in hypothyroidism resolves in the euthyroid state. J Clin Endocrinol Metab 1985;61: 454–456.

24. Wolf M, Ingbar SH, Moses AC. Thyroid hormone and growth hormone interact to regulate insulin-like growth factor-I messenger ribonucleic acid and circulating levels in the rat. Endocrinology 1989; 125:2905–2914.

25. Chernausek SD, Underwood LE, Utiger RD, Van Wyk JJ. Growth hormone secretion and plasma somatomedin-C in primary hypothyroidism. Clin Endocrinol (Oxf) 1983;19:337–344.

26. Brent GA. The molecular basis of thyroid hormone action. N Engl J Med 1994;331:847–853.

27. Britto JM, Fenton AJ, Holloway WR, Nicholson GC. Osteoblasts mediate thyroid hormone stimulation of osteoclastic bone resorption. Endocrinology 1994;134:169–176.

28. Heyerdahl S, Ilicki A, Karlberg J, Kase BF, Larsson A. Linear growth in early treated children with congenital hypothyroidism. Acta Paediatr 1997;86:479–483.

29. Casado de Frias E, Ruibal JL, Reverte F, Bueno G. Evolution of height and bone age in primary congenital hypothyroidism. Clin Pediatr (Phila) 1993;32:426–432.

30. Martha PM Jr, Gorman KM, Blizzard RM, Rogol AD, Veldhuis JD. Endogenous growth hormone secretion and clearance rates in normal boys, as determined by deconvolution analysis: relationship to age, pubertal status, and body mass. J Clin Endocrinol Metab 1992;74:336–344.

31. Tanner JM, Whitehouse RH, Hughes PC, Carter BS. Relative importance of growth hormone and sex steroids for the growth at puberty of trunk length, limb length, and muscle width in growth hormone-deficient children. J Pediatr 1976;89:1000–1008.

32. Keenan BS, Richards GE, Ponder SW, Dallas JS, Nagamani M, Smith ER. Androgen-stimulated pubertal growth: the effects of testosterone and dihydrotestosterone on growth hormone and insulin-like growth factor-I in the treatment of short stature and delayed puberty. J Clin Endocrinol Metab 1993;76: 996–1001.

33. Metzger DL, Kerrigan JR. Estrogen receptor blockade with tamoxifen diminishes growth hormone secretion in boys: evidence for a stimulatory role of endogenous estrogens during male adolescence. J Clin Endocrinol Metab 1994;79:513–518.

34. Metzger DL, Kerrigan JR. Androgen receptor blockade with flutamide enhances growth hormone secretion in late pubertal males: evidence for independent actions of estrogen and androgen. J Clin Endocrinol Metab 1993;76:1147–1152.

35. Smith EP, Boyd J, Frank GR, et al. Estrogen resistance caused by a mutation in the estrogen-receptor gene in a man [see comments] [published erratum appears in N Engl J Med 1995 Jan 12;332 (2):131]. N Engl J Med 1994;331:1056–1061.

36. Morishima A, Grumbach MM, Simpson ER, Fisher C, Qin K. Aromatase deficiency in male and female siblings caused by a novel mutation and the physiological role of estrogens. J Clin Endocrinol Metab 1995;80:3689–3698.

37. Grumbach MM, Auchus RJ. Estrogen: consequences and implications of human mutations in synthesis and action. J Clin Endocrinol Metab 1999;84:4677–4694.

38. Murashita M, Tajima T, Nakae J, Shinohara N, Geffner ME, Fujieda K. Near-normal linear growth in the setting of markedly reduced growth hormone and IGF-1. A case report. Horm Res 1999;51:184–188.

39. Geffner ME, Bersch N, Kaplan SA, et al. Growth without growth hormone: evidence for a potent circulating growth factor. Lancet 1986;1:343–347.

40. Sandberg DE, Brook AE, Campos SP. Short stature: a psychosocial burden requiring growth hormone therapy? Pediatrics 1994;94:832–840.

41. Bercu BB. The growing conundrum. Growth hormone treatment of the non-growth hormone deficient child [editorial; comment] [see comments] [published erratum appears in JAMA 1996 Dec 18;276 (23): 1878]. JAMA 1996;276:567–568.

42. Downie AB, Mulligan J, Stratford RJ, Betts PR, Voss LD. Are short normal children at a disadvantage? The Wessex growth study. BMJ 1997;314:97–100.

43. Sandberg DE, MacGillivray MH, Clopper RR, Fung C, LeRoux L, Alliger DE. Quality of life among formerly treated childhood-onset growth hormone-deficient adults: a comparison with unaffected siblings. J Clin Endocrinol Metab 1998;83:1134–1142.

44. Samaras TT, Elrick H, Storms LH. Height, health and growth hormone. Acta Paediatrica 1999;88: 602–609.

45. Pozo J, Argente J, Barrios V, Gonzalez-Parra S, Munoz MT, Hernandez H. Growth hormone secretion in children with normal variants of short stature. Horm Res 1994;41:185–192.

46. Boguszewski CL, Carlsson B, Carlsson LM. Mechanisms of growth failure in non-growth-hormone deficient children of short stature. Horm Res 1997;48:19–22.

46a. Ranke MB, Graver ML, Kistner K, Blum WF, Wollman HA. Spontaneous adult height in idiopathic short stature. Hormone Res 1995;44:152–157.

47. Albertsson-Wikland K, Boguszewski M, Karlberg J. Children born small-for-gestational age: postnatal growth and hormonal status. Horm Res 1998;49:7–13.

48. Hintz RL, Attie KM, Baptista J, Roche A. Effect of growth hormone treatment on adult height of children with idiopathic short stature. Genentech Collaborative Group. N Engl J Med 1999;340:502–507.

49. LaFranchi S, Hanna CE, Mandel SH. Constitutional delay of growth: expected versus final height. Pediatrics 1991;87:82–87.

50. Acampora D, Mazan S, Tuorto F, et al. Transient dwarfism and hypogonadism in mice lacking Otx1 reveal prepubescent stage-specific control of pituitary levels of GH, FSH and LH. Development 1998; 125:1229–1239.

51. Clayton PE, Shalet SM, Price DA, Addison GM. Growth and growth hormone responses to oxandrolone in boys with constitutional delay of growth and puberty (CDGP). Clin Endocrinol (Oxf) 1988;29: 123–130.

52. Blizzard RM, Martha PM, Kerrigan JR, Mauras N, Rogol AD. Changes in growth hormone (GH) secretion and in growth during puberty. J Endocrinol Invest 1989;12:65–68.

53. Stanhope R, Buchanan CR, Fenn GC, Preece MA. Double blind placebo controlled trial of low dose oxandrolone in the treatment of boys with constitutional delay of growth and puberty. Arch Dis Child 1988;63:501–505.

54. Bramswig JH, Fasse M, Holthoff ML, von Lengerke HJ, von Petrykowski W, Schellong G. Adult height in boys and girls with untreated short stature and constitutional delay of growth and puberty: accuracy of five different methods of height prediction. J Pediatr 1990;117:886–891.

55. Ferrandez Longas A, Mayayo E, Valle A, Soria J, Labarta JI. Constitutional delay in growth and puberty: a comparison of final height achieved between treated and untreated children. J Pediatr Endocrinol Metab 1996;9:345–357.

56. Herber SM, Milner RDG. Growth hormone deficiency presenting under age 2 years. Arch Dis Childhood 1984;59:557–560.

57. Rose SR, Ross JL, Uriarte M, Barnes KM, Cassorla FG, Cutler GB Jr. The advantage of measuring stimulated as compared with spontaneous growth hormone levels in the diagnosis of growth hormone deficiency. N Engl J Med 1988;319:201–207.

58. Donaldson DL, Pan F, Hollowell JG, Stevenson JL, Gifford RA, Moore WV. Reliability of stimulated and spontaneous growth hormone (GH) levels for identifying the child with low GH secretion. J Clin Endocrinol Metab 1991;72:647–652.

59. Ghigo E, Bellone J, Aimaretti G, et al. Reliability of provocative tests to assess growth hormone secretory status. Study in 472 normally growing children. J Clin Endocrinol Metab 1996;81:3323–3327.

60. Rosenfeld RG, Albertsson-Wikland K, Cassorla F, et al. Diagnostic controversy: the diagnosis of childhood growth hormone deficiency revisited. J Clin Endocrinol Metab 1995;80:1532–1540.

61. Guyda HJ. Four decades of growth hormone therapy for short children: what have we achieved? J Clin Endocrinol Metab 1999;84:4307–4316.

62. Maheshwari HG, Silverman BL, Dupuis J, Baumann G. Phenotype and genetic analysis of a syndrome caused by an inactivating mutation in the growth hormone-releasing hormone receptor: dwarfism of Sindh. J Clin Endocrinol Metab 1998;83:4065–4074.

63. Phillips JAD, Hjelle BL, Seeburg PH, Zachmann M. Molecular basis for familial isolated growth hormone deficiency. Proc Natl Acad Sci USA 1981;78:6372–6375.

64. Cogan JD, Phillips JA III, Schenkman SS, Milner RD, Sakati N. Familial growth hormone deficiency: a model of dominant and recessive mutations affecting a monomeric protein. J Clin Endocrinol Metab 1994;79:1261–1265.

65. Takahashi Y, Shirono H, Arisaka O, et al. Biologically inactive growth hormone caused by an amino acid substitution. J Clin Invest 1997;100:1159–1165.
66. Laron Z, Pertzelan A, Mannheimer S. Genetic pituitary dwarfism with high serum concentation of growth hormone: a new inborn error of metabolism? Isr J Med Sci 1966;2:152–155.
67. Rosenbloom AL, Savage MO, Blum WF, Guevara-Aguirre J, Rosenfeld RG. Clinical and biochemical characteristics of growth hormone receptor deficiency (Laron syndrome). Acta Paediatr Suppl 1992; 383:121–124.
68. Goddard AD, Dowd P, Chernausek S, et al. Partial growth-hormone insensitivity: the role of growth-hormone receptor mutations in idiopathic short stature. J Pediatr 1997;131:S51–S55.
69. Sanchez JE, Perera E, Baumbach L, Cleveland WW. Growth hormone receptor mutations in children with idiopathic short stature. J Clin Endocrinol Metab 1998;83:4079–4083.
70. Kojima M, Hosoda H, Date Y, Nakazato M, Matsuo H, Kangawa K. Ghrelin is a growth-hormone-releasing acylated peptide from stomach. Nature 1999;402:656–660.
71. Woods KA, Camacho-Hubner C, Savage MO, Clark AJ. Intrauterine growth retardation and postnatal growth failure associated with deletion of the insulin-like growth factor I gene [see comments]. N Engl J Med 1996;335:1363–1367.
72. Momoi T, Yamanaka C, Kobayashi M, et al. Short stature with normal growth hormone and elevated IGF-I. Eur J Pediatr 1992;151:321–325.
73. Bierich JR, Moeller H, Ranke MB, Rosenfeld RG. Pseudopituitary dwarfism due to resistance to somatomedin: a new syndrome. Eur J Pediatr 1984;142:186–188.
74. Dattani MT, Martinez-Barbera JP, Thomas PQ, et al. Mutations in the homeobox gene HESX1/Hesx1 associated with septo-optic dysplasia in human and mouse. Nat Genet 1998;19:125–133.
74a. Thomas PQ, Dattani MT, Brickman JM, McNay D, Warne G, Zacharin M, et al. Heterozygous HESX1 mutations associated with isolated congenital pituitary hypoplasia and septo-optic dysplasia. Hum Mol Genet 2001;10:39–45.
75. Gage PJ, Camper SA. Pituitary homeobox 2, a novel member of the bicoid-related family of homeobox genes, is a potential regulator of anterior structure formation. Hum Mol Genet 1997;6:457–464.
76. Netchine I, Sobrier M, Krude H, et al. Mutations in LHX3 result in a new syndrome revelaed by combined pituitary hormone deficiency. Nature Genet 2000;25:182–186.
76a. Pernasetti F, Toledo SP, Vasilyeu VV, Hayashida CY, Cogan JD, Ferrari C, et al. Impaired adrenocorticotropin-adrenal axis in combined pituitary hormone deficiency caused by a two-base pair deletion (301–302 del AG) in the prophet of Pit-1 gene. J Clin Endocrinol Metab 2000;85:390–397.
77. Pfaffle R, Kim C, Otten B, et al. Pit-1: clinical aspects. Horm Res 1996;45:25–28.
78. Birnbacher R, Riedl S, Frisch H. Long-term treatment in children with hypopituitarism: pubertal development and final height. Horm Res 1998;49:80–85.
79. August GP, Julius JR, Blethen SL. Adult height in children with growth hormone deficiency who are treated with biosynthetic growth hormone: the National Cooperative Growth Study experience. Pediatrics 1998;102:512–516.
80. Pantsiouou S, Stanhope R, Uruena M, Preece MA, Grant DB. Growth prognosis and growth after menarche in primary hypothyroidism. Arch Dis Child 1991;66:838–840.
81. Rivkees SA, Bode HH, Crawford JD. Long-term growth in juvenile acquired hypothyroidism: the failure to achieve normal adult stature. N Engl J Med 1988;318:599–602.
82. Kerrebijn KF, Kroon JPD. Effect of height of corticosteroid therapy in asthmatic children. Arch Dis Child 1968;43:556–561.
83. Allen DB. Growth suppression by glucocorticoid therapy. Endocrinol Metab Clin North Am 1996;25: 699–717.
84. Chang KC, Miklich DR, Barwise G, Chai H, Miles-Lawrence R. Linear growth of chronic asthmatic children: the effects of the disease and various forms of steroid therapy. Clin Allergy 1982;12:369–378.
85. Avioli LV. Glucocorticoid effects on statural growth. Br J Rheumatol 1993;32(Suppl) 2:27–30.
86. Lai HC, FitzSimmons SC, Allen DB, et al. Risk of persistent growth impairment after alternate-day prednisone treatment in children with cystic fibrosis. N Engl J Med 2000;342:851–859.
87. Rivkees SA, Danon M, Herrin J. Prednisone dose limitation of growth hormone treatment of steroid-induced growth failure. J Pediatr 1994;125:322–325.
88. Simons FE. A comparison of beclomethasone, salmeterol, and placebo in children with asthma. Canadian Beclomethasone Dipropionate-Salmeterol Xinafoate Study Group. N Engl J Med 1997;337:1659–1665.
89. Verberne AA, Frost C, Roorda RJ, van der Laag H, Kerrebijn KF. One year treatment with salmeterol compared with beclomethasone in children with asthma. The Dutch Paediatric Asthma Study Group. Am J Respir Crit Care Med 1997;156:688–695.

90. Heuck C, Wolthers OD, Kollerup G, Hansen M, Teisner B. Adverse effects of inhaled budesonide (800 micrograms) on growth and collagen turnover in children with asthma: a double-blind comparison of once-daily versus twice-daily administration. J Pediatr 1998;133:608–612.

91. Welch MJ. Inhaled corticosteroids and growth in children [see comments]. Pediatr Ann 1998;27:752–758.

92. Wang X, Zuckerman B, Coffman GA, Corwin MJ. Familial aggregation of low birth weight among whites and blacks in the United States [see comments]. N Engl J Med 1995;333:1744–1749.

93. Leger J, Noel M, Limal JM, Czernichow P. Growth factors and intrauterine growth retardation. II. Serum growth hormone, insulin-like growth factor (IGF) I, and IGF-binding protein 3 levels in children with intrauterine growth retardation compared with normal control subjects: prospective study from birth to two years of age. Study Group of IUGR. Pediatr Res 1996;40:101–107.

94. Cance-Rouzaud A, Laborie S, Bieth E, et al. Growth hormone, insulin-like groeth factor-1 and insulin-like growth factor binding protein-3 are regulated differently in small-for-gestational-age and appropriate-for-gestational-age neonates. Biol Neonate 1998;73:347–355.

95. Barker DJ. The fetal origins of diseases of old age. Eur J Clin Nutr 1992;46(Suppl)3:S3–S9.

96. Houang M, Morineau G, le Bouc Y, Fiet J, Gourmelen M. The cortisol-cortisone shuttle in children born with intrauterine growth retardation. Pediatr Res 1999;46:189–193.

97. Karlberg J, Albertsson-Wikland K. Growth in full-term small-for-gestational-age infants: from birth to final height [published erratum appears in Pediatr Res 1996 Jan;39 (1):175]. Pediatr Res 1995;38:733–739.

98. Karlberg JPE, Albertsson-Wikland K, Kwan EYW, Lam BCC, Low LCK. The timing of early postnatal catch-up growth in normal, full-term infants born short for gestational age. Hormone Res 1997;48:17–24.

99. Sas T, de Waal W, Mulder P, et al. Growth hormone treatment in children with short stature born small for gestational age: 5-year results of a randomized, double-blind, dose-response trial. J Clin Endocrinol Metab 1999;84:3064–3069.

100. Shiang R, Thompson LM, Zhu YZ, et al. Mutations in the transmembrane domain of FGFR3 cause the most common genetic form of dwarfism, achondroplasia. Cell 1994;78:335–342.

101. Lemyre E, Azouz EM, Teebi AS, Glanc P, Chen MF. Bone dysplasia series. Achondroplasia, hypochondroplasia and thanatophoric dysplasia: review and update. Can Assoc Radiol J 1999;50:185–197.

102. Eiholzer U, Bachmann S, L'Allemand D. Growth hormone deficiency in Prader-Willi syndrome. Endocrinologist 2000;10:50S–56S.

103. Rao E, Weiss B, Fukami M, et al. Pseudoautosomal deletions encompassing a novel homeobox gene cause growth failure in idiopathic short stature and Turner syndrome. Nat Genet 1997;16:54–63.

104. Belin V, Cusin V, Viot G, et al. SHOX mutations in dyschondrosteosis (Leri-Weill syndrome). Nat Genet 1998;19:67–69.

105. Binder G, Schwarze CP, Ranke MB. Identification of short stature caused by SHOX defects and therapeutic effect of recombinant human growth hormone. J Clin Endocrinol Metab 2000;85:245–249.

106. Haverkamp F, Wolfle J, Zerres K, et al. Growth retardation in Turner syndrome: aneuploidy, rather than specific gene loss, may explain growth failure. J Clin Endocrinol Metab 1999;84:4578–4582.

107. Cacciari E, Mazzanti L. Final height of patients with Turner's syndrome treated with growth hormone (GH): indications for GH therapy alone at high doses and late estrogen therapy. Italian Study Group for Turner Syndrome. J Clin Endocrinol Metab 1999;84:4510–4515.

108. Carel JC, Mathivon L, Gendrel C, Ducret JP, Chaussain JL. Near normalization of final height with adapted doses of growth hormone in Turner's syndrome. J Clin Endocrinol Metab 1998;83:1462–1466.

109. de Muinck Keizer-Schrama S, Van den Broeck J, Sas T, Hokken-Koelega A. Final height of growth hormone-treated GH-deficient children and girls with Turner's syndrome: the Dutch experience. The Dutch Advisory Group on Growth Hormone. Horm Res 1999;51:127–131.

110. Van den Broeck J, Van Teunenbroek A, Hokken-Koelega A, Wit JM. Efficacy of long-term growth hormone treatment in Turner's syndrome. European Study Group. J Pediatr Endocrinol Metab 1999;12:673–676.

111. Chernausek SD, Attie KM, Cara JF, Rosenfeld RG, Frane J. Growth hormone therapy of Turner syndrome: the impact of age of estrogen replacement on final height. Genentech, Inc., Collaborative Study Group. J Clin Endocrinol Metab 2000;85:2439–2445.

112. Widdowson EM. Mental contentment and physical growth. Lancet 1951;16:1316.

113. Green WH, Campbell M, David R. Psychosocial dwarfism: a critical review of the evidence. J Am Acad Child Psychiatry 1984;23:39–48.

114. Powell GF, Brasel JA, Blizzard RM. Emotional deprivation and growth retardation simulating idiopathic hypopituitarism. I. Clinical evaluation of the syndrome. N Engl J Med 1967;276:1271–1278.

115. Hernandez RJ, Poznanski AK, Hopwood NJ, Kelch RP. Incidence of growth lines in psychosocial dwarfs and idiopathic hypopituitarism. Am J Roentgenol 1978;131:477–479.

116. Peck MN, Lundberg O. Short stature as an effect of economic and social conditions in childhood. Social Sci Med 1995;41:733–738.

117. Rochiccioli P, Messina A, Tauber MT, Enjaume C. Correlation of the parameters of 24-hour growth hormone secretion with growth velocity in 93 children of varying height. Horm Res 1989;31:115–118.

118. Dickerman Z, Loewinger J, Laron Z. The pattern of growth in children with constitutional tall stature from birth to age 9 years. A longitudinal study. Acta Paediatr Scand 1984;73:530–536.

119. Lecointre C, Toublanc JE. Psychological indications for treatment of tall stature in adolescent girls. J Pediatr Endocrinol Metab 1997;10:529–531.

120. Binder G, Grauer ML, Wehner AV, Wehner F, Ranke MB. Outcome in tall stature. Final height and psychological aspects in 220 patients with and without treatment. Eur J Pediatr 1997;156:905–910.

121. Weimann E, Bergmann S, Bohles HJ. Oestrogen treatment of constitutional tall stature: a risk-benefit ratio. Arch Dis Child 1998;78:148–151.

122. Drop SL, De Waal WJ, De Muinck Keizer-Schrama SM. Sex steroid treatment of constitutionally tall stature. Endocr Rev 1998;19:540–558.

123. Bartsch O, Weschke B, Weber B. Oestrogen treatment of constitutionally tall girls with 0.1 mg/day ethinyl oestradiol. Eur J Pediatr 1988;147:59–63.

124. Weimann E, Brack C. Severe thrombosis during treatment with ethinylestradiol for tall stature. Horm Res 1996;45:261–263.

125. de Waal WJ, Torn M, de Muinck Keizer-Schrama SM, Aarsen RS, Drop SL. Long term sequelae of sex steroid treatment in the management of constitutionally tall stature. Arch Dis Child 1995;73:311–315.

126. Bettendorf M, Heinrich UE, Schonberg DK, Grulich-Henn J. Short-term, high-dose testosterone treatment fails to reduce adult height in boys with constitutional tall stature. Eur J Pediatr 1997;156:911–915.

127. Hindmarsh PC, Pringle PJ, Di Silvio L, Brook CG. A preliminary report on the role of somatostatin analogue (SMS 201-995) in the management of children with tall stature. Clin Endocrinol (Oxf) 1990;32: 83–91.

128. Tauber MT, Harris AG, Rochiccioli P. Clinical use of the long acting somatostatin analogue octreotide in pediatrics. Eur J Pediatr 1994;153:304–310.

129. Holl RW, Bucher P, Sorgo W, Heinze E, Homoki J, Debatin KM. Suppression of growth hormone by oral glucose in the evaluation of tall stature. Horm Res 1999;51:20–24.

130. Rieu M, Kuhn JM, Bricaire H, Luton JP. Evaluation of treated acromegalic patients with normal growth hormone levels during oral glucose load. Acta Endocrinol (Copenh) 1984;107:1–8.

131. Pieters GF, Hermus AR, Smals AG, Kloppenborg PW. Paradoxical responsiveness of growth hormone to corticotropin-releasing factor in acromegaly. J Clin Endocrinol Metab 1984;58:560–562.

132. Felix IA, Horvath E, Kovacs K, Smyth HS, Killinger DW, Vale J. Mammosomatotroph adenoma of the pituitary associated with gigantism and hyperprolactinemia. A morphological study including immunoelectron microscopy. Acta Neuropathol 1986;71:76–82.

133. Abe T, Tara LA, Ludecke DK. Growth hormone-secreting pituitary adenomas in childhood and adolescence: features and results of transnasal surgery. Neurosurgery 1999;45:1–10.

134. Asa SL, Kovacs K, Horvath E, et al. Human fetal adenohypophysis. Electron microscopic and ultrastructural immunocytochemical analysis. Neuroendocrinology 1988;48:423–431.

135. Stratakis CA, Carney JA, Lin JP, et al. Carney complex, a familial multiple neoplasia and lentiginosis syndrome. Analysis of 11 kindreds and linkage to the short arm of chromosome 2. J Clin Invest 1996; 97:699–705.

136. Casey M, Mah C, Merliss AD, et al. Identification of a novel genetic locus for familial cardiac myxomas and Carney complex. Circulation 1998;98:2560–2566.

137. Gadelha MR, Prezant TR, Une KN, et al. Loss of heterozygosity on chromosome 11q13 in two families with acromegaly/gigantism is independent of mutations of the multiple endocrine neoplasia type I gene. J Clin Endocrinol Metab 1999;84:249–256.

138. Gadelha MR, Une KN, Rohde K, Vaisman M, Kineman RD, Frohman LA. Isolated familial somatotropinomas: establishment of linkage to chromosome 11q13.1-11q13.3 and evidence for a potential second locus at chromosome 2p16-12. J Clin Endocrinol Metab 2000;85:707–714.

139. Manski TJ, Haworth CS, Duval-Arnould BJ, Rushing EJ. Optic pathway glioma infiltrating into somatostatinergic pathways in a young boy with gigantism. Case report. J Neurosurg 1994;81:595–600.

140. Fuqua JS, Berkovitz GD. Growth hormone excess in a child with neurofibromatosis type 1 and optic pathway tumor: a patient report. Clin Pediatr (Phila) 1998;37:749–752.

141. Duchowny MS, Katz R, Bejar RL. Hypothalamic mass and gigantism in neurofibromatosis: treatment with bromocriptine. Ann Neurol 1984;15:302–304.

142. Daughaday WH. Pituitary gigantism. Endocrinol Metab Clin North Am 1992;21:633–647.

143. Cuttler L, Jackson JA, Saeed uz-Zafar M, Levitsky LL, Mellinger RC, Frohman LA. Hypersecretion of growth hormone and prolactin in McCune-Albright syndrome. J Clin Endocrinol Metab 1989;68: 1148–1154.

144. Lyons J, Landis CA, Harsh G, et al. Two G protein oncogenes in human endocrine tumors. Science 1990;249:655–659.

145. Boggild MD, Jenkinson S, Pistorello M, et al. Molecular genetic studies of sporadic pituitary tumors. J Clin Endocrinol Metab 1994;78:387–392.

146. Losa M, von Werder K. Pathophysiology and clinical aspects of the ectopic GH-releasing hormone syndrome. Clin Endocrinol (Oxf) 1997;47:123–135.

147. Nanto-Salonen K, Koskinen P, Sonninen P, Toppari J. Suppression of GH secretion in pituitary gigantism by continuous subcutaneous octreotide infusion in a pubertal boy. Acta Paediatr 1999;88:29–33.

148. Gelber SJ, Heffez DS, Donohoue PA. Pituitary gigantism caused by growth hormone excess from infancy. J Pediatr 1992;120:931–934.

149. Eastman RC, Gorden P, Roth J. Conventional supervoltage irradiation is an effective treatment for acromegaly. J Clin Endocrinol Metab 1979;48:931–940.

150. Ritzen EM, Wettrell G, Davies G, Grant DB. Management of pituitary gigantism. The role of bromocriptine and radiotherapy. Acta Paediatr Scand 1985;74:807–814.

151. Whitehead EM, Shalet SM, Davies D, Enoch BA, Price DA, Beardwell CG. Pituitary gigantism: a disabling condition. Clin Endocrinol (Oxf) 1982;17:271–277.

152. Carani C, Qin K, Simoni M, et al. Effect of testosterone and estradiol in a man with aromatase deficiency. N Engl J Med 1997;337:91–95.

153. Wollschlaeger K, Nieder J, Koppe I, Hartlein K. A study of fetal macrosomia. Arch Gynecol Obstet 1999;263:51–55.

154. Pinar H, Pinar T, Singer DB. Beta-cell hyperplasia in macrosomic infants and fetuses of nondiabetic mothers. Pediatr Dev Pathol 2000;3:48–52.

155. Silverman BL, Rizzo TA, Cho NH, Metzger BE. Long-term effects of the intrauterine environment. The Northwestern University Diabetes in Pregnancy Center. Diabetes Care 1998;21(Suppl)2:B142–B149.

156. Pettenati MJ, Haines JL, Higgins RR, Wappner RS, Palmer CG, Weaver DD. Wiedemann-Beckwith syndrome: presentation of clinical and cytogenetic data on 22 new cases and review of the literature. Hum Genet 1986;74:143–154.

157. Caspary T, Cleary MA, Perlman EJ, Zhang P, Elledge SJ, Tilghman SM. Oppositely imprinted genes p57 (Kip2) and igf2 interact in a mouse model for Beckwith-Wiedemann syndrome. Genes Dev 1999; 13:3115–3124.

158. Grandjean V, Smith J, Schofield PN, Ferguson-Smith AC. Increased IGF-II protein affects p57kip2 expression in vivo and in vitro: implications for beckwith-wiedemann syndrome. Proc Natl Acad Sci USA 2000;97:5279–5284.

159. Weaver DD, Graham CB, Thomas IT, Smith DW. A new overgrowth syndrome with accelerated skeletal maturation, unusual facies, and camptodactyly. J Pediatr 1974;84:547–552.

160. Dumic M, Vukovic J, Cvitkovic M, Medica I. Twins and their mildly affected mother with Weaver syndrome. Clin Genet 1993;44:338–340.

161. Sotos JF. Overgrowth. Section VI. Genetic syndromes and other disorders associated with overgrowth. Clin Pediatr (Phila) 1997;36:157–170.

162. Pilia G, Hughes-Benzie RM, MacKenzie A, et al. Mutations in GPC3, a glypican gene, cause the Simpson-Golabi-Behmel overgrowth syndrome. Nat Genet 1996;12:241–247.

163. Pellegrini M, Pilia G, Pantano S, et al. Gpc3 expression correlates with the phenotype of the Simpson-Golabi-Behmel syndrome. Dev Dyn 1998;213:431–439.

164. Sotos JF. Overgrowth. Section V. Syndromes and other disorders associated with overgrowth. Clin Pediatr (Phila) 1997;36:89–103.

165. Hersh JH, Cole TR, Bloom AS, Bertolone SJ, Hughes HE. Risk of malignancy in Sotos syndrome. J Pediatr 1992;120:572–574.

166. Agwu JC, Shaw NJ, Kirk J, Chapman S, Ravine D, Cole TR. Growth in Sotos syndrome. Arch Dis Child 1999;80:339–342.

167. Winship IM. Sotos syndrome: autosomal dominant inheritance substantiated. Clin Genet 1985;28: 243–246.

168. Maroun C, Schmerler S, Hutcheon RG. Child with Sotos phenotype and a 5:15 translocation. Am J Med Genet 1994;50:291–293.

169. Schrander-Stumpel CT, Fryns JP, Hamers GG. Sotos syndrome and de novo balanced autosomal translocation (t (3;6) (p21;p21)). Clin Genet 1990;37:226–269.

170. Haeusler G, Guchev Z, Kohler I, Schober E, Haas O, Frisch H. Constitutional chromosome anomalies in patients with cerebral gigantism (Sotos syndrome). Klin Padiatr 1993;205:351–353.

171. Faivre L, Viot G, Prieur M, et al. Apparent sotos syndrome (cerebral gigantism) in a child with trisomy 20p11.2-p12.1 mosaicism. Am J Med Genet 2000;91:273–276.

172. Lipscomb KJ, Clayton-Smith J, Harris R. Evolving phenotype of Marfan's syndrome. Arch Dis Child 1997;76:41–46.

173. Ramirez F, Gayraud B, Pereira L. Marfan syndrome: new clues to genotype-phenotype correlations. Ann Med 1999;31:202–207.

174. Pyeritz RE. The Marfan syndrome. Annu Rev Med 2000;51:481–510.

175. Grieco AJ. Homocystinuria: pathogenetic mechanisms. Am J Med Sci 1977;273:120–132.

176. Cacciari E, Salardi S. Clinical and laboratory features of homocystinuria. Haemostasis 1989;19:10–13.

177. Ratcliffe SG, Butler GE, Jones M. Edinburgh study of growth and development of children with sex chromosome abnormalities. IV. Birth Defects Orig Artic Ser 1990;26:1–44.

178. Stewart DA, Bailey JD, Netley CT, Park E. Growth, development, and behavioral outcome from mid-adolescence to adulthood in subjects with chromosome aneuploidy: the Toronto Study. Birth Defects Orig Artic Ser 1990;26:131–188.

179. Robinson A, Bender BG, Linden MG. Summary of clinical findings in children and young adults with sex chromosome anomalies. Birth Defects Orig Artic Ser 1990;26:225–228.

180. Sotos JF. Genetic disorders associated with overgrowth. Clin Pediatr (Phila) 1997;36:39–49.

181. Ratcliffe SG, Pan H, McKie M. The growth of XXX females: population-based studies. Ann Hum Biol 1994;21:57–66.

182. Itu M, Neelam T, Ammini AC, Kucheria K. Primary amenorrhoea in a triple X female. Aust NZJ Obstet Gynaecol 1990;30:386–388.

4

Adult Growth Hormone Deficiency

Zehra Haider, MD and James W. Edmondson, MD

INTRODUCTION

Adult-onset growth hormone deficiency (GHD) is a rare disease with an exact incidence that is not currently known, but indirect estimates based on the incidence of pituitary tumors suggest an incidence of 10 people per million annually *(1)*. Over the last decade the adverse metabolic and psychological sequelae of adult GHD have been increasingly recognized, and the benefits of GH replacement demonstrated in randomized trials. These trials are limited to patients with severe GHD; thus the effects of GH replacement are most clearly established in patients with more severe GHD.

CAUSES OF GH DEFICIENCY

GHD in adults most commonly results from pituitary or peripituitary tumors and their treatment *(2)*. Pituitary adenoma is the most common cause of adult hypopituitarism *(3)* It can also be owing to craniopharyngioma or other tumors in the hypothalamic-pituitary area, as well as to cranial irradiation for leukemia, retinoblastoma, medulloblastoma, other head and neck tumors, such as optic glioma. Cranial trauma and congenital malformations including suprasellar arachnoid cyst, hydrocephalus, cleft lip, and palate, and other midline defects can also lead to GHD. In 22% of cases, GHD in adulthood is idiopathic. Sporadic and familial cases exist, in isolation or sometimes in association with idiopathic diabetes insipidus. The causes of adult-onset GHD are listed in Table 1.

Clinical Description

Figure 1 outlines the effects of GHD. GHD in adults results in alterations in body composition, including reduced lean body mass and bone mineral density, increased fat mass, thin and dry skin, reduced sweating, and reduced muscle strength and exercise performance.

From: *Contemporary Endocrinology: Developmental Endocrinology: From Research to Clinical Practice*
Edited by: E. A. Eugster and O. H. Pescovitz © Humana Press Inc., Totowa, NJ

Table 1
Causes of Growth Hormone
Deficiency in Adults

Tumors
    Pituitary tumors
    Meningioma
    Craniopharyngioma
    Germinoma
    Rathke's cleft cyst
Infiltrative diseases
    Histiocytosis
    Sarcoidosis
Trauma
    Head trauma
Vascular injury
    Apoplexy
    Sheehan's syndrome
Cranial irradiation
    Pituitary irradiation
    Brain irradiation
    Head and neck tumors
Idiopathic
Autoimmune

In severe adult-onset GHD, vitality, energy, and physical mobility are markedly decreased. There is an impaired sense of well-being, emotional liability, feelings of social isolation, and disturbances in sexual function, despite adequate correction of other hormone deficiencies. These symptoms tend to be more severe in adult-onset disease as compared to childhood onset deficiency. The probability of GHD increases with other coexisting hormone deficiencies, in patients with organic pituitary disease. The presence of three or four other pituitary hormonal deficits is almost always associated with GHD. The probability of GHD is reduced to about 45% if no other pituitary hormonal abnormality is demonstrable in a patient with a known pituitary lesion. Partial GHD may also exist in adulthood but treatment benefits in such conditions have not been definitely established. The clinical features of GHD are listed in Table 2. Biochemical effects of growth hormone are listed in Table 3.

Diagnostic Testing

Since the typical concentrations of GH in blood are at the lower limit of detection for current GH assays, the diagnosis of GHD in adults relies on the results of GH provocative testing. There is reasonable agreement that only a single GH provocative study is required to diagnose severe GHD in patients with panhypopituitarism, as severe GHD is almost inevitable. In contrast, if GH status is to be defined accurately, the teenager with a putative diagnosis of isolated GHD requires at least two studies to assess GH secretory status at the attainment of final height *(4)*. However, the optimum strategy of investigation is less clear in those patients with partial hypopituitarism in whom there are only one or two additional pituitary-hormone deficits. Diagnostic investigation for GHD should be con-

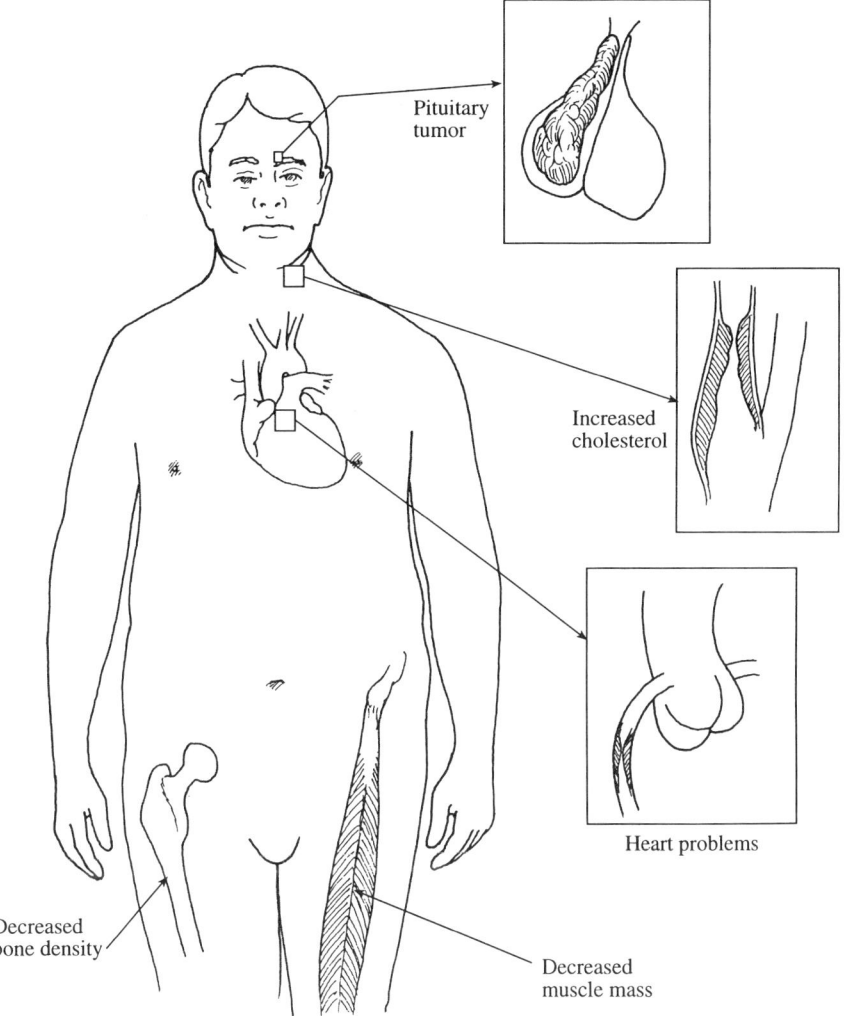

Fig. 1. Clinical features of adult growth hormone deficiency: pre-growth-hormone replacement.

sidered in patients with hypothalamic-pituitary (H-P) disease caused by an adenoma or by radiation or surgery for pituitary disease; and in childhood onset GHD occurring prior to adulthood. A subnormal response to provocative stimuli serves as the basis of establishing a diagnosis of GHD. Insulin-like growth factor-1 (IGF-1) levels and insulin-like-growth factor binding protein-3 (IGFBP-3) are both dependent on GH secretion but are not always reliable markers for GHD in adulthood *(5)*. In the absence of malnutrition, hepatic disease, poorly controlled diabetes mellitus, and hypothyroidism, a low IGF-1 level may be suggestive of GHD, particularly if two or more pituitary hormone deficiencies are present.

INSULIN TOLERANCE TEST

Insulin tolerance testing (ITT) is considered the diagnostic test of choice in adults. This diagnostic modality best distinguishes between GHD and the reduced GH secretion

Table 2
Clinical Features of Growth Hormone Deficiency

Symptoms	Signs
Abnormal body composition	Thin dry skin
Reduced lean body mass	Cool peripheries
Abdominal obesity	Reduced muscle strength
Low energy	Obesity
Poor temperature control	Reduced exercise performance
Reduced strength and exercise capacity	Poor venous access
Impaired psychological well-being	Depression
Depressed mood	Emotional lability
Emotional lability	
Anxiety	
Feelings of social isolation	

Table 3
Biochemical Effects
in Growth Hormone Deficiency

Lipids
   Increased total cholesterol
   Elevated LDL cholesterol
   Increased apolipoprotein B
   Decreased HDL cholesterol
   Increase triglycerides
Reduced bone mineral density

that can be associated with normal aging and obesity. Achieving adequate hypoglycemia is important to the test validity. Since some patients develop profound hypoglycemia in response to insulin, this test is contraindicated in patients with coronary artery disease, generalized debility, and seizure disorders. The ITT should be performed in specialized endocrine units with experience in ITT and in treating hypoglycemia. Initially, 0.05U/Kg of body weight of human synthetic regular insulin is injected intravenously, and serum samples are collected from an indwelling catheter every 15–30 min for a total of 90 min. Blood-glucose levels are monitored serially with bedside glucose monitoring. Keeping a supply of 50% dextrose at the study site is an absolute requirement. It is important to confirm that blood sugar has fallen to a value less than 50 mg/dl by sending blood samples to the laboratory for blood-glucose analysis. Following the establishment of hypoglycemia, glucose can be administered without compromising the validity of the study. Failure to achieve adequate hypoglycemia (serum glucose levels below 50 mg/dl) warrants repeat testing with 0.1 U/Kg intravenous regular insulin; in obese individuals insulin doses of 0.15–0.2 U/Kg may be required. Severe GHD is defined as a peak GH response to hypoglycemia of <3 micrograms/L (normal response being >5 micrograms/L). This criterion has been established by the Growth Hormone Research Society and is widely accepted in Europe (6). Food and Drug Administration (FDA) guidelines accept levels below 5 micrograms/L (by radioimmunoassay) or <2.5 micrograms/L (by immuno-radiometric assay).

Other provocative testing modalities include GH responses to levodopa, arginine, growth hormone-releasing hormone (GHRH), glucagon, and clonidine. At present combined administration of arginine and GHRH is the most promising alternative to ITT. The clonidine test is less useful in adults than in children. Studies that do not depend on the establishment of hypoglycemia have the attractiveness of being far safer for patients and are expected to replace the ITT, provided acceptable diagnostic sensitivity and specificity criteria can be established.

GROWTH HORMONE THERAPY

Since 1996 GH has been used in the United States not only in GHD adults but also in adults with catabolic illnesses, such as burn injuries and AIDS. There are also multiple unestablished assertions that GH treatment prevents and reverses aging. The starting dose of GH replacement therapy in adults is 3–4 micrograms/kg once a day, by subcutaneous injection. The United States FDA recommends a maximal daily dose of 25 micrograms/kg for adults up to 35 yr of age, and 12.5 micrograms/kg for older individuals. The Growth Hormone Research Society favors a starting dose of 150–300 micrograms/d regardless of weight. GHD patients should be evaluated at monthly or bimonthly intervals, and the GH dose adjusted to maintain a target IGF-1 level in the upper half of the age- and gender-adjusted reference range. IGF-1 levels are useful in following the adequacy of treatment even though this test is not very reliable for screening or the initial diagnosis of GHD. Figure 2 depicts the effects of GH on various parts of the body.

Effects of GH on Body Composition

Prolonged GHD is associated with an abnormal fat-distribution pattern (7). There is an increase in total body fat in GHD states (8). Body fat was found to be 6–8 kg higher in GHD adults than in controls. In males the fat-deposition pattern is characterized by excessive subcutaneous fat accumulation in the breast and abdominal areas. This pattern is less well-defined in females. Using a wide range of measurement techniques, these results have been confirmed by other investigators (9–12). The fat-mass distribution has been assessed in a number of studies by waist/hip ratios, skin-fold thickness (13), computed tomography (CT) scan (14), and MRI (15) with consistent results. The abdominal distribution has been associated with an increased risk of mortality and morbidity from cardiovascular disease.

Lean body mass (LBM) is significantly lower in GHD adults. Thigh-muscle area was significantly smaller in GHD patients than in controls, when expressed per kilogram body weight. Initial studies demonstrated a mean reduction in LBM of 7–8%, corresponding to approx 4 kg lean tissue (8). These results were confirmed by the subsequent studies (16–18).

Fluid Volume

Radioisotope dilution technique and bioimpedance measurements indicate that total body water is reduced in adult-onset GHD (12,13). There is a reduction in the extracellular water (19,20). Reduced plasma volume and total blood volume contributes to the reduced extracellular water (20,21).

GH is a lipolytic hormone and enhances the lipolytic response of adipocytes to beta adrenergic stimuli (22). GH replacement therapy has resulted in a mean reduction in fat

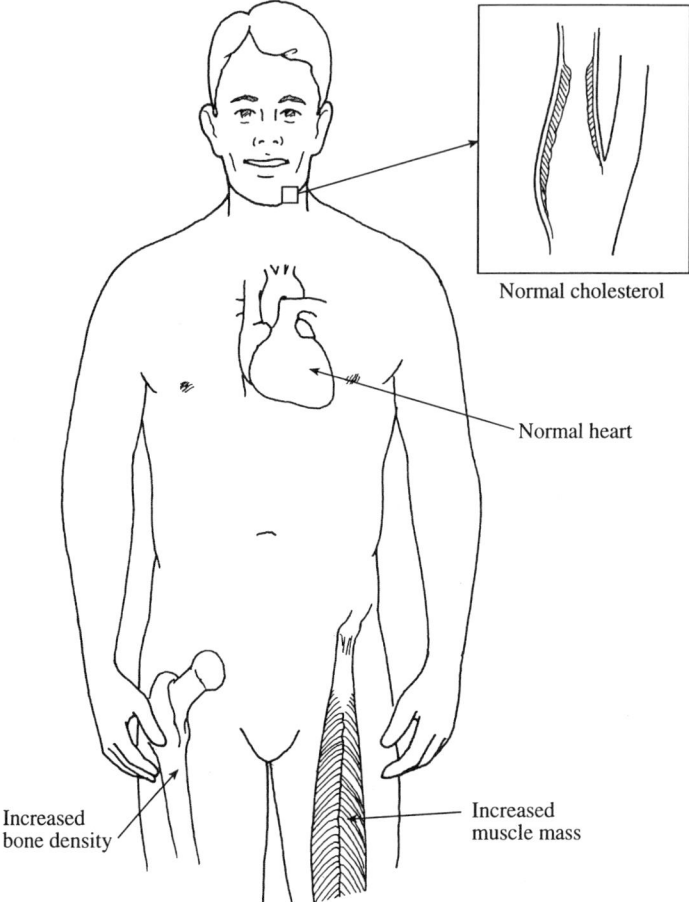

Fig. 2. Post-growth-hormone replacement.

mass of approx 4–6 kg in GHD adults *(23,24)*. Anthropometric measurements indicate that the most important change occurs in the abdominal region. The reduction in abdominal fat mass is mainly due to reduction in visceral fat mass. Solomon et al. *(25)* and Jorgensen et al. *(26)* noted a 10% increase in LBM, an increase in leg-muscle volume, a decrease in subcutaneous fat, and a decrease in total body fat of approx 5 kg after treatment with rhGH for a period of 4–6 mo in GHD adults. In the first 4–6 wk, GH therapy produces a maximal increase in total body water, thereafter changes are negligible. A longer study has shown that an increase in plasma volume occurs after at least 3 wk of GH replacement therapy *(20)*. In a recent study, GH therapy resulted in a 400-mL increase in total blood volume after 3 mo of treatment *(27)*. The mechanism underlying this sodium and water retention by GH treatment is not established. Alterations in renin-angiotensin, plasma renin activity, atrial natriuretic peptide, and renal tubular sodium absorption have been suggested *(28)*.

Bone Density

Bone mineral density (BMD) is significantly decreased in adults with GHD *(29)*. Long-standing GHD in 36 adults demonstrated that 17% had reduced vertebral height, consistent with prevalent vertebral fracture, and an additional 19% had density features of osteopenia *(30)*. In a retrospective analysis of 89 adult patients with GHD, the fracture rate was significantly higher (245 vs 12%) than that in a control population *(31)*. These data suggest that adults with GHD are at increased risk of osteoporotic fractures. In addition, markers of bone resorption have are increased in patients with multiple pituitary deficiencies, but not in patients with isolated GHD. The role of GH in maintaining bone mass in adults is inadequately understood. Age at onset rather than duration of the deficiency seems to be important in determining the degree of reduction in BMD. In adult-onset GHD, a reduction in bone density of the lumbar spine compared to age-matched normal adults has been described *(32)*. GH replacement has not been shown to increase bone mass in the short term (3–6 mo). After starting GH replacement therapy, a rapid increase in plasma (osteocalcin, bone alkaline phosphates, and carboxyl-terminal propeptide of type I procollagen) and urinary markers (deoxypyridinoline, pyridinoline, and cross-linked telopeptide of type I collagen) of bone turnover, presenting an overall picture of increased bone remodeling, has been noted *(33)*. Bone mineral content increases progressively with prolonged GH treatment, and, after 18 mo of therapy, a 5.7% increase in the lumbar spine density has been reported *(34)*. Histology of transiliac bone biopsies of 36 patients with GHD after 6–12 mo of GH treatment showed an increase in cortical thickness, increased bone formation, and decreased bone resorption. It is not known whether GH replacement therapy is capable of normalizing BMD in GHD subjects, but the initial observations are promising.

Lipid Metabolism

Adult patients with GHD have increased morbidity and mortality, which is thought to be of cardiovascular origin *(3)*. GHD adults have increased levels of total cholesterol, low-density lipoproteins (LDL), and triglycerides, which, along with an increased waist to hip ratio, contribute to this morbidity risk. Cuneo et al. showed in 1993 that treatment with recombinant human. GH over a 6-mo period resulted in decreases in total cholesterol level, LDL cholesterol level, LDL:HDL cholesterol ratio, apo B level, and apo B:A-1 ratio. In this study no changes in high-density lipoproteins (HDL) and apo A-1 levels were noted *(35)*. In 1998, Leese et al. reported that in GHD adults, rhGH replacement resulted in a reduction in HDL cholesterol concentration, but they were unable to demonstrate alterations in other aspects of the lipid profile, including serum Lp(a) *(36)*. The only exception to the trend of normalization after GH replacement is Lp(a), a proposed independent risk factor for the development of atherosclerosis and myocardial infarction *(37,38)*. Lp(a) levels increased in all studies except one. The significance of this observation is not yet clear.

GH directly stimulates the release of free fatty acids within the first weeks of treatment. Free fatty acids are either oxidized in the peripheral tissues or taken up by the liver and re-estrified into the triglycerides. LDL-C clearance is regulated by the availability of hepatic LDL receptors. It has been shown that the administration of GH leads to upregulation of hepatic LDL receptors and therefore to increased clearance of LDL-C. Patients with GHD are a heterogeneous group, in terms of their serum lipids who may respond in diverse ways. The lipid response to rhGH replacement may depend on genetic factors controlling lipoprotein metabolism. Lipid profiles should be carefully monitored in patients at high risk of cardiovascular disease after starting rhGH, since a reduction in HDL may occur. The overall effect on cardiovascular events remains to be demonstrated.

Physical Performance

The changes in body composition occurring in GHD with reduced LBM result in a mild-to-moderate reduction in muscle strength. Isometric quardriceps force has been shown to be decreased in GHD adults compared with that in matched normal controls *(39)*. GH treatment improves physical performance in GHD adults *(40)*. An increase in muscle strength has been shown in hip flexors and knee extensors *(41)* during GH replacement. Several studies have shown an increase in exercise capacity assessed by bicycle ergometry *(17)*. The optimal regimen for increasing muscle function in the GHD adult should include GH replacement in combination with exercise, including endurance training, which improves neural activation and may further stimulate the autocrine/paracrine actions of IGF-1 in muscle. In GH-deficient adults, 2 yr of GH treatment has been shown to increase both isometric and isokinetic muscle strength in proximal muscle groups *(42)*. This effect first appeared after 12–24 mo of treatment, but was sustained over time. After GH treatment for up to 6 mo, maximum oxygen uptake increased significantly *(27)*, and reached predicted value. An increase in erythrocyte mass/oxygen transport capacity due to a stimulatory effect of IGF-I on erythropoiesis may also contribute to an increased exercise capacity *(43–45)*.

The anabolic action of GH is not restricted to GHD, as GH treatment has been shown to increase fat-free mass in athletes, healthy young untrained men, and elderly men *(46)*. However factors other than anabolic ones, stimulated by exercise, may be of more importance to muscle strength in GH-sufficient adults.

Cardiovascular System

Mortality in hypopituitary patients is nearly twice as high as age-matched controls, with this excess mortality risk secondary to cardiovascular death *(3)*. These findings were confirmed by Erfurth et al. *(47)*, who found a standardized mortality ration (SMR) of 1.74 for cardiovascular disease among 344 patients with hypopituitarism in the south of Sweden compared with that in the healthy population in the same area. The main causes of death were myocardial infarction, cardiac failure, and cerebrovascular accidents. The data support that hypothesis that long-standing GHD in adulthood predisposes to the development of premature atherosclerosis. Reduced arterial compliance is noted among patients with hypopituitarism, a finding that may be related to the increased prevalence of elevated LDL cholesterol levels in these patients. Other risk factors for premature vascular disease include increased fibrinogen levels and plasminogen activator inhibitor activity *(48)*. Prolonged GHD may ultimately result in cardiac failure due to dilated cardiac myopathy. GHD patients have significantly lower values of interventricular septum and left ventricular posterior wall thickness, resulting in a smaller left ventricular mass index.

The left ventricular end-diastolic and end-systolic diameters are unaffected, but ejection phase indices are lower. After 6 mo of replacement therapy with rhGH, there were no significant changes in either cardiac function or structure, as measured by echocardiography. The only observed changes were a modest, insignificant increase in left ventricular mass, as expressed per body surface area. Previously, an increase in left ventricular myocardial mass as well as an increase in stroke volume after 6 mo of therapy with rhGH, in GHD adults had been reported *(49)*. Other cardiac parameters (left ventricular end systolic diameter, fractional shortening, and wall thickness) were not significantly different.

The fact that treatment with rhGH does not change the cardiac structure, but does affect cardiac stroke volume might be explained by the effect of GH on muscle-fiber metabolism.

At present, data on the effects of growth hormone on the heart are scarce. The results presently available suggest the response of cardiac muscle to GH is time- and dose- dependent. Long-term effects of GH on cardiac function are presently unknown; however, GH replacement should be aimed at restoring somatic deficiency, including cardiac size and function, and treatment should be carefully monitored to prevent the cardiac complications of GH excess.

Endothelial Function

Atherosclerosis begins long before the appearance of overt disease. Endothelial dysfunction is an early and potentially reversible event in the pathogenesis of atherosclerosis, predisposing to thrombosis, leukocyte adhesion, and smooth-muscle proliferation within the arterial wall. GHD with hypopituitarism is associated with a number of atherogenic risk factors, including reduced exercise capacity, insulin resistance, and detrimental body composition. Flow-mediated dilatation of the brachial artery is significantly impaired in GHD adults compared to age- and sex-matched controls. In contrast, glyceryl trinitrate-mediated dilatation or endothelium-independent vasodilatation was similar in both groups (50). Endothelial dysfunction in hypopituitary adults with GHD may be a consequence of the metabolic and physiologic abnormalities associated with the condition, supporting the view that adult GHD is a pro-atherogenic state.

Metabolism

ENERGY EXPENDITURE

Recent studies have shown that resting energy expenditure (REE) in adults with GHD is lower than predicted values corrected for age, height, and weight (51,52). GH replacement in GHD results in rapid and large increases in REE. Restoration of LBM accounts for much of the increase in REE along with direct increase in cellular metabolism. GH treatment of the GHD adults results in an increase in circulating T3 levels in patients receiving T4 replacement and those with normal thyroid function (53,54). This indicates that GH is a physiological regulator of thyroid function in general and of peripheral conversion of T4 in particular.

Protein Metabolism

Studies of protein metabolism in adults with GHD have shown reduced protein flux and synthesis. A 6-mo open study was performed with GH replacement in eight adults with GHD using [15N] glycine as a tracer. There was increased protein synthesis at 1 mo, with no protein change in protein breakdown. The effect was no longer evident after 3, 6, or 9 mo of GH therapy. Beshyah et al. (55) used L-[1-13C] leucine to study protein metabolism and compared 16 adults with GHD with 20 matched controls. The patients had decreased oxidation, protein synthesis, and leucine flux. Six months of GH therapy demonstrated a nonsignificant increase in protein flux, oxidation, and synthesis. In another randomized, double-blind, placebo-controlled trial of the effect of GH replacement on protein metabolism, a 245 increase in protein synthesis at 2 mo was demonstrated with no change in protein degradation (56). It is evident from the studies that GH replacement increases protein synthesis for the first few months, with a return to baseline rates after 6 mo, probably due to a new baseline rate of metabolism.

Carbohydrate Metabolism

GHD patients have altered body composition, with an increase in central obesity. The fasting insulin levels are above the normal reference range. In a double-blind, placebo-controlled, crossover study, the effects of 6 mo of GH replacement on glucose metabolism were studied. After 6 wk of GH therapy, fasting glucose levels and plasma insulin concentrations were elevated, but both had returned to baseline at 26 wk *(57)*. This reflected a short-term reduction of insulin-stimulated glucose utilization, directed by GH, with reversal of these changes with time, perhaps as a result of altered body composition. GH replacement also demonstrated increased fasting glucose, insulin, and C peptide as well as increase in first and second phases of insulin secretion after 1 wk of GH therapy *(58)*. Even after 3 mo, the fasting plasma insulin and C peptide levels remained elevated. GHD leads to hyperinsulinemia with insulin resistance. GH therapy has been demonstrated to further increase insulin resistance over a period of 1–6 wk of treatment, but although carbohydrate metabolism returns to baseline at 3 mo of GH replacement, hyperinsulinemia persists.

Leptin

Leptin is a hormonal product of adipose tissue, expression of which reflects the body status of nutritional reserves. Leptin is one of the metabolic signals capable of regulating GH secretion. In rats it was demonstrated that central injection of leptin increased pituitary GH mRNA levels by 53.2% and hypothalamic GHRH mRNA by 61.8%, and reduced somatostatin mRNA levels by 41.5% *(59)*. Addition of leptin along with GHRH to anterior pituitary cells in culture does not alter basal GH release or the GH-releasing activity of GHRH. Thus, leptin appears to act on hypothalamic GH-regulatory hormones and may be a critical hormonal signal of nutritional status in the neuroendocrine regulation of pulsatile GH secretion.

GH treatment is associated with a reduction in fat mass in healthy and GHD adults. A direct effect of GH on adipose cells and stimulation of lipolysis seem to be the underlying mechanism for this effect. Leptin is released from adipose tissue and may be involved in signaling information about adipose tissue stores to the brain. However, in GHD adults, treatment with GH for 4 mo had no independent effect on either serum leptin or leptin gene expression *(60)*. Fasting reduced leptin levels in both GHD and healthy subjects but no independent effect of GH suppression or GH substitution on serum leptin was found during fasting.

Skin

Skin thickness and total skin collagen are reduced in hypopituitary adults. An increase in skin thickness was demonstrated after GH treatment in normal elderly males *(61)*. The sweat-secretion rate in response to pilocarpine iontophoresis was significantly lower in GHD adults than in age- and sex-matched control subjects and with treatment it increased significantly *(62)*. Impaired ability to dissipate heat by sweating, after heat stress or exercise in GHD patients, may be an important contributory factor to their reduced exercise capacity *(63)*.

Role of GH in Immunity

IGF-1 receptors are expressed on human peripheral blood B cells, T cells, natural killer (NK) cells, and monocytes. Animal studies have confirmed the role of GH in the modulation of both humoral and cell-mediated immunity. Immunity is usually not compromised in adults with GHD.

Quality of Life

Patients with GHD report lower self-perceived health status and lower levels of psychological well-being. They perceive themselves to be unstable, more socially isolated, less energetic, with a poorer level of general health and self-control, less vitality, and more anxiety than individuals without GHD. A disturbed sex life was reported in another study *(64)*. Rosen et al. used the Nottingham Health Profile (NHP) and compared psychological well-being in 86 adults with GHD with age-matched controls. The GHD patients reported less energy, greater emotional liability, and a greater sense of social isolation than the control subjects *(65)*. Using the Assessment of Growth Hormone Deficiency in Adults (AGHDA), a self-administered questionnaire designed specifically to evaluate quality of life in GHD adults *(66)* it was shown that GHD patients not receiving GH replacement therapy had a high AGHDA score, indicating a low health-related quality of life that is maintained over time. Treatment with rhGH for 12 mo significantly improved the quality of life in GHD adults in terms of energy, pain and emotional reaction *(67)*.

Other Uses of Growth Hormone in Adults

The FDA of the United States has approved GH for use in cachectic and wasting patients with AIDs because it increases LBM and decreases fat mass. No survival benefit is conferred by GH therapy in patients suffering from AIDS. GH therapy has been used, in high doses, in critically ill patients, in an intensive care setting but was associated with increased mortality *(68)*. Among survivors, the length of stay in intensive care and in the hospital and the duration of mechanical ventilation were prolonged. Thus GH is contraindicated in the ICU setting. The use of GH in obesity, osteoporosis, muscular dystrophy, and infertility has shown no consistent benefit. No improvement in muscle strength and exercise tolerance was documented after using GH in elderly ambulatory patients. There is no added benefit to exercise alone, when given short-term to athletes for increased strength and endurance. Recently rhGH has been shown to be beneficial in the treatment of patients with chronically active Crohn's disease. At 4 mo, the Crohn's Disease Activity Index score decreased by a mean of 143 points in the GH group, as compared with a decrease of 19 points in the placebo group *(69)*.

SIDE EFFECTS OF GH THERAPY

GH side effects usually result from excess replacement. In contrast to children, side effects of GH treatment in adults are relatively common. Patients most at risk are older and obese with a greater response to provocative testing, and the largest IGF-1 rise after GH replacement. The side effects include sodium and water retention, weight gain, dependent edema, occasional carpal tunnel syndrome, and arthralgia or myalgia, which appear to be dose-dependent effects. There was no significant change in blood pressure after 3 yr of treatment. Usually daily doses of 6–26 microgram/kg produced side effects and reduction by 25 or 50% led to resolution of these effects. There is no proven increase in the incidence of any malignancy with GH treatment, nor is there an enhancement of pituitary-tumor recurrence *(70)*. A baseline scan is recommended before starting treatment, but there is no need for an intensified follow-up, other than regular serial imaging for residual tumor.

Table 4
Side Effects
of Growth Hormone Replacement

Common
  Headache
  Edema
  Arthralgia
  Myalgia
  Carpal and tarsal tunnel syndrome
Uncommon
  Tinnitus
  Hypertension
  Atrial fibrillation
  Benign intracranial hypertension
  Raynaud's phenomenon
  Gynecomastia

Table 5
Contraindications
to Growth Hormone Therapy

Active malignancy
Benign intracranial hypertension
Proliferative diabetic retinopathy
Pregnancy

GH therapy is associated with hyperinsulinemia and elevated Lp(a) levels, which may increase the risk of cardiovascular complications (71). GH-induced atrial fibrillation and hypertension have been reported, but are rare occurrences. Some patients may experience headache and tinnitus. Gynecomastia rarely can occur in elderly men. The side effects of GH are outlined in Table 4. Contraindications to GH treatment include active malignancy, benign intracranial hypertension, and proliferative or proliferative diabetic retinopathy. GH treatment has not been approved for use in pregnancy. Contraindications of growth therapy are listed in Table 5.

CONCLUSION

The existence of an adult GHD syndrome is no longer hypothetical (72). It has been established that short-term GH replacement therapy improves the abnormalities in body composition and metabolism and that physical performance and well-being can be increased. With prolonged treatment, initially induced beneficial changes are preserved and some may even become more pronounced (73). At this point GH use has only been shown to be beneficial as replacement therapy. Other uses are under investigation and may yield added beneficial results. Because GH replacement therapy has been administered for only about 11 yr in adults, the long-term benefits and outcomes are not yet known. More long-term trials of GH treatment are needed in the future in order to clarify whether GH replacement decreases mortality rate and morbidity in GHD adults.

GH therapy is expensive, at a cost of $4500–5000 per year in the United States. In many developed countries, people are being denied access to appropriate hormone replacement purely on the basis of cost *(74)*. Even in the US, adult endocrinologists are still reluctant to treat GHD. We believe that the evidence now indicates that GH replacement therapy is merited for all patients with documented GHD.

REFERENCES

1. Carrol PV, Christ ER, et al. Growth hormone deficiency in adulthood and the effects of growth hormone replacement: a review. J Clin Endocrinol Metab 1998;83:382–395.
2. Sonksen PH. Replacement therapy in hypothalamo-pituitary insufficiency after childhood: management in the adult. Horm Res 1990;33(Suppl 4):45–51.
3. Rosen T, Bengtsson BA. Premature mortality due to cardiovascular disease in hypopituitarism. Lancet 1990;336:285–288.
4. Shalet SM, Toogood AA, Rahim A, Brennan BMD. The diagnosis of growth hormone deficiency in children and adults. Endocr Rev 1998;19:203–223.
5. Hoffman DM, O'Sullivan AJ, Baxter RC, Ho KKY. Diagnosis of growth hormone deficiency in adults. Lancet 1994;343:1064-1068 [Erratum, Lancet 1994;344:206.]
6. Consensus guidelines for the diagnosis and treatment of adults with growth hormone deficiency: summary statement of the Growth Hormone Research Society Workshop on Adult Growth Hormone Deficiency. J Clin Endocrinol Metab 1998;83:379–381.
7. De Boer H, Block GJ, Voerman HJ, De Vries PMJM, van der Veen EA. Body composition in adult growth hormone deficient men, assessed by anthropometry and bioimpedance analysis. J Clin Endocrinol Metab 1992;75:833–837.
8. Salomon F, Cuneo RC, Hesp R, Sonksen PH. The effects of treatment with recombinant human growth hormone on body composition and metabolism in adults with growth hormone deficiency. N Engl J Med 1989;321:1797–1803.
9. Snel YE, Doerga ME, Brummer RJ, Zelissen PM, Zonderland ML, Koppeschaar HP. Resting metabolic rate, body composition and related hormonal parameters in growth hormone deficient adults before and after growth hormone replacement therapy. Eur J Endocrinol 1995;133:445–450.
10. Hoffman DM, O'Sullivan AJ, Freund J, Ho KK. Adults with growth hormone deficiency have abnormal body composition but normal energy metabolism. J Clin Endocrinol Metab 1995;80:72–77.
11. Beshyah SA, Freemantle C, Thomas E. Abnormal body composition and reduced bone mass in growth hormone deficient hypopituitary adults. Clin Endocrinol (Oxf) 1995;42:179–189.
12. Rosen T, Bosaeus I, Tolli J, Lindstedt G, Bengtsson BA. Increased body fat mass and decreased extracellular fluid volume in adults with growth hormone deficiency. Clin Endocrinol (Oxf) 1993;38:63–71.
13. Amato G, Carella C, Fazio S. Body composition, bone metabolism, and heart structure and function in growth hormone-deficient adults before and after GH replacement therapy at low doses. J Clin Endocrinol Metab 1993;77:1671–1676.
14. Bengtsson BA, Eden S, Lonn L. Treatment of adults with growth hormone deficiency with recombinant human GH. J Clin Endocrinol Metab 1993;76:309–317.
15. Snel YE, Doerga ME, Brummer RM, Zelissen PM, Koppeschaar HP. Magnetic resonance imaging-assessed adipose tissue and serum lipid and insulin concentrations in growth hormone-deficient adults. Effect of growth hormone replacement. Arterioscler Thromb Vasc Biol 1995;15:1543–1548.
16. Whitehead HM, Boreham C, McIlrath EM. Growth hormone treatment of adults with growth hormone deficiency: results of a 13-month placebo controlled cross-over study. Clin Endocrinol (Oxf) 1992;36: 45–52.
17. Binnerts A, Swart GR, Wilson JHP. The effect of growth hormone administration in growth hormone deficient adults on bone, protein, carbohydrate and lipid homeostasis, as well as body composition. Clin Endocrinol (Oxf) 1992;37:79–87.
18. Chong PKK, Jung RT, Scrimgeour CM, Rennie MJ, Peterson CR. Energy expenditure and body composition in growth hormone deficient adults on exogenous growth hormone. Clin Endocrinol (Oxf) 1994; 40:103–110.
19. De Boer H, Blok GJ, Voerman HJ, de Vries P, Popp-Snijders C, van der Veen E. The optimal growth hormone replacement dose in adults, derived from bioimpedance analysis. J Clin Endocrinol Metab 1995; 80:2069–2076.

20. Moller J, Frandsen E, Fisker S, Jorgensen JOL, Christiansen JS. Decreased plasma and extracellular volume in growth hormone-deficient adults and the acute and prolonged effects of GH administration: a controlled experimental study. Clin Endocrinol (Oxf) 1996;44:533–539.

21. Christ ER, Cummings MH, Pearson TC, Sonksen PH, Russell-Jones DL. Effects of growth hormone deficiency on plasma volume and red cell mass. Endocrinol Metab 1997;4(Suppl)A:60.

22. Beauville M, Harant I, Crampes F, Riviere D, Tauber MT, Tauber JP, Garrigues M. Effect of long term rhGH administration in GH-deficient adults on fat cell epinephrine response. Am J Physiol 1992;263: E467–E472.

23. Johansson G, Rosen T, Lindstedt G, Bosaeus I, Bengtsson BA. Effect of two years of growth hormone treatment on body composition and cardiovascular risk factors in adults with growth hormone deficiency. Endocrinol Metab 1996;4(Suppl A):3–12.

24. Orme SM, Sebastian JP, Oldroyd B. Comparison of measures of body composition in a trial of low dose growth hormone replacement therapy. Clin Endocrinol (Oxf) 1992;37:453–459.

25. Solomon F, Cuneo Rc, Hesp R, Sonksen PH. The sffects of treatment with recombinant human growth hormone on body composition and metabolism in adults with growth hormone deficiency. N Engl J Med 1989;321:1797–1803.

26. Jorgensen JOL, Pederson SA, Theusen L, Jorgensen J, Ingemann-Hansen T, Skakkebaek NE, Christiansen JS. Beneficial effects of growth hormone treatment in growth hormone deficient adults. Lancet 1989;1: 1221–1225.

27. Christ E, Cummings MH, Westwood NB. The importance of growth hormone in the regulation of erythropoiesis, red cell mass, and plasma volume in adults with growth hormone deficiency. J Clin Endocrinol Metab 1997;82:2985–2990.

28. Hoffman DM, Crampton L, Sernia C, Nguyen TV, Ho KKY. Short term growth hormone treatment of GH-deficient adults increases body sodium and extracellular water, but not blood pressure. J Clin Endocrinol Metab 1996;81:1123–1128.

29. De Boer H, Blok GJ, Van Lingen A, Teule GJJ, Lips P, van der Veen EA. The consequences of childhood-onset growth hormone deficiency for adult bone mass. J Bone Miner Res 1994;9:1319–1326.

30. Wuster CHR, Slenczka E, Ziegler R. Increased prevalence of osteoporosis and arteriosclerosis in patients with conventionally substituted pituitary insufficiency: is there a need for additional growth hormone substitution? Klin Wochenschr 1991;69:769–773.

31. Rosen T, Wilhelmsen L, Landin-Wilhelmsen K. Increased fracture rate in adults with growth hormone deficiency. Endocrinol Metab 1996;3(Suppl A):121.

32. Holmes SJ, Economou G, Whitehouse RW, Adams JE, Shalet SM. Reduced bone mineral density in patients with adult onset growth hormone deficiency. J Clin Endocrinol Metab 1994;78:669–674.

33. Beshyah SA, Thomas E, Kyd P, Sharp P, Fairney A, Johnston DG. The effect of growth hormone replacement therapy in hypopituitary adults on calcium and bone metabolism. Clin Endocrinol (Oxf) 1994;40:383–391.

34. Vandeweghe M, Taelman P, Kaufman JM. Short and long term effects of growth hormone treatment on bone turnover and bone mineral content in adult growth hormone deficient males. Clin Endocrinol (Oxf) 1993;39:409–415.

35. Cuneo R, Salomon F, Watts G, Hesp R, Sonksen P. Growth hormone treatment improves serum lipids and lipoproteins in adults with growth hormone deficiency. Metabolism 1993;42:1519–1523.

36. Leese GP, Wallymahmed M, VanHeyningen C, Tames F, Wieringas G, MacFarlane IA. HDL-cholesterol reductions associated with growth hormone replacement. Clin Endocrinol 1998;49:673–677.

37. Armstrong VM, Cremer P, Eberle E. The association between serum Lp(a) concentrations and angiographically assessed coronary atherosclerosis. Atherosclerosis 1986;62:249–257.

38. Bostom AG, Cupples LA, Jenner JL. Elevated plasma lipoprotein(a) and coronary heart disease in men aged 55 years and younger. A prospective study. J Am Med Assoc 1996;276:544–548.

39. Cuneo RC, Salomon F, Wiles CM. Skeletal muscle performance in adults with growth hormone deficiency. Horm Res 1990;33(Suppl 4):55–60.

40. Cuneo RC, Saloman F, Wiles CM, Hesp R, Sonksen PH. Growth hormone treatment in growth hormone deficient adults.II.Effects on exercise performance. J Appl. Physiol 1991;70:695–700.

41. Jorgensen JOL, Pedersen SA, Theusen L, Jorgensen J, Moller J, Muller J, et al. Long term growth hormone treatment in growth hormone deficient adults. Acta Endocrinol (Copenh) 1991;125:449–453.

42. Johannsson G, Grimby G, Sunnerhagen KS, Bengtsson BA. Two years of growth hormone (GH) treatment increase isometric and isokinetic muscle strength in GH-deficient adults. J Clin Endocrinol Metab 1997;82:2877–2884.

43. Jepson JH, McGary EE. Hemopoiesis in pituitary dwarfstreated with human growth hormone and testosterone. Blood 1972;39:238–248.

44. Claustres M, Chatelain P, Sultan C. Insulin-like growth factor-1 stimulates human erythroid colony formation in vitro. J Clin Endocrinol Metab 1987;65:78–82.

45. Merchav S, Tatarsky I, Hochberg Z. Enhancement of erythropoises in vitro by human growth hormone is mediated by insulin-like growth factor-1. Br J Hematol 1988;70:267–271.

46. Yarasheski KE, Zachwieja JJ, Campbell JA, Bier DM. Effect of growth hormone and resistance exercise on muscle growth and strength in older men. Am J Physiol 1995;268:E268–E276.

47. Erfurth EM, Buelow B, Mikozy Z, Nordstroem CH, Hagmar L. Increased cardiovascular mortality in patients with hypopituitarism. Endocrinol Metab 1996;3(Suppl A):121.

48. Johansson JO, Landin K, Tengborn L, Rosen T, Bengtsson BA. High fibrinogen and plasma activator inhibitor activity in growth hormone-deficient adults. Atheroscler Thromb 1994;14:434–437.

49. Cuneo RC, Salomon F, Wilmshurst P, et al. Cardiovascular effects of growth hormone treatment in growth-hormone-deficient adults: stimulation of renin-aldosterone system. Clin Sci 1991;81:587–592.

50. Evans LM, Davies JS, Goodfellow J, Rees JAE, Scanlon MF. Endothelial dysfunction in hypopituitary adults with growth hormone deficiency. Clin Endocrinol 1999;50:457–464.

51. Salomon F, Cuneo RC, Umpleby AM. Interactions of body fat and muscle mass with substrate concentrations and fasting insulin levels in adults with growth hormone deficiency. Clin Sci 1994;87:201–206.

52. Snel YEM, Doerga ME, Zonderland ML. Resting metabolic rate in growth hormone deficient adults. Proceedings of the 4th International Meeting on Growth Hormone Deficiency in Adults. 1993, p. 48.

53. Jorgensen JOL, Moller J, Laursen T. Growth hormone administration stimulates energy expenditure and extrathyroidal conversion of thyroxine to triiodothyronine in a dose-dependent manner and suppresses circadian thyrotrophin levels: studies in GH-deficient adults. Clin Endocrinol (Oxf) 1994;41:609–614.

54. Jorgensen JOL, Pedersen SA, Laurberg P. Effects of growth hormone therapy on thyroid function of growth hormone deficient adults with and without concomitant thyroxine-substituted central hypothyroidism. J Clin Endocrinol Metab 1989;69:1127–1132.

55. Beshyah SA, Sharp PS, Gelding SV. Whole-body leucine turnover in adults on conventional treatment for hypopituitarism. Acta Endocrinol (Copenh) 1993;129:158–164.

56. Russell-Jones DL, Weissberger AJ, Bowes SB. The effects of growth hormone on protein metabolism in adult growth hormone deficient patients. Clin Endocrinol (Oxf) 1993;38:427–431.

57. Fowelin J, Attvall S, Lager I, Bengtsson BA. Effects of treatment with recombinant human growth hormone on insulin sensitivity and glucose metabolism in adults with growth hormone deficiency. Metab Clin Exp 1993;42:1443–1447.

58. O'Neal DN, Kalfas A, Dunning PL. The effect of 3 months of recombinant human growth hormone (GH) therapy on insulin and glucose mediated glucose disposal and insulin secretion in GH-deficient adults: a minimal model analysis. J Clin Endocrinol Metab 1994;79:975–983.

59. Cocchi D, De Gennaro Colonna V, Bagnasco M, Bonacci D, Muller EE. Leptin regulates GH secretion in the rat by acting on GHRH and somatostainergic functions. J Endocrinol 1999;162(1):95–99.

60. Kristensen K, Pedersen SB, Fisker S, Norrelund H, Rosenfalck AM, Jorgensen JO, Richelsen B. Serum leptin levels and leptin expression in growth hormone-deficient and healthy adults: influence of GH treatment, gender, and fasting. Metab Clin Exp 1998;47(12):1514–1519.

61. Rudman D, Feller AG, Nagraj HS. Effects of human growth hormone in men over 60 years old. N Engl J Med 1990;323:1–6.

62. Pedersen SA, Welling K, Michaelsen KF. Reduced sweating in adults with growth hormone deficiency. Lancet 1989;2:681–682.

63. Juul A, Behrenscheer A, Tims T. Impaired thermoregulation in adults with growth hormone deficiency during heat exposure and exercise. Clin Endocrinol 1993;38:237–244.

64. Rosen T, Wilhelmsen L, Wiklund I, Bengtsson BA. Decreased psychological well-being in adult patients with growth hormone deficiency. Clin Endocrinol 1994;40:111–116.

65. Stabler B, Turner JR, Girdler SS, Light KC, Underwood LE. Reactivity to stress and psychological adjustments in adults with pituitary insufficiency. Clin Endocrinol (Oxf) 1992;6:467–473.

66. Holmes SJ, McKenna SP, Doward LC, Hunt SM, Shalet SM. Development of a questionnaire to assess the quality of life of adults with growth hormone deficiency. Endocrinol Metab 1995;2:63–69.

67. Cuneo RC, Judd S, Wallace JD, Perry-Keene D, Burger H, LimTio S, et al. The Australian multicenter trial of growth hormone (GH) treatment in GH-deficient adults. J Clin Endocrinol Metab 1998;83:107–116.

68. Takala J, Ruoken E, Webster NR, et al. Increased mortality associated with growth hormone treatment in critically ill adults. N Engl J Med 1999;341:785–792.

69. Slonim AE, Bulone L, Damore M, Goldberg T, Wingertzahn MA, McKinley MJ. A preliminary study of growth hormone therapy for Crohn's disease. N Engl J Med 2000;342:1633–1637.

70. Blethen SL, Allen DB, Graves D, August G, Moshang T, Rosenfeld R. Safety of recombinant deoxyribonucleic acid-derived growth hormone: The National Cooperative Growth Study Experience. J Clin Endocrinol Metab 1996;81:1704–1710.

71. Reaven GM. Role of insulin resistance in human disease. Diabetes 1988;37:1595–1607.

72. Cuneo RC, Salomon F, Mcgauley GA, Sonksen PH. The growth hormone deficiency syndrome in adults. Clin Endocrinol (Oxf) 1992;37:387–397.

73. Jorgensen JOL, Theusen L, Muller J, Ovesen P, Skakkebaek NE, Christiansen JS. Three years of growth hormone treatment in growth hormone-deficient adults: near normalization of body composition and physical performance. Eur J Endocrinol 1994;130:224–228.

74. Simpson H, Sonksen P. Therapeutic contraversy: treatment of growth hormone deficiency in adults. J Clin Endocrinol Metab 2000;85:933–942.

III THYROID

5

Molecular Mechanisms of Thyroid Gland Development

Insights from Clinical Studies and from Mutant Mice

Guy Van Vliet, MD

CONTENTS

INTRODUCTION: CONGENITAL HYPOTHYROIDISM, A KEY TO UNDERSTAND THYROID GLAND DEVELOPMENT

As in many other fields of biomedical research, the careful description of congenital disorders affecting the development of the thyroid ("experiments of nature") is an absolute prerequisite and an invaluable tool for generating hypotheses about the molecular mechanisms involved at various stages of the differentiation, migration, and growth of the gland *(1)*. Several genes involved not only in thyroid function, but also in the organogenesis of the gland have been identified in the past few years (reviewed in ref. *2*).

From: *Contemporary Endocrinology: Developmental Endocrinology: From Research to Clinical Practice*
Edited by: E. A. Eugster and O. H. Pescovitz © Humana Press Inc., Totowa, NJ

Renewed interest in the molecular pathophysiology of congenital hypothyroidism (CH), a common disorder affecting about 1 in 4000 newborns, has led to the generation of several mouse knockouts and to the identification of a small number of single gene defects in humans (reviewed in ref. *3*). Even though a better understanding of CH in molecular terms will probably have no impact on treatment, it will be important for genetic counseling in these families. Furthermore, it may shed light on other, more complex and less easily treatable, congenital malformations.

CH is a heterogeneous condition, which is usually classified on the basis of the level of the defect and of its transient or permanent nature. When the hypothyroidism results from a defect in the thyroid itself, it is called primary. On the other hand, secondary (pituitary defects) and tertiary (hypothalamic defects) are often grouped together under the designation "central hypothyroidism." Transient causes of primary (transplacental transfer of antithyroid drugs or of thyroid-stimulating hormone [TSH]-receptor blocking antibodies, chronic iodine deficiency, and/or acute iodine overload) or of central congenital hypothyroidism (immaturity of the hypothalamo-pituitary control mechanisms) will not be considered further in this chapter. Because the vast majority of cases of permanent CH are of the primary type, the focus of this review will be on the development of the thyroid itself. However, new mechanisms of central hypothyroidism that have contributed to our understanding of the role of TSH in the development of the thyroid will also be briefly discussed.

The causes of permanent primary CH fall under two broad categories: the most frequent, accounting for ~80% of cases, is called thyroid dysgenesis (a category including defective thyroid migration, resulting in ectopic tissue, and complete absence of thyroid or athyreosis) and is in general considered sporadic with a female predominance. However, in a large series, we have recently shown *(4)* that the female predominance was only significant for ectopy: in athyreosis, as in dyshormonogenesis, a known autosomal recessive condition (*see* below), the proportion of girls is not significantly different from 0.5, suggesting that a proportion of athyreoses may have autosomal recessive mechanisms. Other recent studies have revealed evidence for genetic transmission in about 2% of cases of thyroid dysgenesis *(5)* (*see* below).

The second cause of permanent primary CH, thyroid dyshormonogenesis, results from a defect in any one of the genes involved in thyroid hormone formation (the sodium/iodide symporter or *NIS*; pendrin or *PDS*; thyroglobulin or *Tg*; the genes responsible for H_2O_2 generation, *ThOX1* and *ThOX2*; and thyroperoxidase or *TPO*), follows an autosomal recessive pattern of inheritance. In the latter situation, the gland is of normal shape and is in the normal position. Because the normal feedback mechanisms are operative, TSH is elevated and goiter often ensues. Thyroid dyshormonogenesis will not be considered in this chapter and the reader is referred to the excellent chapter by Refetoff et al. *(6)*.

There is some confusion in the nomenclature regarding thyroid dysgenesis; because the lateral lobes of the gland develop only if the medial anlage has reached its normal position, an ectopic thyroid is by definition "hypoplastic" (hence the hypothyroidism). However, as discussed below, the mechanisms leading to defective or aberrant migration of the anlage differ from those leading to hypoplasia of a normally located gland *(7)*. Therefore, it is essential to specify whether a hypoplastic gland is ectopic or orthotopic. However, this is not always done and makes the interpretation of some studies difficult. A further challenge in this area is that the distinction between the presence of a small ectopic gland and complete absence of any thyroid tissue is difficult to make in humans;

technetium scintigraphy remains the gold standard, but up to 50% of CH newborns with no uptake on scintiscan have detectable plasma thyroglobulin levels *(8)* and the percentage of CH cases with detectable thyroid tissue varies considerably between centers and even within a center over time *(9)*. It is therefore likely that patients labeled as "athyreotics" in the past would be reclassified as "ectopics," and this may be important in the study of family pedigrees extending over several generations (*see* below). Furthermore, a patient with a severely hypoplastic and hypofunctional orthotopic gland may present with "apparent athyreosis" on scintigraphy *(7)*.

FORMATION AND MIGRATION OF THE THYROID ANLAGE

In human embryos, the median thyroid primordium, a round thickening of the pharyngeal floor, is visible on day 16–17 of gestation (E 8.5 in the mouse). These cells migrate caudally, while multiplying, and reach the normal adult position in front of the thyroid cartilage at 6–7 wk (E 13–14 d in the mouse). The thyroid-specific genes *Tg*, *Tpo*, and TSH receptor (*Tshr*) then begin to be expressed and the typical follicular architecture develops progressively until birth *(2)*.

The lateral lobes of the thyroid develop from the 4th and 5th pharyngeal pouches, which connect with the medial anlage at about 6 wk only if the latter has reached its normal position; if migration is incomplete or "excessive" (as in the case of mediastinal thyroids), the ectopic tissue will have a round, and not a bilobed appearance. This likely reflects the fact that the vascularization of the lateral lobes, which originates from the medial anlage *(10)*, develops only when it has reached the normal position.

Interestingly, when migration of the medial anlage is incomplete, no orthotopic thyroid tissue will be present, whereas when the migration is excessive (e.g., with ectopic thyroid tissue found in the mediastinum), there is also an orthotopic gland of normal shape and size. Accordingly, patients with only ectopic tissue in the sublingual area will have congenital hypothyroidism (although it has been estimated that a small proportion [1.6%] may have a normal TSH in the neonatal period *[11]*). Conversely, patients with mediastinal thyroid tissue are euthyroid and are usually diagnosed later in life, often because of compression of adjacent organs or by incidental finding on an imaging study *(12)*. The occurrence of ectopic thyroid tissue in the mediastinum likely results from the fact that migration of the thyroid anlage and of the embryonic heart occur at the same time during embryogenesis (5–7 wk in humans) and that the heart may be "pulling" some thyroid tissue during its caudal migration *(13)*.

It is noteworthy that, contrasting with these findings of macroscopic ectopies, microscopic thyroid remnants have been found in the tongue, in addition to a normal gland, in 10% of routine autopsies in one study *(14)*. Interestingly, this was found in an equal number of men and women, whereas the finding of only sublingual uptake on scintigraphy in CH has a clear female predominance *(4)*. Aside from incomplete or excessive migration of the median anlage along the midline, a few cases of lateral thyroid ectopies, with no thyroid tissue in the normal location, have been described *(15)*. These observations demonstrate that differentiated thyroid follicular cells can arise from the lateral anlage as well *(16)*. The fact that hyperthyroidism *(15)* and papillary cancer *(16a)* occur in patients with only ectopic thyroid tissue shows that ectopic thyroid cells can have full growth and functional potential. Moreover, the plasma concentrations of thyroxine in children with ectopic glands studied after treatment withdrawal at ages 1–11 yr are correlated to plasma thyroxine at diagnosis in the newborn period *(17,18)*. This suggests that the postnatal survival of ectopic thyroid cells is normal.

ORIGIN OF THE CALCITONIN-PRODUCING CELLS (C-CELLS)

Aside from follicular cells, the second major epithelial cells of the thyroid are parafollicular or calcitonin-producing C cells, which are of neural-crest origin and migrate to the ultimobranchial bodies *(16)*. These paired structures, which are closely associated with parathyroid IV and with thymus IV, derive from the fourth and fifth pharyngeal pouches and fuse with the lateral thyroid lobes. In the postnatal human thyroid, C cells are present throughout the gland (hence the need for near-total thyroidectomy in individuals bearing *ret* mutations associated with multiple endocrine neoplasia type 2 or familial medullary thyroid carcinoma), although they are more abundant at the point of fusion with the ultimobranchial body *(19)*.

ROLES OF TRANSCRIPTION FACTORS
IN THYROID DIFFERENTIATION AND MIGRATION

Three transcription factors are expressed, starting at E 8.5 in the mouse, in the bud that forms at that age in the floor of the primitive pharynx. These are thyroid transcription factors-1 and-2 (Ttf-1 and Ttf-2) and Pax-8. While these three transcription factors are often called thyroid-specific, they are not completely so, as will be illustrated later.

TTF-1 mRNA encodes a protein which binds DNA through a highly conserved 61 amino-acid homeodomain. *TTF-1* maps to chromosome 14q13 and contains three exons and two introns. Expression studies in mice have shown that Ttf-1 mRNA can be detected not only in the thyroid, but also in the lung and in some regions of the forebrain and in the infundibulum and posterior pituitary; however, the anterior pituitary does not express *Ttf-1*. Ttf-1 increases the expression of *Tpo*, *Tg*, and *Tshr*, three genes whose protein products are essential for thyroid hormone biosynthesis *(20)*. In adult lung, Ttf-1 also increases the expression of surfactant protein *(6)*.

TTF-2 belongs to a family of proteins that bind DNA through a conserved 100-amino acid domain with a winged-helix structure, which is named a fork-head domain. The TTF-2 protein is coded for by a gene that is located on chromosome 9q22 and contains a single exon. In the mouse, *Ttf-2* shows a restricted tissue distribution, being expressed in the thyroid and in most of the foregut endoderm, the craniopharyngeal endoderm involved in the formation of the palate, and in Rathke's pouch. The human cDNA was cloned from a skin cDNA library. In the adult thyroid, Ttf-2 is involved in the stimulation of Tg transcription by insulin and possibly by TSH *(6)*.

PAX-8 is a protein belonging to the large family of transcription factors that bind DNA via a highly conserved paired domain. *PAX-8* maps to chromosome 2q12-14 and contains at least 10 exons. It is expressed in both the kidney and the thyroid. In the adult thyroid, it activates transcription of *Tg*, *Tpo*, and *Nis (21)*.

TTF-1 KNOCKOUT MICE
AND THE SEARCH FOR *TTF-1* MUTATIONS IN HUMANS

Ttf-1 −/− mice are alive until E 19.5. At birth, they are stillborn, but their weight is only reduced to ~85% of that of normal littermates. They have normal parathyroid glands, but

Table 1
Haploinsufficiency for the Chromosomal
Region Containing *TTF-1*, *PAX-9*, and Unknown Genes

Patient (ref.)	Deletion	First TSH (mIU/L)	First T4 (nmol/L)	2nd TSH (mIU/L)	2d T4 (nmol/L)	Thyroid Scan (^{99m}Tc)	Other features
1	14q13-21	60	114	48	179	↓ Uptake	–Neonatal RDS
(24)	(de novo)	(at 15 h)	(at 15 h)	(at 19 d)	(at 19 d)	Normal size	–Nl brain MRI
2	14q12-13.3	16	—	45.6	80	Normal	–RDS (at 10 yr)
(25)	(inherited)	(at 5 d)		(at 8 mo)	(at 8 mo)		–Cerebral atrophy
3	14q12-13.3	16	—	7.4	118	Not reported	–RDS (died at 3 yr)
(25)	(Patient 2's sister)	(at 5 d)	—	(at 1 yr)	(at 1 yr)		–Cerebral atrophy

no detectable thyroid gland epithelium at any location along the head and neck; not only are thyroid follicular cells absent, but C-cells cannot be detected either *(20)*; this contrasts with the situation observed in humans with athyreosis *(10)* and with *pax-8 –/–* mice (*see* below). In addition, these animals lack lung parenchyma, with only a rudimentary bronchial tree. Lastly, they have severe malformations of the forebrain and no anterior or posterior pituitary tissue. These findings are consistent with the expression pattern of *Ttf-1* in thyroid and lung, and the absence of anterior pituitary shows that "induction" by the adjacent *Ttf-1*-expressing infundibulum is required for the development of this tissue. In contrast to the complete absence of the thyroid, the adrenal glands are detectable, but atrophic most likely from lack of ACTH stimulation. Heterozygous *Ttf-1 +/-* mice are born and develop normally.

In 76 children with thyroid dysgenesis, no mutations in *TTF-1* were found *(22,23)*. Given the severity of the *Ttf-1 –/–* phenotype in mice, it is possible that *TTF-1* mutations in humans are lethal. On the other hand, three children (including two sisters) (*see* Table 1) with a combination of mild primary CH associated with a thyroid of normal size and location, severe respiratory distress (although occurring at various ages), and developmental delay (with or without cerebral atrophy) had a heterozygous deletion of the chromosomal region encompassing the *TTF-1* locus *(24,25)*. The deleted region (14q13-21 and 14q12-13.3, respectively) contains other developmental genes such as *PAX-9*, so the phenotype of these patients could be due in part to haploinsufficiency for genes other than *TTF-1*. Lastly, the appropriate elevations in plasma TSH in these children suggests that pituitary thyrotroph function is normal, which contrasts with the absence of pituitary of *Ttf-1 –/–* mice.

TTF-2 KNOCKOUT MICE
AND *TTF-2* MUTATIONS IN HUMANS

Unlike *Ttf-1 –/–* mice, *Ttf-2 –/–* mice are born alive but they die within 48 h, probably because of an inability to suckle due to a severe cleft lip and palate. Heterozygous *Ttf-2 +/–* mutants show no overt phenotype. Again, the cleft palate of homozygous *Ttf-2 –/–* animals is consistent with the expression pattern described earlier. The most interesting aspect of the thyroid phenotype of *Ttf-2 –/–* mice is that 50% of the litters have complete absence of thyroid tissue, while the other 50% have an ectopic gland in the sublingual region. This demonstration that a single molecular lesion can lead to either phenotype shows that multiple genetic or stochastic factors are involved in thyroid morphogenesis

Table 2
Athyreosis (A) and Thyroid Ectopy (E): Distinct Entities or Part of a Spectrum?

Distinct entities	References	Part of a spectrum	References
–Different sex ratios	(4)	–ttf-2 -/- mice: can have A or E	(26)
–TSHR inactivation can lead to A,		–Occurrence of A and E in	
not to E	(7)	same pedigree	(5)

(26). It is also the most convincing evidence that athyreosis and ectopy could be considered as part of a spectrum; however, there are other clinical and molecular arguments for considering athyreosis and ectopy separately; Table 2 summarizes these two contradictory lines of evidence.

In humans, Bamforth et al. (27) had described a syndrome of athyreosis, cleft palate, choanal atresia, bifid epiglottis, and kinky hair in two brothers from nonconsanguineous parents; the mother was euthyroid but had unilateral choanal atresia. Buntincx et al. (28) later reported a girl with a similar constellation of findings. In the boys initially reported by Bamforth et al. (27), a homozygous missense mutation at a highly conserved residue (Ala65Val) in TTF-2 was subsequently found. In vitro, this mutation results in normal nuclear expression of the mutant protein, but with a dramatic reduction of DNA binding and of transactivation of a reporter gene (29). In another child with athyreosis and cleft palate but with other malformations (dextrocardia and imperforated anus) and without kinky hair, Devos et al. (4) found a normal TTF-2 coding sequence. Although cleft palate is not common in children with thyroid dysgenesis, the prevalence and phenotypic spectrum of abnormalities in TTF-2 structure or function remain to be determined.

PAX-8 KNOCKOUT IN MICE
AND PAX-8 MUTATIONS IN HUMANS

The thyroids of newborn Pax-8 –/– mice are composed almost exclusively of C-cells and have a complete absence of follicular cells. In contrast to what one might have expected from the expression pattern of Pax-8, no renal anomaly is observed; this may be due to partially redundant functions of Pax-2 and Pax-5 in this organ. Consistent with the absence of thyroid follicular cells, growth retardation becomes apparent 1 wk after birth. Plasma T4 is greatly reduced at 2 wk and, unless rescued by thyroxine treatment, Pax-8 –/– mice die after weaning. Pax-8 +/- mice have no obvious phenotype, although their plasma TSH is more frequently elevated than in wild-type animals (30). In contrast, there is a thyroid phenotype with heterozygous PAX-8 mutations in humans.

In a series of 145 patients with thyroid dysgenesis, Macchia et al. (31) found three subjects with abnormal SSCP profiles. The heterozygous mutations found were de novo in two females and inherited from the mother in a brother and a sister. Another pedigree has been recently reported by Vilain et al. (21). The four different Pax-8 mutations and their phenotype are presented in Table 3. The patients described by Macchia et al. (31) had thyroid hypoplasia (but the fact that the gland was ectopic was specified in only one of the sporadic cases), or "cystic thyroid remnants." In the pedigree described by Vilain et al. (21), the daughter had an orthotopic gland and the mother had apparent athyreosis on technetium scan, but orthotopic hypoplasia with cystic rudiments on ultrasound. Pedigree

Table 3
Spectrum of Heterozygous PAX-8 Mutations in Humans

Mutation	Phenotype	References
Arg108STOP	Hypoplasia and ectopy, TSH 44.9 mUI/L at 20 d	(31)
Arg31His	Hypoplasia (location?), TSH > 200 mUI/L at 10 d	(31)
Arg62Leu	–Mother: hypoplasia, TSH not done, diagnosed at 10 yr	(31)
	–Son: severe hypoplasia w/cystic rudiment, TSH 167 mUI/L at 7 d	
	–Daughter: mild hypoplasia, TSH 176 mUI/L at 10 wk	
Cys57Tyr	–Daughter: ^{99m}Tc: orthotopic hypoplasia, TSH > 100 mUI/L at 32 d	(21)
	–Mother: ^{99m}Tc: no uptake (at 9 mo)	
	–U/S: orthotopic hypoplasia w/ cystic rudiments (at 23 yr)	

analysis was interpreted as suggestive of a dominant transmission with variable penetrance. A complete discussion of the possible reasons for the effect of heterozygous mutations in humans, which contrasts with the euthyroidism of *Pax-8* +/− mice, is beyond the scope of this review. It may be related to the difference between the inbred background of laboratory mice vs the genetic heterogeneity of human populations. Alternatively, it may be due to species differences in gene-dosage effects or in monoallelic expression *(21).*

INACTIVATION
OF THE TSH RECEPTOR IN MICE AND MEN

Several lines of evidence suggest that inactivation of the TSH receptor should not interfere with thyroid-gland differentiation and migration, but may result in hypoplasia of an orthotopic gland. First, expression of the TSH receptor by thyroid follicular cells only begins after the gland has reached its final position (reviewed in ref. *3*). Second, patients with severe congenital TSH deficiency or unresponsiveness always have an orthotopic gland, although the gland may be so small and hypoactive that it may be missed on echographic or even on nuclear medicine studies. The most convincing demonstration of this stems from the observation of a severely hypothyroid infant who was later found to have a mutation inactivating beta-TSH and who had no detectable technetium uptake in the basal state; however, after stimulation with exogenous TSH, the gland was of normal shape and in the normal position, albeit small *(32).*

On the other hand, the concept that unresponsiveness to TSH could result in congenital hypothyroidism was proposed by Stanbury et al. in 1968 *(33)* on the basis of the observation of a severely hypothyroid child without goiter or thyroiditis whose thyroid failed to respond to TSH in vivo or in vitro. In 1994, Stein et al. *(34)* reported that the congenital hypothyroidism of the *hyt/hyt* mouse, a naturally occurring mutant, was due to a homozygous mutation inactivating the TSH receptor. These mice have small orthotopic thyroids, with a disorganized follicular architecture. In 1995, Sunthornthepvarakul et al. *(35)* reported the first description of mutations inactivating the TSH receptor in humans. The phenotype of these three affected sisters was relatively mild, with high plasma TSH but normal plasma thyroxine and no signs and symptoms of hypothyroidism. Four families with five similarly affected patients were described in 1996 by De Roux et al. *(36).* Subsequently however, three pedigrees with severe TSH resistance and apparent athyreosis

Table 4
Spectrum of Mutations Inactivating TSHR in Humans

	High TSH, Normal T4 (Refs.)	High TSH, Low T4 (Refs.)	"Apparent athyreosis" (Refs.)	Total
Compound heterozygotes	I167D/P162A (35)	C390W/ Frameshift (39)	G>C+3IVS6 /delAC655 (7)	7
	Q324stop/D410N (36)	R109Q/ W546stop (40)		
	C41S/F525L (36)			
	C390W/W546stop (36)			
Homozygotes	P162A (36)	T477I (41)	A553T (37) R609stop (38)	4
Total	5	3	3	11

(no technetium uptake, but normal plasma thyroglobulin concentrations and definitive presence of small thyroid lobes on ultrasound) were reported (7,37,38). In other pedigrees still, the phenotype is intermediate with overt hypothyroidism but detectable thyroid tissue on imaging (39–41). In all reported pedigrees with TSH resistance from mutations inactivating TSHR, the inheritance pattern is autosomal recessive and the majority of patients are compound heterozygotes (Table 4). This suggests that a heterozygous state for *TSHR* mutations may be relatively common. This autosomal recessive pattern contrasts with the dominant transmission of non-TSHR related TSH resistance, a generally mild phenotype that has not been reported to present with apparent athyreosis (42).

OTHER CANDIDATE GENES, MOLECULAR INTERACTIONS, AND ANATOMIC VARIANTS

Aside from *TTF-1*, *TTF-2*, *PAX-8*, and *TSHR*, it is likely that mutations in other genes will be found to be responsible for some cases of thyroid dysgenesis. Apparent athyreosis may occur as the result of an inactivating mutation in *NIS*, in which isotope studies will show no uptake and which may present without goiter (43). The spectrum of thyroid dysgenesis should be expanded to include agenesis of one of the thyroid lobes, most often on the left ("hemiagenesis"). This condition, which is found on routine ultrasound in 1 in 500 normal children (44), has been reported in siblings (45,46), in mothers (47), and in the monozygotic twin (48) of patients with thyroid ectopies. Thyroid hemiagenesis is part of the phenotype of *Hoxa3* mice (49) and may be observed in the Di George syndrome (50).

Thyroid dysgenesis is associated with a five-fold increase in incidence of atrial or ventricular septal defects (4). While this may result from an environmental insult occurring during wk 5–7 of embryonic life (the time during which migration of the thyroid and septation of the heart occur), it may also indicate that genes involved in both thyroid and heart development are involved. Dominant transmission of septation defects due to mutations in *NKX 2.5* have been described (51); while the affected patients were not reported to have a thyroid phenotype, it is noteworthy that *NKX 2.5* is homologous to *TTF-1*.

Because of the different sex ratios we found in ectopies and athyreoses, we have proposed the following multistep mechanism: if a molecular event arresting thyroid-cell

Table 5
Mutations, Knockouts, and Thyroid Dysgenesis in Mice and Humans

	Mice (Refs.)	*Humans (Refs.)*
ttf-1/TTF-1	Athyreosis (+ absence of C-cells) (recessive, homozygote) *(20)*	Deletion? (Heterozygote) *(24,25)*
ttf-2/TTF-2	Athyreosis or ectopy +Cleft palate (Recessive, homozygote) *(26)*	Athyreosis +Cleft palate +Kinky hair (Recessive, homozygote) (29)
pax-8/PAX-8	Athyreosis (c-cells present)–ectopic (Recessive, homozygote) *(30)*	–Hypoplasia –Orthotopic –Cystic rudiments (Dominant, heterozygous) (*see* Table 3)
tshr/TSHR	Orthotopic hypoplasia (Recessive, homozygote) *(34)*	–Normal gland –Orthotopic hypoplasia –Apparent athyreosis (*see* Table 4)

migration occurs with equal frequency in male and female embryos, but the ectopic cells are more prone to disappear (through apoptosis or other mechanisms) in male fetuses, then there would be a predominance of females with ectopies, but not athyreosis, at birth *(4)*. After birth, however, it appears that the survival of ectopic thyroid cells is normal *(17,18)*.

Because the vast majority of patients with thyroid dysgenesis have not been found to harbor mutations in the coding sequences of the genes discussed earlier, it may be that they have polymorphisms that, in isolation, have no consequences, but that, in certain combinations, result in thyroid dysgenesis. Some evidence for polygenic transmission has recently been reported *(52)*. Along the same line, cross-breeding experiments of mice heterozygous for *Ttf-1*, *Ttf-2*, and *Pax-8* knock-outs, to explore this concept of gene team interactions, are underway.

EVIDENCE FOR AND AGAINST
GENETIC TRANSMISSION OF THYROID DYSGENESIS

Aside from scattered case reports of familial occurrence *(45,46,53,54)*, including in two daughters of consanguineous parents *(55)*, thyroid dysgenesis has always been considered as a sporadic entity. Because of the mental deficiency that was commonly seen before the era of neonatal screening for CH 15–25 yr ago, some have argued that thyroid dysgenesis was only apparently sporadic because of decreased reproductive fitness of affected CH individuals in earlier generations *(31)*. In the pre-screening era, 60% of CH patients had an IQ above 70 *(56)* and whether this would in itself result in a reduced rate of reproduction is controversial *(57)*. Recently, Castanet et al. *(5)* undertook a systematic reassessment of the heritability of thyroid dysgenesis. In a survey by questionnaire of pediatricians caring for CH patients with thyroid dysgenesis in France, they found that 2% of cases had an affected relative. This is 15 times higher than what would be expected by chance alone.

Pedigree analysis showed different patterns with affected siblings, parents, or distant relatives. The authors considered that their findings were most compatible with autosomal dominant transmission and variable penetrance.

While the aforementioned is strongly suggestive of a genetic component in a few percent of cases of thyroid dysgenesis, the fact remains that the vast majority of cases appear truly sporadic. Another argument against genetic transmission stems from observations in monozygotic twins: the vast majority of the reported pairs are discordant for thyroid dysgenesis, including the three most recently studied in whom monozygosity had been established at the DNA level by analysis of microsatellite markers *(58;* and our own unpublished observations).

CONCLUSION

Considerable progress in our understanding of the molecular mechanisms of thyroid-gland development has been made over the last few years through knockout experiments and through the careful identification and phenotypic characterization of naturally occurring mutations. However, a great many questions remain unanswered. Thyroid dysgenesis is a heterogeneous condition, with clinical and molecular evidence that athyreosis and ectopy should be considered separately; thus, the sex ratio in athyreosis would be compatible with autosomal recessive mechanisms, whereas the clear predominance of females in ectopy is not compatible with simple dominant transmision. On the other hand, some molecular lesions can give rise to both phenotypes (as in *Ttf-2* knockout mice), but some other lesions (i.e., inactivation of *TSHR*) can only lead to apparent athyreosis. Single gene defects may ultimately be identified in some cases while polygenic inheritance will be documented in others. In the vast majority, epigenetic mechanisms, somatic mutations occurring early in embryogenesis or postzygotic stochastic events are likely responsible for thyroid dysgenesis *(59).*

ACKNOWLEDGMENTS

Research on pediatric thyroid diseases at the Sainte-Justine Hospital is supported by its Research Center and by the Blouin-MacBain Foundation. I would like to thank Drs. Jean-Pierre Chanoine, Samuel Refetoff, and Gilbert Vassart for helpful discussions.

REFERENCES

1. Refetoff S. How clinical observations of a congenital disease can be translated in molecular biology terms. In: Querido A, van Es LA, Mandema E, eds. The Discipline of Medicine: Emerging Concepts and Their Impact Upon Medical Research and Medical Education. Elsevier Science Publishers b.v., Amsterdam, 1994, pp. 43–54.
2. Damante G, Tell G, Di Lauro R. A unique combination of transcription factors controls differentiation of thyroid cells. Prog Nucleic Acid Res Mol Biol 2000;66:307–356.
3. Macchia PE. Recent advances in understanding the molecular basis of primary congenital hypothyroidism. Mol Med Today 2000;6:36–42.
4. Devos H, Rodd C, Gagné N, Laframboise R, Van Vliet G. A search for the possible molecular mechanisms of thyroid dysgenesis: sex ratios and associated malformations. J Clin Endocrinol Metab 1999;84: 2502–2506.
5. Castanet M, Lyonnet S, Bonaïti-Pellié C, Polak M, Czernichow P, Léger J. Familial forms of thyroid dysgenesis among infants with congenital hypothyroidism. N Engl J Med 2000a;343:441–442.
6. Refetoff S, Dumont JE, Vassart G. Thyroid disorders. In: Scriver CR, Beaudet AL, Sly WS, Valle D, eds. The Metabolic and Molecular Basis of Inherited Disease, 8th ed. McGraw-Hill, New York, 2001, pp. 4029–4076.

7. Gagné N, Parma J, Deal C, Vassart G, Van Vliet G. Apparent athyreosis contrasting with normal plasma thyroglobulin levels and associated with mutations in the thyrotropin receptor gene. are athyreosis and ectopic thyroid distinct entities? J Clin Endocrinol Metab 1998;83:1771–1775.

8. Mitchell ML, Hermos RJ. Measurement of thyroglobulin in newborn screening specimens from normal and hypothyroid infants. Clin Endocrinol 1995;42:523–527.

9. Van Vliet G. Neonatal hypothyroidism: treatment and outcome. Thyroid 1999;9:79–84.37.

10. Chanoine JP, Toppet V, Body JJ, Van Vliet G, Lagasse R, Bourdoux P, et al. Contribution of thyroid ultrasound and serum calcitonin to the diagnosis of congenital hypothyroidism. J Endocrinol Invest 1990;13:97–102.

11. Gillis D, Brjnac L, Perlman K, Sochett EB, Daneman D. Frequency and characteristics of lingual thyroid not detected by screening. J Pediatr Endocrinol Metab 1998;11:229–233.

12. Wick MR. Mediastinal cysts and intrathoracic thyroid tumors. Sem Diagn Pathol 1990;7:285–294.

13. Pintar JE. Normal development of the hypothalamic-pituitary-thyroid axis. In: Braverman LE, Utiger RD, eds. Werner and Ingbar's The Thyroid, 8th ed. Lippincott Williams & Wilkins, Philadelphia, PA, 2000, pp. 7–19.

14. Sauk JJ. Ectopic lingual thyroid. J Path 1970;102:239–243.

15. Kumar R, Gupta R, Bal CS, Khullar S, Malhotra A. Thyrotoxicosis in a patient with submandibular thyroid. Thyroid 2000;10:363–365.

16. Williams ED, Toyn CE, Harach HR. The ultimobranchial body and congenital thyroid abnormalities in man. J Pathol 1989;159:135–141.

16a. Zink A, Raue F, Hoffmann R, Ziegler R. Papillary carcinoma in an ectopic thyroid. Horm Res 1991;35: 86–88.

17. Grant DB, Hulse JA, Jackson DB, Leung SP, Ng WK. Ectopic thyroid: residual function after withdrawal of treatment in infancy and later childhood. Acta Paediatr Scand 1989;78:889–892.

18. Léger J, Czernichow P. Secretion of hormones by ectopic thyroid glands after prolonged thyroxine therapy. J Pediatr 1990;116:111–114.

19. Capen CC. Anatomy. In: Braverman LE, Utiger RD, eds. Werner and Ingbar's The Thyroid, 8th ed. Lippincott Williams & Wilkins, Philadelphia, PA, 2000, pp. 20–43.

20. Kimura S, Hara Y, Pineau T, et al. The T/ebp null mouse: thyroid-specific enhancer-binding protein is essential for the organogenesis of the thyroid, lung, ventral forebrain and pituitary. Genes Dev 1996;10: 60–69.

21. Vilain C, Rydlewski C, Duprez L, et al. Autosomal dominant transmission of congenital thyroid hypoplasia due to a loss-of-function mutation of PAX8. J Clin Endocrinol Metab 2001;86:234–238.

22. Lapi P, Macchia PE, Chiovato L, et al. Mutations in the gene encoding thyroid transcription factor-1 (TTF-1) are not a frequent cause of congenital hypothyroidism (CH) with thyroid dysgenesis. Thyroid 1997;7:383–387.

23. Perna MG, Civitareale D, De Filippis V, Sacco M, Cisternino C, Tassi V. Absence of mutations in TTF-1 gene in patients with thyroid dysgenesis. Thyroid 1997;7:377–381.

24. Devriendt K, Vanhole C, Matthijs G, de Zegher F. Deletion of thyroid transcription factor 1 gene in an infant with neonatal thyroid dysfunction and respiratory failure (letter). N Engl J Med 1998;338: 1317–1318.

25. Iwatani N, Mabe H, Devriendt K, Kodama M, Miike T. Deletion of NKX2.1. gene encoding thyroid transcription factor-1 in two siblings with hypothyroidism and respiratory failure. J Pediatr 2000;137:272–276.

26. De Felice M, Ovitt C, Biffali E, et al. A mouse model for hereditary thyroid dysgenesis and cleft palate. Nature Genet 1998;19:395–398.

27. Bamforth JS, Hughes IA, Lazarus JH, Weaver CM, Harper PS. Congenital hypothyroidism, spiky hair, and cleft palate. J Med Genet 1989;26:49–60.

28. Buntincx IM, Van Overmeire B, Desager K, Van Hauwaert J. Syndromic association of cleft palate, bilateral choanal atresia, curly hair, and congenital hypothyroidism. J Med Genet 1993;30:427–428.

29. Clifton-Bligh RJ, Wentworth JM, Heinz P, et al. Mutation of the gene encoding human TTF-2 associated with thyroid agenesis, cleft palate and choanal atresia. Nature Genet 1998;19:399–401.

30. Mansouri A, Chowdhury K, Gruss P. Follicular cells of the thyroid gland require Pax8 gene function. Nature Genet 1998;19:87–90.

31. Macchia PE, Lapi P, Krude H, et al. PAX8 mutations associated with congenital hypothyroidism caused by thyroid dysgenesis. Nature Genet 1998;19:83–86.

32. Heinrichs C, Parma J, Scherberg NH, et al. Congenital central isolated hypothyroidism caused by abnormal TSH due to a homozygous mutation in the TSH-beta subunit gene. Thyroid 2000;10:387–391.

33. Stanbury JB, Rocmans P, Buhler UK, Ochi Y. Congenital hypothyroidism with impaired thyroid response to thyrotropin. N Engl J Med 1968;279:1132–1136.
34. Stein SA, Oates EL, Hall CR, et al. Identification of a point mutation in the thyrotropin receptor of the hyt/hyt hypothyroid mouse. Mol Endocrinol 1994;8:129–138.
35. Sunthornthepvarakul T, Gottschalk M, Hayashi Y, Refetoff S. Brief Report: resistance to thyrotropin caused by mutations in the thyrotropin-receptor gene. N Engl J Med 1995;332:155–160.
36. De Roux N, Misrahi R, Brauner R, et al. Four families with loss-of-function mutations of the thyrotropin receptor. J Clin Endocrinol Metab 1996;81:4229–4235.
37. Abramovicz MJ, Duprez L, Parma J, Vassart G, Heinrichs C. Familial congenital hypothyroidism due to inactivating mutation of the thyrotropin receptor causing profound hypoplasia of the thyroid gland. J Clin Invest 1997a;99:3018–3024.
38. Tiosano D, Pannain S, Vassart G, et al. Hypothyroidism in an inbred kindred with congenital thyroid hormone and glucocorticoid deficiency is due to a mutation producing a truncated thyrotropin receptor. Thyroid 1999;9:887–894.
39. Biebermann H, Schöneberg T, Krude H, Schultz G, Gudermann T, Grüters A. Mutations of the human thyrotropin receptor gene causing thyroid hypoplasia and persistent congenital hypothyroidism. J Clin Endocrinol Metab 1997;82:3471–3480.
40. Clifton-Bligh RJ, Gregory JW, Ludgate M, et al. Two novel mutations in the thyrotropin (TSH) receptor gene in a child with resistance to TSH. J Clin Endocrinol Metab 1997;82:1094–1100.
41. Tonacchera M, Agretti P, Pinchera A, et al. Congenital hypothyroidism with impaired thyroid response to thyrotropin (TSH) and absent circulating thyroglobulin: evidence for a new inactivating mutation of the TSH receptor gene. J Clin Endocrinol Metab 2000;85:1001–1008.
42. Xie J, Pannain S, Pohlenz J, et al. Resistance to thyrotropin (TSH) in three families is not associated with mutations in the TSH receptor or TSH. J Clin Endocrinol Metab 1997;82:3933–3940.
43. Kosugi S, Bhanaya S, Dean HJ. A novel mutation in the sodium/iodide symporter gene in the largest family with iodide transport defect. J Clin Endocrinol Metab 1999;84:3248–3253.
44. Shabana W, Delange F, Freson M, Osteaux M, De Schepper J. Prevalence of thyroid hemiagenesis: ultrasound screening in normal children. Eur J Pediatr 2000;159:456–458.
45. Orti E, Castells S, Qazi QH, Inamdar S. Familial thyroid disease: lingual thyroid in two siblings and hypoplasia of a thyroid lobe in a third. J Pediatr 1971;78:675–677.
46. Rosenberg T, Gilboa Y. Familial thyroid ectopy and hemiagenesis. Arch Dis Childhood 1980;55:639–641.
47. Cassio A, Cacciari E, Bal M, Colli C. Thyroid morphological findings in the mothers of infants with congenital hypothyroidism. Arch Dis Childhood 1997;77:185.
48. McLean R, Howard N, Murray IPC. Thyroid dysgenesis in monozygotic twins: variants identified by scintigraphy. Eur J Nucl Med 1985;10:346–348.
49. Manley NR, Capecchi MR. *Hox* Group 3 paralogs regulate the development and migration of the thymus, thyroid and parathyroid glands. Dev Biol 1998;195:1–15.
50. Scuccimari R, Rodd C. Thyroid abnormalities as a feature of Di George syndrome: a patient report and review of the literature. J Pediatr Endocrinol Metab 1998;11:273–276.
51. Schott JJ, Benson DW, Basson CT, et al. Congenital heart disease caused by mutations in the transcription factor *NKX2.5*. Science 1998;281:108–111.
52. Castanet M, Léger J, Lyonnet S, Pelet A, Czernichow P, Polak M. Linkage analysis of two candidate genes in familial thyroid dysgenesis. Horm Res 2000b;53(Suppl 2):10 (abstract).
53. Kaplan M, Kauli R, Raviv U, Lubin E, Laron Z. Hypothyroidism due to ectopy in siblings. Am J Dis Child 1977;131:1264–1265.
54. Goujard J, Safar A, Rolland A, Job JC. Épidémiologie des hypothyroïdies congénitales malformatives. Arch Fr Pédiatr 1981;38:875–879.
55. El-Desouki MI, Al-Herbish AS, Al-Juryyan NA. Familial occurrence of hypothyroidism due to a lingual thyroid. Clin Nuc Med 1999;24:421–423.
56. Klein RZ, Mitchell ML. Neonatal screening. In: Braverman LE, Utiger RD, eds. Werner and Ingbar's The Thyroid, 8th ed. Lippincott Williams & Wilkins, Philadelphia, PA, 2000, pp. 973–977.
57. Herrnstein RJ, Murray C. The Bell Curve. Intelligence and Class Structure in American Life. Simon and Schuster, New York, 1994.
58. Bargagna S, Chiovato L, Dinetti D, et al. Neuropsychological development in a child with early-treated congenital hypothyroidism as compared with her unaffected identical twin. Eur J Endocrinol 1997;136:100–104.
59. Abramowicz MJ, Vassart G, Refetoff S. Probing the cause of thyroid dysgenesis. Thyroid 1997b;7:325–326.

6   Fetal-Perinatal Thyroid Physiology

Delbert A. Fisher, MD

CONTENTS

INTRODUCTION
ROLE OF THE PLACENTA
HYPOTHALAMIC-PITUITARY-THYROID EMBRYOGENESIS
MATURATION OF THYROID FUNCTION
THYROID HORMONE METABOLISM
THYROID HORMONE ACTIONS
NEONATAL ADAPTATION
REFERENCES

INTRODUCTION

Many of the hormones important for normal growth and development during childhood are of limited significance for fetal growth and maturation. Until recent years, thyroid hormones were included in this category, but it is now clear that thyroid hormones, while having little impact on fetal growth, have an important role in fetal central nervous system (CNS) maturation *(1)*. Iodine deficiency, genetic, or autoimmune disorders associated with combined maternal and fetal hypothyroidism leads to cretinism and mental deficiency of the offspring *(2–4)*. Mild subclinical maternal hypothyroidism due to autoimmune thyroid disease also has been associated with reduced IQ of offspring with or without transient neonatal hypothyroidism *(5)*. The precise timing and the mechanism(s) of the thyroid hormone effect(s) on CNS maturation remain unclear. Much of our information regarding ontogenesis of the hypothalamic-pituitary-thyroid system has been developed in the rodent and ovine species in which the timing of parturition relative to the events of CNS maturation differ. The rodent is an altricial species in which CNS maturation is a predominantly postnatal event; the ovine precocial species delivers relatively mature neonates capable of homeothermy and early mobility. Relative CNS maturation in the human newborn is more advanced than in rodents and less advanced than in ovine neonates. Nonetheless, the similarities of thyroid system ontogenesis in these and the human species have provided important insights and understanding and have allowed detailed characterization of fetal and perinatal thyroid physiology.

From: *Contemporary Endocrinology: Developmental Endocrinology: From Research to Clinical Practice*
Edited by: E. A. Eugster and O. H. Pescovitz © Humana Press Inc., Totowa, NJ

ROLE OF THE PLACENTA

Fetal development is dependent on the placenta, which serves nutritive, excretory, and endocrine-metabolic roles. With regard to thyroid function, the placenta provides a relative barrier between the maternal and fetal systems *(1)*. The mammalian placenta is freely permeable to iodide, relatively impermeable to thyroid hormones, and impermeable to thyroid-stimulating hormone (TSH). Placental tissue is endowed with a mixture of type II and type III iodothyronine monodeiodinases (MDI); the type II MDI deiodinates thyroxine (T4) to active triiodothyronine (T3) while the type III MDI deiodinates T3 to inactive diiodothyronine (T2) and T4 to inactive reverse triiodothyronine (rT3). Placental T4 to T3 conversion may be important for local paracrine action of T3, but the net effect of inherent placental membrane characteristics and the MDI activities is to limit access of most bioactive maternal T4 and T3 to the fetal compartment. Placental iodothyronine monodeiodination also serves to provide a supplemental source of iodide for fetal thyroid hormone synthesis. Thyroxine monodeiodination in human placental tissue is incomplete, however, and significant maternal to fetal transport of intact T4 has been documented both early (6–11 wk) in gestation, prior to the onset of fetal thyroid function, and at term *(6)*. Precise quantification of maternal to fetal transport has not been possible, but at term in the athyroid human fetus, the average cord serum T4 concentration approximates 4 µg/dL (50 nmol/L), whereas the normal mean level is about 11 µg/dL (140 nmol/L) *(7)*.

The placenta also is permeable to thyrotropin-releasing hormone (TRH), but maternal serum TRH concentrations are very low and little, if any, maternal TRH reaches the fetus. However, placental tissue produces TRH in significant quantities as does fetal gastrointestinal tissue, especially pancreas *(8,9)*. Additionally, TRH degrading activity in fetal serum is low or absent in contrast to maternal or postnatal serum so that fetal serum TRH concentrations are relatively high *(9)*. The significance of the fetal extrahypothalamic TRH production remains unclear, but a contributory effect to maintenance of the relatively high TSH levels in fetal serum during the third trimester has been postulated. Additionally, the large amounts of chorionic gonadotropin (hCG) produced by the placenta, with peak blood levels at the end of the first trimester, have inherent, low level (0.06%) TSH bioactivity, which transiently increases maternal serum free T4 and decreases TSH concentrations at this time *(10,11)*. These maternal changes usually are minimal however; serum free T4 and TSH remain within the normal range and there is little influence of hCG on fetal thyroid function.

HYPOTHALAMIC-PITUITARY-THYROID EMBRYOGENESIS

The human fetal forebrain and hypothalamus begin to differentiate by 3 wk of gestation *(12)*. The hypothalamic nuclei, median eminence, and supraoptic tract are identifiable by 15–18 wk and significant concentrations of TRH and dopamine are detectable at this time. The anterior pituitary hormones, including TSH, can be identified in serum during the second trimester and concentrations increase progressively from midgestation to term. Forebrain and hypothalamic development are dependent on a series of homeodomain proteins or transcription factors (Fig. 1). Mutations of one of three homeobox genes, sonic hedgehog (SHH), SIX-3, and ZIC-2 have been identified in familial and sporadic holoprosencephaly *(13–15)*. HESX-1 homeobox gene mutations have been described in siblings with septo-optic dysplasia involving midline brain defects and pituitary hypoplasia *(16)*.

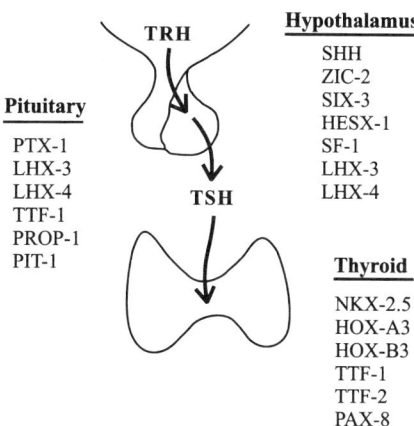

Fig. 1. Genetic factors associated with hypothalamic-pituitary-thyroid maturation. See text for details.

Other homeodomain genes involved in hypothalamic development in the rodent include SF-1, LHX-3, and LHX-4; the latter are LIM class homeodomain factors *(17)*.

Anatomically, the pituitary gland develops from two anlagen: 1) an evagination of the floor of the primitive forebrain; and 2) Rathke's pouch, a ventral pouch from the ectoderm of the primitive oral cavity. The latter is visible by 5 wk, evolving to a morphologically mature pituitary gland by 14–15 wk. The pituitary-portal blood vessels are present by this time and further mature through 30–35 wk *(12)*. In rodent models the Rathke's pouch gene and pituitary homeobox (PTX-1) gene are early factors in a cascade of determinants programming pituitary embryogenesis *(17)* (Fig. 1). Later factors in the cascade include TTF-1, LHX-3, LHX-4, Prop-1, and Pit-1 *(12,17,18)*. TTF-1 knockout leads to pituitary gland as well as thyroid aplasia. LHX-3 and LHX-4 also are essential for normal pituitary embryogenesis. Prop-1 and Pit-1 are terminal factors in the cascade, programming development and function of pituitary cells producing growth hormone, prolactin, TSHβ, and the growth hormone-releasing hormone (GHRH) receptors *(12,18)*. Mutations of Prop-1 or Pit-1 have been described in patients with familial hypopituitarism *(12)*.

Thyroid gland embryogenesis begins at 2–3 wk gestation as a medial outpouching from the floor of the primitive pharynx *(19)*. This precursor of the thyroid hormone-producing follicular cells descends and merges with bilateral evaginations of the fourth pharyngeal pouches, which give rise to the parafollicular calcitonin-secreting C cells. Thyroid-gland embryogenesis and descent into the anterior neck are largely complete by 10–12 wk gestation, at which time tiny follicle precursors, iodine uptake, TSH receptors, and thyroglobulin and thyroid peroxidase mRNA and protein can be demonstrated. Thyroid hormonogenesis is detected by 11–12 wk coincident with the appearance of TSH in the fetal circulation. Thyroid embryogenesis in the rodent is dependent on production of a programmed sequence of homeobox and transcription factors, including thyroid transcription factors 1 and 2 (TTF-1, TTF-2) and PAX-8 *(20–25)* (Fig. 1). NKX-2.5 appears to play a role in regulation of TTF-1, and HOX-A3 and HOX-B3 are important in expression of TTF-1 and PAX-8 *(26–28)*. Targeted disruption of TTF-1 in mice leads to thyroid-gland aplasia *(29)*. PAX-8 gene disruption results in a small thyroid gland composed almost exclusively of C cells *(25)*. TTF-2 null mice manifest thyroid aplasia or an ectopic, sublingual thyroid gland *(30)*. Mutations in these genes, however, account for less than 5% of human thyroid dysgenesis *(24)*.

MATURATION OF THYROID FUNCTION

The secretion of TSH and thyroid hormones is limited until midgestation, at which time fetal thyroid iodine uptake and serum T4 concentrations begin to increase (31–33). Serum TSH levels increase progressively from low values at 16–18 wk to concentrations at term approximating 10 mU/L. Total T4 levels increase to levels approximating 10 µg/dL (129 nmol/L) at term (34). This increase in serum total T4 concentration is due largely to increasing serum thyroxine binding globulin (TBG) concentrations as hepatic TBG synthesis and secretion mature to plateau levels at 35–36 wk gestation. However, free T4 concentrations also increase progressively during the latter half of gestation, reaching values of 1.0–1.5 ng/dL (13–19 pmol/L) at term, indicative of a progressive increase in fetal thyroid T4 secretion in response to the increasing serum TSH concentrations (35).

Negative feedback control of TSH secretion is observed as early as 20 wk gestation, but maturation of pituitary thyroid regulation is a prolonged and complex process involving hypothalamic TRH secretion, pituitary thyrotroph-cell TRH receptors, thyrotroph nuclear T3 receptors and pituitary T4 MDI activity for T4 to T3 conversion (35). The net result of these maturational events is a progressive maturation of the fetal serum free T4/TSH ratio from 15.0 at midgestation to 4.7 at term and 2.9 at 2–3 mo of age (34). The progressive increase in fetal serum free T4 concentration during the latter half of gestation in the fetal sheep model appears to be due both to increasing fetal serum TSH and to progressive maturation of thyroid follicular-cell TSH responsiveness (36). Whether the latter is due to increasing TSH receptor number of postreceptor responsiveness is not clear.

Thyroid-gland maturation also includes development of the thyroid follicular-cell capacity to autoregulate iodine uptake, independent of serum TSH levels. This autoregulatory mechanism is mediated via the follicular-cell membrane sodium/iodine symporter protein (37,38). In the mature gland, the thyroid follicular-cell iodide-uptake rate increases progressively as serum iodide levels decrease. This capacity develops progressively in the fetal gland, presumably due to maturation of factors modulating cell-membrane symporter number and/or function. The response of thyroid follicular cells to increased iodide concentrations, in addition to reduced iodide-symporter transport, includes decreased thyroglobulin iodination and turnover (39,40). Immaturity of thyroid autoregulation by the fetal thyroid follicular cell predisposes to iodine-induced blockade of thyroid function, and there are many reports of iodine or iodine-containing compounds, such as radiographic contrast agents, producing transient hypothyroidism in the human fetus and neonate (41).

THYROID HORMONE METABOLISM

Thyroid hormones undergo several types of biochemical transformation in tissues (1,42). These include deiodination (to T3 or rT3 and subsequently to T2, T1, and T0), side-chain modifications (from an alanine moiety to thyroacetic or thyropropionic acid), and sulfate or glucuronide conjugation. Sequential monodeiodination is the most important pathway, and all of these modifications except T4 to T3 conversion lead to hormone inactivation. Characteristics and localization of the monodeiodinase enzymes (MDI-1, MDI-II, and MDI-III) are shown in Table 1 (1,42). MDI-I predominantly expressed in liver, kidney, and thyroid tissues is the major factor regulating serum active T3 concentrations in the adult. MDI-II activity, located predominantly in brain, pituitary, brown adipose tissue, keratinocytes, and placenta regulates T3 production in these adult tissues and is impor-

Table 1
Iodothyronine Monodeiodinase Enzymes

Enzyme	Major issue	Preferred substrates	Products
Type I	Liver, kidney, thyroid	rT3, T4, T2S, rT3S	T2, T3, T1S, T2S
Type II	Brain, pituitary, brown adipose tissue keratinocytes, placenta	T4S, T3S, T4, rT3	rT3S, T2S, T3, T2
Type III	Placenta, brain, epidermis	T4, T3	RT3, T2

tant in pituitary T4 feedback modulation of TSH secretion and brown adipose tissue thermogenesis. MDI-III, present in most adult tissues, functions largely to inactivate thyroid hormones via inner ring monodeiodination of T4 to reverse T3 and T3 to T2.

Fetal thyroid hormone metabolism is characterized by relatively low liver and kidney MDI-I, active placental, liver, brain, and skin MDI-III, and significant MDI-II activities in brain and placenta *(1,43–45)*. Studies in fetal rodents and sheep have shown MDI-III activity, predominantly in placenta and fetal membranes, accounting for the high concentrations of rT3 in fetal serum and amniotic fluid *(1,43)*. Human fetal serum T3 concentrations are low or undetectable until 28–30 wk gestation, due to low MDI-I activity prior to 25–30 wk and active T3 deiodination to T2 by MDI-III in the placenta *(1,46)*. MDI-II activity is present early in fetal brain and matures progressively in brown adipose tissue and probably pituitary during the latter half of gestation. MDI-II activity increases in response to hypothyroxinemia, and it has been shown in rodents that brain T3 levels are maintained in the hypothyroid fetus by increased brain MDI-II activity, providing protection from the damaging effects of hypothyroxinemia *(47)*.

Sulfation of the iodothyronines due to sulfotransferase activities in liver and other tissues is a normal process, particularly in liver, but the iodothyronine sulfates are preferred substrates for MDI-I and facilitate monodeiodinative deactivation of thyroid hormones *(42)*. As a result, levels of iodothyronine sulfates in adult serum are low. In fetal serum, in contrast, concentrations of iodothyronine sulfates are high, and plasma production rate studies in fetal sheep have shown that these sulfates are the predominant thyroid hormone metabolites *(48)*. This appears to be due both to high tissue sulfotransferase and low MDI-I enzyme activities *(43,46,48)*. Thus, fetal thyroid hormone metabolism is characterized by predominant inactivation of hormone activity. Plasma production rates for rT3, T4S, rT3S, and T3S in near-term fetal sheep average 5,10,12, and 2 (total 29) µg/kg/d, whereas T4 and T3 production average 40 and 2 µg/kg/d, respectively *(48)*. Thus, fetal production of inactive metabolites (29 µg/kg/d) greatly exceeds production of active T3 (2 µg/kg/d). The pattern of change in fetal and neonatal T4, T4S. T3, T3S, and rT3 concentrations is shown in Fig. 2.

THYROID HORMONE ACTIONS

Thyroid hormone effects are mediated predominantly via nuclear thyroid hormone protein receptors (TR), which act as DNA binding transcription factors regulating gene transcription. There are two mammalian genes that code for TR, TRα, and TRβ, and alternative splicing of expressed mRNA species leads to production of several TR isoforms *(49–51)*. The major isoforms, TRα1, TRα2, TRβ1, and TRβ2, are developmentally regulated and

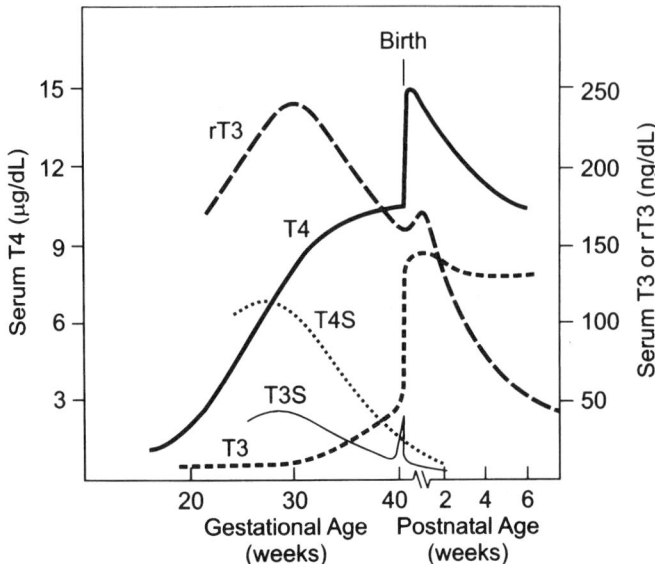

Fig. 2. Maturation of thyroid hormone metabolism in the fetal-neonatal period. Serum T4 levels increase progressively during the latter half of gestation due to increasing serum thyroxine binding globulin concentrations and increased T4 secretion. Fetal serum rT3 levels peak at 30 wk and fall thereafter while serum T3 concentrations increase after 30 wk. These changes are due to decreasing iodothyronine monodeiodinase (MDI) type III and increasing type I activities in placenta and fetal tissues. The levels of sulfated metabolites shown here as T4S and T3S tend to parallel fetal serum rT3 levels. The TSH surge peaking 30 minutes after birth (not shown) stimulates thyroid T4 and T3 secretion and neonatal T4 and T3 concentrations peak at 3–4 d of age. Postnatal serum T3 levels remain relatively high due to increased MDI-I activity. Reverse T3 (rT3) levels fall progressively to postnatal values due to placental separation and decreasing MDI-III activity.

are present in varying concentrations ratios in adult tissues *(49–51)*. In rodent species, hepatic TR binding activity matures during the first 3–5 wk of extrauterine life, a period roughly equivalent to the last trimester of human fetal development *(2,51)*. TR binding in brain and pituitary cells appears earlier; TRα isoforms are present in these tissues during fetal life while TRβ isoforms appear during the early neonatal period. In the fetal/neonatal rat, thyroid hormone effects on thermogenesis, hepatic enzyme activities, skin and brain maturation, and growth hormone (GH) metabolism mature predominantly during the first 4 postnatal wk *(2,52)*.

In fetal sheep, maturation of most thyroid hormone actions occurs in utero and during the perinatal period *(52)*. TR binding develops during the latter two-thirds of gestation. Brain TR are present at midgestation and decrease in number during the first 2–3 postnatal mo. Hepatic TR mature during the last trimester. Thyroid hormone actions on brain maturation, carcass and bone growth, skin maturation, hair growth, and TSH secretion appear near midgestation. Effects on cardiac atrial natriuretic hormone and cardiac output appear near term. Effects on cardiac and lung adrenergic receptors and hepatic epidermal growth-factor receptors appear during the neonatal period *(43,52)*.

In the human fetus, low levels of T4 binding have been detected in brain tissue at 10 wk gestation, and hepatic, cardiac, and lung TR binding are observed at 16–18 wk *(53,54)*. However, information is limited regarding the timing of appearance of thyroid hormone postreceptor effects in the human fetus. The length, weight, appearance, behavior, biochemical parameters, extrauterine adaptation, and early neonatal course of the athyroid human neonate usually are normal *(31,55–58)*. Growth of the human fetus is programmed by a complex interplay of genetic, nutritional, hormonal, and growth factors largely independent of thyroid hormones. However, bone maturation in the athyroid newborn is delayed somewhat in 50–60% of cases with delayed epiphyseal maturation in the lower extremities and delayed cerebral fontanelle closure *(31,55,56)*. Serum TSH concentrations are elevated in the hypothyroid fetus by 20–24 wk gestation, indicating the presence of a negative feedback effect of T3 on TSH synthesis and secretion.

Congenitally hypothyroid neonates with marked hypothyroxinemia (<30 nmol/L, 2.3 µg/dL) may manifest prolonged physiological jaundice, feeding difficulty, umbilical hernia, and macroglossia, but the classical clinical manifestations of congenital hypothyroidism appear progressively during the early months of life. These include soft-tissue myxedema, delayed bone and body growth, metabolic derangements, and retarded CNS development *(59)*. The lack of or minimal clinical manifestations of thyroid-hormone deficiency in most athyroid human neonates has been attributed to the limited maternal to fetal placental transfer of thyroxine coupled with the localization of MDI-II enzyme activity in fetal brain tissue *(6–8,47)*. MDI-II is modulated by thyroid hormone; high concentrations suppress and low concentrations stimulate MDI-II activity. Thus, in the hypothyroid fetal rat brain MDI-II activity is increased and T3 concentrations in brain tissue are normal in the face of low fetal serum thyroxine concentrations *(47)*.

Thyroid hormone effects on thermogenesis are mediated via brown adipose tissue (BAT), which is prominent in subscapular and perirenal areas in the mammalian fetus and neonate, and the ability of human infants to maintain body temperature in the immediate extrauterine environment is BAT-dependent *(60)*. BAT tissue is characterized by high concentrations of mitochondria and the oxidative degradation of substrate, predominantly lipid, in BAT mitochondria maintains a proton gradient across the mitochondrial membrane that provides for the phosphorylation of nucleotides and storage of energy as ATP *(60)*. Heat production in BAT is stimulated by catecholamines via β adrenergic receptors and is thyroid hormone-dependent. The uncoupling protein, thermogenin, unique to BAT, is located on the inner mitochondrial membrane and uncouples phosphorylation by dissipating the proton gradient created by the mitochondrial respiratory chain. The type II MDI in BAT mediates local T4 to T3 conversion and thermogenin expression. Full thermogenin expression in BAT requires both catecholamine and T3 stimulation *(60)*. The volume and functional activity of fetal BAT, including MDI-II activity and thermogenin levels, increase progressively with fetal age, and BAT thermogenic activity is maximal in the perinatal period *(43,60–62)* (Fig. 3). BAT thermogenesis is immature in small premature infants, and BAT tissue mass decreases in the neonatal period in full-term infants as the capacity for nonshivering thermogenesis develops in other tissues.

The important role of thyroid hormones is CNS maturation has long been recognized, but the precise timing of this dependency and the mechanism(s) remains unclear. The events of nervous-system development are programmed from early embryogenesis through 3–4 yr of age including neurogenesis, gliogenesis, neural cell migration, neuronal differentiation, dendritic and axonal growth, synaptogenesis, myelination, and neurotransmitter synthesis *(2,63)*. These events, as other fetal developmental events, involve a temporally controlled, cascading, genetic transcriptional program. Thyroid hormones have been shown to stimulate a number of developmentally regulated nervous-tissue genes, including neurogranin,

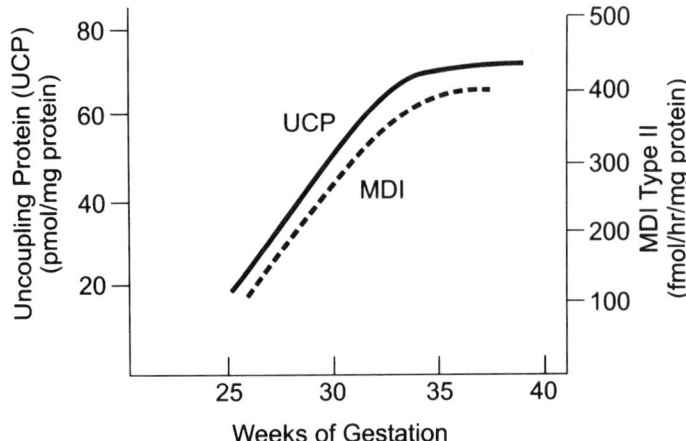

Fig. 3. Maturation of uncoupling protein (UCP) and iodothyronine monodeiodinase (MDI) activities in human fetal brown adipose tissue (BAT). The volume and functional activity of BAT increase progressively with fetal age. Full UCP (thermogenin) expression in BAT and optimal heat production require both catecholamine and thyroid hormone (T3) stimulation in the neonatal period.

specific myelin genes, and several Purkinje-cell protein genes, but the role of these factors in the CNS developmental program remains undefined *(2,53,63–65)*. Available evidence suggests that deficiency or excess of thyroid hormones alters the timing or synchronization of the CNS developmental program, presumably by initiating critical homeobox or other genetic CNS maturation events. Thyroid hormones primarily affect neuronal differentiation, neuronal arborization, and synaptogenesis.

Human neuronal proliferation in the cochlea, basal ganglia, and cerebral hemispheres is temporally localized largely to the second trimester of gestation; cellular differentiation manifested by increasing brain weight and protein content is most rapid during the third trimester and early postnatal period *(2,63)*. Studies of the timing of iodine supplementation in pregnant women in geographical areas of severe iodine deficiency have suggested a critical period of thyroid hormone action for subsequent CNS maturation during a narrow interval of time at the beginning of the third trimester of gestation *(66)*. This critical period has been likened to the irreversible thyroid-dependent action of thyroid hormone initiating tadpole metamorphosis *(67)*. Recent studies of the dose and timing of thyroid hormone therapy in infants with congenital hypothyroidism suggest a second critical period of thyroid hormone action during the very early neonatal period *(68)*. Early third-trimester thyroid hormone deficiency in the fetus produces more severe neurological abnormalities, whereas later third-trimester and neonatal/postnatal thyroid hormone deficiency is more characteristically associated with mental deficiency reflected in IQ deficit *(67)* (Fig. 2). These concepts are illustrated in Fig. 4.

Interestingly, TRβ knockout mice, while showing hearing impairment, exhibit neither morphological nor functional abnormalities of brain development, suggesting that the TRα receptor and other coacting nuclear transcription factors are the more important mediators of the thyroid effects on CNS maturation *(51,53)*. The large literature describing TRβ gene mutations and failure to identify TRα gene mutations in patients with thyroid hormone resistance suggests that TRα gene mutations are lethal in humans.

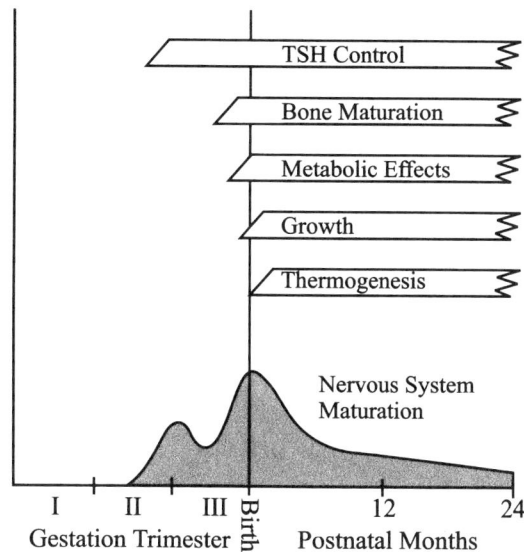

Fig. 4. Maturation of thyroid hormone actions in the human fetus and infant. The timing of onset of thyroid hormone effects on TSH control, bone maturation, carcass growth, and on metabolism and thermogenesis are illustrated. There appears to be two critical windows of brain maturative dependency on thyroid hormone: one at the beginning of the third trimester and one during the early neonatal period, both illustrated on the horizontal axis showing the pattern of brain thyroid dependency peaking at birth and extending to 24–36 postnatal mo (labeled nervous-system maturation). See text for further details.

Hypothroxinemia in pregnant women has been reported to be associated with impaired neuropsychological development of their offspring. Mean full-scale IQ values in a recent study of children from a series of 48 untreated hypothyroxinemic pregnant women averaged 7 points lower than values in 124 matched control children *(5)*. The neonatal thyroid screening results were normal in all of the children. The serum free T4 and TSH concentrations during pregnancy in these affected women averaged 0.7/ng/dL and 13.2 mU/L vs 0.97 ng/dL and 1.4 mU/L in the control population. Thus, the hypothyroidism was subclinical (TSH elevation alone) or relatively mild. The mechanism of this effect of hypothyroxinemia on offspring IQ is obscure. Any protective effect of compensatorily increased fetal brain type II MDI activity on IQ seems to have been absent or ineffective. Most of the affected women had high serum levels of anti-thyroid peroxidase autoantibodies suggesting that the hypothyroidism was due to autoimmune thyroiditis *(5)*. The role of the autoimmune disease in fetal-brain maturation and IQ is not known. Maternal autoimmune disease has been reported to increase the incidence of miscarriage, suggesting some compromise of placental function, but procoagulant autoantibodies are not involved *(68,69)*.

NEONATAL ADAPTATION

Term Infants

The changes in thyroid function associated with extrauterine adaptation of term infants are summarized in Table 2 *(31,46,71)*. Delivery of the term fetus into the extrauterine environment is associated with a transient, marked increase in serum TSH (the neonatal TSH surge) stimulated by neonatal cooling. This TSH surge, which peaks during the first

30 min at a secretory rate approximating 3 mU/L/min, stimulates thyroidal T4 and T3 secretion and increased serum T4 and T3 concentrations peaking at 24–36 h of postnatal life *(72)*. Umbilical-cord occlusion triggers activation of BAT thermogenesis, at least in part, by removing placental inhibitors. Both placental inhibitors and low fetal oxygen levels limit in utero catecholamine release and BAT thermogenesis. One of the placental inhibiting factors appears to be adenosine, which suppresses BAT thermogenesis; the levels of adenosine rapidly fall after umbilical-cord occlusion *(73)*.

In addition to the stimulation of BAT thermogenesis in the newborn term infant, there is a dramatic and permanent increase in serum T3 and free T3 concentrations (T3 increases from 50–150 ng/dL during the first 36–48 h of postnatal life) *(31,70)* (Fig. 2). This is due to increased secretion as well as decreased placental degradation. Serum rT3 concentrations decrease rapidly during the first few postnatal days *(46)*. The postnatal progressive increase in serum T3 concentrations to levels characteristic of the extrauterine state is largely due to increased activity of hepatic type I MDI. This increased activity is developmentally regulated in part by the maturational increase in free T4 concentrations, which stimulates activity of the hepatic enzyme (Fig. 2).

After the first 1–2 h, serum TSH concentrations decrease progressively from the early TSH peak, falling to permanent values characteristic of the extrauterine environment and significantly below cord-blood concentrations. The mechanism(s) for this permanent reduction in serum TSH concentration remain unclear. The high neonatal free T4 and free T3 concentrations play a role, but newborn serum TSH concentrations remain at the new, lower plateau level even after the transient neonatal hyperthyroxinemic state has resolved *(35)*. A resetting of the hypothalamic-pituitary setpoint for free T4 feedback control of TSH must be involved. Umbilical-cord cutting also removes the placental source of TRH production *(71)*. Whether this affects the TSH feedback control system is not known.

Finally, transition to the extrauterine environment and umbilical-cord cutting is associated with a progressive decrease in production and concentrations of inactive thyroid hormone analogs. These include rT3, and the sulfated metabolites T4S, T3S, rT3S, and T2S *(46,74,75)*. This process occurs over several days to weeks and involves changes in activities of the monodeiodinase enzymes and presumably the tissue levels of sulfotransferase enzymes. The net effect is decreased production of bioinactive thyroid hormone analogs and increased production of active T3.

Premature Infants

Preterm infants are delivered before full maturation of the hypothalamic-pituitary-thyroid system. They have qualitatively similar but quantitatively decreased changes in serum TSH and iodothyronine concentrations in the neonatal period *(71)* (Table 2). The serum TSH response to parturition is attenuated, and serum T4 concentrations remain below those in full-term infants during the first few weeks of life. An abrupt early neonatal (2–4 h) increase in serum T3 concentrations also occurs in premature infants, but the increments are smaller and serum T3 concentrations increase only slowly to the concentrations found in term infants. The timing of the decrease of the serum rT3 is similar to that in term infants (*see* Fig. 3) *(71,75)*.

Relative to term infants at birth, serum TBG and total T4 concentrations in premature infants are lower, tissue type I monodeiodinase activities and serum T3 levels are lower, TRH and free T4 concentrations are lower, bioinactive thyroid hormone analog levels are higher, BAT thermogenic mechanisms are immature, and tissue thyroid hormone response

Table 2
Changes in Thyroid Function at Birth

Changes	Term	Premature
Transient		
Neonatal TSH surge	Marked	Attenuated
Increased T4, T3 secretion	Marked	Reduced, prolonged
Stimulation of BAT thermogenesis	Marked	Attenuated
Permanent		
Decreased tissue MDI, type III	Rapid	Slower
Increased tissue MDI, type I	Rapid	Slower
Increased serum T3	Abrupt	Prolonged
Decreased serum rT3	Rapid	Slower
Decreased sulfated analogue levels	Rapid	Slower
Decreased serum TSH	Rapid	Rapid

systems are variably immature *(71)*. The extent of these immaturities is related inversely to gestation age. All but the largest premature infants are relatively hypothyroxinemic with serum levels of TBG, T4, and free T4 directly related to gestation age at birth. Free T4 concentrations in the more immature 25- to 27-wk infants are twofold to threefold lower than values in term infants *(76,77)*. This gestation age-related hypothyroxinemia is referred to as the "hypothyroxinemia of prematurity." The mechanisms vary in degree in larger and smaller premature infants, but include low TBG concentrations, decreased T4 secretion largely resulting from inefficient thyroid-gland synthesis, and decreased TSH secretion and action probably are involved *(76,78–80)*.

In very low birthweight (VLBW) premature infants (<27 wk gestation), the TSH surge and the early thyroidal response are limited and followed by a progressive decrease in serum T4 and free T4 concentrations with nadir values at 1–2 wk postnatal age *(74)*. The decrease in serum total T4 concentrations is due to a transient decrease in TBG, which reflects neonatal morbidity *(78,80)*. Serum TSH levels do not usually increase in response to the transient hypothyroxinemia, and serum free T4 levels re-equilibriate to cord-blood values by 3–4 wk *(77,80)*. These very premature infants manifest a negative iodine balance during the early postnatal weeks, suggesting that they are unable to adapt to the extrauterine environment with augmentation of thyroidal iodine uptake and increased T4 secretion as do the larger infants *(71,79)*.

The nosology of thyroid function disorders in premature infants is summarized in Table 3. The prevalences of permanent congenital primary and hypothalamic-pituitary hypothyroidism are similar in premature and full-term infants and require prompt treatment. Transient primary hypothyroidism, characterized by low free T4 and elevated TSH concentrations also should be treated. The prevalence of transient hypothalamic-pituitary hypothyroidism and the criteria for diagnosis in VLBW infants are not well defined. Data of van Wassenaer and coworkers have shown that a serum free T4 level, measured by immunoassay, below 10 pmol/L (0.78 ng/dL) will trigger an increase in serum TSH concentration in most VLBW infants, and Rooman et al. have reported a prevalence of free T4 concentrations below 10 pmol/L in VLBW infants approximating 5–10% *(76,80)*.

Table 3
Thyroid Function Disorders in Hypothyroxinemic Premature Infants

Thyroid dysfunction	Prevalence
Hypothyroxinemia, physiologic	70%
Transient hypothyroidism	
Primary	0.12–0.41%
Secondary-tertiary	? 5–10%, VLBW
Permanent hypothyroidism	
Primary	1 in 4000
Secondary-tertiary	1 in 25,000–29,000
Nonthyroidal illness	30% LBW, 60% VLBW

In a placebo-controlled treatment study of VLBW infants, van Wassenaer et al. showed that a subgroup of 13 VLBW infants 25–26 wk gestation age manifested a higher DQ at 24 mo than 18 placebo-control infants *(77)*. The VLBW infant cohorts were small, however, and the results must be considered preliminary.

These studies suggest a prevalence of transient hypothalamic-pituitary hypothyroidism in VLBW infants of 5–10% defined by a serum free T4 concentration below 10 pmol/L (0.78 ng/dL) by immunoassay. The impact on brain maturation of the transient hypothyroxinemia is not clear, but the preliminary treatment results suggest that treatment is not harmful and may be beneficial. Van Wassenaer administered a thyroxine dose of 8 micrograms/kg/d given parenterally. Earlier dosage studies suggest that a 4–5 microgram/kg parenteral dose or a 5–6 microgram/kg oral dose of Na-l-thyroxine provides adequate replacement *(71)*. Treatment duration in the study of van Wassenaer et al. was 6 wk, but 4 wk would seem adequate.

REFERENCES

1. Burrow GN, Fisher DA, Larsen PR. Maternal and fetal thyroid function. N Engl J Med 1994;331:1072–1078.
2. Oppenheimer JH, Schwartz HL. Molecular basis of thyroid hormone dependent brain development. Endocr Rev 1997;18:462–475.
3. de Zegher F, Pernasetti F, Vanhole C, Devlieger H, Vanden Berghe G, Martial JA. The prenatal tole of thyroid hormone evidenced by fetomaternal Pit-1 deficiency. J Clin Endocrinol Metab 1995;80:3127–3130.
4. Yasuda T, Ohnishi H, Wataki K, Minagawa M, Minamitani K, Niimi H. Outcome of a baby born from a mother with acquired juvenile hypothyroidism having undetectable thyroid hormone concentraitons. J Clin Endocrinol Metab 1999;84:2630–2632.
5. Haddow JE, Palomaki GE, Allan WC, Williams JR, Knight GJ, Gagnon J, et al. Maternal thyroid deficiency during pregnancy and subsequent neuropsychological development of the child. N Engl J Med 1999;341:549–555.
6. Contempre B, Jauniaux E, Calvo R, Jurkovic D, Campbell S, Morreale de Escobar G. Detection of thyroid hormones in human embryonic cavities during the first trimester of pregnancy. J Clin Endocrinol Metab 1993;77:1719–1722.
7. Vulsma T, Gons MH, De Vijlder JJM. Maternal fetal transfer of thyroxine in congenital hypothyroidism due to a total organification defect or thyroid agenesis. N Engl J Med 1989;321:13–16.
8. Roti E, Gnudi A, Braverman LE. The placental transport, synthesis, and metabolism of hormones and drugs which affect thyroid function. Endocr Rev 1983;4:131–149.
9. Polk DH, Reviczky A, Lam RW, Fisher DA. Thyrotropin-releasing hormone in the ovine fetus: ontogeny and effect of thyroid hormone. Am J Physiol 1991;260:E53–E58.

10. Ballabio M, Poshyachinda M, Ekins RP. Pregnancy-induced changes in thyroid function: role of human chorionic gonadotropin as putative regulator of maternal thyroid. J Clin Endocrinol Metab 1991; 73:824–831.

11. Kennedy RL, Darne J, Cohn M. Human chorionic gonadotropin may not be responsible for thyroid-stimulating activity in normal pregnancy serum. J Clin Endocrinol Metab 1992;74:260–265.

12. Grumbach MM, Gluckman PD. The human fetal hypothalamus and pituitary gland: the maturation of neuroendocrine mechanisms controlling secretion of fetal pituitary growth hormone, prolactin, gona-dotropins, adrenocorticotropin-related peptides and thyrotropin. In: Tulchinsky D, Little AB, eds. Maternal Fetal Endocrinology, 2nd ed. WB Saunders, Philadelphia, PA, 1994, pp. 193–261.

13. Roessler E, Belloni E, Gaudenz K, Jay P, Berta P. Mutations in the human Sonic hedgehog gene cause holoprosencephaly. Nature Genet 1996;14:353–356.

14. Wallis DE, Roessler E, Hehr U, Nanni L, Wiltshire T, Richieri-Costa A, et al. Mutations in the home-odomain of the human SIX-3 gene cause holoprosencephaly. Nature Genet 1999;22:196–198.

15. Brown SA, Warburton D, Brown LY, Yu CY, Roeder ER, Stengel-Rutkowski S, et al. Holopros-encephaly due to mutation in ZIC2, a homologue of drosphila odd paired. Nature Genet 1998;20:180–183.

16. Dattani MT, Martinez-Barbera JP, Thomas PQ, Brickman JM, Gupta R, Krauss S, et al. HESX1: a novel homeobox gene implicated in septo-optic dysplasia. Horm Res 1998;50(Suppl 3):8 Abstr 06.

17. Lanctôt C, Gauthier Y, Drouin J. Pituitary homeobox (Ptx-1) is differentially expressed during pituitary development. Endocrinology 1999;140:1416–1422.

18. Wu W, Cogan JD, Pfaffle RM, Dasen JS, Frisch H, O'Connell SM, et al. Mutations in PROP-1 cause familial combined pituitary hormone deficiency. Nature Genet 1998;18:147–149.

19. Pintar JE. Normal development of the hypothalamic-pituitary-thyroid axis. In: Braverman LE, Utiger RD, eds. The Thyroid, 7th ed. Lippincott-Raven, Philadelphia, PA, 1996, pp. 6–18.

20. Missero C, Cobellis G, DeFelice, DiLauro R. Molecular events involved in differentiation of thyroid follicular cells. Mol Cell Endocrinol 1998;140:37–43.

21. Lazzaro F, Price M, De Felice M, Di Lauro R. The transcription factor TTF-1 is expressed at the onset of thyroid and lung morphogenesis and in restricted regions of the foetal brain. Development 1991;113: 1093–1104.

22. Plachov D, Chowdhury K, Walther C, Simon D, Guenet JL, Gruss P. Pax8, a murine paired box gene expressed in the developing excretory system and thyroid gland. Development 1990;110:643–651.

23. Zannini M, Avantaggiato V, Biffali E, Arnone MI, Sato K, Pischetola M, et al. TTF-2, a new forkhead protein, shows a temporal expression in the developing thyroid which is consistent with a role in con-trolling the onset of differentiation. EMBO J 1997;16:3185–3197.

24. Macchia PE, De Felice M, Di Lauro R. Molecular genetics of congenital hypothyroidism. Curr Opin Gen Dev 1999;9:289–294.

25. Mansouri A, Chowdhury K, Gruss P. Follicular cells of the thyroid gland require Pax8 gene function. Nature Genet 1998;19:87–90.

26. Manley NR, Capecchi MR. HOX group 3 paralogs regulate the development and migration of the thy-mus, thyroid and parathyroid gland. Dev Biol 1998;195:1–15.

27. Guazzi S, Lonigro R, Pintonello L, Boncinelli E, Di Lauro R, Mavilio F. The thyroid transcription factor-1 gene is a candidate target for regulation by Hox proteins. EMBO J 1994;13:3339–3347.

28. Lints TJ, Parsons LM, Hartley L, Lyons I, Harvey RP. Nkx-2.5: a novel murine homeobox gene expressed in early heart progenitor cells and their myogenic descendants. Development 1993;119:419–431.

29. Kimura S, Hara Y, Pineau T, Fernandez-Salguero P, Fox CH, Ward JM, Gonzales FJ. The T/ebp null mouse: thyroid-specific enhancer-binding protein is essential for the organogenesis of the thyroid, lung, ventral forebrain, and pituitary. Genes Dev 1996;10:60–69.

30. De Felice M, Ovitt C, Biffali E, Rodriquez-Mallon A, Arra C, Anastassiadis K, et al. A mouse model for hereditary thyroid dysgenesis and cleft palate. Nature Genet 1998;19:395–398.

31. Fisher DA, Klein AH. Thyroid development and disorders of thyroid function in the newborn. N Engl J Med 1981;304:702–712.

32. Fisher DA. Thyroid function in premature infants: the hypothyroxinemia of prematurity. Clin Perinatol 1998;25:999–1014.

33. Fisher DA, Brown RS. Thyroid physiology in the perinatal period and during childhood. In: Braverman LE, Utiger RD, eds. The Thyroid: A Fundamental and Clinical Text, 8th ed. JB Lippincott, Philadelphia, PA, 2000, pp. 959–972.

34. Thorpe-Beeston JG, Nicolaides KH, McGregor AM. Fetal thyroid function. Thyroid 1992;2:207–217.

35. Fisher DA, Nelson JC, Carlton EI, Wilcox RB. Maturation of human hypothalamic-pituitary-thyroid function and control. Thyroid 2000;10:229–234.

36. Klein AH, Fisher DA. Thyrotropin releasing hormone stimulated pituitary and thyroid gland responsiveness and 3,5,3'-triiodothyronine suppression in fetal and neonatal lambs. Endocrinology 1980;106: 697–701.

37. Dai G, Levy O, Carrasco N. Cloning and characterization of the thyroid iodide transporter. Nature 1996; 379:458–460.

38. Verkataraman GM, Yatin M, Ain KB. Cloning of the human sodium-iodide symporter promotor and characterization in a differentiated human thyroid cell line, KAT-50. Thyroid 1998;8:63–69.

39. Uyttersprot N, Pelgrims N, Carrasco N, Gervy C, Maenhaut C, Dumont JE, Miot F. Moderate doses of iodide in vivo inhibit cell proliferation and the expression of thyroperoxidase and Na/I symporter mRNA in dog thyroid. Mol Cell Endocrinol 131, 1997;131:195–203.

40. Penel C, Rognoni JB, Bastiani P. Thyroid autoregulation: impact of thyroid structure and function in rats. Am J Physiol 1987;16:E165–E172.

41. Theodoropoulos T, Braverman LE, Vagenakis AG. Iodide induced hypothyroidism: a potential hazard during perinatal life. Science 1979;205:502–503.

42. Larsen PR, Davies TF, Hay ID. The thyroid gland. In: Wilson JD, Foster DW, Kronenberg HM, Larsen PR, eds. Williams Textbook of Endocrinology, 9th ed. WB Saunders, Philadelphia, PA, 1998, pp. 389–515.

43. Fisher DA, Polk DH, Wu SY. Fetal thyroid metabolism: a pluralistic system. Thyroid 1994;4:367–371.

44. Koopdonk-Kool JM, De Vijlder JJM, Veenboer GJM, Ris-Stalpers C, Kok JH, Vulsma T, et al. Type II and type III deiodinase in human placenta as a function of gestational age. J Clin Endocrinol Metab 1996;81:2154–2158.

45. Richard K, Huine R, Kaptein E, Sanders JP, Van Toor H, De Herder WW, et al. Ontogeny of iodothyronine deiodinases in human liver. J Clin Endocrinol Metab 1998;83:2868–2874.

46. Santini F, Chiovata L, Ghirri P, Lapi P, Mammoli C, Montanelli L, et al. Serum iodothyronines in the human fetus and the newborn: evidence for an important role of placenta in fetal thyroid hormone homeostasis. J Clin Endocrinol Metab 1999;84:493–498.

47. Calvo R, Obregon MJ, Ruiz de Ona C, Escobar del Rey F, Morreale de Escobar G. Congenital hypothyroidism as studied in rats: crucial role of maternal thyroxine but not of 3,5,38-triiodothyronine in the protection of the fetal brain. J Clin Invest 1990;86:889–899.

48. Polk DH, Reviczky A, Wu SY, Huang WS, Fisher DA. Metabolism of sulfoconjugated thyroid hormone derivatives in developing sheep. Am J Physiol 1994;266:E892–E896.

49. Lazar M. Thyroid hormone receptors: multiple forms, multiple possibilities. Endocr Rev 1993;14:348–399.

50. Hsu JH, Brent GA. Thyroid hormone receptor gene knockouts. Trends Metab 1998;9:103–112.

51. Forrest D, Golarai G, Connor J, Curran T. Genetic analysis of thyroid hormone receptors in development and disease. Rec Prog Horm Res 1996;51:1–22.

52. Polk DH, Cheromcha D, Reviczky AL, Fisher DA. Nuclear thyroid hormone receptors: ontogeny and thyroid hormone effects in sheep. Am J Physiol 1989;256:E543–E549.

53. Bernal J, Pekonen F. Ontogenesis of nuclear 3,5,3' triiodothyronine receptors in human fetal brain. Endocrinology 1984;114:677–679.

54. Gonzales LA, Ballard PL. Identification and characterization of nuclear 3,5,3' triiodothyronine binding sites in fetal human lung. J Clin Endocrinol Metab 1981;53:21–28.

55. LaFranchi SH, Hanna CE, Krainz PL, Skeels MR, Miyahara RS, Sesser DE. Screening for congenital hypothyroidism with specimen collection at two time periods. Results of the Northwest Regional screening program. Pediatrics 1985;76:734–740.

56. Grant DB, Smith I, Fuggle PW, Tokar S, Chapple J. Congenital hypothyroidism detected by neonatal screening: relationship between biochemical severity and early clinical features. Arch Dis Childhood 1992;67:87–90.

57. Leger J, Czernichow P. Congenital hypothyroidism, decreased growth velocity in the first weeks of life. Biol Neonate 1989;55:218–223.

58. Grant DB. Growth in early treated congenital hypothyroidism. Arch Dis Childhood 1994;70:464–468.

59. Delange F. Neonatal screening for congenital hypothyroidism. Results and perspectives. Horm Res 1997; 48:51–61.

60. Silva JE, Rabelo R. Regulation of the uncoupling protein gene expression. Eur J Endocrinol 1997;136: 251–264.

61. Klein AH, Reviczky A, Chou P, Padbury J, Fisher DA. Development of brown adipose tissue thermogenesis in the ovine fetus and newborn. Endocrinology 1983;112:1662–1666.

62. Obregon MJ, Calvo R, Hernandez A, Escobar del Rey F, Morreale de Escobar G. Regulation of uncoupling protein messenger ribonucleic acid and 5'-deiodinase activity by thyroid hormones in fetal brown adipose tissue. Endocrinology 1996,137:4721–4729.

63. Porterfield SP, Hendrich CE. The role of thyroid hormones in prenatal and neonatal neurological development-current perspectives. Endocrine Rev 1993;14:94–106.

64. Farwell AP, Tranter P, Leonard JL. Thyroxine-dependent regulation of integrin-laminin interactions in astrocytes. Endocrinology 1995;136:3909–3915.

65. Sandhofer C, Schwartz HL, Mariash CN, Forrest D, Oppenheimer JH. Beta receptor isoforms are not essential for thyroid hormone-dependent acceleration of PCP-2 and myelin basic protein gene expression in the developing brains of neonatal mice. Mol Cell Endocrinol 1998;137:109–115.

66. Cao XY, Jiang XM, Dou ZH, Rakeman MA, Zhang ML, O'Donnell K, et al. Timing of vulnerability of the brain to iodine deficiency in endemic cretinism. N Engl J Med 1994;331:1739–1744.

67. DeLong GR, Xue-Yi C, Xin Min J, Zhi-Hong D, Rakeman MA, Ming-Li Z, et al. Iodine supplementation of a cross-section of iodine deficient pregnant women: does the human fetal brain undergo metamorphosis? In: Stanbury JB, Delange F, Dunn JT, Pandav CS, eds. Iodine in Pregnancy. Oxford University Press, Calcutta, India, 1998, pp. 55–78.

68. Bongers-Schokking JJ, Koot HM, Wiersma D, Yerkerk PH, DeMuinck Keizer-Schrama SMPF. Influence of timing and dose of thyroid hormone replacement on development in infants with congenital hypothyroidism. J Pediatrics 2000;136:292–297.

69. Stagnaro Green A, Roman SH, Cohen RH, El-Harazy E, Alvarez-Marfany M, Davies TF. Detection of at risk pregnancy by means of highly sensitive assays for thyroid autoantibodies. JAMA 1990;264:1422–1425.

70. Bossen SS, Steck T. Thyroid antibodies and their relation to antithrombin antibodies, anticardiolipin antibodies, and lupus anticoagulant in women with recurrent spontaneous abortions. Eur J Obstet Gynecol Reprod Biol 1997,74:139–143.

71. Fisher DA. The hypothyroxinemia of prematurity. Clin Perinatol 1998;25:999–1014.

72. de Zegher F, Vanhole C, Van den Berghe G, Devlieger H, Eggermont E, Veldhuis JD. Properties of thyroid stimulating hormone and cortisol secretion by the human newborn on the day of birth. J Clin Endocrinol Metab 1994;79:576–581.

73. Gunn TR, Gluckman PD. Perinatal thermogenesis. Early Hum Dev 1995;42:169–183.

74. Chopra IJ, Wu SY, Chua Teca GN, Santini F. A radioimmunoassay for measurement of 3,5,3' triiodothyronine sulfate: studies in thyroidal and nonthyroidal diseases, pregnancy, and neonatal life. J Clin Endocrinol Metab 1992;75:189–194.

75. Oddie TH, Bernard B, Klein AH, Fisher DA. Comparison of T4, T3, rT3, and TSH concentrations in cord blood and serum of infants up to 3 months of age. Early Hum Dev 1979;3:239–244.

76. Rooman RP, Du Caju MVL, Op De Beeck L, Docx M, Van Reempts P, Van Acker KJ. Low thyroxinemia occurs in the majority of very preterm newborns. Eur J Pediatr 1996;155:211–215.

77. Van Wassenaer AG, Kok JH, De Vijlder JJM, Briet JM, Smit BJ, Tamminga P, et al. Effects of thyroxine supplementation on neurologic development in infants born at less than 30 weeks gestation. N Engl J Med 1997;336:21–26.

78. Frank JE, Faix JE, Hermos RJ, Mullaney DM, Rojan DA, Mitchell ML, Klein RZ. Thyroid function in very low birthweight infants: effects on neonatal hypothyroidism screening. J Pediatr 1996;128:548–554.

79. Ares S, Escobar-Morreale H, Quero J, Duran S, Presas MJ, Herruzo R, Morreale de Escobar G. Neonatal hypothyroxinemia: effects of iodine intake and of premature birth. J Clin Endocrinol Metab 1997;82:1704–1712.

80. Van Wassenaer AG, Kok JH, Dekker FW, De Vijlder JJM. Thyroid function in very preterm infants: Influences of gestational age and disease. Pediatric Res 1997;42:604–609.

7

Thyroid Disorders in Children and Adolescents

Scott A. Rivkees, MD

Contents

INTRODUCTION

In children, thyroid disorders have a range of presentations, including asymptomatic thyromegally, behavioral disturbances, lassitude, and growth retardation. The hyperthyroid state is often much more symptomatic than the hypothyroid state, although physical abnormalities are apparent in both conditions. Surprisingly, thyroid disorders are often insidious in onset and difficult to recognize, even in the face of gross biochemical disturbances. Detection of thyromegaly and thyroid masses can also be elusive if time is not taken to properly examine the thyroid. Recognizing thyroid disorders in children thus requires a keen eye and a strong element of suspicion.

EVALUATION OF THYROID FUNCTION

Physical Evaluation of the Thyroid Gland

Because thyroid disease can present with isolated thyromegaly, evaluation of the thyroid should be included in routine examinations and can be accomplished rapidly. Evaluation of the thyroid also provides important clues about causes of hyper- and hypothyroidism.

The thyroid can be visualized by having the patient look to the ceiling and swallow. As the thyroid moves, the margins of the gland are viewed to estimate size and symmetry. Next, the thyroid should be palpated to assess size, consistency, and symmetry. This is best done while standing behind the patient and palpating with the finger tips, starting in the midline and moving laterally.

From: *Contemporary Endocrinology: Developmental Endocrinology: From Research to Clinical Practice*
Edited by: E. A. Eugster and O. H. Pescovitz © Humana Press Inc., Totowa, NJ

The texture of the thyroid should also be assessed to determine if it is smooth or irregular. Attention should also be directed to determine if there are any nodules, which may be firm or soft. If any asymmetry or abnormal thyroid fullness is noted, ultrasonographic evaluation is recommended *(1)*, as pathological thyroid nodules may feel like normal tissue.

To assess gland size, one may estimate the size of each thyroid lobe relative to that of a teaspoon (5 gm) or a tablespoon (15 gm). Generally, until the end of puberty, gland size (in gms) approximates the patient's age in years × 0.5–0.7 *(2)*. Thus, each thyroid lobe of a 10-yr-old will be about one-half of a teaspoon for a total gland size of 5-7 gms *(2)*.

To follow changes in thyroid size, the outline of the thyroid gland can also be traced. This is done by drawing on the patient's neck with a felt-tipped marker, rubbing an alcohol pad on a small sheet of paper, and then placing the paper on the neck. The outline of the thyroid will then be transferred to the paper, which can be kept in the medical record.

For newborns and young infants, the thyroid can be examined by placing the infant spine on the parent's lap, with the head toward the parent's knees. The head can then be gently tipped backward exposing the neck, allowing the thyroid to be palpated.

If the examiner can palpate each ring of the trachea from the sternal notch to above the larynx, this suggests the absence of pretracheal thyroid tissue, which occurs if there is failure of thyroid formation or migration. Failure to detect pre-tracheal thyroid tissue in older children warrants visual examination of the base of the tongue for ectopic thyroid tissue. When a sublingual thyroid gland is discovered late in childhood or in adolescence, the tissue should be palpated with a gloved finger during regular office visits since nodules and malignancies may develop in ectopic thyroid glands *(3,4)*. In contrast, when an ectopic thyroid is detected in infancy and replacement therapy is started, the residual thyroid tissue becomes atrophic and does not present long-term problems.

Interpretation of Thyroid Function Tests

Approximately 97% of the thyroid hormone released from the thyroid gland is thyroxine (T4) *(5)*. After its release, less than 1% of T4 remains free, whereas the remainder circulates bound to the proteins thyroglobulin (TBG, 70%), prealbumin (transthyretin, 10%) and albumin (15–20%) *(5)*. Thyroid function can therefore be assessed by measurement of total-T4 and total-T3 and levels, along with indices that reflect thyroid hormone-binding proteins (T3- or T4- resin uptake) *(5)*. Measurement of free T4 (FT4; or unbound T4 levels) is used to assess thyroid hormone status without confounding influences of carrier proteins.

When FT4 values are normal, yet total T4 values are high, familial dysalbuminemic hyperthyroxinemia (FDH) needs to be considered *(6,7)*. This autosomal dominant disorder is most commonly seen in Hispanic individuals and can be diagnosed by thyroid hormone binding protein electrophoresis. If FT4 values are normal, but total T4 values are low, TBG deficiency needs to be considered. TBG deficiency is an X-linked disorder that may be associated with color-blindness *(8)*. In these and other conditions affecting thyroid hormone binding, treatment is not needed and the patient should be educated about the condition to avoid treatment by unsuspecting practitioners.

Whereas T4 is much more abundant in the circulation, triiodothyronine (T3) is the more metabolically active thyroid hormone. T3 is produced peripherally from T4 and can be secreted by the thyroid. A metabolically inactive form of T3, reverse T3, is also produced and is elevated in conditions such as the "euthyroid-sick syndrome" *(9)*.

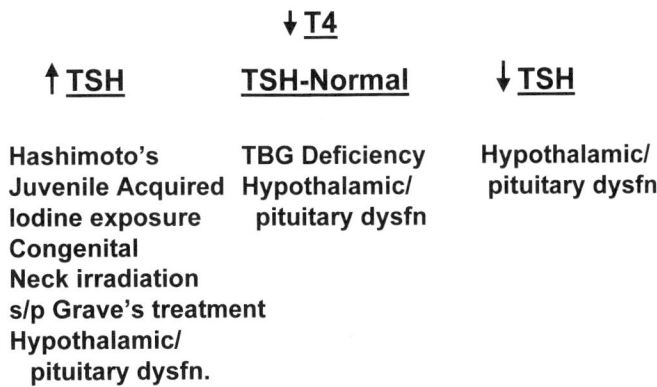

Fig. 1. Causes of hypothyroxinemia.

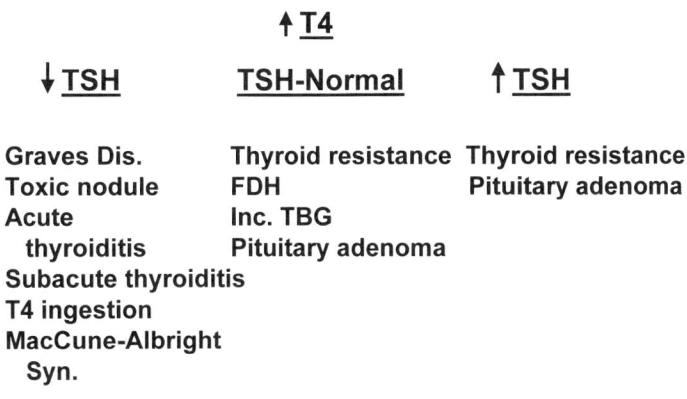

Fig. 2. Causes of hyperthyroxinemia.

With the development of the ultra-sensitive thyrotroponin (TSH) assays, assessment of TSH has greatly improved the evaluation of thyroid status *(10)*. TSH levels will help distinguish many thyroid disorders presenting with either low (Fig. 1) or high (Fig. 2) T4 levels in most cases. TSH values within the normal range for assay are indicative of a euthyroid state if the hypothalamic pituitary axis is intact. Elevations of TSH generally indicate primary thyroid dysfunction; suppressed TSH values indicate hyperthyroidism. When both FT4 and TSH levels are elevated, TSH producing pituitary adenomas and thyroid hormone resistance need to be considered.

HYPOTHYROIDISM

Disorders of the thyroid lead to hypothyroidism much more commonly than hyperthyroidism. Surprisingly, hypothyroidism may be "silent," with symptoms elicited only in retrospect. In the extreme, hypothyroidism can be associated with cold intolerance, bardycardia, carotenemia, coarse and brittle hair, dry skin, pallor, and myxedema. Surprisingly, these symptoms may not be distressing, allowing prolonged hypothyroidism to escape detection.

The most common causes of hypothyroidism in children result from autoimmune processes leading to Hashimoto's thyroiditis. Autoimmune thyroiditis also leads to juvenile acquired hypothyroidism that can present with growth failure. Hypothyroidism in children also results from iodine exposure or hypothalamic/pituitary dysfunction. Other causes of hypothyroidism include exogenous goitrogens, cystinosis, acute thyroiditis, and thyroid irradiation during cancer treatment, which are topics covered elsewhere. Hypothyroidism in the newborn is also a serious health concern and is detected by newborn screening programs.

Hashimoto's Thyroiditis

Autoimmune thyroiditis with thyroid enlargement is one of the most common presentations of childhood thyroid disease *(11,12)*. Associated with by antibodies against thyroglobulin and peroxidase *(12,13)*, there is lymphocytic infiltration of the thyroid gland resulting in thyromegaly. Depending on the nature of antithyroid antibodies, Hashimoto's disease may be associated with a euthyroid state, hypothyroidism, or transient hyperthyroidism *(14)*.

Hashimoto's may rarely present in very young infants *(15)*, yet typically presents in adolescents, affecting females more than males *(12)*. The thyroid gland is usually diffusely enlarged and may have a "cobblestone" feel. There may be asymmetric thyroid enlargement, mimicking a thyroid nodule. The presence of antithyroid antibodies and the absence of nodules on ultrasound can distinguish inflammation from other pathological processes.

Untreated, Hashimoto's thyroiditis can result in progressive thyromegaly and hypothyroidism *(12)*. Treatment with levo-thyroxine will prevent hypothyroidism and TSH elevations that stimulate gland enlargement. When T4 levels are modestly depressed (>5 ug/dl) or normal, treatment can be initiated with 1–2 ug/kg/d of levo-thyroxine. If profound hypothyroidism is present, pseudotumor cerebri may develop when children are treated with conventional doses *(16)*. Thus, treatment is often initiated with one-third to one-half of the usual dose of levo-thyroxine. After 2–4 wk, the patient can be advanced to conventional doses. However, we have also seen children with profound hypothyroidism develop pseudotumor cerebri on low doses of levo-thyroxine.

Although it was suggested that there are differences between proprietary and generic forms of levo-thyroxine, available evidence shows that this is not the case *(17)*. It has also been suggested that hypothyroidism in adolescents can be treated with a single dose given weekly *(18)*. Yet, this approach is not recommended, as thyroid hormone levels are high shortly after the dose and are low by the week's end *(18)*. Treatment of congenital hypothyroidism with weekly doses of levo-thyroxine also can result in mental retardation *(19)*.

Uncommonly, patients may present with Hashitoxicosis, in which immunological destruction of thyroid tissue results in the release of preformed thyroid hormone leading to elevated T4 levels *(13,20)*. In comparison with Graves' disease, hyperthyroidism is transient, eye findings are not seen, radionuclide uptake is low, and elevated levels of thyroidstimulating immunoglobulins are not present *(20)*.

Hashimoto's thyroiditis may be associated with other autoimmune diseases, including diabetes mellitus, adrenal insufficiency, vitiligo, and hypoparathyroidism *(21,22)*. Autoimmune thyroiditis is also seen in patients with inflammatory bowel disease and juvenile arthritis *(23,24)*. Annual surveillance of thyroid gland size and TSH levels should thus be considered for children with other autoimmune problems, and clinicians should be vigilant for signs of hyper- or hypothyroidism. Conversely, children with autoimmune thyroiditis should be watched for signs of diabetes mellitus and Addison's disease.

Juvenile Acquired Hypothyroidism

When autoimmune thyroiditis occurs during childhood, resulting in juvenile-acquired hypothyroidism, severe hypothyroidism can be well-tolerated. Thus, prolonged hypothyroidism may not be detected until children are evaluated for growth failure *(25,26)*.

Because untreated infantile hypothyroidism is associated with mental retardation, it is often assumed that juvenile hypothyroidism is associated with learning problems and poor academic performance. Yet, this is not the case. Children with juvenile hypothyroidism can be successful academically.

Children with severe hypothyroidism may manifest cold intolerance, decreased frequency of bowel movements, and decreased physical activity *(25–27)*. Bardycardia, facial puffiness, delayed reflexes, and carotenemia may be present. In comparison with Hashimoto's thyroiditis, the thyroid gland is either small or only modestly enlarged *(25,26)*. Antithyroid antibodies are usually present, suggesting an autoimmune basis *(26)*.

Although it is commonly believed that hypothyroidism is a cause of obesity, these patients are generally not overweight, and body mass index (BMI) values are similar before and after treatment *(28)*. Treatment of slipped capital femoral epiphyses may also antedate the detection of hypothyroidism *(29)*.

Some children with juvenile hypothyroidism may present with signs of puberty without pubic hair *(30–32)*. Boys may present with testicular enlargement and girls may present with menarche with or without breast development *(30,32)*. With treatment of the hypothyroid state, these characteristics may regress *(25)*. Available evidence suggests that the hypothyroid state leads to increased gonadotropin secretion triggering gonadal activity *(30,33)*. However, in some children puberty may develop within a year or two of treatment onset, which may limit catch-up growth *(25)*.

Because juvenile hypothyroidism may not be recognized until there is a sizable statural deficit *(25)*, unfortunately, the lost height is usually not regained *(25)*. When presenting with growth failure, children with juvenile hypothyroidism manifest very low T4 values that are often less than 2 mg/dl, and profoundly elevated TSH levels that are greater than 250 uU/mL *(25)*. Hypercholesterolemia and anemia may be present *(25)*.

The magnitude of the statural deficit is proportional to the duration of hypothyroidism, which can be estimated as the difference between the chronological and bone ages *(25)*. When treated with conventional doses of levo-thyroxine, accelerated skeletal maturation is observed with the skeletal age advancing disproportionately faster than gains in height *(25)*. Thus, predicted heights fall and genetic growth potential is not achieved.

Because of the poor outcomes of patients with hypothyroidism, we have treated these patients with low doses of levo-thyroxine (0.25–0.5 ug/kg/d; i.e., 50 ug for a 10-yr-old). Interestingly, we find that on low-dose levo-thyroxine, T4 values normalize (6–7 ug/dl) within 2 mo, and TSH levels normalize or remain only modestly elevated. When serial bone ages have been obtained, we have not observed the disproportionate advancement of skeletal age seen with conventional therapy. However, we do not know if this approach leads to more favorable height outcomes. It has also been suggested that treating these children with LHRH-analogs will lead to improved long-term growth *(34,35)*. Yet, we have found that catch-up growth slows markedly in some hypothyroid children on LHRH analog therapy, and predicted adult heights fall. Because the loss in adult height is proportional to the duration of hypothyroidism *(25)*, early detection of this disorder is the best intervention for preventing statural deficits *(36)*.

Iodine-Induced Hypothyroidism

Iodine is a trace element that is essential for thyroid hormone formation. Recommended dietary iodine intake is about 8 ug/kg, or 100–150 ug/d for adolescents and adults *(37)*. Although modest iodine intake is essential for thyroid function, high-level iodine exposure results in an acute block in the release of preformed thyroid hormone and impaired thyroid hormone synthesis, a phenomena referred to as the Wolf-Chaikoff effect *(38)*. When suspected, iodine-induced hypothyroidism can be diagnosed by detecting high iodine levels in urinary samples *(39)*.

In children, iodine can be absorbed through the skin, and iodine-induced hypothyroidism has been observed after cutaneous iodine or betadine use *(39–42)*. We have also observed iodine-induced suppression of thyroid hormone production in children with central lines, in which regular cleansing of the insertion site with iodine was included in central line care. Neonatal hypothyroidism has also been associated with maternal providone exposure at the time of delivery *(40)*.

In preterm infants, iodine-induced hypothyroidism warrants special attention, as it has been suggested that cutaneous iodine exposure is a major cause of hypothyroidism in premature babies *(41)*. Fortunately, recent studies show that the incidence of iodine-induced hypothyroidism is low in the United States *(43)*.

Significant iodine exposure also occurs from Amiodarone, an antiarrhythmic drug that contains 37% iodine *(44)*. Hypothyroidism occurs in 10% of individuals treated with this compound *(45)*. Amiodarone can also reach the fetus by transplacental passage and induce fetal hypothyroidism *(44)*.

In addition to iodine excess, iodine deficiency also leads to hypothyroidism. It is estimated that more than one billion people worldwide are at risk for iodine deficiency *(46)*. Clinically, iodine deficiency is associated with goiter, hypothyroidism *(46)*, and endemic cretinism *(47,48)*. In the United States, there are geographical areas of iodine deficiency *(49,50)*. However, with the prevalent use of iodized salt, iodine deficiency has been markedly reduced, and hypothyroidism and goiter due to iodine deficiency are rare *(49)*. Of note, the iodine intake in the United States has declined over the past decade, an issue that may have future clinical implications *(49)*.

Hypothalamic/Pituitary Dysfunction

Central hypothyroidism should be considered in children with a history of head trauma, brain tumors, meningitis, central nervous system (CNS) irradiation, or congenital nervous-system malformations. Central hypothyroidism has also been associated with the use of retinoid X receptor-selective ligands in the treatment of lymphomas *(51)*.

In contrast to primary hypothyroidism, the diagnosis of hypothyroidism secondary to hypothalamic/pituitary dysfunction may be difficult to establish. Often circulating levels of T4 are in the low-normal range and TSH levels may be low, normal, or elevated *(52,53)*. FT4 values, however, are usually low.

Whereas congenital central hypothyroidism will be diagnosed in states that perform T4 screening, neonatal screening programs that rely on TSH determinations will not detect this condition *(54)*. Central hypothyroidism should therefore be suspected in infants with cholestasis, poor growth, hypoglycemia, structural nervous system problems, or pituitary insufficiency *(55)*. When interpreting neonatal T4 values, care should also be taken to use infant thyroid hormone values, as infantile T4 levels are higher than those seen in adults *(56)*.

When central hypothyroidism is suspected, the thyrotrophin-releasing hormone (TRH) test will help distinguish pituitary (secondary) and hypothalamic (tertiary) hypothyroidism *(53,57)*. CNS imaging should also be performed to look for congenital malformations or hypothalamic/pituitary lesions. Care should be taken to look of other pituitary hormone deficiencies, especially abnormalities of the hypothalamic/pituitary/adrenal and growth hormone (GH) axes.

Treatment consists of replacement therapy with levo-thyroxine. Interestingly, some children with central hypothyroidism require doses lower than those used to treat primary hypothyroidism *(58)*. Because TSH values will not be helpful in guiding treatment, measurement of FT4 levels is recommended *(58)*.

Congenital Hypothyroidism

Congenital hypothyroidism is the most common preventable form of mental retardation and when treated early and appropriately is usually associated with a good outcome. In North America, the incidence of congenital hypothyroidism is about 1 in 4,000 live births *(59,60)*.

In about 40% of infants with congenital hypothyroidism the thyroid gland is not present. Interestingly, mutations in genes responsible for the development of thyroid follicular cells (TITF1, TITF2, PAX8, and TSHR) have been discovered in some athyroitic children *(61)*. In 30% of infants there is defective thyroid migration resulting in ectopic or sublingual thyroid tissue. In 10% of infants, enzymatic defects in thyroid hormone production are present. Less commonly, transplacental-transferred thyroid blocking immunoglobulins impair fetal and neonatal thyroid function *(59)*. Mutations in the TSH receptor have also been described in infants with congenital hypothyroidism presenting with TSH elevation, normal T4 levels, and normal-size thyroid glands *(62)*.

Newborn Screening

Because the clinical features of congenital hypothyroidism are usually subtle *(63)*, if present at all, detection of congenital hypothyroidism is dependent on newborn screening programs *(64)*. In some states, T4 is measured in all samples and TSH is measured in samples with T4 values in the bottom 10% in each run, or in samples with T4 values less than 9 ug/dl. In other programs, TSH alone is measured.

An advantage of programs that include T4 measurements in newborn screening is the ability to detect both primary and hypothalamic/pituitary hypothyroidism. The rare infant with hypothalamic/pituitary hypothyroidism may therefore elude detection in states relying on TSH screening. Testing for hypothyroidism is therefore indicated if there is prolonged jaundice, signs of anterior pituitary insufficiency, including hypoglycemia, cyptorchidism, a small phallus, diabetes insipidus, CNS abnormalities, or midline defects.

Because of the surge in TSH levels within 12 h of birth and a rise in T4 levels 24 h later, the discharge of infants within 24–48 h of birth portends special problems for newborns screening programs. Newborn T4 and TSH values thus need to be interpreted relative to age, and second samples are needed in most infants *(65)*. In addition to evaluating the thyroid axis, a repeat sample after the child has begun protein-containing feeds is crucial in detecting inborn errors of metabolism, such as phenylketonuria

Children with Down syndrome also require repeat screening for congenital hypothyroidism. The incidence of congenital hypothyroidism in infants with Down syndrome is nearly 1 in 140 and elevations in TSH may not be apparent initially *(66,67)*. Thus, we obtain repeat samples at 1–2 mo of age even if initial screening laboratory tests are normal.

EVALUATION OF INFANTS

If a newborn is found to have an abnormal newborn screening test result, repeat thyroid function tests should be promptly obtained. Fortunately, many hospital and commercial laboratories provide test results the same day the sample is obtained. However, if a delay in obtaining laboratory results is anticipated, treatment should be initiated while awaiting the results of confirmatory tests.

If the child has biochemical evidence of hypothyroidism, it is important to look for severe hyperbilirubinemia, hypoglycemia, or hypothermia that may warrant immediate medical attention. Care should also be taken to assess if other congenital problems are present, as cardiac disease may be present in 3–7% of infants with congenital hypothyroidism *(68,69)*.

To assess the duration of hypothyroidism, we are fond of obtaining an A-P radiographic view of the knee and a lateral foot. Generally, five ossification centers are present in term infants (proximal tibia, appears between 34–39 wk postconception; distal femur, 31–34 wk; calcaneus, 22–25 wk; talus, 25–31 wk; cuboid 31–48 wk) *(70)*. In addition to providing an index of the magnitude of intrauterine hypothyroidism, the size of the femoral ossification center has been show to correlate with intellectual prognosis, as infants with absent or small femoral ossification centers are at higher risk for learning problems than infants without markedly delayed skeletal maturation *(71)*.

Thyroid scanning is also recommended to determine the location of thyroid tissue. This can be accomplished easily with an intramuscular injection of 99Te-pertechnetate followed by imaging 60 min later. If there is athyrosis or an ectopic thyroid gland, lifelong replacement therapy will be needed. Recently, thyroglobulin levels have been shown to distinguish athyrosis from other forms of congenital hypothyroidism *(72)*. Ultrasound has also proven to be useful in detecting thyroid tissue in some neonates *(73,74)*. However, ultrasonography may not detect ectopic tissue *(74)*.

TREATMENT

When congenital hypothyroidism is detected, the goal is the rapid normalization of thyroid function. This approach is rooted in the results of studies showing more favorable neurological outcomes in infants with more rapid normalization of circulating T4 levels *(75,76)*. Whereas treating juveniles with low-doses of levo-thyroxine may be advantageous, this approach cannot be justified in infants.

Current recommendations are to treat with 10–16 ug/kg/d of levo-thyroxine, which corresponds with a daily dose of 37.5 ug for term infants *(76)*. When the initial T4 value is <5 ug/dl, initial treatment with higher doses (50 ug for term infants) of levo-thyroxine has been recommended *(77,78)*. When treated in this manner, T4 values usually normalize within 1 wk of therapy *(75)*. In contrast, when treatment is initiated with 6–8 ug/kg/d (25 ug for term infants), up to 4 wk are needed to reach desired T4 levels *(75)*.

After doses of thyroid hormone are given, 30% increases in FT4 levels are seen within 5 h and are associated with 40% decreases in TSH levels by 6 h *(79)*. Thus, TSH determinations obtained 4–8 h after medication may slightly underestimate mean levels. Consideration of the timing of doses is also needed if there is monitoring of treatment by FT4 levels *(79)*.

Although thyroxine is transmitted to the nursing infant in breast milk *(80)*, the amount of thyroid hormone consumed by the infant is generally insufficient *(80–84)*. Thus, breast-fed infants should be treated in a standard manner. Because soy proteins can bind thyroid hormone, soy-based formulas should be avoided in infants taking levo-thyroxine *(85,86)*. Iron supplements, above and beyond that provided in infant formulas, may also interfere with thyroxine absorption and should be given at a different time of the day than when levo-thyroxine is given *(87)*. This is an important issue as anemia is more commonly seen in infants with congenital hypothyroidism *(88)*.

Treatment goals are to maintain T4 values in the upper half of the normal range for age (10–16 ug/dl) *(75,76)*. If the TSH is greater than 10 uU/mL after 1 mo of age, the dose may be increased further. On occasion, high T4 values may be seen in infants treated with standard or even relatively low doses of levo-thyroxine *(89,90)*. T3 levels are normal in these infants, symptoms of hyperthyroidism are not seen, and outcome is not adversely affected *(89,90)*. It has also been suggested that outcomes are more favorable in infants in which T4 values were maintained between 15 and 20 ug/dl *(91)*. However, if there are symptoms of hyperthyroidism including tachycardia, weight loss, frequent bowel movements, and irritability, the thyroxine dose should be reduced.

In some infants, there is transient resistance to thyroid hormone *(92,93)*. Recent evidence, suggests that thyroid hormone resistance is present in 10% of infants with congenital hypothyroidism *(94)*. If there is resistance to thyroid hormone resulting in TSH elevations, this condition is usually transient.

Follow-up blood testing is frequent for the infant with congenital hypothyroidism. In 1993 *(76)*, it was recommended that thyroid hormone levels be obtained every month for the first 6 mo, every 2 mo for the next 6 mo, every 3 mo until 2 yr of age, and every 4 mo until 3 yr of age. Reevaluation of these recommendations has found them to be justified *(95)*.

With proper treatment the growth of children with congenital hypothyroidism is normal *(96,97)*. Delays in skeletal maturation are also markedly reduced by 2 yr of age *(96,98)*.

If there is a question as to whether an infant with ectopic thyroid tissue will need prolonged therapy, medication can be stopped after 3 yr of age and serial thyroid hormone indices assessed. However, even in children with borderline hypothyroidism in the neonatal period, persistent hypothyroidism is usually found after 3 yr of levo-thyroxine replacement therapy *(99)*. Occasionally an adolescent taking medication for congenital hypothyroidism will question the need for continued therapy. Before these individuals leave the shelter of their parent's home, medication can be stopped and thyroid indices measured to demonstrate the need of continued treatment.

OUTCOME

The long-term intellectual function of children diagnosed and treated early for congenital hypothyroidism is usually good and mental retardation is prevented. However, it is increasingly apparent that thyroid hormone plays an important role in fetal nervous system development, and some children with congenital hypothyroidism will have long-term learning problems despite prompt and appropriate therapy. This notion is supported by recent studies showing that maternal hypothyroidism during early gestation is associated with reduced intelligence quotients *(100,101)*.

Studies performed more than a decade ago failed to find differences among affected individuals and sibling in intelligence quotients and the need for special education *(102)*. Yet, several subsequent studies have found reduced intelligence quotients and neuropsychological problems in 10–15% of children with congenital hypothyroidism *(103–106)*. The risk for neurocognitive problems is greatest in infants with low T4 values and delayed skeletal maturation at birth *(106,107)*. The proportion of children needing special education also appears to be higher if there is a history of severe congenital hypothyroidism *(107)*.

A higher incidence of sensory-neural hearing loss is seen in children with congenital hypothyroidism *(108)*. Thus, hearing screening should be considered for children with congenital hypothyroidism if there are language or learning problems. If school difficulties are detected, noncompliance may be a cause and improvement in thyroid control will be associated with improvement in psychometric test scores *(109)*.

PRETERM INFANTS

Premature infants present special concerns for newborn screening programs (*see* Chapter 8). T4 values usually remain less than 10 ug/dl until after 32 wk postconception *(110,111)*. Thus, hypothyroxinemia is usually present in premature infants. However, when FT4 values are measured in accurate reference laboratories, values are normal and TSH levels are not elevated *(56,112)*.

Currently, controversy exists regarding whether preterm infants with low T4 values should be treated *(110)*. A higher incidence of cerebral palsy has been noted in infants with lower total-T4 values than in infants with higher levels *(113)*. However, these observations may reflect a greater degree of illness in the babies with lower total T4 levels rather than effects of hypothyroidism. When infants with low T4 levels are studied, FT4 values are normal *(112)*. Furthermore, in a controlled clinical study, the preterm infants receiving thyroid hormone had higher mortality and complication rates than untreated control infants *(114)*.

When serial thyroid function tests are monitored in preterm infants, 1 in 500 babies will develop biochemical evidence of primary hypothyroidism *(115)*. Thus, thyroid function should be assessed in the latter part of the first week of life, and again at 2, and 4–6 wk of age *(115)*. If primary hypothyroidism develops, the infant should be treated.

HYPERTHYROIDISM

Hyperthyroidism occurs less commonly in children than hypothyroidism, yet is far more symptomatic *(116,117)*. Graves' disease is the most common cause of childhood thyrotoxicosis and is characterized by diffuse goiter, hyperthyroidism, and occasionally ophthalmopathy. Other causes of hyperthyroidism in children include autonomously functioning thyroid nodules, neonatal thyrotoxicosis, and infections of the thyroid. Hyperthyroidism also results from thyroid hormone ingestion, McCune-Albright syndrome, struma ovarii, TSH-producing pituitary adenomas, and nephritis, which are topics discussed elsewhere. Epidemic hyperthyroidism has also been seen when thyroid tissue has been inadvertently included in meat products *(118)*. In contrast to these disorders, thyroid hormone resistance may appear like hyperthyroidism, yet is best left untreated.

Graves' Disease

Graves' disease is of autoimmune basis and involves stimulation of the TSH receptor by thyrotropin receptor antibodies (TRAbs) or thyroid-stimulating immunoglobulins (TSI) *(119)*. In 90% of cases, elevated levels of TRAbs can be detected *(119)*. When thyroid scanning is performed, uptake of 99Te-pertechnetate or radioiodine is usually diffusely elevated.

Because Graves' disease is uncommon in childhood, hyperthyroidism is often unexpectedly discovered when the child or adolescent is evaluated for nonspecific complaints after being symptomatic for months. One of the most distressing symptoms is the inability to concentrate, and school performance often deteriorates as Graves' disease is developing. Other symptoms include palpitations, increased bowel movement frequency, nocturia, tiredness, and poor exercise tolerance *(120)*.

The thyroid gland is usually symmetrically enlarged and smooth, and either firm or soft. Care should be taken to determine if an isolated thyroid nodule is present, as autonomously functioning nodules may produce hyperthyroidism. Tachycardia is usually present, and heart rate may provide the best index of the hyperthyroid state *(120)*. Reflexes are brisk and the patient is usually fidgety *(120)*. The patient may be thin and appear tired *(120)*. Clinicians should therefore consider hyperthyroidism when children are evaluated for tachycardia, weight loss, dyspnea, or attention deficit/hyperactivity disorders.

Graves' disease is often associated with eye findings that are less dramatic in children than in adults *(120)*. Proptosis may be present along with fullness of the palpebrae and redness of the conjunctiva. The degree of proptosis can be followed accurately using a Hurtle Ophthalmometer. Occasionally, eye disease may antedate the development of overt hyperthyroidism.

Biochemically, the cardinal feature of hyperthyroidism is a suppressed TSH *(121)*. T4 and T3 levels are generally elevated, but in some cases only elevations in T3 are observed *(122)*. Elevation in T4 and T3 levels can also be seen in the syndrome of thyroid hormone resistance. However, with thyroid hormone resistance, TSH levels are not suppressed *(121)*. TSH producing pituitary adenomas *(123)* also need to be considered if T4 and T3 levels are high and TSH levels are not suppressed.

Because Graves' disease only rarely spontaneously resolves within a short period, treatment of hyperthyroidism is essential. Current treatment approaches include surgery, antithyroid drugs, and radioiodine. The risks and benefits of each approach need to be considered by physician and patient in developing a treatment strategy (Fig. 3).

THYROIDECTOMY

Whereas subtotal (partial) thyroidectomy was advocated in previous years for children and adults *(124,125)*, total (near-total) thyroidectomy is now recommended to reduce the risk of recurrent hyperthyroidism *(126,127)*. In preparation for surgery, the child should be rendered euthyroid or hypothyroid. This is typically done with either propylthiouracil (PTU) or methimazole (MMI). One week before surgery, iodine is added to cause the gland to become firmer and less vascular, facilitating surgery.

Complication rates are comparable following subtotal or total thyroidectomy *(128)*. Reported in-hospital mortality rates are 0.5% for adults and 0.08% (1 death in about 1,000 operations) for children *(129)*. The most frequent nonlethal complications include pain and transient hypocalcemia *(129)*. Less common problems (1–4%) include hemorrhage, permanent hypoparathyroidism, and vocal-cord paralysis *(129)*.

Surgery is especially useful for the patient with a large thyroid gland (>100 gm) and in individuals who have not gone into remission with drug therapy and do not desire radioiodine. Yet, because of increasing use of radioiodine, less thyroid surgery is now performed and fewer surgeons can develop and maintain their skills than in the past *(130)*. Thus, surgery should only be performed by surgeons with expertise in performing thyroidectomies in children.

GRAVES DISEASE TREATMENTS

	MEDICAL	SURGERY	RADIOIODINE
LONG TERM (CURE) REMISSION RATES	20-30%	90-95%	80-90%
MINOR SIDE EFFECTS	20-30% RASH/URTICARA ARTHRALGIA LEUKOPENIA	100%, POST-OPERATIVE PAIN 5 %, TRANSIENT HYPOCALCEMIA	5%, THYROID PAIN
MAJOR SIDE EFFECTS	0.8% SEVERE HEPATITIS[a] AGRANULOCYTOSIS	1-5% VOCAL CORD PARESIS 1-5%, HYPOPARA- THYROIDISM	0.01%, THYROID STORM
REPORTED MORTALITY	3 CHILDREN	1/1000 CHILDREN	NONE
LONG-TERM THYROID CANCER RISKS[b]	0.3%	0.03%	0.05%[c]

a. Risk of severe hepatitis is associated with PTU.
b. Collaborative Thyrotoxicosis Study Group data.
c. There is a theoretical risk of higher thyroid cancer rates in young children treated with low 131-iodine doses.

Fig. 3. Effectiveness and side effects of treatments for Graves' disease.

ANTITHYROID DRUGS

Despite disappointing long-term rates of remission and the risk of minor and major side effects, treatment with antithyroid drugs remains the first line of therapy for children with Graves' disease in many centers. Mainstays of antithyroid therapy include the thionamide derivatives PTU and MMI. MMI is 10-fold more potent than PTU and has a longer half-life *(131)*. Recommended doses for initial therapy are 5–10 mg/kg/d for PTU and 0.5–1.0 mg/kg/d for MMI. Yet, even lower doses may be effective for induction or maintenance therapy.

To control the hyperthyroid state, PTU and MMI are typically given every 8 h. Once-a-day dosing, though, may bring remission as rapidly as divided doses and is especially well suited for maintenance therapy *(132,133)*. Because MMI pills (5 or 10 mg) are smaller than PTU tablets (50 mg), and fewer MMI pills are generally needed, MMI is more convenient to take than PTU. Another advantage of MMI is the much lower risk of severe hepatitis than with PTU use *(134)*.

Although MMI and PTU promptly inhibit hormone formation, they do not inhibit thyroid hormone release. Thus, levels of circulating thyroid hormones may remain elevated for several weeks as stored hormone is released. Until circulating levels of thyroid hormones normalize, the signs and symptoms of hyperthyroidism may be controlled with beta blockers such as atenolol (25 or 50 mg, QD or BID) or propranolol (2.5–10 mg BID or TID). Please note that if the child has reactive airway disease, beta blocker therapy may trigger acute exacerbations of asthma. Iodine drops are also a useful adjunct for treatment of severe hyperthyroidism by acutely blocking hormone release and controlling hyperthyroidism more rapidly than PTU or MMI alone *(135)*.

After initiation with PTU or MMI, maximal clinical responses are seen after 4–6 wk, at which time biochemical hypothyroidism often develops and the thionamide dose can be reduced 30–50%. If hypothyroidism develops, the dose of MMI or PTU can be reduced further, or levo-thyroxine given *(136)*.

Despite the common use of PTU or MMI in treating childhood Graves' disease, these medications have toxicity. More than 25% of children treated with PTU or MMI will develop minor complications and up to 1% of children will develop serious complications *(137, 138)*. Minor complications include elevations in liver enzymes (28%), leukopenia (25%), rashes (9%), granulocytopenia (4.5%), arthritis (2.4%), and lymphadenopathy (2%). Serious complications include agranulocytosis (0.4%) and hepatitis (0.45%).

Agranulocytosis is usually reversible when the drug is stopped and is rarely fatal *(134, 139)*. Severe hepatitis, however, may not be reversible and may progress to end-stage liver disease requiring transplantation *(140)*. In children and adults, deaths due to PTU-induced liver failure have been reported *(134,138)*. As noted earlier, severe hepatotoxicity appears to be a complication of PTU, but not of MMI therapy *(134)*.

In children, remission rates after several years of drug therapy are usually less than 30% *(138,141,142)*. It has also been suggested that after 2 yr of treatment, remission rates in children are 25%, and 4 yr of drug therapy are needed to achieve remission in 50% *(143)*. However, most reports do not show such favorable outcomes *(138)*. When responses to medical therapy between prepubertal and pubertal children are compared, remission rates are much less in prepubertal (17%) than in pubertal children (30%) *(144)*. Thus, prepubertal children have a lower chance of spontaneous remission.

Radioactive Iodine

The use of radioiodine to treat Graves' disease was introduced by Chapman and coworkers more than 50 years ago *(145,146)*. In comparison with other forms of treatment, radioiodine is the simplest and most cost-effective treatment of Graves' disease *(147)*. Treatment is achieved when 131-iodine is trapped in thyroid cells, leading to thyroid cell destruction by internal radiation. It has been suggested that doses (administered activities) delivering 300–400 Gy (30,000–40,000 cGy or rads; 360–480 uCi/gm) are required to ablate the thyroid gland *(148,149)*. However, doses delivering 120–200 cGy (150–250 uCi/gm) to the thyroid are more commonly used and may result in complete or partial destruction of the thyroid *(150)*.

The details of 131-iodine therapy for childhood Graves' disease have been reported in more than 1,000 children with 131-iodine doses ranging from 100–400 uCi/gm of thyroid tissue *(138)*. Long-term cure rates are higher in patients treated with larger rather than with smaller amounts of radioiodine *(151)*. In children treated with a single dose of 150–200 uCi/gm thyroid, hyperthyroidism persists in 5–20%, and 60–90% become hypothyroid *(138)*. Hypothyroidism usually occurs within 2–6 mo of treatment. If hyperthyroidism persists, additional courses of 131-iodine are indicated. After repeated treatments, 6–12 mo may pass before hypothyroidism develops *(152)*.

Importantly, responses to 131-iodine therapy are much less favorable in patients with large rather than with small glands *(149,151)*. Thus, we usually recommend surgery when the thyroid is >100 gms. To determine thyroid volume in this setting, ultrasound is very useful (volume = 0.52 [length × depth × width]) *(153)*. We have also found less favorable responses in children with 24-h radioiodine (123-iodine) uptake values that are very high (>90%), possibly because of rapid iodine turnover. It has recently been suggested that adjunctive treatment with lithium during radioiodine decreases iodine turnover and increases radioiodine effectiveness in adults *(154)*.

Recent discussions have focused on the association of 131-iodine therapy of Graves' disease with the development or progression of ophthalmopathy in adult patients *(155)*. In contrast to adults, children rarely develop severe ophthalmopathy and proptosis is generally mild. Of 87 children treated with 131-iodine for Graves' disease at one center, eye signs improved in 90% of children, did not change in 7.5%, and worsened in 3%, which was not different from the drug-treatment group *(156)*. In the unusual setting where there is severe eye disease, adjunctive prednisone therapy or surgery should be considered *(157,158)*.

Studies involving children show that thyroid cancer risks are not increased if adequate doses of radioiodine are used to treat Grave's disease *(138,159)*. Yet, if low doses of radioiodine are given, the risk of thyroid neoplasia is increased *(138)*. There are four reported cases of thyroid malignancy in children previously treated with 131-iodine (5-yr-of-age at treatment with 50 uCi/gm; 9-yr of age at treatment with 5.4 mCi; 11-yr of age at treatment with 1.25 mCi; 16 yr of age at treatment with 3.2 mCi) *(138)*. All of these individuals were treated with low doses of 131-iodine.

In contrast, there is currently no evidence that children treated with high doses of radioiodine have increased risks of thyroid cancer *(138)*. We therefore believe that relatively high doses of 131-iodine should be used in children. Based on the data of Peters *(160)* (Fig. 4), we now aim for absorbed doses of 200–300 Gy (240–360 uCi/gm of tissue [*161*]) to make patients hypothyroid.

Although radioiodine is being used in progressively younger ages, we do not know if there is an age below which high-dose 131-iodine therapy should be avoided. Risks of thyroid cancer after external irradiation are highest in children less than 5 yr of age and progressively decline with advancing age *(138,162)*. Thus, if thyroid tissue remains in young children after radioiodine treatment, there is a risk of thyroid cancer. It may therefore be prudent to avoid radioiodine therapy in children less than 5 yr. However, children as young as 1 yr of age have been treated with radioiodine with excellent outcomes *(156)*.

Neonatal Thyrotoxicosis

Thyrotoxicosis in the neonate is a severe and life-threatening condition that can be associated with lasting neurological problems *(163)*. If a mother has Graves' disease, there is a 1 in 80 chance that TRAbs will be transferred to the fetus, resulting in intrauterine or neonatal hyperthyroidism *(164)*. Rarely, neonatal thyrotoxicosis will persist like the Graves' disease seen in older children *(165)*.

If a mother with Graves' disease is taking antithyroid medications during pregnancy, fetal thyroid hormone synthesis will be inhibited, preventing the development of intrauterine hyperthyroidism *(165)*. However, the infant may be born with a goiter and hypothyroidism *(166)*. At birth, circulating levels of T4 may be low and TSH elevated. In most cases the effects of antithyroid drugs wane and thyroid function normalizes within a week *(164)*. Yet, if there has been significant transplacental passage of TRAbs, thyrotoxicosis will develop *(164,167)*.

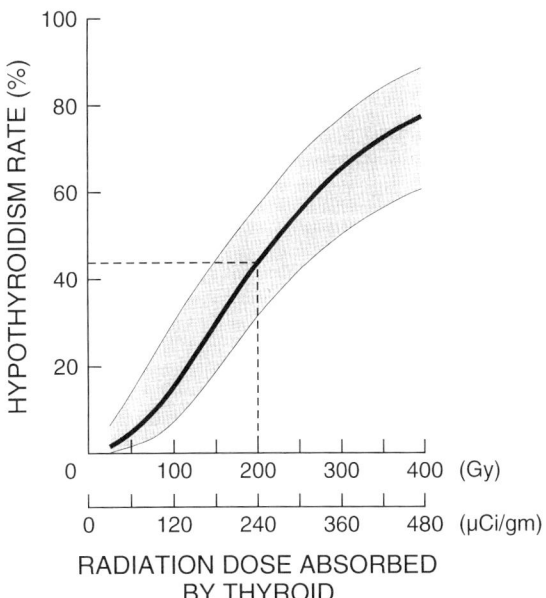

Fig. 4. Relationship between the amount of 131-iodine absorbed by the whole thyroid per gm of thyroid tissue and the incidence of hypothyroidism after treatment of Grave's disease. Data adapted from Peters and co-workers *(160)*. Data assumes effective T1/2 of 6 d, uniform distribution of 131-iodine in thyroid tissue, and 24-h retention of 100 uCi/g with an absorbed β dose of 83.2 Gy *(161)*.

If a mother with a history of Graves' disease is not taking antithyroid drugs during pregnancy, the fetus may develop intrauterine hyperthyroidism *(163)*. If not recognized, this may result in profound intrauterine thyrotoxicosis and growth retardation *(163)*. Such infants have prematurely fused cranial sutures, advanced skeletal ages, long-term learning problems, and mental retardation *(163,168)*. If fetal hyperthyroidism is recognized prenatally by the presence of fetal tachycardia (heart rate >160 after 22 wk), treatment of the mother with antithyroid drugs will reduce intrauterine thyrotoxicosis *(165,169,170)*.

Treatment of thyrotoxic infants consists of antithyroid medications (PTU 5–10 mg/kg/d or MMI 0.5–1.0 mg/kg/d) and beta-blockade (propranolol 1 mg/kg/d). Lugol's solution or saturated potassium iodide may be given (1–2 drops every 8 h) for 7–10 d to more rapidly control biochemical hyperthyroidism. After approximately 2 wk of antithyroid drug therapy, thyroid hormone levels will decline. When thyroid hormone levels fall below normal (8 ug/dl), supplementary levo-thyroxine (37.5 ug/d for term infants) is added to prevent hypothyroidism. As TRAbs are cleared from the infants circulation, spontaneous recovery begins within 3 mo and is usually complete by 6 mo *(163,167)*. Thus, treatment can be weaned after 3 mo. Monitoring the infant's TRAb levels is also a useful predictor of when antithyroid medication can be weaned *(171,172)*.

Infectious Thyroiditis

Occasionally a child will present with hyperthyroidism, tenderness over the thyroid gland, and fever due to bacterial infection on the thyroid, a condition referred to as acute thyroiditis *(173,174)*. This is usually associated with a fistula connecting the piriform sinus on the left side of the pharynx to the thyroid *(174,175)*. Fevers can be high, and erythrocyte sedimentation rates and white counts elevated. Ultrasonography may reveal a local abscess. In contrast with Graves' disease, there is reduced uptake for 99Te-pertechnetate or radioiodine when thyroid scanning is performed.

The offending bacteria consist of Hemophyllus influenza, oral flora, group A Streptococcus, or Staphylococcus *(174)*. Thus, treatment with a beta-lactamase-resistant antibiotic is recommended. For severe cases, hospitalization and intravenous antibiotic administration is indicated, as there may be lymphatic drainage into the mediastinal region. Surgical drainage is needed if a localized abscess develops and the response to antibiotics is poor *(174,175)*.

Because the infectious process results in destruction of thyroid tissue, there may be release of preformed thyroid hormone and hyperthyroidism during infection. The hyperthyroid state is usually transient and treatment with antithyroid drugs is not indicated *(174)*. If the patient becomes symptomatic, beta-blockers may be used.

After the child has recovered, a pharyngeogram is indicated to test for a patent piriform sinus tract. Occasionally, the tract may close as the result of the infection. However, if the tract persists and acute thyroiditis recurs, resection is needed *(174)*.

Viral infections of the thyroid may occur and result in subacute thyroiditis *(173)*. In comparison with acute thyroiditis, subacute thyroiditis may be less severe *(173,176)*. However, there may be fever, thyroid tenderness, and hyperthyroidism that may last for several weeks *(177)*. Because it is difficult to clinically distinguish bacterial and viral thyroid infections, antibiotic treatment is indicated when infectious thyroiditis is suspected.

Thyroid Hormone Resistance

Thyroid hormones exert their effects by binding to specific nuclear receptors to regulate cellular gene expression *(178,179)*. When the thyroid hormone receptor is mutated, impaired tissue responsiveness results leading to thyroid enlargement, elevated levels of T4 and T3 tachycardia, and behavioral problems *(180,181)*. In contrast with Graves' disease, TSH levels are normal or slightly elevated.

The most common forms of thyroid hormone resistance are caused by mutations of the thyroid hormone receptor beta gene *(181)*. More than 75 mutations have been identified, resulting in impaired affinity for T3 *(181)*. Mutant thyroid hormone receptors also block the function of normal thyroid hormone receptors *(180,181)*. Thus, thyroid hormone resistance is a dominant-negative mutation, and inheritance is autosomal dominant *(181)*. Detection of thyroid hormone resistance in the index case may therefore lead to diagnosing the condition in other family members.

Most individuals with resistance to thyroid hormone have generalized thyroid hormone resistance (GRTH) *(182)*. These individuals are eu-metabolic and asymptomatic, with TSH levels in the normal range. In contrast, some individuals will have isolated pituitary thyroid hormone resistance (PRTH). These individuals have symptoms of hyperthyroidism, as they are sensitive to the effects of increased thyroid hormone levels *(183,184)*. Resistance to thyroid hormone can also be associated with CNS problems. About 50% of individual with resistance to thyroid hormone will have attention deficit hyperactivity disorder and a minority will have mental retardation *(184,185)*.

Because individuals compensate for thyroid hormone resistance by secreting more thyroid hormone, treatment is not necessary *(181,186)*. However, patients with thyroid

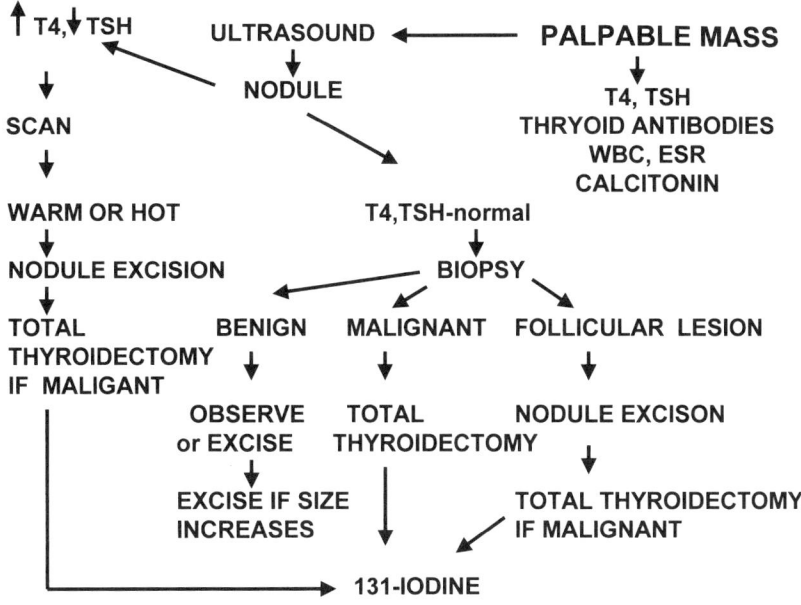

Fig. 5. Algorithm for the diagnosis and treatment of palpable thyroid nodules.

hormone resistance may be improperly diagnosed as having Graves' disease and ablation of the thyroid performed. In this situation, replacement therapy with large doses of exogenous thyroid hormone is needed.

With the earlier recognition of resistance to thyroid hormone due to newborn screening, the issue of whether children with resistance to thyroid hormone should be treated prenatally or during infancy has been raised *(181,186)*. Treatment is generally reserved for infants with elevated TSH levels, growth failure, seizures, and developmental delay *(181,186)*.

THYROID MASSES

One area of distinction between adult and pediatric endocrinology is in the evaluation and treatment of thyroid nodules. The risk of malignancy is far greater in a child or adolescent with a thyroid nodule than an adult *(187–189)*. Thus, evaluation and treatment of thyroid nodules in pediatric patients involves biopsy and/or surgical resection *(190)* (Fig. 5). Fortunately, if a thyroid malignancy is present, the prognosis is usually excellent *(191)*.

Thyroid Tumors

Although the incidence of malignancy in thyroid nodules in children has fallen over the past few decades, malignancy is present 20% of the time when a nodule is present *(187–189)*. Nonmalignant thyroid nodules include follicular adenomas, inflammatory rests, cysts, multinodular goiters, granulomatous disorders, and abscesses *(187–189)*. Of the malignant tumors, papillary and follicular carcinomas predominate *(189)*. Less common cancers include anaplastic, insular, and squamous lesions. Rarely sarcomas treatments and lymphoma are detected in the thyroid.

Medullary carcinoma of the thyroid also occurs in children, usually in the setting of Multiple Endocrine Neoplasia syndromes (MEN IIa or IIb) or familial medullary carcinoma of the thyroid *(192)*. If there is a history of MEN IIa or IIb, or familial medullary carcinoma of the thyroid, testing for mutations in the RET oncogene should be preformed early in infancy. If the child has a mutation, total thyroidectomy before 5 yr of age is recommended *(193–195)*.

The likelihood that a thyroid nodule is present needs to be considered when there is asymmetrical fullness in the thyroid, or the gland appears to be symmetrically enlarged and antithyroid antibodies are not present *(190)*. Ultrasonography can determine if a thyroid mass is present. If a nodule is seen, radionuclide scanning using either 99Te-pertechnetate or radioiodine is used to assess if the nodule has the capacity to trap iodine (a warm or hot nodule) or is nonfunctional (a cold nodule) *(1)*. Calcitonin determination is also useful in determining if a medullary thyroid carcinoma is present *(14)*.

The risk of malignancy is higher when the age is young, there is a history of radiation exposure, and the nodule is large *(196,197)*. However, cancers are seen in small nodules (<1.0 cm), and nodule size does not distinguish between malignant and benign disease in children *(197)*.

Whereas the latency time between radiation exposure and the development of thyroid cancer is generally more than 10 yr *(198)*, children exposed to radiation after the explosion at the Chernobyl nuclear power plant developed thyroid cancers with much shorter latency periods *(199)*. The risk of thyroid cancer and nodules is also higher in children who have received head and neck radiation therapy for Hodgkin's disease *(200)*. Thus, radiation-exposed children need close follow-up.

Hyperfunctioning Nodules

Warm or hot nodules lead to excessive production of thyroid hormone and can be associated with clinical and biochemical hyperthyroidism *(201)*. Interestingly, activating mutations of the TSH receptor and G_s have been discovered in hyperfunctioning nodules *(202,203)*. Whereas it is possible to ablate hyperfunctioning nodules with radioiodine, surgical excision of hyperfunctioning nodules in children and adolescents is recommended, since radiation-exposed normal thyroid tissue will remain after the hyperfunctioning nodule is ablated. Although the risk of malignancy in hyperfunctioning nodules is low, thyroid cancers have also been described in warm nodules *(204,205)*.

Nonfunctioning (Cold) Nodules

Nonfunctioning nodules are far more common than hyperfunctioning nodules and are more likely to be malignant *(190)*. Thus, percutaneous or excisional biopsy is indicated if a cold-nodule is detected. Thyroid biopsies are painful without local anesthesia. Yet by instilling local lidocaine, excellent local anesthesia can be obtained allowing repeated biopsy. For small nodules (<1.0 cm), ultrasound-guided biopsy may be needed. Even if a thyroid biopsy is not suggestive of a thyroid malignancy, excision of the nodule may still be recommended, as the incidence of malignancies in childhood thyroid nodules is about 20% and biopsies may miss malignant tissue *(206,207)*.

If cytology indicates a papillary or undifferentiated thyroid carcinoma, total thyroidectomy is performed along with lymph-node dissection *(191,196,208)*. However, if cytology indicates a follicular lesion, only the nodule is removed and formal pathological examination is performed *(209)*. If pathology indicates a follicular neoplasm, a total thyroidectomy is performed several weeks later *(209)*. This approach reflects the difficulty in determining if cancer is present in a follicular lesion by cytology *(209)*.

If excision is not performed and a benign lesion is suspected, some clinicians will treat with levo-thyroxine to suppress TSH and monitor nodule size by ultrasound *(210,211)*. However, the utility of this approach has been recently questioned *(211,212)*. If nodular enlargement occurs during observation, excision is indicated. Fortunately, if a malignancy is present in a "watched" nodule, most thyroid neoplasms grow slowly and are not aggressive *(196,213)*.

Thyroid Cancer Treatment

A large body of evidence shows excellent long-term outcomes when thyroid cancers are treated with total thyroidectomy and 131-iodine *(191,214,215)*. Thus, total thyroidectomy and 131-iodine administration is recommended when papillary or follicular carcinoma is detected. 131-iodine also improves the long-term outcome of aggressive insular tumors *(216)* and medullary tumors that can trap iodine *(217,218)*. Depending on the nature of the tumor, doses ranging from 30–200 mCi of radioiodine are used *(214)*.

After radioiodine treatment, patients need to be treated with relatively high doses of levo-thyroxine to lower TSH secretion *(191)*. Measurement of thyroglobulin levels should be performed at 4- to 6-mo intervals, and 131-iodine scanning should be considered annually *(191)*. Measurement of calcitonin is also indicated in patients with medullary carcinoma *(219)*. Increasing cancer-marker levels are indicative of recurrent disease that may require additional 131-iodine treatment or surgical resection *(191,220)*.

Fortunately, cure rates for most thyroid malignancies are excellent in children. When papillary and follicular lesions are treated with total thyroidectomy and radioiodine, complete cure is the rule rather than the exception *(191,196,213,221)*. Even when metastatic disease is seen at presentation, cure rates are greater than 70% for the most common thyroid malignancies *(196,213)*.

SUMMARY

Coupling clinical observation with diagnostic testing can identify disorders of the thyroid axis in most children. However, thyroid disorders are often insidious in onset and may escape early clinical detection. Effective treatments are now available for most forms of thyroid diseased that affect children.

REFERENCES

1. Mirk, P, Rufini, V, Summaria V, Salvatori M. Diagnostic imaging of the thyroid: methodology and normal patterns. Rays 1999;24:215–228.
2. Ueda D. Normal volume of the thyroid gland in children. J Clin Ultrasound 1990;18:455–462.
3. Hopwood NJ, Carroll RG, Kenny FM, Foley TP Jr. Functioning thyroid masses in childhood and adolescence. Clinical, surgical, and pathologic correlations. J Pediatr 1976;89:710–718.
4. Page CP, Kemmerer WT, Haff RC, Mazzaferri EL. Thyroid carcinomas arising in thyroglossal ducts. Ann Surg 1974;180:799–803.
5. Kaplan MM. Clinical perspectives in the diagnosis of thyroid disease. Clin Chem 1999;45:1377–1383.
6. Ruiz M, Rajatanavin R, Young RA, et al. Familial dysalbuminemic hyperthyroxinemia: a syndrome that can be confused with thyrotoxicosis. N Engl J Med 1982;306:635–639.
7. Farror C, Wellby ML, Beng C. Familial dysalbuminaemic hyperthyroxinaemia and other causes of euthyroid hyperthyroxinaemia. J R Soc Med 1987;80:750–752.
8. Nikolai TF, Seal US. X-chromosome linked inheritance of thyroxine-binding globulin deficiency. J Clin Endocrinol Metab 1967;27:1515–520.

9. De Groot LJ. Dangerous dogmas in medicine: the nonthyroidal illness syndrome. J Clin Endocrinol Metab 1999;84:151–164.

10. Squire CR, Fraser WD. Thyroid stimulating hormone measurement using a third generation immunometric assay. Ann Clin Biochem 1995;32:307–313.

11. Lafranchi S. Thyroiditis and acquired hypothyroidism. Pediatr Ann 1992;21:29, 32–39.

12. Rapoport B. Pathophysiology of Hashimoto's thyroiditis and hypothyroidism. Annu Rev Med 1991;42: 91–96.

13. Fisher DA, Pandian MR, Carlton E. Autoimmune thyroid disease: an expanding spectrum. Pediatr Clin North Am 1987;34:907–918.

14. Pacini F, Fontanelli M, Fugazzola L, et al. Routine measurement of serum calcitonin in nodular thyroid diseases allows the preoperative diagnosis of unsuspected sporadic medullary thyroid carcinoma. J Clin Endocrinol Metab 1994;78:826–829.

15. Foley TP Jr, Abbassi V, Copeland KC, Draznin MB. Brief report: hypothyroidism caused by chronic autoimmune thyroiditis in very young infants. N Engl J Med 1994;330:466–468.

16. Van Dop C, Conte FA, Koch TK, Clark SJ, Wilson-Davis SL, Grumbach MM. Pseudotumor cerebri associated with initiation of levothyroxine therapy for juvenile hypothyroidism. N Engl J Med 1983; 308:1076–1080.

17. Dong BJ, Hauck WW, Gambertoglio JG, et al. Bioequivalence of generic and brand-name levothyroxine products in the treatment of hypothyroidism. JAMA 1997;277:1205–1213.

18. Sekadde CB, Slaunwhite WR Jr, Aceto T Jr, Murray K. Administration of thyroxin once a week. J Clin Endocrinol Metab 1974;39:759–764.

19. Rivkees SA, Hardin DS. Cretinism after weekly dosing with levothyroxine for treatment of congenital hypothyroidism. J Pediatr 1994;125:147–149.

20. Carnell NE, Valente WA. Thyroid nodules in Graves' disease: classification, characterization, and response to treatment [published erratum appears in Thyroid 1998 Nov;8(11):1079]. Thyroid 1998;8: 647–652.

21. Case records of the Massachusetts General Hospital. Weekly clinicopathological exercises. Case 15-1985. Cardiopulmonary arrest in a 14-year-old girl. N Engl J Med 1985;312:976–983.

22. Ahonen P, Myllarniemi S, Sipila I, Perheentupa J. Clinical variation of autoimmune polyendocrinopathy-candidiasis-ectodermal dystrophy (APECED) in a series of 68 patients. N Engl J Med 1990;322: 1829–1836.

23. Mihailova D, Grigorova R, Vassileva B, et al. Autoimmune thyroid disorders in juvenile chronic arthritis and systemic lupus erythematosus. Adv Exp Med Biol 1999;455:55–60.

24. Jarnerot G, Azad Khan AK, Truelove SC. The thyroid in ulcerative colitis and Crohn's disease. II. Thyroid enlargement and hyperthyroidism in ulcerative colitis. Acta Med Scand 1975;197:83–87.

25. Rivkees SA, Bode HH, Crawford JD. Long-term growth in juvenile acquired hypothyroidism: the failure to achieve normal adult stature. N Engl J Med 1988;318:599–602.

26. Sklar CA, Qazi R, David R. Juvenile autoimmune thyroiditis. Hormonal status at presentation and after long-term follow-up. Am J Dis Child 1986;140:877–880.

27. Abbassi V, Rigterink E, Cancellieri RP. Clinical recognition of juvenile hypothyroidism in the early stage. Clin Pediatr (Phila) 1980;19:782–786.

28. Smith S, Rivkees SA. Influence of thyroid hormone status on body mass index in children. Unpublished.

29. Guiral J, Fisac R, Martin-Herraez A, Garcia-Velazquez J. Slipped capital femoral epiphysis in primary juvenile hypothyroidism. Acta Orthop Belg 1994;60:343–345.

30. Anasti JN, Flack MR, Froehlich J, Nelson LM, Nisula BC. A potential novel mechanism for precocious puberty in juvenile hypothyroidism. J Clin Endocrinol Metab 1995;80:276–279.

31. Rao NS, Sriprakash ML, Dash RJ. Primary juvenile hypothyroidism with precocious puberty, galactorrhoea and multicystic ovaries. J Assoc Physicians India 1987;35:161–163.

32. Piziak VK, Hahn HB Jr. Isolated menarche in juvenile hypothyroidism. Clin Pediatr (Phila) 1984;23: 177–179.

33. Pringle PJ, Stanhope R, Hindmarsh P, Brook CG. Abnormal pubertal development in primary hypothyroidism. Clin Endocrinol (Oxf) 1988;28:479–486.

34. Watanabe T, Minamitani K, Minagawa M, et al. Severe juvenile hypothyroidism: treatment with GH and GnRH agonist in addition to thyroxine. Endocr J 1998;45(Suppl):S159–S162.

35. Minamitani K, Murata A, Ohnishi H, Wataki K, Yasuda T, Niimi H. Attainment of normal height in severe juvenile hypothyroidism. Arch Dis Child 1994;70:429–430; discussion 430–431.

36. Fisher DA. Catch-up growth in hypothyroidism [editorial]. N Engl J Med 1988;318:632–634.
37. Mitchell HS. Recommended dietary allowances up to date. J Am Diet Assoc 1974;64:149–150.
38. Woeber KA. Iodine and thyroid disease. Med Clin North Am 1991;75:169–178.
39. Bona G, Chiorboli E, Rapa A, Weber G, Vigone MC, Chiumello G. Measurement of urinary iodine excretion to reveal iodine excess in neonatal transient hypothyroidism. J Pediatr Endocrinol Metab 1998;11:739–743.
40. Koga Y, Sano H, Kikukawa Y, Ishigouoka T, Kawamura M. Effect on neonatal thyroid function of povidone-iodine used on mothers during perinatal period. J Obstet Gynaecol 1995;21:581–585.
41. l'Allemand D, Gruters A, Beyer P, Weber B. Iodine in contrast agents and skin disinfectants is the major cause for hypothyroidism in premature infants during intensive care. Horm Res 1987;28:42–49.
42. Gordon CM, Rowitch DH, Mitchell ML, Kohane IS. Topical iodine and neonatal hypothyroidism. Arch Pediatr Adolesc Med 1995;149:1336–1339.
43. Brown RS, Bloomfield S, Bednarek FJ, Mitchell ML, Braverman LE. Routine skin cleansing with povidone-iodine is not a common cause of transient neonatal hypothyroidism in North America: a prospective controlled study. Thyroid 1997;7:395–400.
44. Grosso S, Berardi R, Cioni M, Morgese G. Transient neonatal hypothyroidism after gestational exposure to amiodarone: a follow-up of two cases. J Endocrinol Invest 1998;21:699–702.
45. Costigan DC, Holland FJ, Daneman D, Hesslein PS, Vogel M, Ellis G. Amiodarone therapy effects on childhood thyroid function. Pediatrics 1986;77:703–708.
46. Delange F. The disorders induced by iodine deficiency. Thyroid 1994;4:107–128.
47. Delange F. Administration of iodized oil during pregnancy: a summary of the published evidence. Bull WHO 1996;74:101–108.
48. Boyages SC, Halpern JP. Endemic cretinism: toward a unifying hypothesis. Thyroid 1993;3:59–69.
49. Lee K, Bradley R, Dwyer J, Lee SL. Too much versus too little: the implications of current iodine intake in the United States. Nutr Rev 1999;57:177–181.
50. Matovinovic I, Trowbridge FL, Nichaman MZ, Child MA. Iodine nutriture and prevalence of endemic goiter in USA. Acta Endocrinol Suppl (Copenh) 1973;179:17–18.
51. Sherman SI, Gopal J, Haugen BR, et al. Central hypothyroidism associated with retinoid X receptor-selective ligands. N Engl J Med 1999;340:1075–1079.
52. Samuels MH, Lillehei K, Kleinschmidt-Demasters BK, Stears J, Ridgway EC. Patterns of pulsatile pituitary glycoprotein secretion in central hypothyroidism and hypogonadism. J Clin Endocrinol Metab 1990;70:391–395.
53. Trejbal D, Sulla I, Trejbalova L, Lazurova I, Schwartz P, Machanova Y. Central hypothyroidism: various types of TSH responses to TRH stimulation. Endocr Regul 1994;28:35–40.
54. Hunter MK, Mandel SH, Sesser DE, et al. Follow-up of newborns with low thyroxine and nonelevated thyroid-stimulating hormone-screening concentrations: results of the 20-year experience in the Northwest Regional Newborn Screening Program. J Pediatr 1998;132:70–74.
55. Hanna CE, Krainz PL, Skeels MR, Miyahira RS, Sesser DE, LaFranchi SH. Detection of congenital hypopituitary hypothyroidism: ten-year experience in the Northwest Regional Screening Program. J Pediatr 1986;109:959–964.
56. Adams LM, Emery JR, Clark SJ, Carlton EI, Nelson JC. Reference ranges for newer thyroid function tests in premature infants. J Pediatr 1995;126:122–127.
57. Persani L. Hypothalamic thyrotropin-releasing hormone and thyrotropin biological activity. Thyroid 1998;8:941–946.
58. Carrozza V, Csako G, Yanovski JA, et al. Levothyroxine replacement therapy in central hypothyroidism: a practice report. Pharmacotherapy 1999;19:349–355.
59. LaFranchi S. Congenital hypothyroidism: etiologies, diagnosis, and management. Thyroid 1999;9:735–740.
60. Klett M. Epidemiology of congenital hypothyroidism. Exp Clin Endocrinol Diabetes 1997;105:19–23.
61. Macchia PE. Recent advances in understanding the molecular basis of primary congenital hypothyroidism. Mol Med Today 2000;6:36–42.
62. Sunthornthepvarakui T, Gottschalk ME, Hayashi Y, Refetoff S. Brief report: resistance to thyrotropin caused by mutations in the thyrotropin-receptor gene. N Engl J Med 1995;332:155–160.
63. Smith DW, Klein AM, Henderson JR, Myrianthopoulos NC. Congenital hypothyroidism: signs and symptoms in the newborn period. J Pediatr 1975;87:958–962.
64. Dussault JH. Screening for congenital hypothyroidism. Clin Obstet Gynecol 1997;40:117–123.

65. Dussault JH. The anecdotal history of screening for congenital hypothyroidism. J Clin Endocrinol Metab 1999;84:4332–4334.

66. Postellon DC, Abdallah A. Congenital hypothyroidism: diagnosis, treatment, and prognosis. Compr Ther 1986;12:67–71.

67. Fort P, Lifshitz F, Bellisario R, et al. Abnormalities of thyroid function in infants with Down syndrome. J Pediatr 1984;104:545–549.

68. Stoll C, Dott B, Alembik Y, Koehl C. Congenital anomalies associated with congenital hypothyroidism. Ann Genet 1999;42:17–20.

69. Law WY, Bradley DM, Lazarus JH, John R, Gregory JW. Congenital hypothyroidism in Wales (1982–1993): demographic features, clinical presentation and effects on early neurodevelopment. Clin Endocrinol (Oxf) 1998;48:201–207.

70. Hall JG, Froster-Iskenius UG, Allanson JE. Handbook of Normal Physical Measurements. Oxford University Press, Oxford, 1989, p. 376.

71. Rovet J, Ehrlich R, Sorbara D. Intellectual outcome in children with fetal hypothyroidism. J Pediatr 1987;110:700–704.

72. Mitchell ML, Hermos RJ. Measurement of thyroglobulin in newborn screening specimens from normal and hypothyroid infants. Clin Endocrinol (Oxf) 1995;42:523–527.

73. Ueda D, Yoto Y, Sato T. Ultrasonic assessment of the lingual thyroid gland in children. Pediatr Radiol 1998;28:126–128.

74. Takashima S, Nomura N, Tanaka H, Itoh Y, Miki K, Harada T. Congenital hypothyroidism: assessment with ultrasound. AJNR Am J Neuroradiol 1995;16:1117–1123.

75. Fisher DA. Clinical review 19: management of congenital hypothyroidism. J Clin Endocrinol Metab 1991;72:523–529.

76. American Academy of Pediatrics AAP Section on Endocrinology and Committee on Genetics, and American Thyroid Association Committee on Public Health: Newborn screening for congenital hypothyroidism: recommended guidelines. Pediatrics 1993;91:1203–1209.

77. Gunn AJ, Wake M, Cutfield WS. High and low dose initial thyroxine therapy for congenital hypothyroidism. J Paediatr Child Health 1996;32:242–245.

78. Fisher DA, Foley BL. Early treatment of congenital hypothyroidism. Pediatrics 1989;83:785–789.

79. Czernichow P, Wolf B, Fermanian J, Pomarede R, Rappaport R. Twenty-four hour variations of thyroid hormones and thyrotrophin concentrations in hypothyroid infants treated with L-thyroxine. Clin Endocrinol (Oxf) 1984;21:393–397.

80. Tenore A. Does breast feeding mitigate short-term and long-term manifestations of congenital hypothyroidism? (Review). Endocrinol Exp 1986;20:267–284.

81. Abbassi V, Steinour TA. Successful diagnosis of congenital hypothyroidism in four breast-fed neonates. J Pediatr 1980;97:259–261.

82. Letarte J, Guyda H, Dussault JH, Glorieux J. Lack of protective effect of breast-feeding in congenital hypothyroidism: report of 12 cases. Pediatrics 1980;65:703–705.

83. Sack J, Katznelson D, Czerniak P, Lunenfeld B. Early detection of thyroid dyshormonogenesis in a breast-fed infant using a filter paper screening method. Monogr Hum Genet 1978;10:185–187.

84. Rovet JF. Does breast-feeding protect the hypothyroid infant whose condition is diagnosed by newborn screening? Am J Dis Child 1990;144:319–323.

85. Jabbar MA, Larrea J, Shaw RA. Abnormal thyroid function tests in infants with congenital hypothyroidism: the influence of soy-based formula. J Am Coll Nutr 1997;16:280–282.

86. Chorazy PA, Himelhoch S, Hopwood NJ, Greger NG, Postellon DC. Persistent hypothyroidism in an infant receiving a soy formula: case report and review of the literature. Pediatrics 1995;96:148–150.

87. Campbell NR, Hasinoff BB. Iron supplements: a common cause of drug interactions. Br J Clin Pharmacol 1991;31:251–255.

88. Franzese A, Salerno M, Argenziano A, Buongiovanni C, Limauro R, Tenore A. Anemia in infants with congenital hypothyroidism diagnosed by neonatal screening. J Endocrinol Invest 1996;19:613–619.

89. Dubuis JM, Glorieux J, Richer F, Deal CL, Dussault JH, Van Vliet G. Outcome of severe congenital hypothyroidism: closing the developmental gap with early high dose levothyroxine treatment. J Clin Endocrinol Metab 1996;81:222–227.

90. Campos SP, Sandberg DE, Barrick C, Voorhess ML, MacGillivray MH. Outcome of lower L-thyroxine dose for treatment of congenital hypothyroidism. Clin Pediatr (Phila) 1995;34:514–520.

91. Heyerdahl S, Kase BF, Lie SO. Intellectual development in children with congenital hypothyroidism in relation to recommended thyroxine treatment. J Pediatr 1991;118:850–857.

92. Cavaliere H, Medeiros-Neto GA, Rosner W, Kourides IA. Persistent pituitary resistance to thyroid hormone in congenital versus later-onset hypothyroidism. J Endocrinol Invest 1985;8:527–532.

93. Heyerdahl S, Kase BF. Significance of elevated serum thyrotropin during treatment of congenital hypothyroidism. Acta Paediatr 1995;84:634–638.

94. Fisher DA. The hypothalamic-pituitary-thyroid negative feedback control axis in children with treated congenital hypothryoidism. J Clin Endocrinol Metab 2000;85:2722–2727.

95. Vogiatzi MG, Kirkland JL. Frequency and necessity of thyroid function tests in neonates and infants with congenital hypothyroidism. Pediatrics 1997;100:E6.

96. Chiesa A, Gruneiro de Papendieck L, Keselman A, Heinrich JJ, Bergada C. Growth follow-up in 100 children with congenital hypothyroidism before and during treatment. J Pediatr Endocrinol 1994;7:211–217.

97. Heyerdahl S, Ilicki A, Karlberg J, Kase BF, Larsson A. Linear growth in early treated children with congenital hypothyroidism. Acta Paediatr 1997;86:479–483.

98. Heyerdahl S, Kase BF, Stake G. Skeletal maturation during thyroxine treatment in children with congenital hypothyroidism. Acta Paediatr 1994;83:618–622.

99. Daliva AL, Linder B, DiMartino-Nardi J, Saenger P. Three-year follow-up of borderline congenital hypothyroidism. J Pediatr 2000;136:53–56.

100. Haddow JE, Palomaki GE, Allan WC, et al. Maternal thyroid deficiency during pregnancy and subsequent neuropsychological development of the child. N Engl J Med 1999;341:549–555.

101. Pop VJ, Kuijpens JL, van Baar AL, et al. Low maternal free thyroxine concentrations during early pregnancy are associated with impaired psychomotor development in infancy. Clin Endocrinol (Oxf) 1999; 50:149–155.

102. Elementary school performance of children with congenital hypothyroidism. New England Congenital Hypothyroidism Collaborative. J Pediatr 1990;116:27–32.

103. Derksen-Lubsen G, Verkerk PH. Neuropsychologic development in early treated congenital hypothyroidism: analysis of literature data. Pediatr Res 1996;39:561–566.

104. Van Vliet G. Neonatal hypothyroidism: treatment and outcome. Thyroid 1999;9:79–84.

105. Dugbartey AT. Neurocognitive aspects of hypothyroidism. Arch Intern Med 1998;158:1413–1418.

106. Rovet JF. Congenital hypothyroidism: long-term outcome. Thyroid 1999;9:741–748.

107. Tillotson SL, Fuggle PW, Smith I, Ades AE, Grant DB. Relation between biochemical severity and intelligence in early treated congenital hypothyroidism: a threshold effect. BMJ 1994;309:440–445.

108. Rovet J, Walker W, Bliss B, Buchanan L, Ehrlich R. Long-term sequelae of hearing impairment in congenital hypothyroidism. J Pediatr 1996;128:776–783.

109. Correlation of cognitive test scores and adequacy of treatment in adolescents with congenital hypothyroidism. New England Congenital Hypothyroidism Collaborative. J Pediatr 1994;124:383–387.

110. Fisher DA. Hypothyroxinemia in premature infants: is thyroxine treatment necessary? Thyroid 1999;9: 715–720.

111. Fisher DA. Thyroid function in premature infants. The hypothyroxinemia of prematurity. Clin Perinatol 1998;25:999–1014.

112. Job L, Emery JR, Hopper AO, et al. Serum free thyroxine concentration is not reduced in premature infants with respiratory distress syndrome. J Pediatr 1997;131:489–492.

113. Vulsma T, Kok JH. Prematurity-associated neurologic and developmental abnormalities and neonatal thyroid function [editorial; comment]. N Engl J Med 1996;334:857–858.

114. Van Wassenaer AG, Kok JH, Briet JM, Pijning AM, de Vijlder JJ. Thyroid function in very preterm newborns: possible implications. Thyroid 1999;9:85–91.

115. Frank JE, Faix JE, Hermos RJ, et al. Thyroid function in very low birth weight infants: effects on neonatal hypothyroidism screening. J Pediatr 1996;128:548–554.

116. Talbot NB, Sobel EH, McArthur JW, Crawford JD. The Thyroid. Functional Endocrinology: From Birth Through Adolescence. Harvard University Press, Cambridge, MA, 1952, pp. 1–51.

117. Wilkins L. Hyperthyroidism. The Diagnosis and Treatment of Endocrine Disorders in Children and Adolescence. 3rd ed. Charles Thomas, Springfield, IL, 1965, pp. 141–150.

118. Hedberg CW, Fishbein DB, Janssen RS, et al. An outbreak of thyrotoxicosis caused by the consumption of bovine thyroid gland in ground beef. N Engl J Med 1987;316:993–998.

119. Ochi Y, Inui T, Kouki T, Yamashiro K, Hachiya T, Kajita Y. Thyroid stimulating immunoglobulin (TSI) in Graves' disease. Endocr J 1998;45:701–708.

120. Saxena KM, Crawford JD, Talbot NB. Childhood thyrotoxicosis: a longer term perspective. BMJ 1964;2:1153–1158.

121. Volpe R. Rational use of thyroid function tests. Crit Rev Clin Lab Sci 1997;34:405–438.

122. Harland PC, McArthur RG, Fawcett DM. T3 toxicosis in children. Acta Paediatr Scand 1977;66:525–528.

123. Cooper DS, Wenig BM. Hyperthyroidism caused by an ectopic TSH-secreting pituitary tumor. Thyroid 1996;6:337–343.

124. Buckingham BA, Costin G, Roe TF, Weitzman JJ, Kogut MD. Hyperthyroidism in children. A reevaluation of treatment. Am J Dis Child 1981;135:112–117.

125. Ching T, Warden MJ, Fefferman RA. Thyroid surgery in children and teenagers. Arch Otolaryngol 1977;103:544–546.

126. Perzik SL. Total thyroidectomy in Graves' disease in children. J Pediatr Surg 1976;11:191–194.

127. Altman RP. Total thyroidectomy for the treatment of Graves' disease in children. J Pediatr Surg 1973; 8:295–300.

128. Miccoli P, Vitti P, Rago T, et al. Surgical treatment of Graves' disease: subtotal or total thyroidectomy? Surgery 1996;120:1020–1024.

129. Foster RS Jr. Morbidity and mortality after thyroidectomy. Surg Gynecol Obstet 1978;146:423–429.

130. Argov S, Duek D. The vanishing surgical treatment of Graves' disease: review of current literature and experience with 50 patients. Curr Surg 1982;39:158–162.

131. Cooper DS. Antithyroid drugs for the treatment of hyperthyroidism caused by Graves' disease. Endocrinol Metab Clin North Am 1998;27:225–247.

132. Greer MA, Meihoff W, Studer H. Treatment of hyperthyroidism with a singe daily dose of propylthiouracil. N Engl J Med 1965;272:888–891.

133. Mashio Y, Beniko M, Ikota A, Mizumoto H, Kunita H. Treatment of hyperthyroidism with a small single daily dose of methimazole. Acta Endocrinol (Copenh) 1988;119:139–144.

134. Cooper DS. The side effects of antithyroid drugs. Endocrinologist 1999;9:457–468.

135. Roti E, Robuschi G, Manfredi A, et al. Comparative effects of sodium ipodate and iodide on serum thyroid hormone concentrations in patients with Graves' disease. Clin Endocrinol (Oxf) 1985;22:489–496.

136. Dallas JS, Foley TP. Hyperthyroidism. In: Lifshitz F, ed. Pediatric Endocrinology. Marcel Dekker, New York, 1996, pp. 401–414.

137. Zimmerman D, Lteif AN. Thyrotoxicosis in children. Endocrinol Metab Clin North Am 1998;27: 109–125.

138. Rivkees SA, Sklar C, Freemark M. Clinical review 99: the management of Graves' disease in children, with special emphasis on radioiodine treatment. [Review] [160 refs]. J Clin Endocrinol Metab 1998;83: 3767–3776.

139. Adorf D, Grajer KH, Kaboth W, Nerl C. Agranulocytosis induced by antithyroid therapy: effects of treatment with granulocyte colony stimulating factor. Clin Invest 1994;72:390–392.

140. Hanson JS. Propylthiouracil and hepatitis. Two cases and a review of the literature. Arch Intern Med 1984;144:994–996.

141. Torring O, Tallstedt L, Wallin G, et al. Graves' hyperthyroidism: treatment with antithyroid drugs, surgery, or radioiodine: a prospective, randomized study. Thyroid Study Group. J Clin Endocrinol Metab 1996;81:2986–2993.

142. Hamburger JI. Management of hyperthyroidism in children and adolescents. J Clin Endocrinol Metab 1985;60:1019–1024.

143. Lippe BM, Landaw EM, Kaplan SA. Hyperthyroidism in children treated with long term medical therapy: twenty-five percent remission every two years. J Clin Endocrinol Metab 1987;64:1241–1245.

144. Shulman DI, Muhar I, Jorgensen EV, Diamond FB, Bercu BB, Root AW. Autoimmune hyperthyroidism in prepubertal children and adolescents: comparison of clinical and biochemical features at diagnosis and responses to medical therapy. Thyroid 1997;7:755–760.

145. Chapman EM. History of the discovery and early use of radioactive iodine. JAMA 1983;250:2042–2044.

146. Chapman EM, Skanse BN, Evans RD. Treatment of hyperthyroidism with radioactive iodine. Radiology 1949;51:558–565.

147. Spencer RP, Kayani N, Karimeddini MK. Radioiodine therapy of hyperthyroidism: socioeconomic considerations. J Nucl Med 1985;26:663–665.

148. Peters H, Fischer C, Bogner U, Reiners C, Schleusener H. Reduction in thyroid volume after radioiodine therapy of Graves' hyperthyroidism: results of a prospective, randomized, multicentre study. Eur J Clin Invest 1996;26:59–63.

149. Peters H, Fischer C, Bogner U, Reiners C, Schleusener H. Treatment of Graves' hyperthyroidism with radioiodine: results of a prospective randomized study. Thyroid 1997;7:247–251.

150. Goolden AWG, Davey JB. The ablation of normal thryoid tissue with iodine-131. British J Radiol 1963;36:340–345.

151. Chiovato L, Fiore E, Vitti P, et al. Outcome of thyroid function in Graves' patients treated with radio-iodine: role of thyroid-stimulating and thyrotropin-blocking antibodies and of radioiodine-induced thyroid damage. J Clin Endocrinol Metab 1998;83:40–46.

152. Leslie WD, Peterdy AE, Dupont JO. Radioiodine treatment outcomes in thyroid glands previously irradiated for Graves' hyperthyroidism. J Nucl Med 1998;39:712–716.

153. Knudsen N, Bols B, Bulow I, et al. Validation of ultrasonography of the thyroid gland for epidemiological purposes. Thyroid 1999;9:1069–1074.

154. Bogazzi F, Bartalena L, Brogioni S, et al. Comparison of radioiodine with radioiodine plus lithium in the treatment of Graves' hyperthyroidism. J Clin Endocrinol Metab 1999;84:499–503.

155. Tallstedt L, Lundell G. Radioiodine treatment, ablation, and ophthalmopathy: a balanced perspective. Thyroid 1997;7:241–245.

156. Safa AM, Schumacher OP, Rodriguez-Antunez A. Long-term follow-up results in children and adolescents treated with radioactive iodine (131I) for hyperthyroidism. N Engl J Med 1975;292:167–171.

157. Wiersinga WM. Preventing Graves' ophthalmopathy. N Engl J Med 1998;338:121–122.

158. Bartalena L, Marcocci C, Bagozzi F, et al. Relation between therapy for hyperthyroidism and the course of Graves' ophthalmopathy. N Engl J Med 1998;338:73–78.

159. Levy WJ, Schumacher OP, Gupta M. Treatment of childhood Graves' disease. A review with emphasis on radioiodine treatment. Cleve Clin J Med 1988;55:373–382.

160. Peters H, Fischer C, Bogner U, Reiners C, Schleusener H. Radioiodine therapy of Graves' hyperthyroidism: standard vs. calculated 131iodine activity. Results from a prospective, randomized, multicentre study. Eur J Clin Invest 1995;25:186–193.

161. Quimby EH, Feitelberg S, Gross W. Radioactive Nuclides in Medicine and Biology. Lea and Febiger, Philadelphia, PA, 1970, p. 129.

162. Ron E, Lubin JH, Shore RE, et al. Thyroid cancer after exposure to external radiation: a pooled analysis of seven studies. Radiat Res 1995;141:259–277.

163. Zimmerman D. Fetal and neonatal hyperthyroidism. Thyroid 1999;9:727–733.

164. Skuza KA, Sills IN, Stene M, Rapaport R. Prediction of neonatal hyperthyroidism in infants born to mothers with Graves disease. J Pediatr 1996;128:264–268.

165. Check JH, Rezvani I, Goodner D, Hopper B. Prenatal treatment of thyrotoxicosis to prevent intrauterine growth retardation. Obstet Gynecol 1982;60:122–124.

166. Refetoff S, Ochi Y, Selenkow HA, Rosenfield RL. Neonatal hypothyroidism and goiter in one infant of each of two sets of twins due to maternal therapy with antithyroid drugs. J Pediatr 1974;85:240–244.

167. McKenzie JM, Zakarija M. Fetal and neonatal hyperthyroidism and hypothyroidism due to maternal TSH receptor antibodies. Thyroid 1992;2:155–159.

168. Daneman D, Howard NJ. Neonatal thyrotoxicosis: intellectual impairment and craniosynostosis in later years. J Pediatr 1980;97:257–259.

169. Bruinse HW, Vermeulen-Meiners C, Wit JM. Fetal treatment for thyrotoxicosis in non-thyrotoxic pregnant women. Fetal Ther 1988;3:152–157.

170. Momotani N, Noh J, Oyanagi H, Ishikawa N, Ito K. Antithyroid drug therapy for Graves' disease during pregnancy. Optimal regimen for fetal thyroid status. N Engl J Med 1986;315:24–28.

171. Tamaki H, Amino N, Iwatani Y, et al. Evaluation of TSH receptor antibody by 'natural in vivo human assay' in neonates born to mothers with Graves' disease. Clin Endocrinol (Oxf) 1989;30:493–503.

172. Sunshine P, Kusumoto H, Kriss JP. Survival time of circulating long-acting thyroid stimulator in neonatal thyrotoxicosis: implications for diagnosis and therapy of the disorder. Pediatrics 1965;36:869–876.

173. Vitti P, Rago T, Barbesino G, Chiovato L. Thyroiditis: clinical aspects and diagnostic imaging. Rays 1999;24:301–314.

174. Jeng LB, Lin JD, Chen MF. Acute suppurative thyroiditis: a ten-year review in a Taiwanese hospital. Scand J Infect Dis 1994;26:297–300.

175. Skuza K, Rapaport R, Fieldman R, Goldstein S, Marquis J. Recurrent acute suppurative thyroiditis. J Otolaryngol 1991;20:126–129.

176. Szabo SM, Allen DB. Thyroiditis. Differentiation of acute suppurative and subacute. Case report and review of the literature. Clin Pediatr (Phila) 1989;28:171–174.

177. Geva T, Theodor R. Atypical presentation of subacute thyroiditis. Arch Dis Child 1988;63:845–846.

178. Brent GA. The molecular basis of thyroid hormone action. N Engl J Med 1994;331:847–853.

179. Lazar MA. Steroid and thyroid hormone receptors. Endocrinol Metab Clin North Am 1991;20:681–695.

180. Chatterjee VK. Resistance to thyroid hormone: an uncommon cause of thyroxine excess and inappropriate TSH secretion. Acta Med Austriaca 1994;21:56–60.

181. Refetoff S. Resistance to thyroid hormone. Curr Ther Endocrinol Metab 1997;6:132–134.

182. Refetoff S. The syndrome of generalized resistance to thyroid hormone (GRTH). Endocr Res 1989;15: 717–743.

183. Beck-Peccoz P, Forloni F, Cortelazzi D, et al. Pituitary resistance to thyroid hormones. Horm Res 1992;38:66–72.

184. Stein MA, Weiss RE, Refetoff S. Neurocognitive characteristics of individuals with resistance to thyroid hormone: comparisons with individuals with attention-deficit hyperactivity disorder. J Dev Behav Pediatr 1995;16:406–411.

185. Hauser P, Zametkin AJ, Martinez P, et al. Attention deficit-hyperactivity disorder in people with generalized resistance to thyroid hormone. N Engl J Med 1993;328:997–1001.

186. Weiss RE, Refetoff S. Treatment of resistance to thyroid hormone: primum non nocere [editorial; comment]. J Clin Endocrinol Metab 1999;84:401–404.

187. Lugo-Vicente H, Ortiz VN. Pediatric thyroid nodules: insights in management. Bol Assoc Med P R 1998;90:74–78.

188. Raab SS, Silverman JF, Elsheikh TM, Thomas PA, Wakely PE. Pediatric thyroid nodules: disease demographics and clinical management as determined by fine needle aspiration biopsy. Pediatrics 1995;95: 46–49.

189. Scott MD, Crawford JD. Solitary thyroid nodules in childhood: is the incidence of thyroid carcinoma declining? Pediatrics 1976;58:521–525.

190. Giuffrida D, Gharib H. Controversies in the management of cold, hot, and occult thyroid nodules. Am J Med 1995;99:642–650.

191. Schlumberger MJ. Papillary and follicular thyroid carcinoma. N Engl J Med 1998;338:297–306.

192. Skinner MA, Wells SA Jr. Medullary carcinoma of the thyroid gland and the MEN 2 syndromes. Semin Pediatr Surg 1997;6:134–140.

193. Giuffrida D, Gharib H. Current diagnosis and management of medullary thyroid carcinoma. Ann Oncol 1998;9:695–701.

194. Gill JR, Reyes-Mugica M, Iyengar S, et al. Early presentation of metastatic medullary carcinoma in multiple endocrine neoplasia, type IIA: implications for therapy. J Pediatr 1996;129:459–464.

195. Heptulla RA, Schwartz RP, Bale AE, Flynn S, Genel M. Familial medullary thyroid carcinoma: presymptomatic diagnosis and management in children. J Pediatr 1999;135:327–331.

196. Feinmesser R, Lubin E, Segal K, Noyek A. Carcinoma of the thyroid in children: a review. J Pediatr Endocrinol Metab 1997;10:561–568.

197. Fowler CL, Pokorny WJ, Harberg FJ. Thyroid nodules in children: current profile of a changing disease. South Med J 1989;82:1472–1478.

198. Ron E, Modan B, Preston D, Alfandary E, Stovall M, Boice JD Jr. Thyroid neoplasia following low-dose radiation in childhood. Radiat Res 1989;120:516–531.

199. Becker DV, Robbins J, Beebe GW, Bouville AC, Wachholz BW. Childhood thyroid cancer following the Chernobyl accident: a status report. Endocrinol Metab Clin North Am 1996;25:197–211.

200. Shafford EA, Kingston JE, Healy JC, Webb JA, Plowman PN, Reznek RH. Thyroid nodular disease after radiotherapy to the neck for childhood Hodgkin's disease. Br J Cancer 1999;80:808–814.

201. Lugo-Vicente H, Ortiz VN, Irizarry H, Camps JI, Pagan V. Pediatric thyroid nodules: management in the era of fine needle aspiration. J Pediatr Surg 1998;33:1302–1305.

202. Tonacchera M, Vitti P, Agretti P, et al. Activating thyrotropin receptor mutations in histologically heterogeneous hyperfunctioning nodules of multinodular goiter. Thyroid 1998;8:559–564.

203. Esapa C, Foster S, Johnson S, Jameson JL, Kendall-Taylor P, Harris PE. G protein and thyrotropin receptor mutations in thyroid neoplasia. J Clin Endocrinol Metab 1997;82:493–496.

204. Vattimo A, Bertelli P, Cintorino M, et al. Hurthle cell tumor dwelling in hot thyroid nodules: preoperative detection with technetium-99m-MIBI dual-phase scintigraphy. J Nucl Med 1998;39:822–825.

205. David E, Rosen IB, Bain J, James J, Kirsh JC. Management of the hot thyroid nodule. Am J Surg 1995; 170:481–483.

206. Taneri F, Poyraz A, Tekin E, Ersoy E, Dursun A. Accuracy and significance of fine-needle aspiration cytology and frozen section in thyroid surgery. Endocr Regul 1998;32:187–191.

207. Caraway NP, Sneige N, Samaan NA. Diagnostic pitfalls in thyroid fine-needle aspiration: a review of 394 cases. Diagn Cytopathol 1993;9:345–350.

208. Ain KB. Papillary thyroid carcinoma. Etiology, assessment, and therapy. Endocrinol Metab Clin North Am 1995;24:711–760.
209. McHenry CR, Sandoval BA. Management of follicular and Hurthle cell neoplasms of the thyroid gland. Surg Oncol Clin N Am 1998;7:893–910.
210. Cooper DS. Clinical review 66: thyroxine suppression therapy for benign nodular disease. J Clin Endocrinol Metab 1995;80:331–334.
211. Gharib H, Mazzaferri EL. Thyroxine suppressive therapy in patients with nodular thyroid disease. Ann Intern Med 1998;128:386–394.
212. Derwahl M, Broecker M, Kraiem Z. Clinical review 101: thyrotropin may not be the dominant growth factor in benign and malignant thyroid tumors. J Clin Endocrinol Metab 1999;84:829–834.
213. Flannery TK, Kirkland JL, Copeland KC, Bertuch AA, Karaviti LP, Brandt ML. Papillary thyroid cancer: a pediatric perspective. Pediatrics 1996;98:464–466.
214. Mazzaferri EL. Thyroid remnant 131I ablation for papillary and follicular thyroid carcinoma. Thyroid 1997;7:265–271.
215. Yeh SD, La Quaglia MP. 131I therapy for pediatric thyroid cancer. Semin Pediatr Surg 1997;6:128–133.
216. Hassoun AA, Hay ID, Goellner JR, Zimmerman D. Insular thyroid carcinoma in adolescents: a potentially lethal endocrine malignancy. Cancer 1997;79:1044–1048.
217. Nieuwenhuijzen Kruseman AC, Bussemaker JK, Frolich M. Radioiodine in the treatment of hereditary medullary carcinoma of the thyroid. J Clin Endocrinol Metab 1984;59:491–494.
218. Nusynowitz ML, Pollard E, Benedetto AR, Lecklitner ML, Ware RW. Treatment of medullary carcinoma of the thyroid with I-131. J Nucl Med 1982;23:143–146.
219. Chi DD, Moley JF. Medullary thyroid carcinoma: genetic advances, treatment recommendations, and the approach to the patient with persistent hypercalcitoninemia. Surg Oncol Clin North Am 1998;7:681–706.
220. Burmeister LA, Goumaz MO, Mariash CN, Oppenheimer JH. Levothyroxine dose requirements for thyrotropin suppression in the treatment of differentiated thyroid cancer. J Clin Endocrinol Metab 1992;75:344–350.
221. Zimmerman D, Hay ID, Gough IR, et al. Papillary thyroid carcinoma in children and adults: long-term follow-up of 1039 patients conservatively treated at one institution during three decades. Surgery 1988;104:1157–1166.

IV

CALCIUM AND BONE

8

Genetic Control of Parathyroid Gland Development and Molecular Insights into Hypoparathyroidism

Michael A. Levine, MD

INTRODUCTION

Normal mineral metabolism and skeletal development depend on an intricate interplay of parathyroid, renal, and skeletal factors. Crucial in this respect is parathyroid hormone (PTH), which is synthesized and secreted from the parathyroid glands and at a rate inversely proportional to the serum-ionized calcium concentration. Hormone secretion is tightly regulated through the interaction of extracellular calcium with specific calcium-sensing receptors (CaSRs) *(1–3)* that are present on the surface of the parathyroid cell. In turn, PTH regulates mineral metabolism and skeletal homeostasis through its actions on specialized target cells in bone and kidney that express the PTH/parathyroid hormone-related peptide (PTHrP) or type 1 PTH receptor. The integrated actions of PTH and 1,25-dihydroxyvitamin D on these target tissues provide a precise system of control and maintain the serum-ionized calcium concentration within a narrow range that is critical for many physiological processes.

Hypoparathyroidism may occur in combination with other endocrine (or nonendocrine) defects or as a solitary endocrinopathy termed "isolated hypoparathyroidism" *(4)*. Molecular genetic studies indicate that hypoparathyroidism is caused by mutations in a variety of genes, including genetic defects that impair synthesis (i.e., *PTH* gene defects) or secretion (i.e., *CASR* gene defects) of PTH as well as defects that impair the embryological

From: *Contemporary Endocrinology: Developmental Endocrinology: From Research to Clinical Practice*
Edited by: E. A. Eugster and O. H. Pescovitz © Humana Press Inc., Totowa, NJ

development of the parathyroid glands. In this chapter we review the genetic defects that have been associated with hypoparathyroidism, and examine the significance of candidate genes that appear critical for the embryological development of the parathyroid glands.

PARATHYROID PHYSIOLOGY AND PATHOPHYSIOLOGY

The concentration of extracellular ionized calcium is tightly regulated by PTH and 1,25-dihydroxyvitamin D (1,25[OH]$_2$D; calcitriol). PTH is synthesized in the four parathyroid glands as a preprohormone (115 amino acids), converted to a prohormone (90 amino acids) as it is transported across the rough endoplasmic reticulum, and stored in secretory granules as the mature 84-amino acid hormone. PTH is secreted at a rate inversely proportional to the ambient serum-ionized calcium concentration. Secretion, as well as synthesis, of PTH is tightly regulated through the interaction of extracellular calcium (and to a lesser extent other divalent cations) with specific CaSRs that are expressed on the surface of parathyroid cells. These receptors are also present on several other cell types that are involved in regulating mineral ion homeostasis (1–3), including the calcitonin-secreting C-cells of the thyroid and renal tubular cells. The CaSR is a member of a large family of plasma-membrane receptors that can bind hormones, neurotransmitter, cytokines, light photons, and taste and odor molecules. These receptors consist of a single polypeptide chain that is predicted by hydrophobicity plots to span the plasma membrane seven times (i.e., heptahelical), forming three extracellular and three or four intracellular loops and a cytoplasmic carboxyl-terminal tail. The heptahelical receptors are coupled by heterotrimeric (αβγ) G proteins (5) to signal effector molecules (e.g., adenylyl cyclase, phospholipase C, potassium channels) that are localized to the inner surface of the plasma membrane (*see* refs. 6,7 for reviews).

Binding of extracellular calcium to the CaSR activates the receptor and facilitates its interaction and activation of G proteins that stimulate phospholipase C activity (G$_q$ and G$_{11}$) and inhibit adenylyl cyclase (G$_i$) (8). Activation of phospholipase C leads to the generation of the second messengers inositol 1,4,5-trisphosphate and diacylglycerol, which increase levels of cytosolic calcium via release from intracellular stores and stimulate protein kinase C (PKC) activity, respectively. These second-messenger systems mediate the parathyroid cell's responses to elevated concentrations of extracellular calcium, which include inhibition of PTH release, suppression of *PTH* gene expression, and accelerated intracellular degradation of PTH. By contrast, PTH secretion is acutely increased when the extracellular calcium concentration is low. Over time, persistent hypocalcemia leads to reduced intracellular degradation of PTH, increased *PTH* gene expression, and enhanced parathyroid-cell proliferation.

PTH has direct effects on bone to regulate calcium exchange at osteocytic sites and to enhance osteoclast-mediated bone resorption. In the kidney, PTH directly enhances distal tubular reabsorption of calcium, decreases the proximal tubular reabsorption of phosphate, and stimulates the metabolic conversion of 25-hydroxyvitamin D (25[OH]D) to 1,25(OH)$_2$D, the active vitamin D metabolite. 1,25(OH)$_2$D acts on bone to enhance bone resorption and on the gastrointestinal mucosa to increase absorption of dietary calcium.

PTH regulates mineral metabolism and skeletal homeostasis through effects on specialized target cells that are present in bone and kidney. PTH action first requires binding of the hormone to specific G protein-coupled receptors that are expressed on the plasma membrane of target cells. The classical PTH receptor is a ~75-kD glycoprotein that is often referred to as the PTH/PTHrP or type 1 PTH receptor (type 1 PTH-r). Molecular cloning of cDNAs encoding PTH receptors from several species *(9–12)* has indicated that the type 1 receptor expressed on bone and kidney cells is identical. The type 1 PTH-r binds both PTH and PTHrP, a factor made by diverse tumors that cause humorally mediated hypercalcemia, with equivalent affinity, which accounts for the similar activities of both hormones. The type 1 PTH-r is most abundantly expressed in the physiological target tissues for PTH action (i.e., kidney and bone), but it is also found in a wide variety of fetal and adult tissues where it appears to mediate the paracrine/autocrine signaling pathways of PTHrP rather than the endocrine actions of PTH. By contrast, a second PTH receptor, termed the type 2 receptor protein, interacts with PTH but not PTHrP *(13,14)*, and has a very restricted tissue distribution that does not include classical PTH target tissues (i.e., bone and kidney). Recently, a hypothalamic peptide termed TIP39 has been identified as the physiological ligand for the type 2 PTH receptor *(14–16)*, but the biological functions mediated by this receptor remain largely unknown.

The type 1 PTH receptor couples to several G proteins *(17)* that activate adenylyl cyclase and phospholipase C. Thus, receptor activation leads to rapid generation of the second messengers cAMP *(18,19)*, inositol 1,4,5-trisphosphate and diacylglycerol *(20,21)*, and cytosolic calcium *(22–25)*.

In states of functional hypoparathyroidism, in which PTH secretion or action is deficient, the normal effects of PTH on bone and kidney are absent. Bone resorption, and release of calcium from skeletal stores, is diminished. Renal tubular reabsorption of calcium is decreased, but because of hypocalcemia and low filtered load, urinary calcium excretion is low. In the absence of PTH action, urinary clearance of phosphate is decreased, and hyperphosphatemia occurs. The deficiency of PTH action and the hyperphosphatemia together impair renal synthesis of $1,25(OH)_2D$, and absorption of calcium from the intestine is markedly impaired. $1,25(OH)_2D$ is also a potent stimulator of bone resorption, and its absence also decreases the availability of calcium from bone.

PARATHYROID CELL DEVELOPMENT AND GROWTH

The parathyroid glands first appear during the fifth wk of gestation in human fetuses *(26)*, which corresponds to d E11.5 in the mouse embryo (Fig. 1). The glands grow to a total parenchymal weight of about 3 µg at a gestational age of 8 wk *(27)*. Weight increases slowly between 8 and 12 wk, but then more rapidly growing to 300 µg by age 18 wk and 4 mg at birth *(27)*. During this time mineralization of the fetal skeleton is provided by active calcium transport from mother to fetus across the placenta, utilizing a calcium pump in the basal membrane of the trophoblast that maintains a 1:1.4 (mother:fetus) calcium gradient throughout gestation *(28)*. PTH and PTHrP share in the regulation of the fetus' unique calcium metabolism, and both hormones are synthesized in the parathyroids. PTHrP is also produced in other fetal tissues (e.g., placenta and liver), and may play the dominant role in maintenance of normal fetal calcium homeostasis, particularly through its unique ability to regulate the placental calcium pump *(29,30)*. The fetal parathyroids, and PTH, are also required for maintenance of normal fetal mineral metabolism, as *Hoxa3*-null mouse fetuses that genetically lack parathyroids (as well as the thymus and other structures derived from the third and fourth pharyngeal arches) have reduced serum calcium, elevated serum phosphate, and reduced calcium in amniotic fluid despite normal plasma

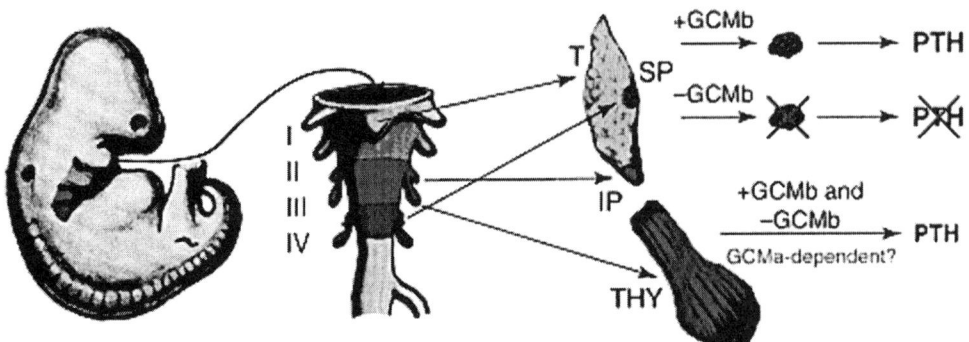

Fig. 1. GCMB and the development of the parathyroid glands. The four entodermal pharyngeal pouches (I-IV) of a 10.5 d postconception (dpc) mouse embryo are shown as well as their derivatives; IP, inferior parathyroid; SP, superior parathyroid; T, thyroid; THY, thymus. Parathyroid development and synthesis of parathyroid hormone (PTH) in the presence (+GCMB) or absence (–GCMB) of GCMB are indicated. Adapted with permission from ref. *(76)*.

PTHrP levels and normal placental calcium transfer *(30)*. Presumably, PTH acts on fetal bone and perhaps kidney to maintain normal serum levels of calcium.

After birth parathyroid growth continues at a rate of about 2.5–3.0 mg/yr. After an apparent second parathyroid growth spurt during adolescence, parathyroid growth continues more slowly until the mature parenchymal weight of approx 85–95 mg is reached at age 30 yr *(27,31)*. Cell turnover in the adult parathyroid gland in humans aged 18–76 yr is approx 5%/yr *(32)*, with cycling cells randomly distributed and without evidence for a separate stem-cell population. These observations indicate that the adult parathyroid gland is a discontinuously replicating or conditionally renewing tissue *(33)*, with an average cell life span of about 20 yr in man. As adult parathyroid cell number does not change, the very slow rate of cell gain must be balanced by a correspondingly slow rate of cell loss. Parathyroid cell loss presumably occurs through apoptosis, and remaining parathyroid cells are somehow triggered from G0 to G1 in order to maintain a stable cell number. Such a compensatory mitotic response typically occurs in endocrine cells under the control of the hypothalamus or the pituitary, but its occurrence in the parathyroid gland, for which no trophic hormone has been identified, suggests the existence of novel proliferative mechanisms. Under special circumstances, the rate of parathyroid cell proliferation can be increased. The parathyroid glands can enlarge greatly during states of chronic hypocalcemia, particularly in renal failure where hyperphosphatemia and low levels of calcitriol accompany hypocalcemia.

MOLECULAR GENETIC
BASIS FOR HYPOPARATHYROIDISM

Hypoparathyroidism is characterized by PTH insufficiency, which can result from: 1) failure of parathyroid development, 2) destruction of parathyroids, and 3) defective or impaired parathyroid cell function (Table 1). Hypoparathyroidism may occur in combination with other disorders, including autoimmune (e.g., autoimmune polyendocrinopathy-candidiasis-ectodermal dystrophy [APECED] syndrome *[34–37]*) or developmental defects (e.g., DiGeorge syndrome (DGS) *(38–42)* or the hypoparathyroidism, sensori-

Table 1
Genetic Causes of Hypoparathyroidism

A. Defective synthesis of parathyroid hormone (MIM 168450)
1. Autosomal dominant mutation in preproPTH gene
2. Autosomal recessive mutation in preproPTH gene
B. Defective secretion of PTH
1. Activating mutation of calcium sensing receptor gene (MIM 145980)
C. Idiopathic hypoparathyroidism
1. Autosomal recessive (MIM 241400)
2. X-linked (MIM 307700)
D. Embryological defects in parathyroid gland development
1. DiGeorge syndrome (del 22q) DGS1; MIM 188400
2. DiGeorge syndrome (del 10p) DGS2; MIM 601362
3. Velocardiofacial syndrome (del 22q) MIM 192430
4. Barakat (HDR) syndrome (*GATA3* mutation) MIM 146255
5. Kenney-Caffey/Sanjad-Sakati syndrome (1q42-q43); MIM 12700; 241410
6. Primary parathyroid aplasia (*GCMB* mutation)
E. Destruction of the parathyroid glands
1. Autoimmune hypoparathyroidism
2. Autoimmune polyglandular syndrome, type 1 (APECED; *AIRE* gene) MIM 240300
F. Metabolic defects and mitochondrial neuromyopathies
1. Kearn-Sayre syndrome (MIM 530000)
2. Pearson syndrome (MIM 557000)
3. t-RNA leu mutations (MIM 590050)
4. Long chain hydroxy acylCoA dehydrogenease deficiency (LCHAD)/Mitochondrial trifunctional protein deficiency (MIM 600890).

neural deafness, renal anomaly (HDR) syndrome *[43]*), or as an isolated endocrinopathy termed isolated hypoparathyroidism (IH) with autosomal or X-linked modes of inheritance *(44)*. Early molecular genetic studies of hypoparathyroidism focused on subjects with autosomal forms of IH, and evaluated the likelihood that mutation of the *PTH* gene was the basis for PTH deficiency *(4)*. These studies identified one family in which IH was likely to be caused by a defect in the *PTH* gene, and confirmed that molecular pathology at additional loci was likely to account for the clinical and genetic heterogeneity of this disorder *(4,44)*. In subsequent work, this mutation was identified as a missense mutation in exon 2 of the *PTH* gene that resulted in the substitution of arginine for cysteine in the hydrophobic core of the signal peptide of the preproPTH molecule *(45)*. This single amino acid substitution impairs proteolytic processing of the mutant protein and interferes with processing of co-expressed wild-type PTH molecules, thus providing a basis for autosomal dominant IH in this family *(46)*. Defects in the *PTH* gene are an uncommon cause of hypoparathyroidism, and additional mutations have been identified in only two other families, both with autosomal recessive forms of IH. In one family affected children were found to be homozygous for a novel mutation in exon 2 that is predicted to disrupt normal processing of the preproPTH molecule. The mutant allele carries a T→C transition in the first base of codon 23 that results in the replacement of serine (TCG) by proline (CCG) at the −3 position of the signal peptide of preproPTH. This change is hypothesized to inhibit cleavage by signal peptidase at the normal position, and thereby lead to rapid degradation of the preproPTH protein in the rough endoplasmic reticulum *(47)*. In a second family *(48)*, hypoparathyroidism occurred in members who were homozygous for a single base transversion (G→C) at the exon 2-intron 2 boundary. This mutation alters the invariant gt dinucleotide of the 5 donor splice site that presumably affects annealing of the U1-snRNP recognition component of the nuclear RNA splicing enzyme. Using a sensitive reverse transcriptase-RT-polymerase chain reaction (PCR) technique, PTH cDNA in affected subjects was found to be 90 bp shorter than the corresponding wild-type form, as exon 1 had been spliced to exon 3 in the mutant PTH mRNA *(48)*. This processing of nascent mRNA results in the deletion of exon 2 from the mature transcript (i.e., exon skipping), thus eliminating both the initiation codon and the signal peptide sequence from the aberrant preproPTH mRNA, and accounts for hypoparathyroidism in this family.

Gain-of-function mutations in the *CASR* gene encoding the CaSR have been identified in many subjects with a mild variant of hypoparathyroidism, termed autosomal dominant hypocalcemia, that is associated with low or low-normal levels of serum PTH and relative hypercalciuria *(49,50)*. Contrasting loss-of-function mutations in the *CASR* gene have been associated with the complementary hypercalcemic syndrome known as familial hypocalciuric hypercalcemia (FHH; also known as familial benign hypocalciuric hypercalcemia [FBHH]) and neonatal severe hyperparathyroidism *(50–52)*.

Defects in the genes encoding PTH and the CaSR impair synthesis (i.e., *PTH* gene defects) or secretion (i.e., *CASR* gene defects) of PTH rather than development of the parathyroid glands *(45,47–50)*. More recently, genes that are important for directing the critical steps in the differentiation of neural-crest cells into parathyroid cells have recently been identified through the complementary approaches of creating genetically modified mice and investigating patients with developmental syndromes. Parathyroid aplasia or dysplasia is a common feature of DGS, the most frequent contiguous gene deletion syndrome in humans. DGS is characterized by a constellation of developmental defects that are thought to result from a disturbance of migration or differentiation of the cervical neural crest into the pharyngeal arches, pouches, and outflow tract. Molecular mapping studies have demonstrated an association between DGS and deletions involving 22q11.21-q11.23 (DGSI) *(38,39,53–58)* in the great majority of patients, but deletions at a second locus at l0p13, termed DGSII, have been found in some patients *(40,41,59)*. Microdeletions in 22q11.21 can be readily identified by fluorescent *in situ* hybridization (FISH), but similar molecular testing for the 10p13 microdeletion is not widely available. Microdeletion of the chromosomal band 22q11.21-q11.23 also occurs in subjects with the velocardiofacial (or Schprintzen) syndrome *(60)*, and it is now believed that DGSI and velocardiofacial syndromes are overlapping disorders that share a common molecular pathophysiology *(61)*. The term "CATCH 22" has been applied to these disorders as a unifying acronym to emphasize the characteristic features: cardiac defects, abnormal facies, thymic aplasia, cleft palate, hypoparathyroidism, and 22 chromosomal deletion. The heterozygous deletion of chromosomal region 22q11.2 is sporadic in most cases of DGSI, but in rare cases the abnormal chromosome is inherited from a mildly affected parent *(62,63)*. Mapping studies of the human DGS deleted region on chromosome 22q11.2 have defined a 250-kb minimal critical region that includes a variety of candidate genes, including a human homolog of a yeast gene, referred to as *UDFIL*, that encodes a protein involved in the degradation of ubiquinated proteins *(42)*. Deletion of the homologous region in the mouse (Df(16)1) causes a very similar disorder *(64)*, and recently, mouse models that closely replicate the

DGS have been generated through targeted ablation of genes within the DGS/Df(16)1. Mice deficient in *Crkol*, a gene expressed in neural-crest cells and that encodes an adapter protein implicated in response to growth factors and focal-adhesion signaling, exhibit defects in multiple cranial and cardiac neural-crest derivatives *(65)*. A similar phenotype occurs in mice deficient in *Tbx1 (66–68)*, a T-box transcription factor that is expressed in nonneural crest-derived cells of head mesenchyme, pharyngeal arches and pouches, and otic vesicles of the embryo. However, the generalized nature of the defects in DGS and these mice suggest that these genes affect neural-crest migration, proliferation, or survival prior to differentiation. By contrast, mice deficient in *Hoxa-3*, a homeodomain transcription factor, have more restricted neural-crest defects that impair development of only thyroid, thymus, and parathyroids *(66,69)*, suggesting that loss of Hoxa-3 affects the intrinsic capacity of this neural-crest-cell population to differentiate and/or to induce proper differentiation of the surrounding pharyngeal arch and pouch tissues.

In addition to these mouse models, molecular genetic studies in patients with the hypo-parathyroidism-deafness-renal anomaly (HDR; also termed Barakat syndrome *[70]*) syndrome have also provided insights into the genetic control of parathyroid development. Patients with HDR have haploinsufficiency of *GATA3 (43)*, a zinc-finger transcription factor that is expressed during human and mouse embryogenesis in the developing kidney, otic vesicle, and parathyroids *(71,72)*. Surprisingly, mice that lack one or both copies of *Gata3* fail to show features of the HDR syndrome despite manifesting other developmental defects *(73)*. Although the *Hox3*, *Gata3*, and DGS genes are involved in parathyroid development, their expression in additional sites and their involvement in development of other tissues suggest that they do not regulate parathyroid-specific gene expression. By contrast, mice deficient in the transcription factor *Gcm2* (glial cell missing, 2), develop hypoparathyroidism but lack defects in other tissues derived from the neural crest or pharyngeal pouches (Fig. 1) *(74)*. The vertebrate GCM transcription factors are a small family of unique proteins that are orthologs of the *gcm* gene originally identified in *Drosophila melanogaster (75,76)*. In the fly, the *gcm* gene is specifically and transiently expressed in the glial lineage and promotes choice between glial vs neuronal fate in a multipotential neural stem cell. Loss-of-function mutations in the *gcm* gene result in conversion of presumptive glial cells into neurons *(75)*. Based on its nuclear localization and sequence specific DNA-binding activity, GCM has been proposed to be a transcriptional activator of glial-specific genes. Two mammalian GCM homologs have been identified, encoded by the *GCMA* and *GCMB* genes. Both genes encode peptides of 504-506 amino acids and contain a number of motifs that are signatures of the GCM family of nuclear transcription factors, including an evolutionarily conserved DNA binding domain in the amino-terminal region, a nuclear-localization signal, and several potential PEST sequences [i.e., a region consisting of the amino acids Pro (P), Glu (E), Ser (S), and Thr (I) that contains phosphorylation sites and is flanked by Lys, Arg, and His], which are typical of proteins displaying a rapid turnover *(75,77–80)*. Despite the significant homology of the GCMA and GCMB proteins to their *Drosophila* ortholog, the unique expression patterns of these two mammalian genes suggest that the roles of these proteins have evolved and diverged significantly from those in the fly. Although GCMB is detectable at low levels in embryonic neural tissues and kidney *(77,80,81)*, transcripts for both GCMA and GCMB are found primarily in non-neural tissues, whereas *GCMA* is most highly expressed in the placenta *(77,79)*, where it plays a critical role in trophoblast differentiation *(82)* and the thymus. By contrast, the *GCMB* gene is expressed predominately, if not exclusively, in the PTH-secreting cells of the developing and mature parathyroid gland *(77)*.

The failure of parathyroid glands to develop in mice in which *Gcm2* has been genetically ablated provides strong evidence that this gene is the master control gene for parathyroid development. Remarkably, levels of circulating PTH in these mice are normal, but apparently insufficient to maintain a normal serum level of calcium. The source of the circulating PTH is the thymus, which contains subcapsular cells that express not only PTH but also CaSR. Although Gcm2 is not present in the thymus, the PTH-positive cells express the closely related gene *Gcm1*, suggesting that this homolog is able to induce development of a parathyroid-like phenotype in these thymic epithelial cells (Fig. 1) *(74)*.

The recent description of a large intragenic mutation in the *GCMB* genes of the proband of an extended kindred with IH indicates that normal function of the *GCMB* genes is similarly required for embryological development of parathyroid glands in humans *(83)*. The parents of the proband as well as several other unaffected relatives were heterozygous for the mutation, indicating that as in the mouse, haploinsufiency of the *GCMB* gene is not associated with a clinical phenotype. These data implicate the *GCMB* gene, located at chromosome 6p23-24 *(80,81)*, as a cause of IH, but the prevalence of *GCMB* gene mutations in IH remains unknown.

HYPOPARATHYROIDISM AS A COMPONENT OF OTHER DEVELOPMENTAL SYNDROMES

Hypoparathyroidism occurs as a variable component of several additional developmental syndromes (Table 1). Hypoparathyroidism is present in more than 50% of patients who have the Kenney-Caffey syndrome, an unusual syndrome characterized by growth retardation, osteosclerosis, and medullary stenosis of tubular bones, and ophthalmic defects *(84,85)*. Recent studies indicate that the Kenney-Caffey syndrome is related to the Sanjad-Sakati syndrome, in which congenital hypoparathyroidism is associated with growth and mental retardation *(86)*. Both of these autosomal recessive disorders are linked to the same 1.0 cM region on chromosome 1q42-q43, and are therefore likely to be allelic *(87,88)*. Hypoparathyroidism also has been described in patients with rare familial syndromes that are associated with collateral developmental defects such as lymphedema, prolapsing mitral valve, brachytelephalangy, and nephropathy *(89)*. Congenital hypoparathyroidism also occurs as a feature of several generalized metabolic defects and mitochondrial neuromyopathies (Table 1). The role of these genetic defects in the etiology of hypoparathyroidism, or in embryological development of the parathyroid glands, remains to be elucidated.

CONCLUSION

Studies of transgenic mice and the identification of mutations in subjects with hypoparathyroidism have resulted in considerable progress towards identifying genes that are required for embryological development of the parathyroid glands. However, the hierarchy of biological action for these various genes, as well as their downstream targets, remains unknown. A more comprehensive understanding of the molecular control of parathyroid embryology will require the functional characterization of these genes as well as identification of additional genes that are essential for parathyroid development.

REFERENCES

1. Hebert SC, Brown EM. The extracellular calcium receptor. [Review] [64 refs]. Curr Opin Cell Biol 1995;7:484–492.
2. Brown EM, Gamba G, Riccardi D, et al. Cloning and characterization of an extracellular Ca^{2+}-sensing receptor from bovine parathyroid. Nature 1993;366:575–580.
3. Chattopadhyay N, Mithal A, Brown EM. The calcium-sensing receptor: a window into the physiology and pathophysiology of mineral ion metabolism. Endocr Rev 1996;17:289–307.
4. Ahn TG, Antonarakis SE, Kronenberg HM, Igarashi T, Levine MA. Familial isolated hypoparathyroidism: a molecular genetic analysis of 8 families with 23 affected persons. Medicine 1986;65:73–81.
5. Neer EJ. Heterotrimeric G Proteins: organizers of transmembrane signals. Cell 1995;80:249–257.
6. Gudermann T, Nurnberg B, Schultz G. Receptors and G proteins as primary components of transmembrane signal transduction. Part 1. G-protein-coupled receptors: structure and function. J Mol Med 1995; 73:51–63.
7. Nurnberg B, Gudermann T, Schultz G. Receptors and G proteins as primary components of transmembrane signal transduction. Part 2. G proteins: structure and function. J Mol Med 1995;73:123–132.
8. Yamaguchi T, Chattopadhyay N, Brown EM. G protein-coupled extracellular Ca^{2+} (Ca^{2+}o)-sensing receptor (CaR): roles in cell signaling and control of diverse cellular functions. Adv Pharmacol 2000; 47:209–53.:209–253.
9. Schipani E, Karga H, Karaplis AC, et al. Identical complementary deoxyribonucleic acids encode a human renal and bone parathyroid hormone (PTH)/PTH-related peptide receptor. Endocrinology 1993; 132:2157–2165.
10. Abou Samra AB, Juppner H, Force T, et al. Expression cloning of a common receptor for parathyroid hormone and parathyroid hormone-related peptide from rat osteoblast-like cells: a single receptor stimulates intracellular accumulation of both cAMP and inositol trisphosphates and increases intracellular free calcium. Proc Natl Acad Sci USA 1992;89:2732–2736.
11. Juppner H, Abou Samra AB, Freeman M, et al. A G protein-linked receptor for parathyroid hormone and parathyroid hormone-related peptide. Science 1991;254:1024–1026.
12. Adams AE, Pines M, Nakamoto C, et al. Probing the bimolecular interaction of parathyroid hormone (PTH) and the human PTH/PTHrP receptor. II. Cloning, characterization of, and photoaffinity cross-linking to the recombinant human PTH/PTHrP receptor. Biochemistry 1995;34:10,553–10,559.
13. Behar V, Pines M, Nakamoto C, et al. The human PTH2 receptor: binding and signal transduction properties of the stably expressed recombinant receptor. Endocrinology 1996;137:2748–2757.
14. Usdin TB, Gruber C, Bonner TI. Identification and functional expression of a receptor selectively recognizing parathyroid hormone, the PTH2. J Biol Chem 1995;270:15,455–15,458.
15. Usdin TB. Evidence for a parathyroid hormone-2 receptor selective ligand in the hypothalamus. Endocrinology 1997;138:831–834.
16. Hoare SR, Clark JA, Usdin TB. Molecular determinants of tuberoinfundibular peptide of 39 residues (TIP39) selectivity for the parathyroid hormone-2 (PTH2) receptor. N-terminal truncation of TIP39 reverses PTH2 receptor/PTH1 receptor binding selectivity. J Biol Chem 2000;275:27,274–27,283.
17. Schwindinger WF, Fredericks J, Watkins L, et al. Coupling of the PTH/PTHrP receptor to multiple G-proteins. Direct demonstration of receptor activation of Gs, Gq/11, and Gi(1) by [alpha-^{32}P]GTP-gamma-azidoanilide photoaffinity labeling. Endocrine 1998;8:201–209.
18. Melson GL, Chase LR, Aurbach GD. Parathyroid hormone-sensitive adenyl cyclase in isolated renal tubules. Endocrinology 1970;86:511–518.
19. Chase LR, Fedak SA, Aurbach GD. Activation of skeletal adenyl cyclase by parathyroid hormone in vitro. Endocrinology 1969;84:761–768.
20. Civitelli R, Reid IR, Westbrook S, Avioli LV, Hruska KA. PTH elevates inositol polyphosphates and diacylglycerol in a rat osteoblast-like cell line. Am J Physiol 1988;255:E660–E667.
21. Dunlay R, Hruska K. PTH receptor coupling to phospholipase C is an alternate pathway of signal transduction in bone and kidney. Am J Physiol 1990;258:F223–F231.
22. Gupta A, Martin KJ, Miyauchi A, Hruska KA. Regulation of cytosolic calcium by parathyroid hormone and oscillations of cytosolic calcium in fibroblasts from normal and pseudohypoparathyroid patients. Endocrinology 1991;128:2825–2836.
23. Civitelli R, Martin TJ, Fausto A, Gunsten SL, Hruska KA, Avioli LV. Parathyroid hormone-related peptide transiently increases cytosolic calcium in osteoblast-like cells: comparison with parathyroid hormone. Endocrinology 1989;125:1204–1210.

24. Reid IR, Civitelli R, Halstead LR, Avioli LV, Hruska KA. Parathyroid hormone acutely elevates intra-cellular calcium in osteoblastlike cells. Am J Physiol 1987;253:E45–E51.

25. Yamaguchi DT, Hahn TJ, Iida-Klein A, Kleeman CR, Muallem S. Parathyroid hormone-activated cal-cium channels in an osteoblast-like clonal osteosarcoma cell line. J Biol Chem 1987;262:7711–7718.

26. Norris EH. Anatomical evidence of prenatal function of the human parathyroid glands. Anat Rec 1946; 96:129–141.

27. Parfitt AM. Parathyroid growth: normal and abnormal. In: Bilezikian JP, Marcus R, Levine MA, eds. The Parathyroids: Basic and Clinical Concepts. Raven Press, New York, 1994, pp. 373–405.

28. Kovacs CS, Kronenberg HM. Maternal-fetal calcium and bone metabolism during pregnancy, puerpe-rium, and lactation. Endocr Rev 1997;18:832–872.

29. Kovacs CS, Lanske B, Hunzelman JL, Guo J, Karaplis AC, Kronenberg HM. Parathyroid hormone-related peptide (PTHrP) regulates fetal-placental calcium transport through a receptor distinct from the PTH/PTHrP receptor. Proc Natl Acad Sci USA 1996;93:15,233–15,238.

30. Kovacs CS, Manley NR, Moseley JM, Martin TJ, Kronenberg HM. Fetal parathyroids are not required to maintain placental calcium transport. J Clin Invest 2001;107:1007–1015.

31. Akerstrom G, Grimelius L, Johansson H, Lundqvist H, Pertoft H, Bergstrom R. The parenchymal cell mass in normal human parathyroid glands. Acta Pathol Microbiol Scand [A] 1981;89:367–375.

32. Wang Q, Palnitkar S, Parfitt AM. The basal rate of cell proliferation in normal human parathyroid tissue: implications for the pathogenesis of hyperparathyroidism. Clin Endocrinol (Oxf) 1997;46:343–349.

33. Wright N, Alison M. The Biology of Epithelial Cell Populations. Clarendon Press, Oxford, 1984.

34. Ahonen P. Autoimmune polyendocrinopathy—candidosis—ectodermal dystrophy (APECED): auto-somal recessive inheritance. Clin Genet 1985;27:535–542.

35. Ahonen P, Myllarniemi S, Sipila I, Perheentupa J. Clinical variation of autoimmune polyendo-crinopathy—candidiasis—ectodermal dystrophy (APECED) in a series of 68 patients. N Engl J Med 1990;322:1829–1836.

36. Scott HS, Heino M, Peterson P, et al. Common mutations in autoimmune polyendocrinopathy—can-didiasis—ectodermal dystrophy patients of different origins. Mol Endocrinol 1998;12:1112–1119.

37. Obermayer-Straub P, Manns MP. Autoimmune polyglandular syndromes. Baillieres Clin Gastroenterol 1998;12:293–315.

38. Greig F, Paul E, DiMartino-Nardi J, Saenger P. Transient congenital hypoparathyroidism: resolution and recurrence in chromosome 22q11 deletion. J Pediatr 1996;128:563–567.

39. Hur H, Kim YJ, Noh CI, Seo JW, Kim MH. Molecular genetic analysis of the DiGeorge syndrome among Korean patients with congenital heart disease. Mol Cells 1999;9:72–77.

40. Monaco G, Pignata C, Rossi E, et al. DiGeorge anomaly associated with 10p deletion. Am J Med Genet 1991;19:215–216.

41. Daw SC, Taylor C, Kraman M, et al. A common region of 10p deleted in DiGeorge and velocardiofacial syndromes. Nat Genet 1996;13:458–460.

42. Yamagishi H, Garg V, Matsuoka R, Thomas T, Srivastava D. A molecular pathway revealing a genetic basis for human cardiac and craniofacial defects. Science 1999;283:1158–1161.

43. Van Esch H, Groenen P, Nesbit MA, et al. GATA3 haplo-insufficiency causes human HDR syndrome. Nature 2000;406:419–422.

44. Thakker RV. The molecular genetics of hypoparathyroidism. In: Bilezikian JP, Marcus R, Levine MA, eds. The Parathyroids: Basic and Clinical Concepts. Academic Press, San Diego, CA, 2001, pp. 779–790.

45. Arnold A, Horst SA, Gardella TJ, Baba H, Levine MA, Kronenberg HM. Mutation of the signal peptide-encoding region of the preproparathyroid hormone gene in familial isolated hypoparathyroidism. J Clin Invest 1990;86:1084–1087.

46. Karaplis AC, Lim SK, Baba H, Arnold A, Kronenberg HM. Inefficient membrane targeting, transloca-tion, and proteolytic processing by signal peptidase of a mutant preproparathyroid hormone protein. J Biol Chem 1995;270:1629–1635.

47. Sunthornthepvarakul T, Churesigaew S, Ngowngarmratana S. A novel mutation of the signal peptide of the preproparathyroid hormone gene associated with autosomal recessive familial isolated hypopar-athyroidism. J Clin Endocrinol Metab 1999;84:3792–3796.

48. Parkinson DB, Thakker RV. A donor splice site mutation in the parathyroid hormone gene is associated with autosomal recessive hypoparathyroidism. Nat Genet 1992;1:149–152.

49. Pearce SH, Williamson C, Kifor O, et al. A familial syndrome of hypocalcemia with hypercalciuria due to mutations in the calcium-sensing receptor [see comments]. N Engl J Med 1996;335:1115–1122.

50. Bai M, Quinn S, Trivedi S, et al. Expression and characterization of inactivating and activating mutations in the human Ca^{2+}o-sensing receptor. J Biol Chem 1996;271:19,537–19,545.
51. Chou YH, Pollak MR, Brandi ML, et al. Mutations in the human Ca(2+)-sensing-receptor gene that cause familial hypocalciuric hypercalcemia. Am J Hum Genet 1995;56:1075–1079.
52. Pollak MR, Chou YH, Marx SJ, et al. Familial hypocalciuric hypercalcemia and neonatal severe hyperparathyroidism. Effects of mutant gene dosage on phenotype. J Clin Invest 1994;93:1108–1112.
53. de la Chapelle A., Herra R, Kiovisto M, Aula P. A deletion in chromosome 22 can cause DiGeorge syndrome. Hum Genet 1981;57:253–256.
54. Kelley RI, Zackai FH, Emanuel BS. The association of the DiGeorge anomalad with partial monosomy of chromosome 22. J Pediatr 1982;101:197.
55. Driscoll DA, Budarf ML, Emanuel BS. A genetic etiology for DiGeorge syndrome: consistent deletions and microdeletions of 22q11. Am J Hum Genet 1991;50:924.
56. Matsuoka R, Kimura M, Scambler PJ, et al. Molecular and clinical study of 183 patients with conotruncal anomaly face syndrome. Hum Genet 1998;103:70–80.
57. Berend SA, Spikes AS, Kashork CD, et al. Dual-probe fluorescence in situ hybridization assay for detecting deletions associated with VCFS/DiGeorge syndrome I and DiGeorge syndrome II loci. Am J Med Genet 2000;91:313–317.
58. Scambler PJ. The 22q11 deletion syndromes. Hum Mol Genet 2000;9:2421–2426.
59. Lai MMR, Scriven PN, Ball C, Berry AC. Simultaneous partial monosomy 10p and trisomy 5q in a case of hypoparathyroidism. J Med Genet 1992;29:586–588.
60. Kelly D, Goldberg R, Wilson D, et al. Confirmation that the velo-cardio-facial syndrome is associated with haplo-insufficiency of genes at chromosome 22q11. Am J Med Genet 1993;45:308–312.
61. Shprintzen RJ. Velocardiofacial syndrome and DiGeorge sequence. J Med Genet 1994;31:423–424.
62. Wilson DI, Cross IE, Goodship JA, et al. DiGeorge syndrome with isolated aortic coarctation and isolated ventricular septal defect in three sibs with a 22q11 deletion of maternal origin. Br Heart J 1991;66: 308–312.
63. De Silva D, Duffty P, Booth P, Auchterlonie I, Morrison N, Dean JC. Family studies in chromosome 22q11 deletion: further demonstration of phenotypic heterogeneity. Clin Dysmorphol 1995;4:294–303.
64. Lindsay EA, Botta A, Jurecic V, et al. Congenital heart disease in mice deficient for the DiGeorge syndrome region. Nature 1999;401:379–383.
65. Guris DL, Fantes J, Tara D, Druker BJ, Imamoto A. Mice lacking the homologue of the human 22q11.2 gene CRKL phenocopy neurocristopathies of DiGeorge syndrome. Nat Genet 2001;27:293–298.
66. Manley NR, Capecchi MR. The role of *Hoxa-3* in mouse thymus and thyroid development. Development 1995;121:1989–2003.
67. Lindsay EA, Vitelli F, Su H, et al. Tbx1 haploinsufficieny in the DiGeorge syndrome region causes aortic arch defects in mice. Nature 2001;410:97–101.
68. Jerome LA, Papaioannou VE. DiGeorge syndrome phenotype in mice mutant for the T-box gene, Tbx1. Nat Genet 2001;27:286–291.
69. Manley NR, Capecchi MR. Hox group 3 paralogs regulate the development and migration of the thymus, thyroid, and parathyroid glands. Dev Biol 1998;195:1–15.
70. Barakat AY, D'Albora JB, Martin MM, Jose PA. Familial nephrosis, nerver deafness, and hypoparathyroidism. J Pediatr 1977;91:61–64.
71. Lakshmanan G, Lieuw KH, Lim KC, et al. Localization of distant urogenital system-, central nervous system-, and endocardium-specific transcriptional regulatory elements in the GATA-3 locus. Mol Cell Biol 1999;19:1558–568.
72. Debacker C, Catala M, Labastie MC. Embryonic expression of the human GATA-3 gene. Mech Dev 1999;85:183–187.
73. Pandolfi PP, Roth ME, Karis A, et al. Targeted disruption of the GATA3 gene causes severe abnormalities in the nervous system and in fetal liver haematopoiesis. Nat Genet 1995;11:40–44.
74. Gunther T, Chen ZF, Kim J, et al. Genetic ablation of parathyroid glands reveals another source of parathyroid hormone. Nature 2000;406:199–203.
75. Hosoya T, Takizawa K, Nitta K, Hotta Y. Glial cells missing: a binary switch between neuronal and glial determination in Drosophila. Cell 1995;82:1025–1036.
76. Wegner M, Riethmacher D. Chronicles of a switch hunt: gcm genes in development. Trends Genet 2001; 17:286–290.
77. Kim J, Jones BW, Zock C, et al. Isolation and characterization of mammalian homologs of the *Drosophila* gene glial cells missing. Proc Natl Acad Sci USA 1998;95:12,364–12,369.

78. Jones BW, Fetter RD, Tear G, Goodman CS. Glial cells missing: a genetic switch that controls glial versus neuronal fate. Cell 1995;82:1013–1023.

79. Altshuller Y, Copeland NG, Gilbert DJ, Jenkins NA, Frohman MA. Gcm1, a mammalian homolog of Drosophila glial cells missing. FEBS Lett 1996;393:201–204.

80. Kammerer M, Pirola B, Giglio S, Giangrande A. GCMB, a second human homolog of the fly glide/gcm gene. Cytogenet Cell Genet 1999;84:43–47.

81. Kanemura Y, Hiraga S, Arita N, et al. Isolation and expression analysis of a novel human homologue of the Drosophila glial cells missing (gcm) gene. FEBS Lett 1999;442:151–156.

82. Schreiber J, Riethmacher-Sonnenberg E, Riethmacher D, et al. Placental failure in mice lacking the mammalian homolog of glial cells missing, GCMa. Mol Cell Biol 2000;20:2466–2474.

83. Ding CL, Buckingham B, Levine MA. Familial isolated hypoparathyroidism caused by a mutation in the gene for the transcription factor *GCMB*. J Clin Invest 2001;108:1215–1220.

84. Thakker RV. Molecular basis of PTH underexpression. In: Bilezikian JP, Raisz LG, Rodan GA, eds. Principles of Bone Biology. Academic Press, San Diego, CA, 1996, pp. 837–851.

85. Franceschini P, Testa A, Bogetti G, et al. Kenny-Caffey syndrome in two sibs born to consanguineous parents: evidence for an autosomal recessive variant. Am J Med Genet 1992;42:112–116.

86. Sanjad SA, Sakati NA, Abu-Osba YK, Kaddoura R, Milner RD. A new syndrome of congenital hypoparathyroidism, severe growth failure, and dysmorphic features. Arch Dis Child 1991;66:193–196.

87. Diaz GA, Gelb BD, Ali F, et al. Sanjad-Sakati and autosomal recessive Kenny-Caffey syndromes are allelic: evidence for an ancestral founder mutation and locus refinement. Am J Med Genet 1999;85: 48–52.

88. Kelly TE, Blanton S, Saif R, Sanjad SA, Sakati NA. Confirmation of the assignment of the Sanjad-Sakati (congenital hypoparathyroidism) syndrome (OMIM 241410) locus to chromosome 1q42-43. J Med Genet 2000;37:63–64.

89. Dahlberg PJ, Borer WZ, Newcomer KL, Yutac WR. Autosomal or X-linked recessive syndrome of congenital lymphedema, hypoparathyroidism, nephropathy, prolapsing mitral valve, and brachytelephalangy. Am J Med Genet 1983;16:99–104.

9 Bone Physiology

Salvatore Minisola, MD
and Lorraine A. Fitzpatrick, MD

CONTENTS

MACROARCHITECTURE OF NORMAL BONE

The skeleton is a specialized structure that serves multiple functions, which are defined as mechanical, protective, and metabolic. The skeleton serves as the support and site of muscle attachment, and in this role, has a mechanical function. The skeleton also protects vital organs and contains bone marrow. For the maintenance of normal calcium-phosphate homeostasis, the skeleton is a metabolic reservoir of these ions, which are essential for numerous functions. The skeleton is comprised of multiple tissues including cartilage, bone, fat, connective tissue, nerves, vessels, and bone marrow. Anatomically, two types of bones are found in the skeleton. Flat bones, such as the skull, scapula, mandible, and ileum are distinctly derived by intramembranous development. Long bones such as the tibia, femur, and humerus are formed by endochondral calcification *(1)*.

If one sections longitudinally through a long bone, there are wider end pieces called the epiphyses and a cylindrical mid-shaft named the diaphyses. The developmental zone

From: *Contemporary Endocrinology: Developmental Endocrinology: From Research to Clinical Practice*
Edited by: E. A. Eugster and O. H. Pescovitz © Humana Press Inc., Totowa, NJ

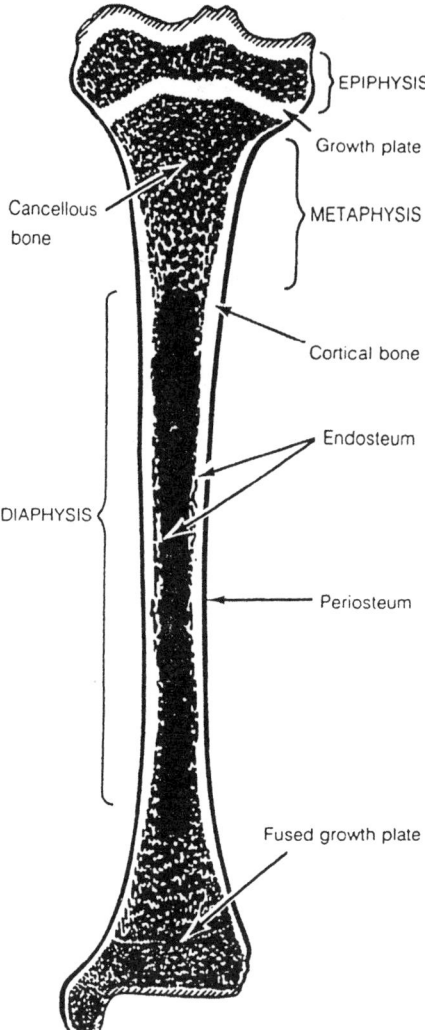

Fig. 1. This drawing represents a longitudinal section through a growing long bone. The two wider extremities are referred to as the epiphyses and the long cylindrical tube in the middle is the midshaft or diaphysis. The zone between, which is usually an area of rapid growth, is referred to as the metaphysis. Adapted with permission from ref. *(59)*.

between them is referred to as the metaphyses (Fig. 1). In long bones, growth occurs in the epiphyses and metaphyses, which are separated by a layer of cartilage, referred to as epiphyseal cartilage or growth plate. The proliferative cells in this layer and the extracellular matrix (ECM), which they secrete, is responsible for longitudinal growth of bone. In long bones, the external part forms a dense, calcified layer of compact bone for cortical bone. As one approaches the metaphyses, cortical bone becomes thinner and the internal space is filled with thin, calcified trabeculae. This type of bone, which is filled with hemopoietic bone marrow, is referred to as cancellous, spongy, or trabecular bone. Owing to the high surface area, this is a metabolically active portion of the skeleton.

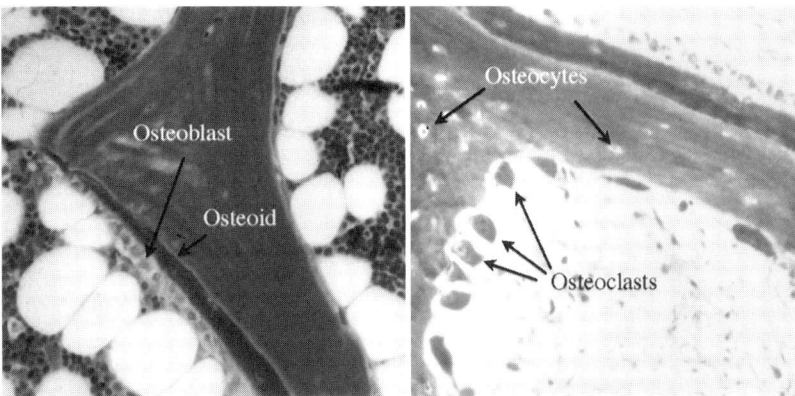

Fig. 2. Left panel, Goldner's-Masson trichrome stain of an undecalcified piece of iliac crest bone. A thick line of osteoid lies adjacent to calcified matrix. Plump osteoblasts line the osteoid surface. Right panel, this panel illustrates osteocytes embedded into the calcified tissue matrix. These are osteoblasts that have been encased in the bone and form an interdigitating network. Osteoclasts are multinucleated cells responsible for the resorption of bone. They are usually morphologically distinct and in this case, sit in scooped out areas referred to as resorption pits or Howship's lacunae.

The calcified portion of bone is in contact with soft tissues in two places. Externally, the periosteal surface is covered by osteogenic cells and layers called the periosteum. Internally, the endosteal surface is coated with cells labeled the endosteum.

Although both cortical and trabecular, or spongy bone, consist of the same cells and matrix elements, there are marked structural and functional differences. Only 15–25% of trabecular bone is calcified per volume compared to 80–90% of the volume of cortical bone. Due to its increased surface area, trabecular bone serves as a metabolic reservoir when compared to cortical bone on a volume basis.

CELLULAR AND MATRIX COMPONENTS

Osteoblasts are cells derived from primitive mesenchymal cells and are responsible for the production of unmineralized bone (osteoid). The osteoblast is characterized by a round nucleus at the base of the cell, basophilic cytoplasm, and due to its secretory function, prominent Golgi complex between the nucleus and the apex of the cell (Fig. 2, left panel). Osteoblasts produce collagenous and noncollagenous proteins (NCPs) that form the structural framework of the skeleton. Osteoblasts regulate bone formation including the synthesis and internal processing of type I collagen and noncollagenous proteins, the secretion and extracellular processing of collagen, the formation of microfibrils, fibrils and fibers from collagen, matrix maturation, and the nucleation of hydroxyapatite crystals resulting in the calcified matrix. Many hormones and growth factors alter the function of osteoblasts *(1)*.

A specific isoform of alkaline phosphatase can be localized in the plasma membrane of the osteoblast. Although its function remains ill-defined, this ectoenzyme is utilized as a histological marker of osteoblasts. Increased levels of alkaline phosphatase are associated with bone formation and can aid in the diagnosis of various metabolic bone diseases and fractures. Elevated alkaline phosphatase activity is a marker of bone formation during growth, diseases with high turnover, or fracture healing.

Osteoblasts become permanently incorporated into osteoid and form an interdigitating network. The osteoblasts, now labeled osteocytes, maintain cellular processes that converse through the mineralized tissue (Fig. 2, right panel). Due to the fact that osteocytes are "entrapped" in calcified bone matrix, studies on the functionality of these cells has been difficult. These cells are thought to be responsible not only for the exchange of nutrients, but also for the regulation of bone resorption and formation in response to mechanical stress and strain. Osteocytes are the most numerous cells in bone (25,000/ mm^3) and modulate signals arising from mechanical loading, which allows the skeleton to grow and adapt efficiently to the body's mechanical needs. Cell-to-cell communication via gap junctions and the generation of molecular signaling pathways, such as nitric oxide and prostaglandins, are methods of communication that the osteocytes invoke. In addition, osteocytes may be influenced by many hormones and cytokines. For example, osteocytes possess receptors for estrogen and parathyroid hormone/parathyroid hormone-related peptide. Apoptosis, or cell death of osteocytes, may be responsible for certain types of bone loss, such as that induced by glucocorticoid usage. Bisphosphonates are a class of drugs that increase bone density. One possible mechanism of action of bisphosphonates is suppression of apoptosis of osteocytes.

Osteoclasts are multinucleated cells that are responsible for bone resorption (Fig. 2, right panel). Osteoclasts are derived from monocyte-macrophage lineage and are formed by the fusion of progenitor cells. Osteoclasts are morphologically distinct as they contain an average of 10–15 nuclei and are highly polarized with a ruffled border that attaches to the bone surface. In the center of the ruffled border is a ring of contractile proteins that attach the cell to the bone surface, sealing off a small bone resorbing compartment. The osteoclasts contain cell surface proteins called integrins that interact with the specific RGD sequence (ARG-GLY-ASP) on several noncollagenous bone-matrix proteins. Osteoclasts are usually found within a lacunae (Howship's lacunae), which results from its own resorptive activity (1).

Striking advances have been made in understanding the molecular mechanisms in the regulation of the interactions among osteoblasts and the hemopoietic osteoclast precursor cells. Osteoprotegerin (OPG) is a naturally occurring protein that inhibits osteoclastogenesis. A transmembrane ligand named RANK-L is expressed on osteoblast and stromal cells and binds to RANK, a transmembrane receptor on hematopoietic osteoclast precursor cells. Interactions between RANK and RANK-L initiates signaling and a gene-expression cascade, which results in differentiation and maturation of osteoclast precursor cells. The resulting osteoclasts are capable of active bone resorption. Osteoprotegerin acts as a decoy receptor, which binds to RANK-L and blocks the RANK-L/RANK interaction. This results in a decrease in the development of osteoclasts. Calciotropic hormones and cytokines, such as vitamin D_3, parathyroid hormone, interleukin-11 (IL-11), and prostaglandin E_2 stimulate osteoclastogenesis through the actions of inhibiting production of OPG and stimulating production of RANK-L. Estrogen inhibits production of RANK-L and RANK-L-stimulated osteoclastogenesis. The understanding provided by the RANK/RANK-L/OPG paradigm in the activation and differentiation of osteoclasts has the potential to develop new therapeutic agents, such as OPG, as a potential for treatment of osteoporosis (2).

MATRIX PROTEINS

The structural framework for calcification and predominant collagen in bone is type I collagen. Type I collagen forms a preferential orientation providing a typical lamellar structure. This is easily identified by polarized light or electron microscopy. Lamellae are parallel when deposited on a flat surface and may form concentric circles when deposited around a channel centered on a blood vessel, such as a Haversian canal. In periods of rapid growth or fracture healing, there is no organization to the collagen and these randomly oriented bundles are referred to as woven bone. Type I collagen is a triple-helical molecule containing two identical α_1 (I) chains and a structurally similar α_2 (II) chain. Alpha chains of collagen are characterized by a GLY-X-Y triplet, which is repeated where X is usually represented by proline. Post-translational modifications include hydroxylation of certain prolyl and lysyl residues, glycosylation of certain lysyl or hydroxylysyl residues with glucose or galactose residues, and formation of intra- and intermolecular covalent cross-links *(3)*. Although bone consists predominantly of type I collagen, trace amounts of type III, V, X, and FACIT collagens may be present during certain stages of bone formation and help regulate fibril diameter. Breakdown products of type I collagen include pyridinoline and deoxypyridinoline. These urinary metabolites are measured to assess bone resorption. Another marker that is part of the amino-terminus of type I collagen is telopeptide (N-telopeptide). N-telopeptide is a serum and urine marker that can be used as a measurement of the breakdown of type I collagen that occurs during bone resorption *(4–6)*.

NCPs are often composed of serum-derived proteins, such as albumin and α_2-hs-glycoprotein. These acidic proteins bind to the bone matrix due to their high affinity for hydroxyapatite. NCPs effect bone mineralization and regulate bone-cell proliferation. Noncollagenous proteins comprise 10–15% of total bone protein content, and frequently their physiologic roles are not well-defined (for review, *see* ref. *7*).

Other parts of the ground substance of bone consist of proteoglycans and glycoproteins that are important to the calcification process and have a high ion-binding capacity. Approximately 10% to 15% of the bone matrix is made up of NCPs, such as osteopontin, osteocalcin, osteonectin, bone sialoprotein, biglycan, and decorin.

Osteonectin is the most abundant NCP produced by bone cells and accounts for approx 2% of the total protein of developing bone in most animal species. Osteonectin is also produced in nonbone tissues that are undergoing rapid proliferation, remodeling, or changes in tissue architecture. Although the function in bone is not well-defined, osteonectin is associated with osteoblast growth, proliferation, and matrix mineralization.

Some of the NCPs contain an RGD sequence and attach to cells via integrins. These NCPs include type I collagen, fibronectin, thrombospondin, vitronectin, fibrillin, osteopontin, bone sialoprotein (BSP), bone acetic glycoprotein-75 (BAG-75), and dentin matrix phosphoprotein-1. Osteopontin and BSP anchor osteoclasts to bone, support cell attachment, and bind calcium with high affinity.

The physiologic role(s) for the γ-carboxylic acid (Gla)-containing proteins is not well-established. Three bone matrix NCPs, matrix Gla protein (MGP), osteocalcin (bone Gla-protein), and protein S are post-translationally modified by the action of vitamin K-dependent γ-carboxylation. The Gla residues enhance binding to calcium. These proteins may function in the inhibition of mineral deposition.

The proteoglycans contain acidic polysaccharide side chains (glycosaminoglycans) attached to a central core protein. In the initial stages of bone formation, versican and hyaluronan are produced and may define the areas that will eventually become mineralized bone. During the process of bone formation, versican is replaced by two small chondroitin sulfate proteoglycans, decorin and biglycan. Decorin may regulate collagen fibrillogenesis and is distributed in the extracellular space of connective tissue and bone *(8)*.

MINERALIZATION OF BONE

In the adult, mineral accounts for 50–70% of bone, 20–40% being comprised of matrix and the remaining 5–10% consists of water. The matrix or osteoid exists because of a lag time of approx 10 d between the period of matrix formation and the calcification process. Type I collagen is the predominant matrix protein, which provides flexibility to bone and is responsible for its structural organization. Mineral is deposited at discrete sites in the collagen matrix, and these crystals enlarge. Mineral deposition is facilitated by membrane-bound extracellular bodies referred to as extracellular matrix (ECM) vesicles, which are released from chondrocytes and osteoblasts. ECM vesicles contain calcium and phosphate ions and provide enzymes to degrade inhibitors of bone mineralization. Their core consists of proteins, acidic phospholipids, calcium, and inorganic phosphate, which induces apatite formation. The crystal lattice begins to form when component ions of the lattice or clusters come together in the right orientation. Nucleation is followed by the addition of ions and ion clusters to the critical nucleus as the crystal grows. Various macromolecules may facilitate the formation of the critical nucleus, and several possible promoters of bone mineral formation have been identified. Important bone mineral nucleators are the phosphoproteins of bone, which include collagen, osteopontin, BSP, and BAG-75. Osteopontin and BSP can inhibit apatite proliferation and growth in solution, and these proteins can all bind calcium in solution or on the apatite crystal surface. Several enzymes that regulate phosphoprotein phosphorylation and dephosphorylation are associated with the mineralization process. Phosphoprotein kinases, which regulate phosphoprotein phosphorylation and alkaline phosphatase, are important enzymes for bone formation. Blocking phosphoprotein phosphorylation in cultured bone cells decreases mineralization rates. Alkaline phosphatase appears to be permissive for the mineralization process, and patients with hypophosphatasia, a deficiency of alkaline phosphatase, have abnormal bone mineralization.

The growth of the bone mineral crystals is governed by collagenous and noncollagenous proteins. A certain dietary cation, such as magnesium and strontium, can be incorporated directly into the bone mineral, substituting for calcium. When this happens, mineral crystals are formed that are smaller and less perfect than those formed in their absence. Carbonate and citrate also form impurities that are absorbed into the surface of bone mineral. Each of these ions make the crystals more soluble, whereas fluoride increases the size and decreases the solubility of apatite crystals *(9)*. Other compounds that bind to the surface of the apatite crystals include the bisphosphonates, which block the dissolution of bone, although there is no change in size of the crystal *(10)*. Tetracycline and other fluorescent compounds chelate calcium and bind with high affinity to the surface of the most recently formed mineral. Tetracycline antibiotics are permanently incorporated into sites of bone formation. This property has allowed histological quantitation of bone formation. Tetracycline is administered at set intervals (3 d on, 12 d off, 3 d on sequence) and a thin fluorescent line is seen at the mineralization front. Tetracycline can be incorporated into growing teeth in pregnant mothers and cause discoloration *(1)*.

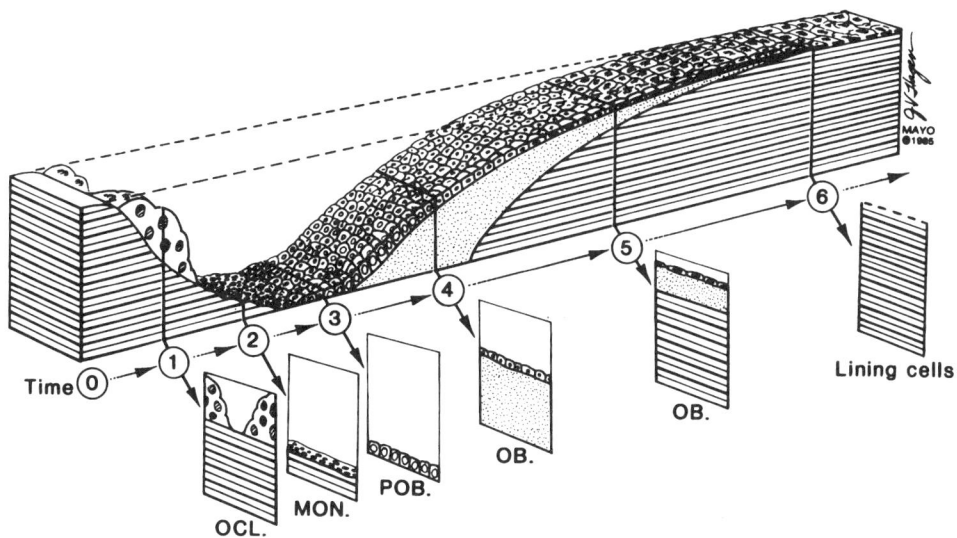

Fig. 3. Longitudinal and cross-sectional representation of the bone remodeling unit. This represents a piece of cancellous bone and five phases are distinguishable: 1, osteoclast-mediated bone resorption; 2, resorption by mononuclear cells; 3, migration of preosteoblasts and differentiation into osteoblasts; 4, osteoid deposition; and 5, mineralization. Abbreviations include MON, mononuclear cells; OB, osteoblasts; OCL, osteoclasts; POB, pre-osteblasts. Reproduced with permission from *(1)*.

The distribution and size of mineral crystals in bone matrix influences the mechanical properties of bone. Bone strength is dependent on bone architecture. Although mechanical strength of bone has correlated with bone mineral density, few studies have related mechanical properties to mineral characteristics. If there are too many crystals or crystals are excessively large, such as occurs in skeletal fluorosis, the bones may become brittle.

BONE REMODELING

Cellular Elements

Cortical bone remodeling occurs in discrete temporal foci that are active for 4–8 mo. According to a model proposed by Parfitt *(11)*, the normal remodeling sequence in bone follows a pattern of quiescence, activation, resorption, reversal, formation, and return to quiescence (Fig. 3). Approximately 80% of trabecular, and 95% of cortical bone surfaces are inactive in the adult. A small area of bone surface may be converted from quiescence to activity, which begins with the recruitment of osteoclast precursors, differentiation of the cells into mature osteoclasts, and osteoclast attachment to bone surfaces. The osteoclasts resorb bone over a specific area. Reversal phase is the time interval between completion of resorption and the initiation of bone formation. This period may last 1–2 wk. Preosteoblasts invade the base of the resorption cavity in response to various growth factors and cytokines. The release of proteins from the bone matrix may also be important in coordinating the activities between the osteoclasts and osteoblasts. The preosteoblasts differentiate into osteoblasts, which are responsible for synthesizing matrix proteins or osteoid. The mineralization process occurs 5–10 d after matrix deposition. The rate of mineral opposition can be measured in vivo after double tetracycline labeling. The mean distance between fluorescent bands divided by the time interval between the midpoints of the tetracycline labels will provide the mineral opposition rate.

A complete remodeling cycle in normal skeleton is 100 d in cortical bone and 200 d in trabecular bone. The activation of osteoclast-mediated bone resorption and osteoblast-induced bone formation is termed "coupling." Changes in bone mass result from an imbalance between the amount of bone resorbed and the amount of bone formed. Many locally produced cytokines and growth factors, as well as polypeptides, steroids, and thyroid hormones, regulate the bone remodeling cycle.

EFFECTS OF PEPTIDE AND STEROID HORMONES

Peptide (parathyroid hormone and calcitonin) and steroid $(1,25(OH)_2$ vitamin D) hormones are essential to the process of bone remodeling. When serum calcium falls, the increase in parathyroid hormone (PTH) directly effects bone by increasing bone resorption and enhancing bone formation. In states of PTH excess, there is a large increase in bone remodeling. PTH stimulates differentiation of progenitor cells to form mature osteoclasts. Bone resorption by the osteoclast and matrix production by the osteoblasts are both enhanced in the presence of PTH. Calcitonin causes contraction of osteoclast cell membranes and this activity correlates with the inhibition of bone resorption. The physiologic role of calcitonin in the adult is not well-established, but is thought that this hormone may regulate bone remodeling in utero. Calcitonin concentrations increase briefly after birth and may be related to the stress of delivery. The early neonatal hypocalcemia that may be seen in stressed infants under conditions of neonatal asphyxia may be associated with an exaggerated calcitonin response.

$1,25(OH)_2$ vitamin D is a potent stimulator of bone resorption. One mechanism by which $1,25(OH)_2$ vitamin D enhances bone resorption is by stimulation of osteoclast progenitors to differentiate. The increase in number and activity of osteoclasts results in increased bone turnover.

Cellular Effects of Estrogen. Estrogen receptors are present on osteoblasts and osteoclasts. In the osteoclast, estrogen increases cell proliferation and enhances expression of genes that encode for growth factors, enzymes, matrix proteins, and cytokines that alter bone remodeling. In cell-culture systems, estrogen inhibits production of cytokines associated with bone resorption such as interleukin (IL)-1, IL-6, and IL-11. Estrogen also stimulates synthesis of transforming growth factor-beta (TGF-β), insulin-like growth factor-1 (IGF-1), and the IGF binding proteins. Proteins involved in bone remodeling, such as bone morphogenic protein-6 and osteoprotegerin, are also regulated by estrogen. In estrogen deficiency, there is an increase in the maturation of osteoclasts and osteoblasts with an overall increase in bone remodeling.

The major action of estrogen on the skeleton is inhibition of bone resorption. Estrogen induces apoptosis and reduces the life-span of the osteoclast. It may be that the synergy of several cytokines enhance osteoclast recruitment, differentiation, and activity. The blockage of the production of cytokines such as the interleukins and tumor necrosis factor-alpha (TNF-α) by osteoblasts prevents bone resorption in an estrogen-deficient state.

EMBRYOLOGY AND DEVELOPMENT

The adult vertebrate skeleton derives from three original embryonic structures: the neural-crest cells, which become the branchial arch derivative of the craniofacial skeleton; the medial region of the somites, constituting the sclerotomes from which vertebrae and axial skeleton develop; and the lateral plate mesoderm, contributing to the skeletal development of the limbs. The patterning of future bones is carried out by mesenchymal cells, which condense and differentiate into bone-forming cells, osteoblasts, chondrocytes, myoblasts, and bone marrow stromal cells including adipocytes. This process is regulated by numerous cytokines, proteins, and transcription factors. Differentiation into osteoblasts occurs in areas of membranous ossification, the process giving rise to flat bones, mainly of the skull, maxilla, mandible, and the subperiosteal thickening of the cortex of long bones. Differentiation into chondrocytes occurs in the remaining skeleton where cartilage models of future bones are formed and subsequently replaced by bone in a process called endochondral ossification.

Membranous Ossification

Mesenchymal cells proliferate and differentiate into preosteoblasts and then into osteoblasts. Regulation of osteoblast differentiation is mediated by local factors such as bone morphogenic proteins, hedgehogs, and the transcription factor, core-binding factor α-1 (Cbfa1) *(12)*. Osteoblasts secrete matrix, forming a branching network of trabeculae, in which the collagen fibers are haphazardly arranged; the osteoblast-derived osteocytes are large and numerous, and calcification proceeds in randomly distributed patches referred to as woven bone. The spaces between the woven bone trabeculae are filled with vascular connective tissue, which will form the hematopoetic bone marrow. The woven bone is remodeled by the osteoclast-osteoblast coordinated activity and eventually replaced by mature lamellar bone.

ENDOCHONDRAL OSSIFICATION

Mesenchymal cells proliferate and differentiate into prechondroblasts and then into chondroblasts while continuing to secrete the cartilaginous matrix. The chondroblasts dwell within lacunae; they are progressively embedded within their own matrix, slowly becoming chondrocytes.

The cartilaginous model continues to grow because the mesenchymal cells proliferate and differentiate at the periphery (appositional growth). There is also synthesis of new matrix between the chondrocytes (interstitial growth).

Endochondral ossification occurs after a series of programmed changes on the pre-existing cartilage. The growth plate of long bones, in which these changes are highly regulated, represents the most studied model of this type of ossification.

Longitudinal Bone Growth. The growth plate in a growing long bone is characterized, from the epiphyseal to the diaphyseal area, by the following zones: 1) the resting zone, closest to the epiphysis, in which chondrocytes are widely separated by cartilage matrix; 2) the proliferative zone, characterized by division of chondrocytes and their alignment in longitudinal columns; and 3) the hypertrophic zone, where chondrocytes become remarkably larger, enlarging their lacunae and then undergo apoptosis. At this level, mineralization of the intercolumnar cartilage matrix in the long axis of bone occurs (zone of provisional calcification). In the zone of endochondral ossification, the cartilage matrix that has been calcified is partially resorbed by osteoclasts and vascular invasion occurs between the longitudinal septa of the remnant calcified cartilage. Once resorption has been completed, osteoblasts differentiate forming a layer of woven bone around the cartilagineous septa.

Table 1
The Effect of Gene Inactivation and/or Activating Mutations
of Proteins Controlling Bone Morphogenesis and Embryologic Development

Protein	Function	Mutation effect
Tyrosine kinase receptor FGFR3	Growth-plate chondrocyte proliferation	Achondroplasia Hypochondroplasia
Parathyroid hormone-related peptide (PTHrP) receptor	Growth-plate chondrocyte hypertrophy	Decreased bone growth and dwarfism
Collagen X	Growth-plate matrix support	Schmid-type metaphyseal chondrodysplasia
Cell-surface receptor Notch1 (and ligands binding to it)	Condensation of paraxial mesoderm cells, segmentation to somites, and mesenchymal-epithelial-cell transformation	Defects in vertebral column
Signaling cytokine sonic hedgehog	Sclerotome-cell differentiation into chondrocytes	Absence of vertebral column and posterior portions of the ribs
TGF-β-homologue (CDMP1)	Limb development	Shortening of distal limb bones
Core-binding factor α-1 (Cbfa1)	Differentiation of osteoblasts	Maturation arrest of bone formation
Transcription factor PAX1	Sclerotome-cell differentiation into chondrocytes	Abnormalities in the vertebral column and neural tube defect
Transcription factor HOXD13	Limb development	Extra fingers
Transcription factor GLI3	Limb development	Extra fingers
Transcription factor LMX-1	Nail and patella development	Nail-patella syndrome

The trabeculae formed by cartilaginous remnants in the central part and by woven bone in the periphery, are known as primary spongiosa. Subequently, these trabeculae are subjected to further remodeling by the sequential action of osteoclasts and osteoblasts and substituted by lamellar bone, constituting the mature trabecular bone of the secondary spongiosa of the metaphysis.

It is now becoming evident that both proliferation and differentiation of growth plate chondrocytes are controlled by a number of signaling molecules. For example, the chondrocyte proliferation may be stopped by local signaling through fibroblast growth factor (FGF) interaction with the cell-surface tyrosine kinase receptor FGFR3. Activating mutations in FGFR3 cause decreased bone growth resulting in achondro- or hypochondroplasia. Other proteins are known to be involved in chondrocyte proliferation and differentiation in growth plates (Table 1).

Formation of Axial Skeleton. At approximately the fourth wk of intra-uterine life, cells of the paraxial mesoderm condense to form the segmented structures called somites on both sides of the neural tube and the notochord. Mesenchymal cells of the somites transform to an epithelial phenotype and those located in the medial area of the structures migrate in a ventral region toward the notochord, giving rise to the sclerotomes. Sclerotome cells differentiate into chondrocytes that will pattern the vertebral bodies. All these steps are controlled by a number of regulatory proteins whose deficiency give rise to specific development defects (Table 1).

THE FORMATION OF THE LIMBS. At approx the second month of intrauterine life, formation of so-called limb buds occurs. Proliferation of mesenchymal cells from the lateral plate mesoderm causes protuberance of the lateral body wall. A group of specialized epithelial cells, called the apical ectodermal ridge, caps the limb bud. Limb development is determined by epithelial-mesenchymal interaction for growth and pattern formation along all three axes: proximal-to-distal, dorsal-to-ventral, and posterior-to-anterior. The development of cartilage model in the proximal-to-distal direction can be represented as a progressive series of bifurcations and segmentations.

Factors produced by the apical ectodermal ridge, mainly including FGFs, control the limb patterning along the proximal-to-distal axis. Furthermore, a number of signaling molecules and transcription factors regulate the patterning of cartilage model. Mutations of the relative genes result in abnormalities in the limb skeleton (Table 1).

BONE ENVELOPES

The concept of bone-surface envelopes was introduced by Frost, who considered bone enclosed by multiple surface systems consisting of anatomically and functionally distinct bone-cell envelopes, each exhibiting different behavior during growth, even in the adult skeleton. The periosteal envelope, or periosteum, covers the skeletal segments on their outer margins: it is fundamentally a forming envelope, involved in the outer volume increase of the skeleton throughout life. The endosteal envelope includes three main subdivisions, which participate at different rates in active bone remodeling throughout life: the endosteal trabecular envelope, which represents the bone cell interface between the marrow cavities and trabecular bone; the cortico-endosteal or innercortical envelope, delimiting the outermost limit of the medullary canal (interrupted by connections of trabeculae to the cortical bone); and the haversian or intracortical envelope, which includes the haversian systems and the walls of Volkmann's canals *(13–15)*.

THE SKELETON IN UTERO: HORMONAL FACTORS

Most of the bone mineral content of the fetus is gained during the last trimester of pregnancy *(16)*. The two major stimuli to bone resorption, PTH and 1,25 (OH_2D), are in relatively low abundance in utero. The parathyroid gland appears to produce parathyroid hormone-related peptides (PTHrP) in preference to PTH in the fetus. Relatively high levels of calcitonin are present from the fetal thyroid gland, which may block the effects of PTH and PTHrP on osteoclasts. Thus, the milieu surrounding the fetus limits bone resorption and a number of hormones may facilitate mineralization. For example, at low levels, PTH may be anabolic to the skeleton. IGF-1 stimulates bone growth and may also augment mineral acquisition *(17)*. In addition, the estrogenic environment of the fetus may enhance bone formation.

Calcium, magnesium, and phosphorus are all actively transported across an uphill gradient across the placenta. In animal models, maternal parathyroidectomy or vitamin D deficiency does not affect this gradient, thus preserving important mineral homeostasis for the fetus.

SKELETAL GROWTH DURING THE FIRST YEAR OF LIFE

Infancy is the period of most rapid growth of the skeleton and body proportions change dramatically. The newborn infant has a large head and limbs relative to the rest of the

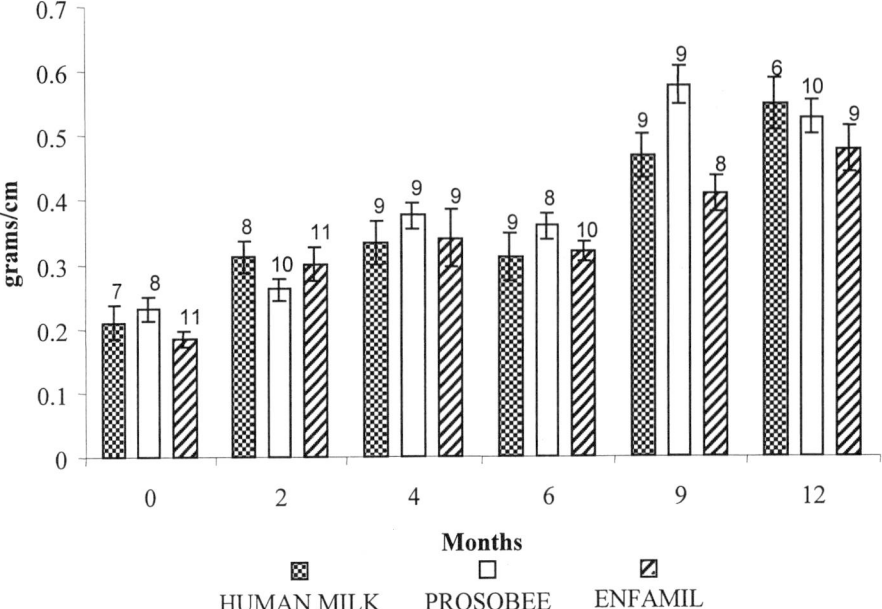

Fig. 4. Bone mineral content in infants being fed three types of formula. Mean values (±SE) of bone mineral content in grams/cm is shown in infants at entry and at 2, 4, 6, 9, and 12 mo of age in infants fed human milk, ProSobee, or Enfamil. The numbers above the bars represent the number of samples. Adapted with permission from ref. *(60)*.

body. Knemometry is a method to accurately determine the length of single bones and can be used to follow growth rates *(18)*.

Nutrition plays a major role in acquisition of skeletal mass during infancy. Infants are fed three types of milk: human milk, cows milk-based formula, and vegetable protein-based formula. There is an increase in bone mineral content over the first year of life in infants fed all three types with no significant difference among the three milks (Fig. 4). The same cannot be said of older soy milk products *(19)*, although newer formulations may have added calcium and/or vitamin D. Human milk is relatively low in calcium and phosphorus (approx 300 and 150 mg/L, respectively). Cow's milk-based formulas and soy protein-based formula have higher amounts of calcium and phosphorus compared to human milk. The infant's digestive system adapts to these differences by increasing the absorption of calcium for human milk (70%) compared to cow's milk (40%). Infant formulas are supplemented with 400 IU vitamin D per quart.

Serum concentrations of $1,25(OH)_2D$ and PTH are comparable in normal children and adults. Growth hormone (GH) and IGF-1, which may contribute to accession of bone mineral, are also increased during childhood. Bone turnover is markedly increased as noted by biochemical markers in bone resorption (pyridinoline crosslinks, N-teleopeptide) and bone formation (bone-specific alkaline phosphatase, osteocalcin). Levels in childhood tend to be double adult levels.

In a classic series of studies by Matkovic, calcium accredation in the skeleton was assessed starting in infancy. From infancy to 1 yr, net absorption of 429 mg/d is required.

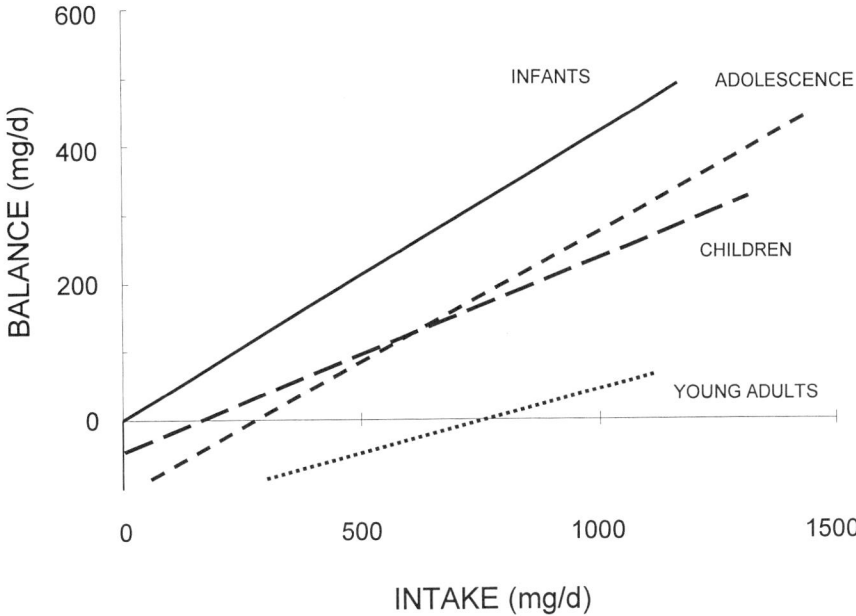

Fig. 5. This figure represents the regression lines for the ascending portion of the relationship of calcium balance vs calcium intake by age group. In each age group, calcium balance is positively correlated with intake. Partial intakes and balances are estimated by fitting the data to two component, split, linear-regression model. Adapted with permission from ref. *(61)*.

At all ages, calcium balance is highly correlated with intake ($r = 0.59$, $p < 0.001$) *(20)*. By re-analyzing numerous balance studies, Matkovic and Heaney have shown that there was a threshold effect for calcium in all ages *(21)*. Absorption efficiency decreases after maximally effective calcium intake is reached (Fig. 5).

BONE REMODELING IN CHILDREN

Growth in children is rapid and from birth to the end of linear growth period at puberty, the healthy child increases in length threefold. There are remarkable changes in the proportions of head size, body, and limb length that occur. The newborn infant has relatively large head and limbs compared to the length of the body. Accurate measurements of growth throughout childhood permit detection of abnormal patterns of growth. Infancy is the period of most rapid skeletal growth and from 3 yr to the onset of puberty, children grow at a slowly decelerated rate (Fig. 6). Prior to puberty, there are no gender differences in bone mass *(22,23)*. During puberty, a sharp increase in growth rate occurs followed by epiphyseal fusion and cessation of growth. The average age for the start of the pubertal growth spurt varies between the sexes and is younger in girls than in boys. In addition, there is a 13 cm mean difference in adult height between men and women, which is due to the fact that the peak velocity and duration of growth spurt are less in girls than in boys. There is a high degree of variability that occurs, making prediction of adult height difficult. In addition, accurate assessment of linear growth in children requires a sophisticated procedure with accurate and technically demanding measurements.

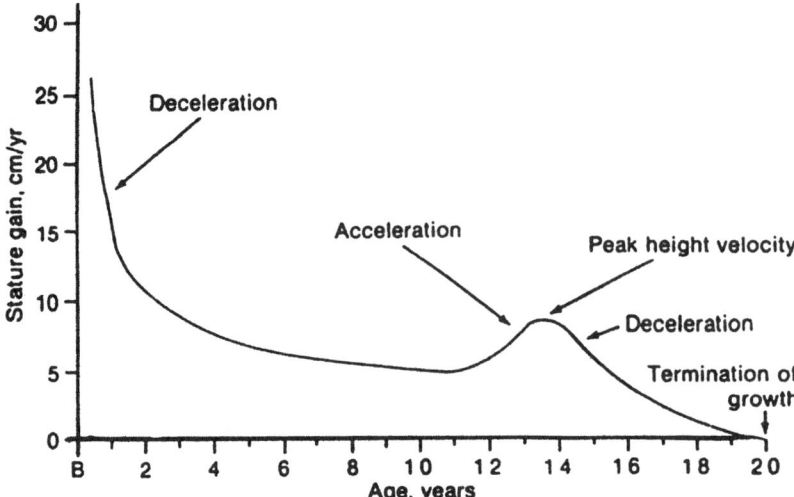

Fig. 6. The age-dependent phases of childhood skeletal growth velocity. Infancy is the period of rapid skeletal growth. From 3 yr to the onset of puberty, children grow at a slowly decelerated rate. During puberty, there is a sharp increase in growth followed by epiphyseal fusion and cessation of growth. Adapted with permission from ref. *(62)*.

Specific developmental stages have been observed and carefully documented for bones of the hand and wrist. By examination of radiographs of the wrist and hand, an average maturation age or "bone age" of the child can be determined *(24,25)*. This information has predictive value for final adult height and can be utilized to assess metabolic disorders that affect skeletal growth.

Linear growth is dependent on the cartilage cells within the epiphyseal growth plate. Columns of chondrocytes grow outward from the epiphyses, and, as they mature, the surrounding matrix mineralizes. Various hormones and local factors will shift the balance between proliferation and maturation. For example, GH and IGF-1 promote proliferation, while thyroid hormone and estrogen induce epiphyseal fusion. Estrogen can be used to limit final adult height, while androgens stimulate proliferation at the epiphyseal plate. Local factors play important roles such as basic fibroblast growth factor (bFGF). An inactivating mutation in the FGF-3 receptor results in achondroplasia and distortion of the epiphyseal plate.

Acquisition of Bone Mineral in Adolescents

Recent studies have provided information regarding active intervention in prepubertal children and adolescents in order to attempt to increase bone mineral density (BMD) with supplemental calcium. In one study in prepubertal children, who received 500 mg or 1000 mg calcium supplements compared to those who were unsupplemented (total intake 888 mg/d), progressive increases in BMD were noted in the supplemented group *(26)*. In certain ethnic groups, low calcium diets are common and calcium absorption is usually markedly increased to compensate. By doubling the calcium intake of Chinese children with the administration of a 300 mg calcium carbonate tablet, Lee et al. showed greater gains of bone mineral content at the 1/3 distal radius site measured by single photon absorptiometry (SPA) *(27)*.

Eighteen months of calcium supplementation of growth at a mean age of 11.9 ± 0.5 yr indicated that bone and whole body BMD by DEXA were increased compared to a placebo-treated group (26). One of the most thorough studies completed was that of Johnston et al., which evaluated 23 pairs of monozygotic twins (28). In 23 twin pairs who went through puberty or were both pubertal during the course of the study, no benefit of calcium supplementation was noted. In 22 prepubertal twin pairs, the twin on supplementation with a mean of 1612 mg of calcium had, on average, 5.1 and 3.8% greater increases in the mid- and distal radius BMD and a 2.8% greater increase in lumbar spine BMD. The control group's daily calcium intake was 908 mg. Bone-turnover markers were reduced in the supplemented prepubertal children. The question remains whether prepubertal supplementation will result in increased bone mass at the time peak bone mass is attained. Even more importantly, will these children have a competitive advantage as adults with a lower threshold for the development of osteoporosis? Currently, retrospective studies of childhood dairy intakes and adult bone mass suggest that there is a positive effect of early calcium supplementation on the skeleton.

ASSESSING BONE MINERAL DENSITY IN CHILDHOOD AND ADOLESCENTS

Normative BMD values are available for children, but the data is difficult to collect in a rigorous manner that accounts for gender, age, height, weight, pubertal status, BMD technique, and site utilized (29,30). Bone length, diameter, and density all contribute to the increased bone mass that occurs during adolescence. Differences in bone mineral content (BMC, g) and BMD (BMC/area, g/cm^2) for any region of interest is highly correlated with age, weight, and height. In adults, BMD is considered as reasonable assessment for changes in volumetric mineral density (grams/cm^3) in adults. This is because shape and volume do not change very much. However, because of rapid changes in a growing child, estimation of volumetric mineral density is difficult. Attempts to correct the areal BMD measurements for bone size may overcorrect with higher than expected values. BMD values are directly dependent on size and thickness of the skeletal tissue and the term bone mineral density without areal qualifications has been widely accepted. However, it is also accepted that neither standard SPA or dual photon absorptiometry (DPA) techniques provide a true measurement of volumetric density.

The biology of BMD is an area of intense investigation. Molgaard et al. examined the role of age, body, size, and pubertal status on bone size and BMD in healthy girls ($n = 201$) and boys ($n = 142$) aged 5–19 yr. BMD was approximated by BMC corrected for whole body bone area and height. BMD was dependent on age and pubertal stage, but weight did not appear to play a substantial role (30).

Bone Mass Velocity by Skeletal Size. A longitudinal study using DXA to measure changes in BMD in children during pubertal maturation indicated that both BMD or content at the lumbar spine and femoral neck increased four- to sixfold over a 3-yr period in females (aged 11–14 yr). In males, these changes occurred over a 4-yr period (aged 13–17 yr) (31) (Fig. 7). During the adolescent growth spurt, a peak velocity of 9 cm/yr is reached in girls and 10.5 cm/yr is reached in boys. Endochondrial growth plates experience accelerated closing leading to a decrease in linear skeletal growth at about age 17 in girls and age 19 yr in boys.

Interestingly, there is an asynchrony between bone mass growth at the lumbar spine and femoral neck and statural height. This occurs when height velocity reaches its greatest rate (11–12 yr in girls and 13–14 yr in boys). At this time, both genders are susceptible

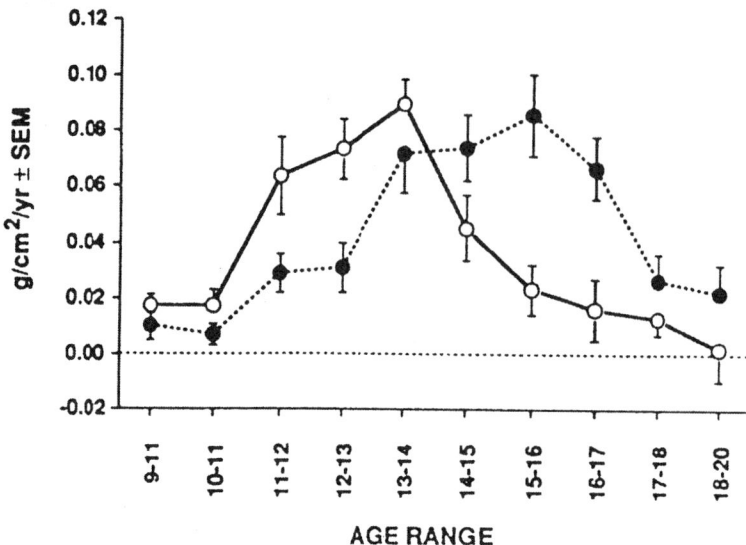

Fig. 7. Using DEXA to measure changes in bone mineral density in children longitudinally, bone mineral density or bone mineral content at the lumbar spine increased three- to sixfold over a 3-yr period in females and over a 4-yr period in males. The results on this graph are presented as yearly increase (% change) in lumbar spine BMD at L2 to L4. Similar findings are present in bone mineral content. Results are represented as mean ± the standard area of the mean. Adapted with permission from ref. *(63)*.

to fracture and the peak of fracture incidence noticed during the second decade of life could be due to fragility that occurs at this time *(23,31,32)*.

Bone Mass Consolidation After Puberty. During puberty, calcium accumulation is intense in the skeleton. While the full-term fetus only contains about 21 grams of calcium, the adult contains about 1000 grams in the skeleton. An increase in calcitriol levels have been described in puberty; it may contribute to the process. During childhood and puberty, well-established markers of bone formation and resorption are markedly increased. It is important to distinguish that high levels of markers such as alkaline phosphatase, osteocalcin, N-telopeptide, and urinary pyridinoline crosslinks may be elevated in children compared to adults and are normal.

Between 17 and 20 yr, mean gains in lumbar spine, femoral neck, and mid-femoral shaft BMD are slight or nonexistent in females *(31)*. In contrast, gain in BMD/BMC was particularly high in adolescent males between the ages of 13–17 yr. There is still a significant bone mass gain in males but not in females in subjects reaching pubertal stage P5 and growing less than 1 cm/yr. Thus, sex differences in the consolidation phase of development of peak bone mass may contribute to gender-related differences in skeletal composition. Between the third and fifth decades of life, little change in bone mass acquisition occurs and bone loss becomes the predominant feature.

HORMONES THAT ALTER SKELETAL GROWTH

Many hormones affect the growth of the skeleton. For example, glucocortical excess, which occurs in Cushing's syndrome, severely limits skeletal growth. However, deficiencies in the production of cortisol do not appear to lead to significant growth failure. The growth hormone insulin-like growth factor (GH IGF-I) axis, the gonadal axis, and the pituitary-thyroid axis are all hormonal systems that have great effects on the skeleton.

GH, or somatotropin, is the major stimulant of growth postnatally. A specific receptor that is part of the cytokine superfamily interacts with GH, which results in the release of IGF-1 (formally called somatomedin-C). IGF-1 resembles proinsulin and may behave in both an endocrine and paracrine manner. The GH IGF-1 system induces proliferation without maturation of the epiphyseal growth plate. GH plays a big role in longitudinal bone growth and is also responsible for attainment of peak bone mass. In young Caucasian men (age 24 ± 1 yr), total body and femoral BMD correlated with nocturnal GH and maximal GH concentrations *(33)*. Growth continues in a linear fashion until the gonadal hormone-mediated epiphyseal closure occurs. Both thyroxine (T4) and trithyroidal thyronine (T3) regulate skeletal growth. Most of the information regarding skeletal regulation by thyroid hormones are due to observations in states of thyroid hormone deficiency. The active metabolite (T3) signals the nuclear receptor of the steroid hormone retinoic acid receptor class. However, T3 is not necessary for both proliferation and maturation of the growth plate.

Sexual dimorphism of the skeletons occurs due to differences of estrogen and testosterone in women and men. During skeletal growth, sex steroids affect the shape, size, and density of the skeleton and influence the formation of both endochondral and intramembranous bone. During the process of endochondrial ossification, a decrease in cartilage expansion results in the normal age-related fall in growth rate. Prior to puberty, bone mass and rates of skeleton growth are comparable in both sexes. The sharp rise of sex steroid production at puberty in concert with GH, thyroid hormone, and cortisol initiates an increased skeletal growth phase which lasts about 2 yr. The adolescent growth phase in girls occurs earlier in years at about age 11 compared to ages 13–14 in boys. The average velocity of linear growth prior to puberty is about 5 cm/yr.

Testosterone and estradiol and their derivatives are important in longitudinal skeletal growth. The epiphyseal growth plate reacts to individual sex hormones but is difficult to sort out their activity from that of the other hormones during puberty such as growth hormone-IGF-1 axis and insulin. In addition, the aromatization of testosterone to estrogens also occurs, confounding the picture of which sex steroid is responsible for epiphyseal closure. The importance of estrogen in the maturation of the human skeleton has recently been recognized with the discovery of two genetic disorders. One patient, a 27-yr-old male, presented with delayed skeletal maturation and incomplete epiphyseal closure. His presentation included tall stature, continued linear growth, progressive genu valgum, and osteoporosis confirmed by dual-energy X-ray absorptiometry. Levels of estradiol, estrone, follicle-stimulating hormone (FSH), and leutinizing hormone (LH) suggested estrogen resistance. The diagnosis was confirmed and was due to a missense mutation in the estrogen receptor *(34)*. Confirmation of the role of estrogen in skeletal maturation was discovered in a second set of patients with aromatase deficiency *(35,36)*. The lack of aromatase suggested that patients were insensitive to estrogen as they were unable to convert androgens to an estrogen. A male patient presented with normal sexual maturity, tall stature, delayed skeletal maturation, eunuchoid proportion, and osteopenia. Plasma levels of testosterone, androstanedione and 5α-dihydrotestosterone were markedly elevated. Administration of exogenous estrogen caused cessation of linear growth and rapid accredation of bone mineral. Estrogen is important for epiphyseal maturation

and fusion, for maintaining normal skeletal proportion, and for accredation and maintenance of bone mineral density and mass.

DETERMINANTS OF PEAK BONE MASS

Recent studies have defined the age when peak bone mass is developed. In the United
States, by age 17, 90% of the BMC has been reached and by 26 yr of age, 99% of peak bone
mass is obtained in women *(37)*. In another study, by age 17 yr, girls had attained 93% of
the adult reference BMC and 94% of volumetric density. Boys lagged behind and attained
86% of adult BMC and volumetric density *(38)*. Family studies have provided insightful
information regarding the genetic determinants of peak bone mass. In twin studies, genetic factors have been proven to account for a larger percentage of the population variability in BMD. For example, BMD at the lumbar spine, femoral neck, and distal forearm
were much more similar in monozygotic twins than in dizygotic twins *(39)* (Fig. 8).

At the lumbar spine, BMD doubles during puberty *(31)*. In male subjects, the bone
growth and accredation sequence is delayed by as much as 2 yr resulting in a prolonged
growth period. As a result, compared to females, men have a larger increase in bone size
and cortical thickness. The gain in statural height and bone mass accredation is asynchro-
nous so that the peak of statural growth velocity precedes peak bone mass. In Caucasian
females with adequate nutrition, peak bone mass is attained prior to the end of the second
decade *(31,40)*. There are multiple determinants of peak bone mass but genetics is responsible for the majority of final bone mineral mass. Specific genetic determinants are not
yet defined although epidemiologic studies in twins indicate that 80% of the variability
in BMD is due to heritable factors. Hormonal status, physical activity, and diet all play
additional roles.

The peak bone mass attained is a significant predictor for the risk of development of
osteoporosis. In Caucasian women aged 18–35 yr, BMD of the hip and spine were positively correlated with weight, body mass index (BMI), height, and level of physical activity.
Dietary intake of calcium positively correlated with BMD at the hip while amenorrhea
of greater than 3 mo duration, caffeine intake, and age negatively correlated with hip
BMD *(41)*. The importance of adequate nutrition cannot be underestimated. Nutritional
deficiency during growth can severely impair bone development and peak bone mass.
Numerous studies have identified the relationship among the levels of protein intake,
calcium-phosphorus metabolism, and BMD on the risk of osteoporotic fracture. In prepubertal identical twins, calcium supplement of 700 mg/d over and above a dietary intake
of 950 mg/d, enhanced the rate of BMD gained *(28)*. Whether supplementation at this age
and its subsequent increase in peak bone mass is maintained throughout life is a question
that remains unanswered.

There is little evidence regarding the effect of exercise on accretion of peak bone mass.
In athletes aged 42–50 yr who had been exercising for over 20 yr, the amount of overall
impact correlated with BMD *(42)*. In a league of prepubertal girls who had at a minimum
of 3 yr of high-level sport training, BMD in gymnasts was statistically higher than in the
control group or in age- or anthropometric-matched swimmers *(43)*. In adolescent males,
BMD, body size and muscle strength are closely related and physical activity is a major
determinant of BMD *(44)*. The minimum (or maximum) amount and the type of exercise
that has the greatest influence in the development of peak bone mass are difficult to assess
in a well-controlled study.

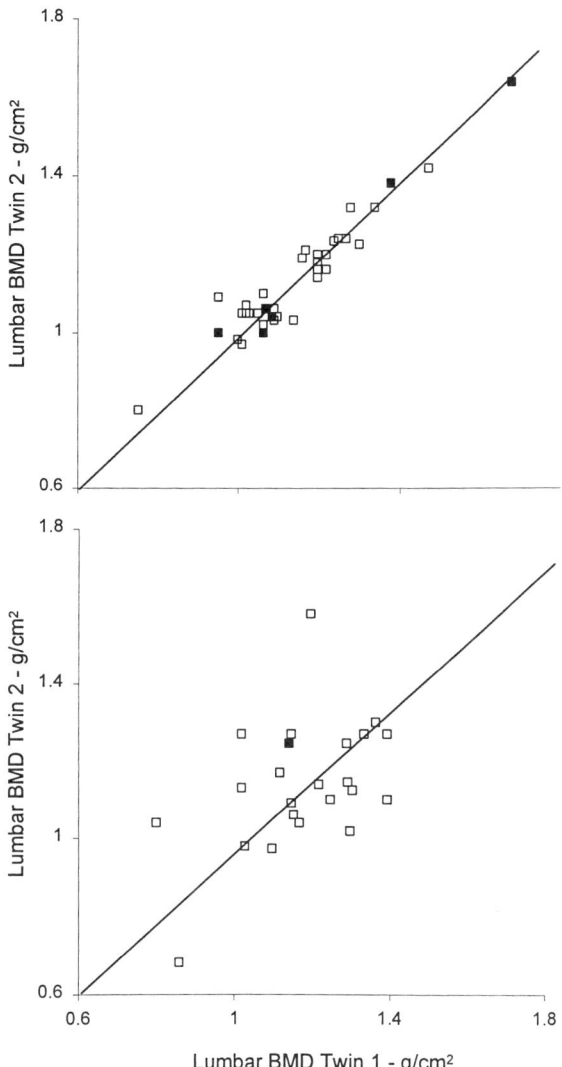

Fig. 8. Genetic basis of bone mineral density. Lumbar spine and proximal femur bone mineral density and areal bone mineral content were measured by proton absorptiometry in 38 monozygotic and 27 dizygotic twin pairs. Bone mineral density was more significantly correlated in monozygotic than in dizygotic twins for the spine and proximal femur. This graph demonstrates the correlation in the lumbar spine BMD between pairs. The line of identity is shown. Adapted with permission from ref. *(64)*.

There are few studies on the role of physical activity during childhood and adolescence on BMD. Mechanical strain plays an important role in skeletal health and several programs have been developed to increase physical activity in adolescents to promote maximal peak bone mass. Some cross-sectional studies have indicated a slightly positive association between physical activity and bone mass values in children and adolescents *(45–47)*. However, some cross-sectional studies did not support the association between exercise and bone mineral accredation and thus, the hypothesis not been confirmed by longitudinal follow-up studies *(48)*.

Nutrition and Bone

Adolescents are greatly influenced by peer pressure and behavioral changes regarding modification of nutrition can be difficult. During puberty, enormous skeletal growth occurs and approx 40% of peak bone mass is gained at this time *(40)*. Bone health during this time period can be compromised due to a lack of appropriate nutrition or by excessive thinness. Excessive exercise or eating disorders can disrupt the hypothalamic-pituitary-ovarian axis *(see* Chapter 16). The lack of sex steroids that occurs can alter bone development in the prepubertal child. In addition, the excessive thinness that can occur can result in less weight load on the skeleton and compromise skeletal growth.

Calcium

The key exogenous determinant of peak bone mass in adolescent women is adequate calcium intake *(49)*. Calcium has an important role in the establishment of peak BMD and this relationship has been confirmed in prospective and observational studies in prepubertal girls. Recommendations of the optimal calcium intake at this age have varied *(see* Table 2). However interventional trials have generally confirmed that calcium attenuates bone loss in calcium-deplete women. Other studies have confirmed that pre-adolescent intake of calcium and magnesium correlates with bone mass as assessed in 18–20 eighteen- to nineteen-yr-olds in a 10-yr longitudinal study. The history of intake in early childhood to age 12 correlates with BMD at the spine, total body, and radius *(50)*.

In postmenopausal women, calcium is an important determinant in attenuating bone loss. This has been more difficult to demonstrate because the relationship between calcium intake and bone density is less definitive due to low bone turnover. Debate has occurred as to whether dietary counseling to increase dairy product intake during adolescence would produce useful changes in BMD. An open, randomized intervention trial investigated the effect of milk supplementation on total body bone mineral acquisition in adolescent girls (mean age 12.3 yr). Subjects received one pint (568 mL) of whole or reduced fat milk daily for 18 mo. In the 80 subjects who completed the trial, baseline intake of milk was 150 mL/d. The intervention group gained 9.6% BMD compared to 8.5% in the control group ($p = 0.017$). No changes were noted in measures of bone turnover markers, height, weight, lean body mass, or fat mass. This study suggests that a relatively simple intervention may enhance bone mineral accreation and increase attainment of peak bone mass in adolescent girls *(51)*. Healthy men and women aged 55–85 were instructed to consume three servings/d of nonfat or 1% milk as part of the daily diet. In the milk-supplemented group, calcium intake increased by 729 ± 45 mg per day. There was a concurrent decrease in serum parathyroid hormone levels and urinary secretion of N-teleopeptide, a marker of bone resorption. Changes in IGF-1 and IGFBP-4 levels were similar to changes seen with calcium supplementation in other prospective studies *(52)*.

Inadequate intake of calcium and vitamin D leads to decreased absorption of these bone-building components. Over time, serum parathyroid hormone levels may rise resulting in increased resorption and bone loss. Supplemental calcium reduces bone loss in middle-aged, postmenopausal women and results in lower rates of vertebral fracture in women with previous vertebral fracture. With aging, absorption of calcium and production of vitamin D declines. Table 2 represents optimal calcium intake as adapted from the National Institutes of Health Consensus Conference.

Vitamin D. Vitamin D is essential in calcium homeostasis and facilitates absorption of dietary calcium. There are many causes of vitamin D deficiency, which include reduced

Table 2
Optimal Calcium Intake

Group	Estimated optimal daily calcium intake (mg/d)
Infants (birth to 6 mo)	400
(6–12 mo)	600
Young children (1–5 yr)	800
Older children (6–10 yr)	800–1200
Adolescents and young adults (11–24 yr)	1200–1500
Women (25–50 yr)	1000
Pregnant or lactating women	1200
Postmenopausal women on estrogen replacement therapy	1000
Postmenopausal women receiving no estrogen replacement therapy	1500
Men (25–65 yr)	1000
Men and women over 65 yr	1500

Table represents optimal calcium intake. Adapted from ref. *(58)*.

synthesis of vitamin D due to liver or kidney disease, low sunlight exposure, or problems with intestinal absorption. Vitamin D status is associated with risk of hip fracture. Infant formula is supplemented with 400 IU vitamin D per quart. Breast milk does not contain very much vitamin D, but vitamin D deficiency in a breast-fed infant is usually only seen during severe maternal vitamin D deficiency. The optimal level of vitamin D for adolescents in order to maximize peak bone mass is difficult to assess. In 21 children, vitamin D metabolites and PTH levels were measured in March and October, before and after supplementation with 40 mcg 25(OH)D for 1 wk. Increase correlations occurred between basal 25(OH)D levels, supplementation-induced and serum PTH and 1,25(OH)$_2$D levels. The authors suggest that the lower limit of 25(OH)D level in children is between 12 and 20 ng/mL. Up to 30% of children have levels below this threshold in winter months *(53)*.

To correlate vitamin D levels with peak bone mass, a cross-sectional study was undertaken in late winter at a latitude of 64 degrees (Reykjavik, Iceland). BMD by DXA was compared with 25(OH) vitamin D levels. No association was found between serum levels of vitamin D and BMD in spite of the fact that 18.5% of the 250 girls had levels of 25(OH) vitamin D less than 25 nmol/L (adult lower level of normal) *(54)*. These two studies illustrate the confusion regarding adequate vitamin D in adolescence. More prospective studies are needed to assess optimal vitamin D and formulate recommendations. Studies are available on the needs of the elderly. In one study, supplemental vitamin D (700 IU) in elderly women without other medical problems slowed bone loss at the femoral neck *(55)*. In a recent study, community-dwelling elderly women who were admitted for a hip replacement were found to have lower levels of 25-hydroxyvitamin D compared to women with osteoporosis who were admitted for elective joint replacement. Even after adjustment for estrogen use and age, parathyroid hormone levels were higher in the osteoporotic group with fracture compared to the osteoporotic women admitted for elective procedures *(56)*.

Vitamins and Micronutrients. There are many constituents of bone matrix, which include vitamins C and K, manganese, copper and zinc. Many of these are co-factors for modification of the bone matrix. It remains uncertain as to whether deficiencies of any of these minerals in humans play a role in the pathogenesis of bone loss. For example, there is no known role for vitamin C in osteoporotic bone fragility even though vitamin C is essential for collagen cross-linking. Gammacarboxylation of bone matrix proteins, particularly osteocalcin, are important mechanisms that distinguish matrix components of bone. Vitamin K is a necessary co-factor but whether vitamin K deficiency causes bone fragility is unknown. It has often been thought that phosphorus, sodium, and protein may influence bone metabolism by their effects on calcium homeostasis. The minimum dose of these micronutrients to cause skeletal damage is unknown. Frequently, factors that maybe thought responsible, such as excessive phosphorus from soda ingestion or increased caffeine intake, may be due simply to calcium insufficiency due to the replacement of milk products by soda or caffeine-containing products *(57)*.

REFERENCES

1. Fitzpatrick LA. Metabolic and nontumorous bone disorders. In: Damjanov I, Linder L, eds. Anderson's Pathology, 10th ed. Mosby-Year Book, St. Louis, MO, 1996, pp. 2574–2611.
2. Roodman GD. Cell biology of the osteoclast. Exp Hematol 1999;27:1229–1241.
3. Lian JB, Stein GS, Canalis E, Gehron-Robey P, Boskey AL. Bone formation: osteoblast lineage cells, growth factors, matrix proteins, and the mineralization process. In: Favus MJ, ed. Primer on the Metabolic Bone Diseases and Disorders of Mineral Metabolism, 4th ed. Lippincott Williams & Wilkins, Philadelphia, PA, 1999, pp. 14–29.
4. Miller PD, Baran DT, Bilezikian JP, Greenspan SL, Lindsay R, Riggs BL, et al. Practical clinical application of biochemical markers of bone turnover: consensus of an expert panel. J Clin Densitometry 1999;2:323–342.
5. de Ridder CM, Delemarre-van de Waal HA. Clinical utility of markers of bone turnover in children and adolescents. Curr Opin Pediatr 1998;10:441–448.
6. Schonau E, Rauch F. Markers of bone and collagen metabolism-problems and perspectives in paediatrics. Horm Res 1997;48:50–59.
7. Gehron Robey P, Boskey AL. The biochemistry of bone. In: Marcus R, Feldman D, eds. Osteoporosis. Raven Press, New York, 1996, pp. 95–184.
8. Donley GE, Fitzpatrick LA. Noncollagenous matrix proteins controlling mineralization: possible role in pathologic calcification of vascular tissue. Trends Cardiovasc Med 1998;8:199–206.
9. Grynpas MD. Fluoride effects on bone crystals. J Bone Miner Res Suppl 1990;1:S169–S175.
10. Fratzl P, Schreiber S, Roschger P, Lafage MH, Rodan G, Klaushofer K. Effects of sodium fluoride and alendronate on the bone mineral in minipigs: a small-angle x-ray scattering and backscattered electron imaging study. J Bone Miner Res 1996;11:248–253.
11. Parfitt AM. Osteonal and hemi-osteonal remodeling: the spatial and temporal framework for signal traffic in adult human bone. J Cell Biochem 1994;55:273–286.
12. Yamaguchi A, Komori T, Suda T. Regulation of osteoblast differentiation mediated by bone morphogenetic proteins, hedgehogs, and Cbfa1. Endocr Rev 2000;21:393–411.
13. Baron R. Anatomy and ultrastructure of bone. In: Forus M, ed. Primer on the Metabolic Bone Diseases and Disorders of Mineral Metabolism, 4th ed. Lippincott Williams & Wilkins, Philadelphia, PA, 1999, pp. 3–10.
14. Olsen RB. Bone morphogenesis and embryologic development. In: Forus M, ed. Primer on the Metabolic Bone Diseases and Disorders of Mineral Metabolism, 4th ed. Lippincott Williams & Wilkins, Philadelphia, PA, 1999, pp. 11–14.
15. Marks SC Jr, Hermey DC. The structure and development of bone. In: Bilezikian JP, Raisz LG, Rodan GA, eds. Principles of Bone Biology. Academic Press, San Diego, CA, 1996, pp. 3–14.
16. Minton SD, Steichen JJ, Tsang RC. Bone mineral content in term and preterm appropriate-for-gestational-age infants. J Pediatr 1979;95:1037–1042.

17. Froesch ER. IGFs: function and clinical importance. J Intern Med 1993;234:533–534.
18. Hermanussen M, Sippell WG, Valk IM. Knemometric monitoring of early effects of human growth hormone on leg length in children with growth hormone deficiency. Lancet 1985;1:1069–1071.
19. Chan GM, Leeper L, Books L. Effects of soy formulas on mineral metabolism in term infants. Am J Dis Child 1987;141:527–530.
20. Matkovic J. Calcium metabolism and calcium requirements during skeletal modeling and consolidation of bone mass. Am J Clin Nutr 1991;54:245S–605S.
21. Matkovic J, Heaney R. Calcium balance during human growth: evidence for threshold behavior. Am J Clin Nutr 1992;55:992–996.
22. Glastre C, Braillon P, David L, Cochat P, Meunier PJ, Delmas PD. Measurement of bone mineral content of the lumbar spine by dual energy X-ray absorptiometry in normal children-Correlations with growth parameters. J Clin Endocrinol Metab 1990;70:1330–1333.
23. Bonjour JP, Theintz G, Buchs B, Slosman D, Rizzoli R. Critical years and stages of puberty for spinal and femoral bone mass accumulation during adolescence. J Clin Endocrinol Metab 1991;73:555–563.
24. Tanner JM, Landt KW, Cameron N, Carter BS, Patel J. Prediction of adult height from height and bone age in childhood. A new system of equations (TW Mark II) based on a sample including very tall and very short children. Arch Dis Child 1983;58:767–776.
25. Young HB, Greulich WW, Gallagher JR, Cone T, Heald F. Evaluation of physical maturity at adolescence. Dev Med Child Neurol 1968;10:338–348.
26. Lloyd T, Andon MB, Rollings N, Martel JK, Landis JR, Demers LM, et al. Calcium supplementation and bone mineral density in adolescent girls. JAMA 1993;270:841–844.
27. Lee WTK, Leung SSF, Fairweather SJ, Leug DM, Tsang HS, Eagles J, et al. True fractional calcium absorption in Chinese children measured with stable isotopes (^{42}Ca and ^{44}Ca). Brit J Nutrit 1994;72:883–897.
28. Johnston CC Jr, Miller JZ, Slemenda CW, Reister TK, Hui S, Christian JC, et al. Calcium supplementation and increases in bone mineral density in children. N Engl J Med 1992;327:82–87.
29. McKay HA, Petit MA, Khan KM, Schutz RW. Lifestyle determinants of bone mineral: a comparison between prepubertal Asian- and Caucasian-Canadian boys and girls. Calc Tissue Int 2000;66:320–324.
30. Molgaard C, Thomsen BL, Michaelsen KF. Influence of weight, age and puberty on bone size and bone mineral content in healthy children and adolescents. Acta Paediatr 1998;87:494–499.
31. Theintz G, Buchs B, Rizzoli R, Slosman D, Clavien H, Sizonenko PC. Longitudinal monitoring of bone mass accumulation in healthy adolescents: evidence for a marked reduction after 16 years of age at the levels of lumbar spine and femoral neck in female subjects. J Clin Endocrinol Metab 1992;75:1060–1065.
32. Landin LA. Fracture patterns in children. Analysis of 8,682 fractures with special reference to incidence, etiology and secular changes in a Swedish urban population 1950–1979. Acta Orthop Scand Suppl 1983;202:1–109.
33. Russell-Aulet M, Shapiro B, Jaffe CA, Gross MD, Barkan AL. Peak bone mass in young healthy men is correlated with the magnitude of endogenous growth hormone secretion. J Clin Endocrinol Metab 1998;83:3463–3468.
34. Smith EP, Boyd J, Frank GR, Takahashi H, Cohen RM, Specker B, et al. Estrogen resistance caused by a mutation in the estrogen-receptor gene in a man. N Engl J Med 1994;331:1056–1061.
35. Conte FA, Greenbach MM, Ito Y, Fisher CR, Simpson ER. A syndrome of female pseudohermaphroditism, hypergonadotropic hypogonadism, and multicystic ovaries associated with missense mutations in the gene encoding aromatase (P450arom). J Clin Endocrinol Metab 1994;78:1287–1292.
36. Morishima A, Grumbach MM, Simpson ER, Fisher C, Qin K. Aromatase deficiency in male and female siblings caused by a novel mutation in the physiological role of estrogen. J Clin Endocrinol Metab 1995;80:3689–3698.
37. Teegarden D, Proulx WR, Martin BR. Peak bone mass in young women. J Bone Miner Res 1995;10:711–715.
38. Magarey AM, Boulton TJ, Chatterton BE, Schultz C, Nordin BE, Cockington RA. Bone growth from 11 to 17 years: relationship to growth, gender and changes with pubertal status including timing of menarche. Acta Paediatr 1999;88:139–146.
39. Pocock NA, Eisman JA, Hopper JL, Yeates MG, Sambrook PN, Eberl S. Genetic determinants of bone mass in adults: a twin study. J Clin Invest 1987;80:706–710.
40. Matkovic V, Jelic T, Wardlaw GM, Ilich JZ, Goel PK, Wright JK. Timing of peak bone mass in caucasian females and its implication for the prevention of osteoporosis: inference from a cross-sectional model. J Clin Invest 1994;93:799–808.

41. Rubin L, Hawker GA, Peltekova VD, Fielding LJ, Ridout R, Cole DEC. Determinants of peak bone mass: clinical and genetic analyses in a young female Canadian cohort. J Bone Miner Res 1999;14:633–643.

42. Dook JE, James C, Henderson NK, Price RI. Exercise and bone mineral density in mature female athletes. Med Sci Sports Exerc 1997;29:291–296.

43. Courteix D, Lespessailles E, Loiseau Peres S, Obert P, Germain P, Benhamou CL. Effect of physical training on bone mineral density in prepubertal girls: a comparative study between impact-loading and non-impact-loading sports. Osteoporos Int 1998;8:152–158.

44. Thorsen K, Nordstrom P, Lorentzon R, Dahlen GH. The relation between bone mineral density, insulin-like growth factor I, lipoprotein (a), body composition, and muscle strength in adolescent males. J Clin Endocrinol Metab 1999;84:3025–3029.

45. Kroger H, Kotaniemi A, Vainio P, Alhava E. Bone densitometry of the spine and femur in children by dual-energy x-ray absorptiometry. Bone Miner 1992;17:75–85.

46. Slemenda CW, Miller JZ, Hui SL, Reister TK, Johnston CC Jr. Role of physical activity in the development of skeletal mass in children. J Bone Miner Res 1991;6:1227–1233.

47. Ruiz JC, Mandel C, Garabedian M. Influence of spontaneous calcium intake and physical exercise on the vertebral and femoral bone mineral density of children and adolescents. J Bone Miner Res 1995;10: 675–682.

48. Grimston SK, Morrison K, Harder JA, Hanley DA. Bone mineral density during puberty in western Canadian children. Bone Miner 1992;19:85–96.

49. Stallings VA. Calcium and bone health in children: a review. Am J Ther 1997;4:259–273.

50. Teegarden D, Lyle RM, Proulx WR, Johnston CC, Weaver CM. Previous milk consumption is associated with greater bone density in young women. Am J Clin Nutr 1999;69:1014–1017.

51. Cadogan J, Eastell R, Jones N, Barker ME. Milk intake and bone mineral acquistion in adolescent girls: randomised, controlled intervention trial. BMJ 1997;315:1255–1260.

52. Heaney RP, McCarron DA, Dawson-Hughes B, Oparil S, Berga SL, Stern JS, et al. Dietary changes favorably affect bone remodeling in older adults. J Am Diet Assoc 1999;99:1228–1233.

53. Docio S, Riancho JA, Perez A, Olmos JM, Amado JA, Gonzalez-Macias J. Seasonal deficiency of vitamin D in children: a potential target for osteoporosis-preventing strategies? J Bone Miner Res 1998;13: 544–548.

54. Kristinsson JO, Valdimarsson O, Sigurdsson G, Franzson L, Olafsson I, Steingrimsdottir L. Serum 25-hydroxyvitamin D levels and bone mineral density in 16-20 year-old girls: lack of association. J Intern Med 1998;243:381–388.

55. Dawson-Hughes B, Harris SS, Krall EA, Dallal GE, Falconer G, Green CL. Rates of bone loss in post-menopausal women randomly assigned to one of two dosages of vitamin D. Am J Clin Nutr 1995;61: 1140–1145.

56. LeBoff MS, Kohlmeier L, Hurwitz S, Franklin J, Wright J, Glowacki J. Occult vitamin D deficiency in postmenopausal US women with acute hip fracture. JAMA 1999;281:1505–1511.

57. Recker, R. R. Combination therapy for osteoporosis. NIH Consensus Conference http://odp.od.nih.gov/consensus/cons/111/osteo_abstract.pdf, 76–77. 2000. 3-27-2000.

58. NIH Consensus Conference. NIH Consensus Development Panel on Optimal Calcium Intake. JAMA 1994;272:1942–1948.

59. Jee WSS. The skeletal tissues. In: Weiss L, ed. Histology, Cell and Tissue Biology. Elsevier Biomedical, New York, 1983, pp. 200–255.

60. Hillman LS, Chow W, Salmons SS, Weaver E, Erickson M, Hansen J. Vitamin D metabolism, mineral homeostasis, and bone mineralization in term infants fed human milk, cow milk-based formula, or soy-based formula. J Pediatr 1988;112:864–874.

61. Matkovic V, Heaney RP. Calcium balance during human growth: evidence for threshold behavior. Am J Clin Nutr 1992;55:992–996.

62. Malina RM, ed. Growth and Development: The First 20 Years in Man. Burgess Publishing Company, Minneapolis, MN, 1975.

63. Theintz G, Buchs B, Rizzoli R, Slosman D, Clavien H, Sizonenko PC, Bonjour JP. Longitudinal monitoring of bone mass accumulation in healthy adolescents: evidence for a marked reduction after 16 years of age at the levels of lumbar spine and femoral neck in female subjects. J Clin Endocrinol Metab 1992;75:1060–1065.

64. Pocock NA, Eisman JA, Hopper JL, Yeates MG, Sambrook PN, Ebert S. Genetic determinants of bone mass in adults. J Clin Invest 1987;80:706–710.

10

Pediatric Bone Disease

Linda Anne DiMeglio, *MD*

Nature is nowhere accustomed more openly to display her secret mysteries than in cases where she shows traces of her workings apart from the beaten path; nor is there any better way to advance the proper cause of medicine than to give our minds to the discovery of the usual law of Nature by careful investigation of cases of rarer forms of disease. For it has been found, in almost all things, that what they contain of useful or applicable nature is hardly perceived unless we are deprived of them, or they become deranged in some way.

—William Harvey, 1657.

INTRODUCTION

Bone is a complex, dynamic tissue, composed of organic (osteoid, mainly collagen) and inorganic (crystalline calcium phosphate) material. Bones begin to form during the embryonic period as centers of endochondral or membranous ossification. Ossification accelerates during the third trimester of pregnancy. By the time of birth, a newborn has about 25 g of skeletal calcium. Bones then continue to model and remodel throughout childhood. Further periods of rapid growth during infancy and adolescence lead to the achievement of peak bone mineral content (BMC) by young adulthood, at which time the average individual has over 1000 g of skeletal calcium.

From: *Contemporary Endocrinology: Developmental Endocrinology: From Research to Clinical Practice*
Edited by: E. A. Eugster and O. H. Pescovitz © Humana Press Inc., Totowa, NJ

Deposition and resorption of bone is under the control of a variety of hormones. Vitamin D and its metabolites promote an adequate dietary supply of calcium and phosphorus, permitting normal mineralization of the osteoid collagen matrix. Vitamin D is synthesized cutaneously from 7-dehydrocholesterol under ultraviolet (UV) light or acquired in the diet primarily from fortified foods. Initially a biologically inactive prohormone, it undergoes two successive hydroxylations before becoming a potent form that binds to the vitamin D receptor in target cells and exhibits biological activity.

The first, 25-hydroxylation, occurs in the liver, and results in the production of $25(OH)_2$ vitamin D. $25(OH)_2$ vitamin D has a half-life of approx 3 wk; its circulating levels reflect vitamin D stores (1). At physiologic concentrations $25(OH)_2D$ does not have demonstrable biological activity, but it does show activity at higher concentrations.

1α-hydroxylation occurs in the proximal renal tubule, and results in the production of $1,25(OH)_2D$. $1,25(OH)_2D$ has a short half-life of approx 4–6 h. It binds to intracellular vitamin D receptors to produce a variety of biologic effects. The vitamin D receptor belongs to the superfamily of trans-acting transcriptional regulatory factors, including the steroid and thyroid hormone receptors. When coupled to $1,25(OH)_2D$ it interacts with the retinoic acid X receptor to bind to vitamin D response elements. This interaction results in alterations of gene transcription, with net effects of stimulation of intestinal calcium and phosphate absorption and enhancement of bone resorption.

Parathyroid hormone (PTH) is produced by the parathyroid glands. It increases serum calcium concentrations. It does this by increasing renal calcium reabsorption, stimulating osteoclast activity and thereby mobilizing calcium from bone, and increasing intestinal calcium absorption by $1,25(OH)_2D$ production. Continuous exposure to high levels of PTH for days leads to osteoclast-mediated bone resorption, whereas chronic intermittent hormone administration appears to have anabolic effects (2).

PTH-related protein (PTHrP) is a second member of the PTH family (3). As a tumor product, it is the predominant cause of hypercalcemia of malignancy, acting in an apparently identical manner to PTH as it acts on the same PTH/PTHrP receptor. Unlike PTH, however, PTHrP is found in many fetal and adult tissues. It appears to have many important physiologic functions, including effects on chondrocyte proliferation and differentiation (4), smooth-muscle relaxation (5), mammary-gland development (6), and central nervous system (CNS) neuron survival (7).

Calcitonin, a peptide hormone secreted by thyroidal C-cells, is involved in regulating osteoclast activity by inhibiting osteoclastic bone resorption and, secondarily, by stimulating renal calcium clearance. In these roles, it acts as a physiologic antagonist to PTH. Like PTHrP, calcitonin has other systemic effects in the brain, gastrointestinal tract, and the immune system (8). It has a more minor role in physiologic bone metabolism than other hormonal mediators such as PTH and $1,25(OH)_2D$.

Another postulated mediator of mineral metabolism is "phosphatonin." Phosphatonin may regulate phosphate concentrations by impairing renal phosphate reabsorption. Phosphatonin is now believed to be the product of the fibroblast growth factor-23 (FGF-23) gene (9). Paracrine factors such as interleukin-1 (IL-1), tumor necrosis factor (TNF), and osteoprotegrin also play distinct roles in bone physiology (10,11). The identities and functions of these factors await full elucidation.

It is important to note that just as the primary hormones of bone mineral metabolism like $1,25(OH)_2D$ and PTH have wide ranging physiologic effects, many hormones that are generally thought of primarily as extra-skeletal physiologic regulators also exert physiologic and pathologic effects on bones. These include (among others) the sex steroids, estrogen and testosterone; glucocorticoids; thyroid hormone and growth hormone (GH). Compared to $1,25(OH)_2D$ and PTH, they typically have more minor physiologic impacts on bone mineral homeostasis. However, some of these hormones have effects that can cause bone pathology (e.g., osteoporosis with glucocorticoid excess) or be exploited for therapeutic benefit (e.g., estrogens in postmenopausal osteoporosis).

EVALUATION OF THE PEDIATRIC PATIENT WITH BONE DISEASE

Evaluation of the child with suspected bone disease involves careful assessment of fracture history, family history, diet history, anthropometric measures, and review of previous studies, including available radiographs. A targeted laboratory assessment, tailored according to the differential diagnosis, is also essential.

The next step in the evaluation may require an assessment of bone mass and/or bone quality. The "gold standard" for bone assessment is bone biopsy. However, this procedure is relatively invasive and often subjectively interpreted. If osteoporotic or osteosclerotic diseases are being considered, there are several noninvasive methods available for the evaluation of bone mineral density (BMD). Noninvasive quantitation of bone mass is important for several reasons. Accurate assessment of BMD allows quantification of the amount of bone deficiency or excess; it also is important for following the treated or untreated child longitudinally.

Evaluations of conventional radiographs are often used. Although radiographs are very useful for many types of bone assessment, they are an insensitive means of examining BMD, as bone mass may have decreased by 30–50% by the time osteoporosis can be appreciated *(12)*. More accurate measures can be obtained using linear absorption methods, computed tomographic procedures, and sonographic procedures.

Dual X-ray absorptiometry (DXA) is the most popular way to assess pediatric BMD. It measures body composition as well as BMDs at multiple sites. It utilizes photon absorption at two different energies to calculate projected amounts of bone mineral, soft tissue, and fat. Frequent studies include assessments of the total body, lumbar spine, proximal femur, and radius. DXA scores are matched for sex and race and either reported as T-scores (comparison to young-adult population at peak lifetime bone mass) or Z-scores (standardized comparison to age-matched population). Z-scores are essential for comparisons in children.

To derive BMD, it is conventional to divide the BMC by the bone area and express the result as an areal BMD. Since absorptiometry cannot determine the depth or thickness of the bone, and the three-dimensional shapes and sizes of children's bones change markedly during growth (and individuals have different rates of skeletal growth and remodeling), areal BMD is limited as a reliable estimate of BMD in children. Total body BMC may be, therefore, more useful for longitudinal or serial pediatric studies *(13)*. Since individual children may vary in their timing of growth and puberty, there is also currently debate and investigation as to whether data for an individual patient should be normalized to age, height, weight, pubertal stage, or skeletal maturity (as assessed by bone age) *(14–16)*.

Quantitative computed tomography (QCT) measures BMC in a well-defined volume of bone. For this reason, QCT is less affected by bone size than DXA measurements. Again, interpretation of QCT measures requires standards by age, sex, and race. Although used in research settings, axial QCT is expensive and involves relatively high amounts of radiation. Therefore, it is not a practical approach for standard clinical monitoring of children with bone disorders. Alternatives to axial QCT include peripheral QCT of the forearm or femur. These studies are of lower cost and radiation exposure; however, pediatric experiences with these applications are limited *(17)*.

Heel (os calcis) quantitative ultrasound measurements are another means of bony assessment *(18)*. Currently, very few normative data are available for ultrasound measurements in children, however, with increased interest in screening using ultrasound technology, normal reference ranges for the pediatric population are being developed. Ultrasound offers a few theoretical advantages over the aforementioned modalities. It is inexpensive, rapid, and does not involve exposure to radiation. It also allows for measurements not only of bone quantity, but also of aspects of bone structure and quality *(19)*.

It is important when choosing diagnostic tests and interpreting any study results to remember that the pediatric skeleton is a dynamic entity. Almost all assessment variables, such as BMD and ultrasound parameters are influenced in varying degrees by physiologic skeletal growth. Available methods for measuring BMC were developed to study the adult skeleton. Since these modalities were designed for adult assessments, special modifications of the equipment, software, or techniques are required for accurate, precise, and interpretable results in the pediatric population.

METABOLIC BONE DISEASES

Rickets: Calcipenic and Phosphopenic

Rickets refers to inadequate bone matrix mineralization in growing bone or osteoid tissue. Since both calcium and phosphorus are needed to form hydroxyapatite, a relative deficiency of either of these minerals can result in rickets. In all rachitic conditions, the growth-plate cartilage hypertrophies in a disorganized fashion with accumulation of osteoid, resulting in long bones with flared, cupped, and frayed distal metaphyses. In children, radiologic evidence of rickets is most often evident on a knee radiograph, since this is the area of most rapid growth. The counterpart of rickets in persons who have completed linear growth is osteomalacia, characterized by excessive amounts of osteoid with widened seams and decreased mineralization.

There are numerous etiologies of rickets in childhood. They include: vitamin D deficiency, hereditary and acquired 1α-hydroxylase deficiency, vitamin D receptor defects, and a variety of types of phosphopenic rickets.

VITAMIN D DEFICIENCY

Vitamin D deficiency can be the result of lack of sun exposure, decreased vitamin D intake, intestinal malabsorption, obstructive jaundice, or increased metabolism as a result of medications (such as anticonvulsants or antituberculous drugs) *(20)*. Disorders that may cause enteric vitamin D malabsorption include celiac disease, regional enteritis, and cystic fibrosis.

During the first half of the 20th century, vitamin D deficient rickets was common; the predominant cause was inadequate UV light exposure. Now, in the United States, primary vitamin D deficiency is relatively rare, since sun exposure is generally adequate and dairy products are D-fortified (10 μg/qt). However, vitamin D deficiency is still experienced in unsupplemented infants who are dark-pigmented or exclusively breast-fed by mothers who are underexposed to sunlight or themselves have osteomalacia *(21)*. These children may manifest with florid rickets (craniotabes, a "rachitic rosary," and thickening of the wrists and ankles) by around 12 mo of age. Children with rickets are often also irritable and inattentive, have weak musculature, and may demonstrate an increased incidence of infections.

In other (especially older) children, the manifestations of rickets can be much more subtle. Diagnosis is made based on history and clinical observation, and then confirmed radiologically and biochemically. Serum calcium may be normal or low; phosphorus is generally low, and alkaline phosphatase levels are elevated. Serum $25(OH)_2$ vitamin D levels are decreased. If severe secondary hyperparathyroidism develops as a response to the hypocalcemia, $1,25(OH)_2D$ levels may be normal or even increased. Treatment consists of administration of vitamin D initially coupled with calcium. Healing is generally detectable radiographically within 1 mo.

At one time, vitamin D deficency was believed to be a major cause of fractures and rachitic bone disease in premature infants *(22)*. However, although premature babies have radiographs that can often look like those of older children with nutritional vitamin D deficiency, premature children have increased serum concentrations of $1,25(OH)_2D$. In infants with overt metabolic bone disease, high serum $1,25(OH)_2D$ concentrations are reduced with calcium and phosphorus supplementation, suggesting that these infants instead have primarily dietary mineral insufficiency *(23)*. Copper deficiency has also been implicated *(24)*.

HEREDITARY DEFICIENCY OF 1α-HYDROXYLASE

A second cause of rickets, deficiency of the 1α-hydroxylase enzyme, is inherited in an autosomal recessive manner. The disease was first described in 1958, when Fraser and Salter coined the name "Vitamin D-dependent rickets" (VDDR) *(25)*. This condition is sometimes also referred to as Pseudovitamin D deficiency. In 1998, Wang et al. identified mutations in the CYP27B1 gene in patients with VDDR *(26)*, and suggested that the disease should therefore be referred to as $25-(OH)_2D$ 1α-hydroxylase deficiency. 1 α-hydroxylase deficiency has a high prevalence in the French Canadian residents of the Saguenay region of Quebec.

Affected patients usually present in the first months of life with hypocalcemic seizures, or later with rickets accompanied by growth retardation, bony pain, and extremity bowing. Since this disease results from defective 1α-hydroxylation of $25(OH)_2D$, a low serum level of $1,25(OH)_2D$, with a normal $25(OH)_2$ vitamin D is characteristic. The biochemical profile mirrors severe vitamin D deficiency, with low serum calcium and phosphate, increased alkaline phosphatase, and secondary hyperparathyroidism. This form of rickets is unresponsive to standard does of vitamin D or $25(OH)_2$ vitamin D. Treatment consists of physiologic doses of $1,25(OH)_2D$ *(27)*. This treatment rapidly reverses all the skeletal and metabolic abnormalities.

ACQUIRED DEFICIENCY OF 1α-HYDROXYLASE

It is important to note that most children with 1α hydroxylase deficiency have the disorder as a result of renal failure (with consequent loss of kidney 1α hydroxylase activity) rather than from an inherited disorder of vitamin D metabolism. Treatment for these children consists of physiologic doses of $1,25(OH)_2D$.

Hereditary Defects in the Vitamin D Receptor

Some children with apparent 1α hydroxylase deficiency fail to improve after treatment with physiologic doses of $1,25(OH)_2D$ *(28)*. These patients characteristically manifest high serum concentrations of $1,25(OH)_2D$ before and during treatment. They have another form of inherited rickets, sometimes referred to as Vitamin D resistant rickets or VDDR Type II. In 1988, Hughes et al. sequenced the vitamin D receptor and found two different mutations in two families with vitamin D resistance *(29)*.

There appear to be two clinical forms of this disease, characterized by the presence or absence of alopecia. The form with alopecia appears to result from deletions of the receptor; the second form is due to inactivating mutations of the 1,25 dihydroxy vitamin D receptor. In both forms patients present with severe rickets, hypocalcemia, hypophosphatemia, elevated serum alkaline phosphatase, normal serum $25(OH)_2D$, markedly elevated $1,25(OH)_2D$, and secondary hyperparathyroidism. This disorder is difficult to treat and is currently managed either with high (3–6 µg/d) doses of $1,25(OH)_2D$ or with a series of calcium infusions followed by high-dose oral calcium (3.5–9 g elemental calcium/m^2/d) *(30)*.

Phosphopenic Rickets

Phosphorous deficiency can be acquired or congenital. Acquired forms of phosphate deficiency include those resulting from use of phosphate-binding antacids or hyperparathyroidism. Dietary phosphate deficiency is rare, seen only in extreme starvation or in inadequately-fed neonates. Congenital forms of phosphate deficiency include X-linked hypophosphatemic rickets (XLH), autosomal dominant hypophosphatemic rickets (ADHR), and hereditary hypophosphatemic rickets with hypercalciuria (HHRH). In the developed world, a large proportion of rickets and osteomalacia is due to isolated renal phosphate wasting disorders. Recently our understanding of these hypophosphatemic, inherited conditions has progressed substantially.

X-Linked Hypophosphatemic Rickets. XLH is an X-linked dominant disorder. It is the most common form of inherited rickets, with an estimated prevalence of 1:20,000 *(31)*. Clinical manifestations are variable, but can include short stature, rickets with resultant varus and valgus deformities of the lower extremities (Fig. 1), enthesopathy (calcification of tendons, ligaments, and joint capsules) and dental abscesses *(32,33)*. Although most children with XLH will have radiographic evidence of rickets, such changes are not omnipresent *(34)*. The disease persists and may progress through adulthood.

All patients have a renal tubular phosphate leak with consequent hypophosphatemia. Laboratory features also include normal serum calcium, normal PTH levels, $1,25(OH)_2D$ levels that are inappropriately normal for the level of phosphorus, and elevated alkaline phosphatase.

Mutations in the *PHEX* gene are responsible for XLH *(35)*. There is no predominant mutation. The PHEX protein is an endopeptidase, which may either activate or degrade a peptide hormone. How loss of PHEX function leads to XLH is not currently known. Although the disease is completely penetrant, disease severity varies widely, even between members of the same family *(36)*. Some persons with XLH have isolated hypophosphatemia; others have severe, disabling bony disease. Since disease severity in XLH is similar between males and females, there appears to be minimal, if any, gene dosage effect *(37)*. There is also no evidence of genetic anticipation, as disease severity does not worsen with succeeding generations of affected individuals *(37)*. Treatment of XLH currently consists of titrated high-dose $1,25(OH)_2D$ coupled with phosphate.

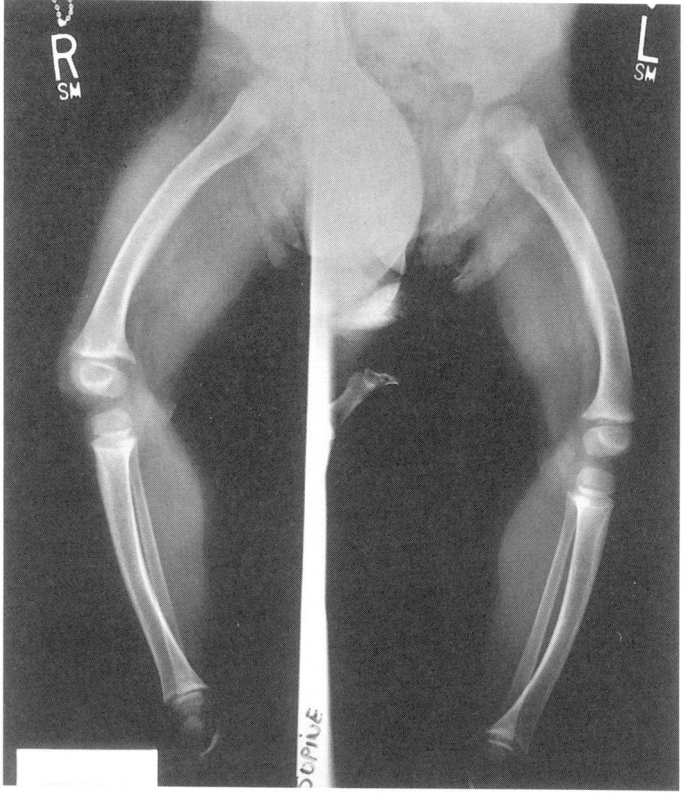

Fig. 1. Supine leg films of an untreated 30-mo-old with XLH. Note bowing of the femurs and tibias. Note also widened epiphyses with fraying.

Autosomal Dominant Hypophosphatemic Rickets (ADHR). In 1971, Bianchine et al. described a family with autosomal dominant renal phosphate wasting *(38)*. Affected family members included the father, one son, and two daughters. The father had isolated renal phosphate wasting, short stature, and an impressive windswept deformity (valgus on one side and varus on the other). He also had a marked tendency to fractures with or without trauma. Otherwise, the clinical course in these individuals appeared similar to that of XLH patients.

ADHR is an autosomal dominant disorder with incomplete penetrance *(39)*. Some individuals have a delayed onset of disease. In those patients who have disease starting from childhood, the clinical features are similar to the rachitic and growth features of XLH. Patients who present as adults have osteomalacia with bone pain, weakness, and fracture, rather than rickets. The laboratory and radiographic features of ADHR are also similar to XLH, including hypophosphatemia with normal serum levels of PTH and $25(OH)_2D$, with inappropriately normal serum $1,25(OH)_2D$. ADHR is due to mutations in phosphatonin, a protein coded for by the FGF-23 gene *(9)*. Phosphatonin mutations result in phosphate wasting.

Hereditary Hypophosphatemic Rickets with Hypercalciuria (HHRH). In 1985, Tieder et al. were the first to describe HHRH in members of a consanguineous Bedouin tribe

(40). Affected members had rickets, short stature, renal phosphate wasting, hypercalciuria with normocalcemia, elevated serum $1,25(OH)_2D$ levels, and suppressed PTH. Initial symptoms of bone pain and lower-extremity deformities generally are present by 6 mo to 7 yr of age. Additional features include short stature and muscle weakness. Persistent hypophosphatemia is felt to be responsible for the reduced bone mineralization and growth. It is now known that disease expression is heterogeneous. Some patients have an intermediate phenotype with idiopathic hypercalciuria, slightly reduced serum phosphate levels, and elevated serum $1,25(OH)_2D$ concentrations without discernible bony disease or growth retardation *(41)*.

Lab abnormalities in HHRH include a decreased tubular resorption of phosphate, resulting in hypophosphatemia with normocalcemia *(40)*. Patients typically demonstrate elevated serum alkaline phosphatase, low to low-normal PTH, and normal serum concentrations of $25(OH)_2D$. In contrast to XLH and ADHR, renal phosphate depletion results in an appropriate increase in serum $1,25(OH)_2D$ concentrations. Excess circulating $1,25 (OH)_2D$ enhances the intestinal calcium and phosphate absorption, increases the renal calcium-filtered load, and suppresses parathyroid-gland function.

Bone biopsies in children with HHRH demonstrate mineralization defects, with irregular mineralization fronts, markedly elevated osteoid surface and seam width, increased number of osteoid lamellae, and prolonged mineralization lag time *(42)*. The HHRH mineralization defect appears to be determined primarily by the degree of hypophosphatemia. Bone parameters are within the normal range in family members with the intermediate phenotype of HHRH.

HHRH is far less prevalent than XLH. The low prevalence may be due partly to under diagnosis, since it shares features of other renal phosphate-wasting disorders and of idiopathic hypercalciuria with bone lesions and stunted growth *(43)*. The gene responsible for HHRH has not yet been identified. The mode of inheritance of HHRH may be heterogeneous *(44)*. A few candidate genes have been proposed and mapped, including the Na^+-phosphate cotransporter gene 1 (NPT1) (6p21.3-p23) *(45)* and NPT2 (5q35) *(46)*. NPT1 and NPT2 are likely candidate genes since both genes are autosomal and expressed predominantly in the kidney. Finding the gene for HHRH will not only help to determine the pathogenesis of the disorder, but will also provide important answers to questions involving the PTH-vitamin D-phosphate feedback loop.

Hypophosphatasia

In 1948 Rathbun coined the term "hypophosphatasia," with a report of a 9-wk-old infant who died from severe rickets, weight loss, and seizures *(47)*. Despite the rachitic appearance, the serum alkaline phosphatase levels were low. Hypophosphatasia is a rare, autosomal recessive disorder, with an estimated general population incidence of 1 in 100,000 births *(48)*. The disease is more common in the Canadian Mennonite population, where the incidence is estimated to be 1:2,500 *(49)*.

Hypophosphatasia is caused by defects in the gene coding for tissue nonspecific (liver/ bone/kidney) alkaline phosphatase (TNALP) on chromosome 1 *(50)*. Even though TNALP is distributed throughout the body, hypophosphatasia primarily affects the skeleton and dentition.

There is a wide, overlapping clinical spectrum with six defined types of disease. Four are defined by age of presentation: perinatal (congenital lethal hypophosphatasia), infantile, juvenile, or adult (hypophosphatasia tarda). The perinatal and infantile forms of the condition are predominantly inherited in an autosomal recessive manner. Individuals demonstrate severe skeletal ossification deficiency with a moth-eaten appearance to the ends of severely shortened long bones. The infantile form can also have hypercalcemia with resultant nephrocalcinosis. The juvenile or adult disorders have milder manifestations (leg bowing and variable short stature) and can be inherited as either autosomal recessive or dominant (48). A fifth form of hypophosphatasia, known as odontohypophosphatasia, presents only with dental disease due to dental cementum hypoplasia. Patients with pseudo-hyophosphatasia have normal in vitro but reduced in vivo alkaline phosphatase activity.

Large quantities of phosphoethanolamine, the substrate for alkaline phosphatase, are found in the urine. Plasma inorganic pyrophosphate and pyridoxal-5-phosphate levels are also high. Serum alkaline phosphatase activity is low. There is no established medical regimen for hypophosphatasia. A variety of treatments have been attempted, including enzyme replacement utilizing weekly infusions of alkaline phosphatase-rich plasma from patients with Paget's disease, yet none has been effective. Traditional therapies for osteoporosis (vitamin D metabolites and calcium supplements) should be avoided because they may worsen hypercalcemia and hypercalciuria (51). Prenatal testing for recognized familial mutations in the TNALP gene is now possible.

OSTEOPOROTIC BONE DISEASES

Albright and Reifenstein defined osteoporosis in 1948, as "There is too little bone in bone" (52). Osteoporosis results from an uncoupling of the processes of bone formation and resorption, resulting in a net excess of resorption. Osteoporosis involves parallel loss of bone mineral and matrix, increasing skeletal porosity, decreasing bone strength, and increasing fracture risk. Children with osteoporosis do not obtain peak bone mass during the first three decades of life. Since they start adult life with a relative bone deficit, they are at increased risk of osteoporotic fractures later in life.

Secondary Forms of Osteoporosis

There are a number of endocrine and nonendocrine disorders that can result in childhood osteoporosis. Endocrine causes include glucocorticoid excess (53), thyrotoxicosis (54), and growth hormone deficiency (GHD) (2,55). Other disease states of childhood have osteoporosis either as a component of the primary disease or as a result of accompanying immobilization or medications. These include many chronic childhood diseases such as juvenile rheumatoid arthritis (56), nephrotic syndrome (57), inflammatory bowel disease (58), gluten enteropathy, diabetes, and cystic fibrosis (59). BMD in children without underlying systemic disease may also correlate with dietary calcium intake, which may be particularly low in children who are lactose intolerant, have milk protein allergies, or are "picky eaters" (60). Adolescents with delayed puberty or secondary amenorrhea, especially when coupled with malnutrition (e.g., anorectics, underweight athletes), are also at risk of failing to reach peak bone mass with subsequent osteoporosis (61).

Osteogenesis Imperfecta

Osteogenesis imperfecta (OI) is an inherited disorder of collagen synthesis, which results in increased bone fragility with ligamentous laxity and, consequently, recurrent

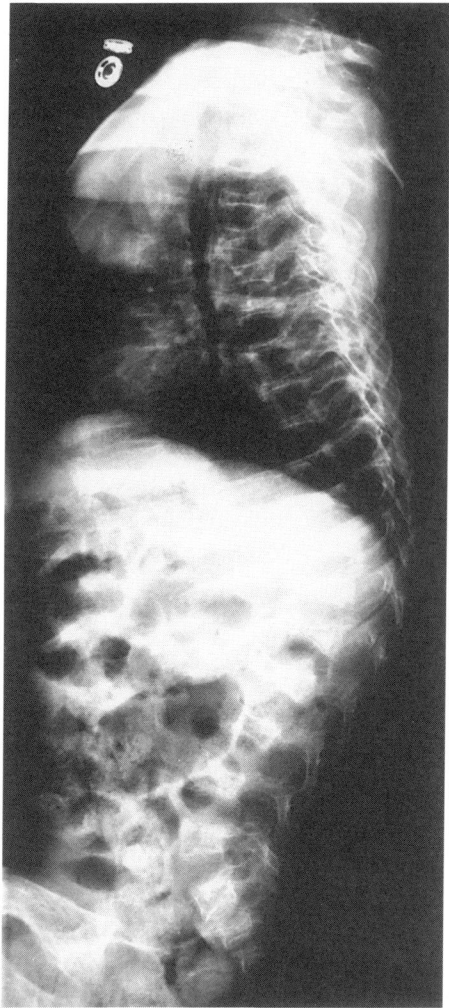

Fig. 2. Lateral spine film of 3-yr-old child with osteogenesis imperfecta, Type III. Note diffuse osseous demineralization, scoliosis, and vertebral compression abnormalities.

fractures (Fig. 2). Persons with severe OI may experience several hundred fractures over a lifetime; others with milder forms may have only a few. OI affects approx 1 in 10,000 persons; due to incomplete reporting, the exact incidence is unknown *(62)*. The best estimates of the total number of persons with OI in the United States suggest a minimum of 20,000 and as many as 50,000.

In the late 1970s, Sillence and colleagues *(63)*, using clinical, radiographic, and inheritance criteria, developed the classification currently used. They separated individuals with OI into types I to IV: Type I, a dominant form with blue sclerae; Type II, a perinatally lethal form; Type III, a progressively deforming form with normal sclerae; and Type IV, a dominant form with normal sclerae. A fifth category (Type V) OI has recently been described *(64)*. Type V separates out those individuals with Type IV OI who have had either an interosseous membrane calcification or a hypertrophic callus formation at a fracture or osteotomy site. These patients also have a visible dense band under the growth plate.

This classification was derived according to phenotype rather than genotype. Yet, it remains the most popular system, since, despite the identification of >300 mutations *(62)*, it remains impossible to predict phenotypes from genotype. Genetic defects are currently technically quite difficult to ascertain. Therefore, many patients with OI remain unclassified by "Type." Even detailed schema probably will never correctly predict the clinical manifestations of OI in every affected individual, because there is often unexplained variability of phenotypic expression between individuals from families with the same genotypic defect *(65)*. How various molecular defects lead to distinctive phenotypes is not well-understood, but variability appears to result from the effects of nongenetic factors (e.g., random developmental events) *(66)* or the interaction of other genes determining disease expression.

Over 90% of patients with OI have mutations in type I collagen. Type I collagen is the major structural protein of the extracellular matrix of tendons, skin, and bone. It is also abundant in lung, dentin, heart valves, fascia, scar tissue, cornea, and liver. A long, rope-like fibril, type I collagen is comprised of two pro α1 chains and one pro 1 α2 chain twisted into a tight left-handed helix *(67)*. Type I OI results from mutations that lead to "functional null" alleles of a Type I collagen gene *(68)*. Types II, III, and IV OI result from a dominant negative effect of a structurally abnormal type I collagen on connective tissue *(69)*. The mutant chain directly disorganizes and weakens the extracellular matrix (ECM).

Patients with OI often, but not uniformly, have a reduced bone mineral density; this, in turn, is associated with an increase in fracture rate. Approximately one-third of patients with OI have dentinogenesis imperfecta Type I *(70,71)*, with dark discoloration of teeth, narrow pulp chambers and a predilection for the enamel to crack off the teeth with subsequent severe attrition of the exposed dentin *(72)*. Persons with OI also have a high frequency of hearing loss, beginning in the late teens, which is usually of a conductive or mixed (conductive/neurologic) type. Hearing loss occurs in about half of all patients by the age of thirty, and in nearly all-older patients *(73)*. Other manifestations of collagen deficiency include ligamentous laxity, joint hypermobility, and vascular fragility. Growth impairment is also a hallmark manifestation of OI. Growth follows relatively consistent patterns according to type of OI. It appears that the etiology of the short stature is multifactorial *(74)*. Abnormal temperature regulation in patients with OI has also been reported *(75)*.

Idiopathic Juvenile Osteoporosis

Idiopathic juvenile osteoporosis is a rare, sporadic disease, most likely of heterogeneous etiology, although the exact pathogenesis is unknown *(76)*. It generally manifests in otherwise healthy children between the ages of 8 and 15 yr. Symptoms may include bone pain, fractures with minor trauma, height loss due to vertebral fractures and kyphoscoliosis, and low BMD. Prolonged disuse may exaggerate this condition. Children with this condition generally experience a spontaneous recovery after puberty, but bony deformities can persist.

Diagnosis at present is made by noting features of the disease and then ruling out other osteoporotic conditions affecting children, especially osteogenesis imperfecta, thyrotoxicosis, Cushing disease, or hematologic malignancies *(2,77)*. This disorder does not have consistent biochemistry, although some children may have decreased levels of 1,25 $(OH)_2D$ *(2,78)*. Rarely, these patients have persistent osteoporosis through adolescence to adulthood.

Treatment of Osteoporotic Bone Diseases

Treatment of osteoporotic bone disease is designed to increase BMD and therefore reduce the risk of fracture. First-line therapy generally consists of optimizing calcium and vitamin D intake. Treatment with vitamin D metabolites has been useful in patients with IJO.

Other agents used for osteoporosis in children include calcitonin and bisphosphonates. Calcitonin can be given by subcutaneous injection or nasal spray. It binds to receptors on the osteoclast surface and reduces osteoclastic bone resorption by diminishing osteoclast numbers, changing osteoclast appearance, reducing resorptive activity, moving osteoclasts away from bone, and increasing apoptosis (79). Calcitonin does increase BMD, particularly in patients with high bone turnover and has some analgesic effect. However, calcitonin's effect on BMD is limited, compared to the efficacy of bisphosphonates.

Bisphosphonates are synthetic, stable analogs of naturally occurring pyrophosphate in which the oxygen that links the phosphates has been replaced by carbon to give a 'P-C-P' structure (80). This backbone renders them resistant to enzymatic degradation. The actual molecular targets of bisphosphonates remain to be identified. At the tissue level, bisphosphonates are adsorbed onto hydroxyapatite crystals in bone mineral (81). There they inhibit osteoclastic bone resorption. Their actions may be also be partially mediated by effects on osteoblasts (82,83). Radiographs of patients on IV bisphosphonate demonstrate multiple dense bands under growth plates corresponding to treatment courses (Fig. 3A). Those on oral bisphosphonate demonstrate a uniform band of subepiphyseal hypermineralization corresponding to the length of therapy (Fig. 3B). Bisphosphonates have been useful in both children and adults in the treatment of various types of osteoporosis (80). Preliminary case series appear to demonstrate that they are safe, effective, and well-tolerated. Further research (including randomized, controlled trials) are in progress.

Recombinant PTH may also prove useful for childhood and adolescent forms of osteoporosis (2). However, concerns about the risk of osteosarcoma development in growing skeletons (as seen in rodent studies) may curtail pediatric investigation in the near future. More preliminary research is needed.

SCLEROSING BONE DISEASES

Several pediatric bone diseases are characterized by an increase in the mass per unit volume of cortical or trabecular bone. Increased mass can result from either excessive formation of new bone or decreased resorption of already-formed bone. It manifests as an increased radiologic bone density. The increases in bone mass can be spotty or diffuse, with bony deposition occurring in the cortex or cancellous trabeculae. If deposition happens in the trabeculae, it can encroach on the medullary spaces leading to decreased blood production. Hyperostosis is often coupled with bone architectural abnormalities, which can subsequently predispose to fracture.

Osteopetrosis

One sclerosing bone disorder is osteopetrosis (marble bone disease), first described by a German radiologist, Heinrich Albers-Schonberg, in 1904 (84). The prevalence of osteopetrosis is unknown, but estimates range from 5.5:100,000 to 1:500,000 (85,86). Resulting from decreased bone resorption relative to bone formation, osteopetrosis manifests with diffuse, symmetric accumulation of excessive bone. Histology reveals pathogno-

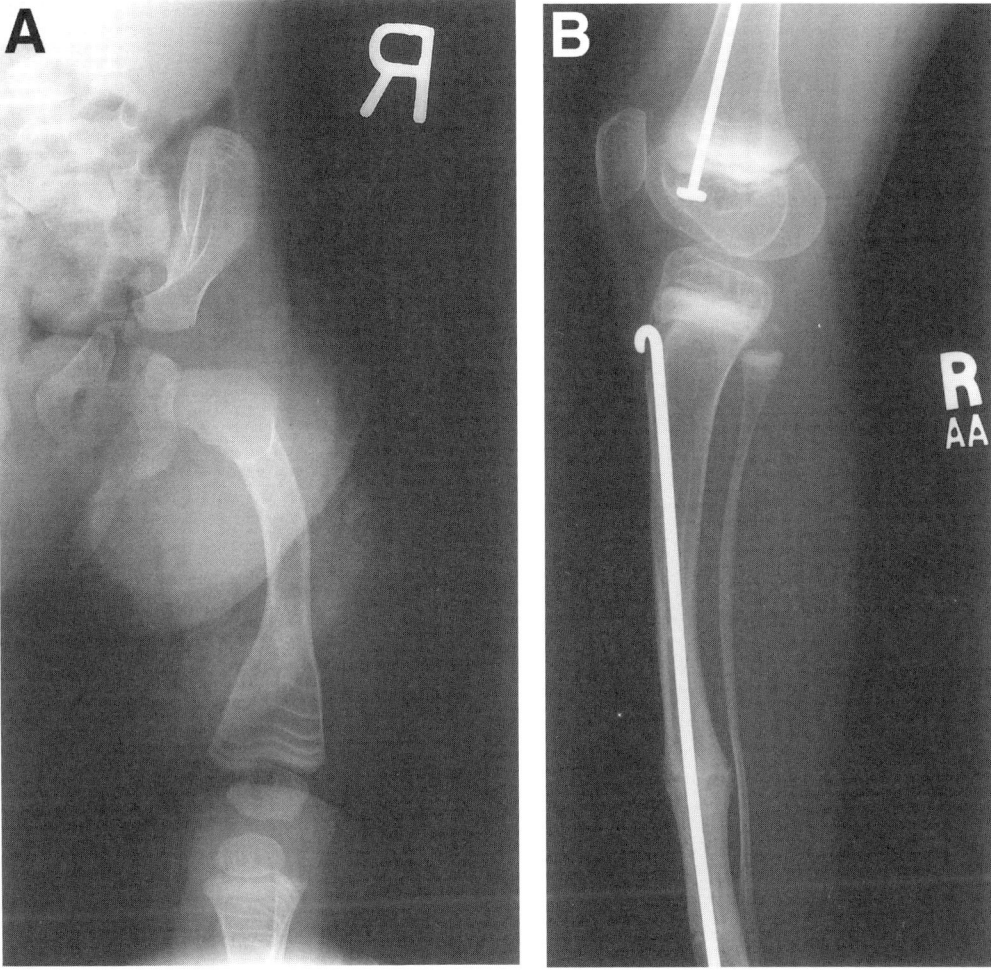

Fig. 3. (A) Right leg and hip film of a 12-mo-old with osteogenesis imperfecta, Type III after seven courses of IV pamidronate. Note diffuse demineralization, bony deformity, and bands of hyper-mineralization corresponding to treatment courses. **(B)** Lateral knee and tibial film of an 8-yr-old with osteogenesis imperfecta, Type III after 11 mo of oral alendronate. Note diffuse demineralization with rods, bony deformity, and healing tibial fractures. Note also subepiphyseal hypermineralization around the knee. The size of these regions corresponds to the time on therapy.

monic remnants of primary spongiosa within bone. Osteosclerosis has numerous deleterious consequences, including a predisposition to fracture, a decreased size of the marrow space of the long bones, and a decrease in the caliber of the various cranial nerve and vascular canals. Laboratory abnormalities include increased levels of tartrate resistant alkaline phosphatase and the creatinine kinase-BB isoenzyme fraction.

Three clinical forms of osteopetrosis have been delineated. All appear to be the result of inherited disorders of osteoclasts. The two major subgroups are an infantile autosomal recessive form and an autosomal dominant form. A third group of patients have intermediate autosomal recessive forms of the disease, including a rare type of osteopetrosis with renal tubular acidosis and cerebral calcifications.

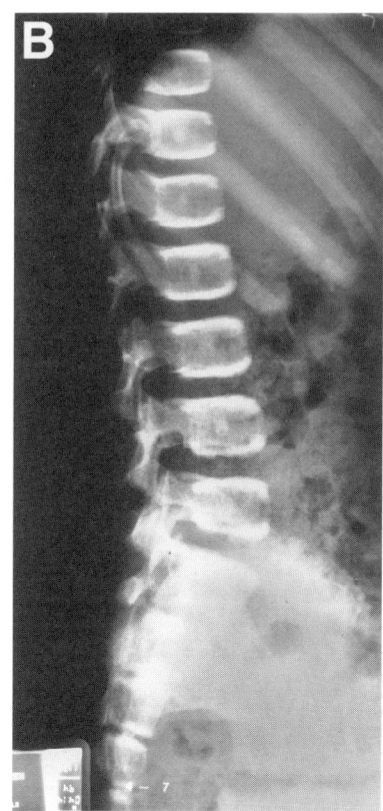

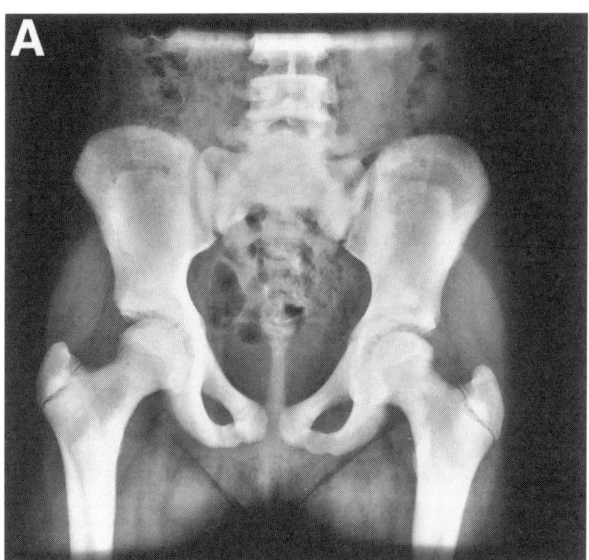

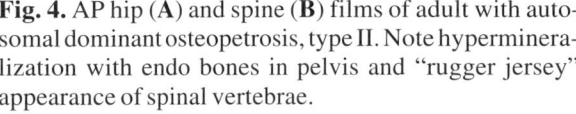

Fig. 4. AP hip (**A**) and spine (**B**) films of adult with auto-somal dominant osteopetrosis, type II. Note hypermineralization with endo bones in pelvis and "rugger jersey" appearance of spinal vertebrae.

The infantile form presents shortly after birth with fractures, hypocalcemia, or with failure to thrive. These children have pancytopenia, hepatosplenomegaly, and recurrent infections from leukopenia. Skull changes can lead to narrowing of the optic and auditory nerve canals, with subsequent blindness and deafness. Untreated infants die within the first few years from hemorrhage or infections. There appears to be significant genetic heterogeneity in this form of osteopetrosis. Two gene mutations that affect osteoclastic function in some individuals have been identified to date. One is in a vacuolar hydrogen ion pump *(87)*; a second is in a chloride channel *(88)*. Both mutations appear to impair osteoclastic ability to acidify extracellular resorption lacunae.

The autosomal dominant form of osteopetrosis is subdivided into two distinct types, type I and type II. Type I has diffuse osteosclerosis including increased skull calvarial thickness *(89)*. On X-ray, a rugger jersey spinal appearance and "endo bones" in the pelvis characterize Type II (Fig. 4).

Persons with Type I osteopetrosis tend to be relatively asymptomatic, without fractures or laboratory abnormalities *(90)*. Type II autosomal dominant osteopetrosis has 75% gene penetrance. Affected individuals have great phenotypic heterogeneity. Although the disorder may be relatively asymptomatic during childhood, many patients with Type II disease have at least one early complication of the disease, which may include pathologic fractures of long bones, bone pain, osteomyelitis (typically mandibular), or cranial-nerve palsies. Rarely, patients may have bone marrow suppression. Although one family with Type II osteopetrosis has demonstrated chromosomal linkage to 1p21 *(91)*, studies on other families have not shown linkage to this site *(92)*. It is likely that there is genetic heterogeneity.

The intermediate forms of osteopetrosis are generally autosomal recessive in inheritance. One intermediate form demonstrates, in addition to osteopetrotic bone disease, renal tubular acidosis, growth failure, dental malocclusion, and intra-cerebral calcifications, with varying degrees of mental retardation. First described in 1972, this form of intermediate osteopetrosis is due to carbonic anhydrase II deficiency *(93)*.

A wide variety of treatments including high dose $1,25(OH)_2D$, steroids, and even thyroid hormone have been utilized for individuals with osteopetrosis. Although $1,25(OH)_2D$ is often used for this condition, no hormonal therapy has proven consistently valuable. Treatment with recombinant human interferon gamma (IFN-γ) ameliorates some symptoms of the disease. Bone-marrow transplantation is curative in some patients and is the therapy of choice for children with severe autosomal recessive osteopetrosis

Pyknodysostosis

Pyknodysostosis is an autosomal-recessive disorder, first described in 1962 *(94,95)*. It is characterized by osteosclerosis with a generalized increase in bone density, short stature, separated cranial sutures, high-arched palate, blue sclerae, a beaked nose, mandibular hypoplasia, truncal deformities including kyphoscoliosis, and progressive phalangeal acroosteolysis. Patients present during infancy or childhood and suffer frequent transverse bone fractures.

This disorder is due to a defect in the gene for cathepsin K, a lysosomal cysteine protease highly expressed in osteoclasts *(96)*. Patients with pyknodysostosis have normal numbers of osteoclasts with typical ruffled borders and clear zones. However, large regions of demineralized bone surround osteoclasts, which have large, abnormal cytoplasmic vacuoles containing bone-collagen fibrils. This histology suggests that these osteoclasts are able to demineralize bone normally, but are then unable to degrade the organic matrix. There is no known therapy for pyknodysostosis.

THE CHONDRODYSPLASIAS

Until 1959, all forms of disproportionate, short-limbed short stature were known as "achondroplasias." Recently, however, it has become possible to group the chondrodysplasias according to the specific causative gene, enzyme, or protein defect or on similar clinical and radiographic manifestations.

FGFR3 Mutations: The Achondroplasias

Achondroplasias, although rare, are the most common nonlethal skeletal dysplasias; their prevalence has been estimated at 2.53/100,000 live births *(97)*. The achondroplasias consist of four phenotypes: achondroplasia, thanatophoric dysplasia, hypochondroplasia, and severe achondroplasia with developmental delay and acanthosis nigricans *(98,99)*. All are the result of autosomal dominant inheritance or sporadic development of mutations in the gene encoding the fibroblast growth factor receptor-3 (FGFR3), a tyrosine kinase receptor, located at 4p16.3 *(100)* These gain-of-function mutations accentuate the physiologic effects of receptor activation on negatively regulating bone growth.

Ninety-seven percent of cases of achondroplasia are due to the same point mutation in nucleotide 1138 causing an Arg→Gly substitution in the receptor's transmembrane domain *(101,102)*. Interestingly, unlike many other pediatric bone diseases, the achondro-plasias demonstrate a very high genotype-phenotype correlation.

The term "a-chondro-plasia" is a misnomer since cartilage does develop, however endochondrally derived bone is underdeveloped in length, resulting in disproportionate short stature. Affected persons have frontal bossing with mid-face hypoplasia, short stature (due to rhizomelic limb shortening), lumbar lordosis, limited elbow extension, genu varum, and trident hands. Children often exhibit true megalencephaly. Disproportion between the skull base and the brain can result in hydrocephalus or brain-stem compression *(103)*. Craniocervical disproportion with cervical-cord compression puts these children at an increased risk of death (as high as 7.5%) *(104)*. Persons with achondroplasia also have an increased incidence of obesity; achondroplasia-specific growth curves have been developed *(105)*. Mean adult height is 131 cm in males and 124 cm in females *(106)*. Leg-lengthening procedures are sometimes done, but pose ethical dilemmas *(107)*.

Homozygosity for the gene defect results in a severe skeletal "double dominant" disorder with radiologic changes qualitatively somewhat different from those of the usual heterozygous achondroplasia *(108)*. This disorder is lethal in the first days to months of life. Early death results from respiratory compromise from a small thoracic cage or spinal compression due to a small foramen magnum and hydrocephalus *(102)*.

Hypochondroplasia has a similar radiologic appearance, yet milder phenotype than achondroplasia *(106)*. It is generally caused by mutations in the tyrosine kinase domain of the FGFR3 gene, although 30–40% of patients do not have a known mutation. Hypochondroplasia often goes undiagnosed. Affected individuals have rhizomelic short-limbed dwarfism that is usually noted around 2 yr of age, broad and stubby hands and feet, and craniofacial abnormalities (macrocephaly with frontal bossing) *(109)*.

Thanatophoric ("death bearing") dysplasia (TD) is generally lethal in the neonatal period from respiratory compromise from a small thoracic cage, lung hypoplasia, and respiratory insufficiency *(106)*. Hydrocephalus is common. Prior to birth, in addition to skeletal abnormalities visible on ultrasound, poor fetal movement and polyhydramnios may be noted. Those few individuals who have survived into early childhood have severe developmental delay. There are two recognized subgroups of patients with TD, known as TD Type 1 and TD Type 2. TD Type 1 patients have severe bowing of the femurs and other tubular bones. TD Type 1 generally results from a variety of missense mutations that create cysteine residues in the extracellular domain of FGFR3 *(110)*; Type 2 is the result of a K650E substitution in the intracellular tyrosine kinase domain of FGFR3. Individuals with TD type 2 have straight femurs, but craniosynostosis of the coronal and lambdoid sutures, resulting in a cloverleaf skull deformity.

A single, specific mutation in the FGFR3 gene (1949 A→T) results in severe achondroplasia with developmental delay and acanthosis nigricans. Persons with this disorder have profound short stature, marked craniofacial characteristics, hydrocephalus, severe developmental delay, seizures, and acanthosis nigricans.

Col2A1 Mutations: Spondyloepiphyseal Dysplasia

Spondyloepiphyseal dysplasia (SED) is the result of autosomal dominant or sporadic mutations in the COL2A1 gene. This disorder is rare (estimated prevalence 1:250,000) and demonstrates poor genotype-phenotype correlation. Persons with SED have shortened trunks relative to limb lengths, abnormal epiphyses, and flattened vertebral bodies.

The range of phenotypes varies, from mild short stature (SED tarda) to variants that are detectable but non-lethal at the time of birth (SED congenita and Kniest dysplasia) to severe growth and pulmonary compromise with early death (achondrogenesis type II or hypochondrogenesis) *(111)*. Other complications of SED can include myopia, vitreal degeneration, retinal detachment, C1-C2 vertebral subluxation with spinal cord compression, and early large joint degenerative disease.

COMP Mutations

The pseudoachondroplasias and multiple epiphyseal dysplasias (MEDs) have distinct phenotypes but are grouped genetically since they both result from dominant-negative mutations in the cartilage oligomeric matrix protein (COMP) gene *(112,113)*. COMP is a large, extra-cellular matrix glycoprotein found in the territorial matrix that surrounds chondrocytes. It is also found in the extracellular matrix of ligaments and tendons, producing ligamentous joint laxity.

PSEUDOACHONDROPLASIA

Pseudoachondroplasia is caused by COMP mutations that result in accumulation of an abnormal form of the glycoprotein *(113)*. The disorder has a prevalence of approximately 1:250,000 persons *(114)*. Individuals with pseudoachondroplasia have normal appearances at birth, but then experience linear growth deceleration between 12 and 24 mo of age. Other clinical and skeletal features include joint laxity, short limbs and digits, various leg and arm deformities (genu valgum, genu varum, windswept deformities), scoliosis, and odontoid hypoplasia. X-rays demonstrate both epiphyseal and metaphyseal changes, vertebral flattening, and anterior vertebral beaking.

MULTIPLE EPIPHYSEAL DYSPLASIA

Individuals with MED demonstrate predominantly epiphyseal X-ray changes. There are two clinical variants, a mild Ribbing type, and a severe Fairbank type. The Fairbank type manifests during childhood with mild short-limbed short stature, some joint pain, and a waddling gait. The Ribbing type may not present until adolescence, where it may resemble bilateral Legg-Perthes disease. Although most cases of MED are due to COMP mutations *(115)*, some MED cases have locus heterogeneity, resulting from mutations in the Type IX collagen genes COL9A2 or COL9A3 *(116)*. It has been suggested that COMP and Type IX collagen may interact functionally in the cartilage matrix, thus explaining the similar phenotypes despite divergent genotypes.

PTH/PTHrP Receptor Mutations:
Jansen Metaphyseal Chondrodysplasia

This disorder is a rare, dominantly inherited metaphyseal chondrodysplasia that results from gain-of-function mutations that of the PTH/PTHrP transmembrane receptor *(117)*. Accentuation of signaling through this receptor causes hypercalcemia and also enhances the terminal differentiation of cartilage cells, slowing bone growth. Affected individuals have severe limb shortening with short stature and leg bowing and an unusual facial appearance consisting of hypertelorism with exophthalmos and a receding chin *(109)*. Occasionally individuals will have club fingers. X-rays demonstrate short, tubular bones with characteristic cupped and ragged metaphyses that develop mottled calcifications with time. The epiphyses are normal.

OTHER BONE DISEASES

Fibrous Dysplasia

Fibrous dysplasia represents about 2.5% of all bone disorders and 7% of all benign bony tumors *(118)*. The hallmark of fibrous dysplasia is fibrous-tissue proliferation in cyst-like spaces, replacing normal bone. The skull, femur, and tibia are the most commonly affected sites. Symptoms are bone pain and repeated fractures. Fibrous dysplasia can be limited to only one bone (monostotic), where it may not produce symptoms and be an incidental finding. However, several bones can be involved (polyostotic). Serum calcium concentrations are normal, but serum alkaline phosphatase and urinary markers of collagen breakdown can be elevated. Hypophosphatemia due to renal phosphaturia is seen commonly *(119)*.

The clinical triad of fibrous dysplasia; café au lait spots, often on the same side as the bone lesions; and endocrine dysfunction, characterized by precocious puberty in girls is known as McCune-Albright syndrome *(120)*. In this condition, the severity of fibrous dysplasia can range from subtle changes, only identifiable by bone scan, to fractures that produce skeletal deformity and significant disability. The clinical manifestations of MAS result from autonomous hyperactivity of tissues that produce products regulated by intracellular accumulation of cyclic adenosine monophosphate (cAMP). Activating mutations of the α-subunit of the stimulatory guanine nucleotide binding protein (Gs) result in constitutive overproduction of cAMP *(121)*. Isolated fibrous dysplasia is also due to mutations in Gsα *(122)*.

Usual treatment for fibrous dysplasia involves preventative orthopedic measures, such as curettage, internal fixation, and bone grafting. Calcitonin and mithramycin therapies have been ineffective. Treatment of the bony lesions of fibrous dysplasia with bisphosphonates has been attempted with promising results *(123)*.

Mucopolysaccharidoses

The mucopolysaccharidoses (MPSs) result from deficiencies of the lysosomal enzymes necessary for glycosaminoglycan (GAG) metabolism *(124)*. Their incidence is estimated to be 1:10,000 individuals. Clinical features reflect lysosomal accumulation of the partially degraded or undegraded complex carbohydrate GAGs. In patients with Hurler (MPS I), Hunter (MPS II), and Sanfilippo (MPS III) syndromes, this excess within marrow cells can lead to dysostosis multiplex, a skeletal change characterized by osteoporosis with coarse trabeculae, macrocephaly with a thickened calvarium and premature lambdoid and sagittal suture closure, a J-shaped sella-turcica, oar-shaped ribs, and widened clavicles *(125)*. The spine demonstrates oval or hook-shaped vertebral bodies with early lumbar kyphosis. These changes are associated with dysplasia of the capital femoral epiphyses, coxa valga, epiphysial and metaphyseal dysplasia, proximal tapering of the second and fifth metacarpals, and dysplasia of long tubular bones. Morquio syndrome (MPS IV) has some different skeletal changes, in particular, central beaking of the flattened vertebral bodies and short, deformed distal ulnae.

Fibrodysplasia Ossificans Progressiva

Fibrosis ossificans progressiva (FOP) is a rare (prevalence of 0.6/million live births), heritable, progressive, disabling disorder of extraskeletal calcification *(126–128)*. It is characterized by great toe malformations (often monophalangic) coupled with recurrent episodes of soft-tissue swelling (often linked to trauma) with consequent heterotopic ossification. Ossification begins at an average age of 5, with early sites at the neck, upper spine, and shoulder *(129,130)*. Children with FOP often have their lesions biopsied initially, in an attempt to exclude malignancy. The bone deposition proceeds in a predictable anatomic pattern: axial to appendicular, cranial to caudad, and proximal to distal. Eventually there is extra-articular bony ankylosis of nearly all joints, rendering movement impossible. Death occurs due to severe restrictive chest-wall disease.

The causal FOP mutation is likely connected in some way to the bone morphogenic protein (BMP) gene family, since Schafritz and colleagues have described selective BMP-4 overexpression in FOP *(131)*. BMP-4, a member of the transforming growth factor-β (TGF-β) superfamily, is a powerful osteogenic morphogen. Yet, the genetic defect in this condition remains unknown; linkage studies have not demonstrated a connection to the BMP-4 containing chromosome 14. Recent studies have shown linkage to two distinct potential genetic regions: 17q21-22, the region of the noggin (NOG) gene (noggin is known to bind and inactivate BMP-4) and 4q27-31, the region of SMAD-1 (a BMP-pathway specific gene involved in signal transduction) *(127,128)*.

CONCLUSIONS

Although this chapter has focused on those pediatric bone diseases with known genetic etiologies, there are many other bony disorders whose underlying etiology remains unknown. This includes disorders as diverse as Ellis-Van Creveld Syndrome and melorheostosis. By furthering our understanding of these disorders, we will enhance our knowledge of normal physiology.

The realm of pediatric bone biology is currently in a state of exponential growth in knowledge and understanding. This has been fueled in part by the increasing interest in preventing medical disorders of later life by recognizing risk factors for adult disease in children and instituting early, effective interventions. Adult osteoporosis has rapidly emerged as a public health problem with an enormous economic impact. It has been estimated that there are 1.5 million fractures annually in the United States, with a resultant health care cost of more than 10 billion dollars *(132)*. Inadequate prepeak bone mineralization is known to increase the risk of osteoporosis later in life. Keeping children's bones healthy is imperative, therefore, for economic as well as medical reasons.

REFERENCES

1. Holick M. The use and interpretation of assays for vitamin D and its metabolites. J Nutr 1990;120(S11): 1464–1469.
2. Neer RM, Arnaud CD, Zanchetta JR, Prince R, Gaich GA, Reginster JY, et al. Effect of parathyroid hormone (1-34) on fractures and bone mineral density in postmenopausal women with osteoporosis. N Engl J Med 2001;344(19):1434–1441.
3. Strewler GJ. The parathyroid hormone-related protein. Endocrinol Metab Clin North Am 2000;29(3): 629–645.
4. Weir EC, Philbrick WM, Amling M, Neff LA, Baron R, Broadus AE. Targeted overexpression of parathyroid hormone-related peptide in chondrocytes causes chondrodysplasia and delayed endochondral bone formation. Proc Natl Acad Sci USA 1996;93:10,240–10,245.
5. Massfelder T, Helwig JJ, Stewart AF. Parathyroid hormone-related protein as a cardiovascular regulatory peptide. Endocrinology 1996;1237:3151–3153.
6. Wysolmerski JJ, Philbrick WM, Dunbar ME, Lanske B, Kronenberg H, Karaplis A, et al. Rescue of the parathyroid hormone-related protein knockout mouse demonstrates that parathyroid hormone-related protein is essential for mammary gland development. Development 1998;125(7):1285–1294.

7. Holt EH, Broadus AE, Brines ML. Parathyroid hormone-related peptide is produced by cultured cere-bellar granule cells in response to L-type voltage-sensitive Ca^{2+} channel flux via a Ca2+/calmodulin-dependent kinase pathway. J Biol Chem 1996;271:28,105–28,111.

8. Pondel M. Calcitonin and calcitonin receptors: bone and beyond. Int J Exp Pathol 2000;81(6):405–422.

9. White KE, Jonnson KB, Carn G, Hampton G, Spector TD, Mannstadt M, et al. The autosomal dominant hypophosphatemic rickets (ADHR) gene is a secreted polypeptide overexpressed by tumors that cause phosphate wasting. J Clin Endocrinol Metab 2001;86(2):497–500.

10. Rifas L. Bones and cytokines: beyond IL-1, IL-6, and TNF-alpha. Calcif Tissue Int 1999;64(1):1–7.

11. Hofbauer LC, Heufelder AE. Osteoprotegerin: a novel local player in bone metabolism. Eur J Endo-crinol 1997;137(4):345–346.

12. Epstein DM, Dalinka MK, Kaplan FS, Arochick JM, Marinelli DL, Kundel HL. Observer variation in the detection of osteopenia. Skeletal Radiol 1986;1986(15):347–349.

13. Nelson DA, Koo WWK. Interpretation of absorptiometric bone mass measurements in the growing skeleton: issues and limitations. Calcif Tissue Int 1999;65(1):1–3.

14. Faulkner RA, Bailey DA, Drinkwater DT, McKay HA, Arnold C, Wilkinson AA. Bone densitometry in Canadian children 8-17 years of age. Calcif Tissue Int 1996;59:344–351.

15. Bailey DA, Faulkner RA, McKay HA. Bone mineral acquisition during the adolescent growth spurt. J Bone Min Res 1996;11:S465.

16. McKay HA, Bailey DA, Mirwald RL, Davison KS, Faulkner RA. Peak bone mineral accrual and age at menarche in adolescent girls: a 6-year longitudinal study. J Pediatr 1998;133(5):682–687.

17. Dyson K, Blimkie CJ, Davison KS, Webber CE, Adachi JD. Gymnastic training and bone density in pre-adolescent females. Med Sci Sports Exerc 1997;29(4):443–450.

18. Hans D, Fuerst T, Uffmann M. Bone density and quality measurement using ultrasound. Curr Opin Rheumatol 1996;8(4):370–375.

19. Gluer CC, Wu CY, Jergas M, Goldstein SA, Genant HK. Three quantitative ultrasound parameters reflect bone structure. Calcif Tissue Int 1994;55:46–52.

20. Harrison HE, Harrison HC. Rickets and osteomalacia. Disorders of calcium and phosphate metabolism in childhood and adolescence. WB Saunders Company, Philadelphia, PA, 1979, pp. 230–249.

21. Kreiter SR, Schwartz RP, Kirkman HN Jr, Charlton PA, Calikoglu AS, Davenport ML. Nutritional rickets in African American breast-fed infants. J Pediatr 2000;137(2):153–157.

22. Seino Y, Ishii T, Shimtsuji T, Ishida M, Yabuuchi H. Plasma active vitamin D concentrations in low birth-weight infants with rickets and its response to vitamin D treatment. Arch Dis Child 1981;56:628–632.

23. Steichen JJ, Tsang RC, Greer FR, Ho M, Hug G. Elevated serum 1,25 dihydroxy vitamin D concentra-tions in rickets of very low-birthweight infants. J Pediatr 1981;99:293–298.

24. Ryan S. Nutritional aspects of metabolic bone disease in the newborn. Arch Dis Childhood: Fetal Neo-natal Ed 1996;74(2):145F–148F.

25. Fraser D, Salter RB. The diagnosis and management of the various types of rickets. Pediatr Clin N Am 1958;5:417–441.

26. Wang JT, Lin C-J, Burridge SM, Fu GK, Labuda M, Portale AA, et al. Genetics of vitamin D 1-alpha-hydroxylase deficiency in 17 families. Am J Hum Genet 1998;63:1694–1702.

27. Delvin EE, Glorieux FH, Marie PJ, Pettifor JM. Vitamin D deficiency: replacement therapy with cal-citriol. J Pediatr 1981;99:26–34.

28. Brooks MH, Bell NH, Love L, Stern PH, Orfei E, Queener SF, et al. Vitamin-D-dependent rickets type II: resistance of target organs to 1,25-dihydroxyvitamin D. N Engl J Med 1978;298:996–999.

29. Hughes MR, Malloy PJ, Kieback DG, Kesterson RA, Pike JW, Feldman D, et al. Point mutations in the human vitamin D receptor gene associated with hypocalcemic rickets. Science 1988;242:1702–1705.

30. Hochberg Z, Tiosano D, Even L. Calcium therapy for calcitriol-resistant rickets. J Pediatr 1992;121(5):803–808.

31. Davies M, Stanbury SW. The rheumatic manifestations of metabolic bone disease. Clin Rheum Dis 1981;7:595–646.

32. Econs MJ, Drezner MK. Bone disease resulting from inherited disorders of renal tubule transport and vitamin D metabolism. In: Favus M, Coe F, eds. Disorders of Bone and Mineral Metabolism. Raven Press, Ltd, New York, 1992, pp. 935–950.

33. Tenenhouse HS, Econs MJ. Mendelian hypophosphatemias. In: Scriver C, Beudet A, Sly W, Valle D, eds. The Metabolic and Molecular Basis of Inherited Disease. McGraw-Hill, New York, 2000, pp. 5039–5068.

34. Econs MJ, Feussner JR, Samsa GP, Effman EL, Vogler JB, Martinez S, et al. X-linked hypophosphate-mic rickets without "rickets." Skeletal Radiol 1991;20:109–114.

35. HYP consortium. A gene (PEX) with homologies to endopeptidases is mutated in patients with X-linked hypophosphatemic rickets. Nat Genet 1995;11:130–136.
36. Winters RW, Graham JB, Williams TF, McFalls VW, Burnett CH. A genetic study of familial hypophosphatemia and vitamin D resistant rickets with a review of the literature. Medicine 1958;37:97–142.
37. Whyte MP, Schrank FW, Armamento-Villareal R. X-linked hypophosphatemia: a search for gender, race, anticipation, or parent of origin effects on disease expression in children. J Clin Endocrinol Metab 1996;81:4075–4080.
38. Bianchine JW, Stambler AA, Harrison H. Familial hypophosphatemic rickets showing autosomal dominant inheritance. Birth Defects: Original Article Series 1971;7:287–295.
39. Econs MJ, McEnery PT. Autosomal dominant hypophosphatemic rickets/osteomalacia: clinical characterization of a novel renal phosphate wasting disorder. J Clin Endocrinol Metab 1997;82:674–681.
40. Tieder M, Modai D, Samuel R, Arie R, Halabe A, Bab I, et al. Hereditary hypophosphatemic rickets with hypercalciuria. N Engl J Med 1985;312:611–617.
41. Tieder M, Modai D, Shaked U, Samuel R, Arie R, Halabe A, et al. "Idiopathic" hypercalciuria and a hereditary hypophosphatemic rickets. Two phenotypical expressions of a common genetic defect. N Engl J Med 1987;316:125–129.
42. Gazit D, Tieder M, Liberman UA, Passi-Even L, Bab IA. Osteomalacia in hereditary hypophosphatemic rickets with hypercalciuria: a correlative clinical-histomorphometric study. J Clin Endocrinol Metab 1991;72:229–235.
43. Tieder M, Arie R, Bab I, Maor J, Liberman UA. A new kindred with hereditary hypophosphatemic rickets with hypercalciuria: implications for correct diagnosis and treatment. Nephron 1992;62:176–181.
44. Proesmans WC, Fabry G, Marchal GJ, Gillis PL, Boullian R. Autosomal dominant hypophosphataemia with elevated serum 1,25 dihydroxyvitamin D and hypercalciuria. Pediatr Nephrol 1987;1:479–484.
45. Chong SS, Kozak CA, Liu L, Kristjansson K, Dunn ST, Bourdeau JE, et al. Cloning, genetic mapping, and expression analysis of a mouse renal sodium-dependent phosphate cotransporter. Am J Physiol 1995;268:F1038–F1045.
46. Kos CA, Tihy F, Econs MJ, Murer H, Lemieux N, Tenenhouse HS. Localization of a renal sodium-phos-phate cotransporter gene to human chromosome 5q35. Genomics 1994;19:176–177.
47. Rathbun J. Hypophosphatasia. Am J Dis Child 1948;75:822–831.
48. Fraser D. Hypophosphatasia. Am J Med 1957;22:730–746.
49. Garcia JV, Jones C, Miller AD. Localization of the amphotropic murine leukemia virus receptor gene to the pericentromeric region of human chromosome 8. J Virol 1991;65:6316–6139.
50. Weiss MJ, Cole DEC, Ray K, Whyte MP, Lafferty MA, Mulivor RA, et al. A missense mutation in the human liver/bone/kidney alkaline phosphatase gene causing a lethal form of hypophosphatasia. Proc Natl Acad Sci USA 1988;85:7666–7669.
51. Whyte MP. Hypophosphatasia. In: Favus MJ, ed. Primer on the Metabolic Bone Diseases and Disorders of Mineral Metabolism. Lippincott, Williams, & Wilkins, Philadelphia, PA, 1999, pp. 337–339.
52. Albright F, Reifenstein EC. The parathyroid glands and metabolic bone disease. William and Wilkins, Baltimore, MD, 1948.
53. Godang K, Ueland T, Bollerslev J. Decreased bone area, bone mineral content, formative markers, and increased bone resorptive markers in endogenous Cushing's syndrome. Eur J Endocrinol 1999;141(2):126–131.
54. Diamond T, Vine J, Smart R, Butler P. Thyrotoxic bone disease in women: a potentially reversible disorder. Ann Intern Med 1994;120:8–11.
55. Wüster C, Abs R, Bengtsson B, Bennmarker H, Feldt-Rasmussen U, Hernberg-Ståhl E, et al. The influence of growth hormone deficiency, growth hormone replacement therapy, and other aspects of hypopituitarism on fracture rate and bone mineral density. J Bone Min Res 2001;16(2):398–405.
56. Hillman L, Cassidy JT, Johnson L, Lee D, Allen SH. Vitamin D metabolism and bone mineralization in children with juvenile rheumatoid arthritis. J Pediatr 1994;124:910–916.
57. Lettgen B, Jeken C, Reiners C. Influence of steroid medication on bone mineral density in children with nephrotic syndrome. Pediatric Nephrol 1994;8:667–670.
58. Issenman RM, Atkinson SA, Rodja C, Fraher L. Longitudinal assessment of growth, mineral metabolism, and bone mass in pediatric Crohn's disease. J Pediatr Gastroenterol Nutr 1994;17:401–406.
59. Bachrach LK, Loutit CW, Moss RB, Marcus R. Osteopenia in adults with cystic fibrosis. Am J Med 1994;96:27–34.
60. Stallings VA. Calcium and bone health in children: a review. Am J Therapeut 1997;4(7-8):259–273.
61. Hergenroeder AC. Bone mineralization, hypothalamic amenorrhea, and sex steroid therapy in female adolescents and young adults. J Pediatr 1995;126(5):683–689.

62. Paterson CR. Osteogenesis imperfecta and other heritable disorders of bone. Balliere's Clin Endocrinol Metab 1997;11(1):195–213.

63. Sillence DO, Senn A, Danks DM. Genetic heterogeneity in osteogenesis imperfecta. J Med Genet 1979;16(2):101–116.

64. Glorieux FH, Bishop NJ, Travers R, Roughley P, Chabot G, Lanoue G, et al. Type V osteogenesis imperfecta (abstract). J Bone Min Res 1997;12(1):S389.

65. Byers PH. Osteogenesis Imperfecta. In: Royce PM, Steinmann BU, eds. Connective Tissue and its Heritable Disorders: Molecular, Genetic, and Medical Aspects. Wyley-Liss, New York, 1993, pp. 317–350.

66. Prockop DJ, Colige A, Helminen H, Khillan JS, Pereira R, Vandenberg P. Mutations in type 1 procollagen that cause osteogenesis imperfecta: effects of the mutations on the assembly of collagen into fibrils, the basis of phenotypic variations, and potential antisense therapies. J Bone Min Res 1993; 8(Suppl) 2:489–492.

67. Minch CM, Kruse RW. Osteogenesis imperfecta: a review of basic science and diagnosis. Orthopedics 1998;21(5):558–567.

68. Barsh GS, David KE, Byers PH. Type I osteogenesis imperfecta: a nonfunctional allele for pro alpha 1 (I) chains of type I procollagen. Proc Natl Acad Sci USA 1982;79(12):3838–3842.

69. Pope F, Nicholls AC, McPheat J, Talmud P, Owen R. Collagen genes and proteins in osteogenesis imperfecta. J Med Genet 1985;22:466–478.

70. Shields ED, Bixler D, El-Kafrawy AM. A proposed classification for heritable human dentine defect with a description of a new entity. Arch Oral Biol 1973;18:543–553.

71. Lukinmaa PL, Ranta H, Ranta K, Kaitila I. Dental findings in osteogenesis imperfecta: I. Occurrence and expression of type I dentinogenesis imperfecta. J Craniofacial Genet Dev Biol 1987;7:115–125.

72. Hartsfield JK Jr. Summary of dental concerns and care for persons with dentinogenesis imperfecta and osteogenesis imperfecta. "Breakthrough," The National Newsletter of the Osteogenesis Imperfecta Foundation, Inc, 1992, pp. 4–5.

73. Pedersen U. Hearing loss in patients with osteogenesis imperfecta. Scand Audiol 1984;13:67–74.

74. Marini JC, Bordenick S, Heavner G, Rose S, Chrousos GP. Evaluation of growth hormone axis and responsiveness to growth stimulation of short children with osteogenesis imperfecta. Am J Med Genet 1993;45(2):261–264.

75. Cropp GJ, Myers DN. Physiological evidence of hypermetabolism in osteogenesis imperfecta. Pediatrics 1972;49(3):375–391.

76. Smith R. Idiopathic juvenile osteoporosis. Am J Dis Child 1979;133:894–900.

77. Krassas GE. Idiopathic juvenile osteoporosis. Ann NY Acad Sci 2000;900:409–412.

78. Marder HK, Tsang RC, Hug G, Crawford AC. Calcitriol deficiency in idiopathic juvenile osteoporosis. Am J Dis Child 1982;136:914–917.

79. Azria M, Copp DH, Zanelli JM. 25 years of salmon calcitonin: from synthesis to therapeutic use. Calcif Tissue Int 1995;57:405–408.

80. Rodan GA. Mechanisms of action of bisphosphonates. Ann Rev Pharmacol Toxicol 1998;38:375–388.

81. Allgrove J. Bisphosphonates. Arch Dis Childhood 1997;76:73–75.

82. Rizzoli R, Fleisch H, Bonjour JP. Role of 1,25-dihydroxyvitamin D_3 on intestinal phosphate absorption in rats with a normal vitamin D supply. J Clin Invest 1977;60:639.

83. Vitte C, Fleisch H, Guenther H. Bisphosphonates induce osteoblasts to secrete an inhibitor of osteoclast-mediated resorption. Endocrinology 1996;137:2324–2333.

84. Albers-Schonberg HE. Projektions: Rontgenbilder einter seltenen Knochenerkrankung. Fortschr Geb Rontgenstrahlen 1903;7:158–159.

85. Stevenson AC. The load of hereditary defects in human populations. Radiat Res 1959;1:306.

86. Bollerslev J. Osteopetrosis. A genetic and epidemiological study. Clin Genet 1987;31:86–90.

87. Frattini A, Orchard PJ, Sobacchi C, Giliani S, Abinun M, Mattsson JP, et al. Defects in TCIRG1 subunit of the vacuolar proton pump are responsible for a subset of human autosomal recessive osteopetrosis. Nat Genet 2000;25:343–346.

88. Kornak U, Kasper D, Bosl MR, Kaiser E, Schweizer M, Schulz A, et al. Loss of the ClC-7 chloride channel leads to osteopetrosis in mice and man. Cell 2001;104:205–215.

89. Bollerslev J, Andersen PE Jr. Radiological, biochemical and hereditary evidence of two types of autosomal dominant osteopetrosis. Bone 1988;9(1):7–13.

90. Bollerslev J, Andersen PE Jr. Fracture patterns in two types of autosomal-dominant osteopetrosis. Acta Orthop Scand 1989;60(1):110–112.

91. Van Hul W, Bollerslev J, Gram J, Van Hul E, Wuyts W, Benichou O, et al. Localization of a gene for autosomal dominant osteopetrosis (Albers-Schonberg disease) to chromosome 1p21. Am J Human Genet 1997;61(2):363–369.

92. White KE, Koller DL, Takacs I, Buckwalter KA, Foroud T, Econs MJ. Locus heterogeneity of autosomal dominant osteopetrosis (ADO). J Clin Endocrinol Metab 1999;84(3):1047–1051.

93. Sly WS, Whyte MP, Sundaram V, Tashian RE, Hewett-Emmett D, Guibaud P, et al. Carbonic anhydrase II deficiency in 12 families with the autosomal recessive syndrome of osteopetrosis with renal tubular acidosis and cerebral calcification. N Engl J Med 1985;313:139–145.

94. Maroteaux P, Lamy M. La pycnodysostose. Presse Med 1962;70:999–1002.

95. Andren L, Dymling JF, Hogeman KE, Wendeberg B. Osteopetrosis acro-osteolytica: a syndrome of osteopetrosis, acro-osteolysis and open sutures of the skull. Acta Chir Scand 1962;124:496–507.

96. Gelb BD, Shi GP, Chapman HA, Desnick RJ. Pycnodysostosis, a lysosomal disease caused by cathepsin K deficiency. Science 1996;273:1236–1238.

97. Martinez-Frias ML, Cereijo A, Bermejo E, Lopez M, Sanchez M, Gonzalo C. Epidemiological aspects of mendelian syndromes in a Spanish population sample: I. Autosomal dominant malformation syndromes. Am J Med Genet 1991;38:622–625.

98. Spranger J. Bone dysplasia 'families'. Pathol Immunopathol Res 1988;7(1-2):76–80.

99. Tavormina PL, Bellus GA, Webster MK, Bamshad MJ, Fraley AE, McIntosh I, et al. A novel skeletal dysplasia with developmental delay and acanthosis nigricans is caused by a Lys650Met mutation in the fibroblast growth factor receptor 3 gene. Am J Hum Genet 1999;64(3):722–731.

100. Shiang R, Thompson LM, Zhu Y-Z, Church DM, Fielder TJ, Mocian M, et al. Mutations in the transmembrane domain of FGFR3 cause the most common genetic form of dwarfism, achondroplasia. Cell 1994;78:335–342.

101. Bellus GA, McIntosh I, Smith EAAAS, Kaitila I, Horton WA. A recurrent mutation in the tyrosine kinase domain of fibroblast growth factor 3 causes hypochondroplasia. Nat Genet 1995;10:357–359.

102. Rousseau F, Bonaventure J, Legeai-Mallet L, Pelet A, Rozet J-M, Maroteaux P, et al. Mutations in the gene encoding fibroblast growth factor receptor-3 in achondroplasia. Nature 1994;371:252–254.

103. Nelson FW, Hecht JT, Horton WA, Butler IJ, Goldie WD, Miner M. Neurological basis of respiratory complications in achondroplasia. Ann Neurol 1988;24:89–93.

104. Hecht JT, Francomano CA, Horton WA, Annegers JF. Mortality in achondroplasia. Am J Hum Genet 1987;41:454–464.

105. Hunter AG, Hecht JT, Scott CI Jr. Standard weight for height curves in achondroplasia. Am J Med Genet 1996;62(3):255–261.

106. Lemyre E, Azouz EM, Teebi AS, Glanc P, Chen MF. Bone dysplasia series. Achondroplasia, hypochondroplasia and thanatophoric dysplasia: review and update. Can Assoc Radiol J 1999;50(3):185–197.

107. Arnott C, Hammond L. Deciding about leg-lengthening. Bull Med Ethics 1993;92:34–36.

108. Patel MD, Filly RA. Homozygous achondroplasia: US distinction between homozygous, heterozygous, and unaffected fetuses in the second trimester. Radiology 1995;196(2):541–545.

109. Lachman RS. Skeletal dysplasias. In: Taybi H, Lachman R, eds. Radiology of Syndromes, Metabolic Disorders, and Skeletal Dysplasias. Mosby, St. Louis, MO, 1996, pp. 745–951.

110. Rousseau F, El Ghouzzi V, Delezoide A, Legeai-Mallet L, Le Merrer M, Munnich A, et al. Missense FGFR3 mutations create cysteine residues in thanatophoric dwarfism type I. Human Molecular Genetics 1996;5:509–512.

111. Beighton P, de Paepe A, Danks D, Finidori G, Gedde-Dahl T, Goodman R, et al. International Nosology of Heritable Disorders of Connective Tissue, Berlin, 1986. Am J Med Genet 1988;29(3):581–594.

112. Hecht JT, Nelson LD, Crowder E, Wang Y, Elder FFB, Harrison WR, et al. Mutations in exon 17B of cartilage oligomeric matrix protein (COMP) cause pseudoachondroplasia. Nat Genet 1995;10:325–329.

113. Briggs MD, Hoffman SMG, King LM, Olsen AS, Mohrenweiser H, Leroy JG, et al. Pseudoachondroplasia and multiple epiphyseal dysplasia due to mutations in the cartilage oligomeric matrix protein gene. Nat Genet 1995;10:330–336.

114. Stevens JW. Pseudoachondroplastic dysplasia: an Iowa review from human to mouse. Iowa Orthop J 1999;19:53.

115. Briggs MD, Mortier GR, Cole WG, King LM, Golik SS, Bonaventure J, et al. Diverse mutations in the gene for cartilage oligomeric matrix protein in a pseudoachondroplasia-multiple epiphyseal dysplasia disease spectrum. Am J Hum Genet 1998;62:311–319.

116. Van Mourik JB, Hamel BC, Mariman EC. A large family with multiple epiphyseal dysplasia linked to COL9A2 gene. Am J Med Genet 1998;77:234–240.

117. Schipani E, Langman CB, Parfitt AM, Jensen GS, Kikuchi S, Kooh SW, et al. Constitutively activated receptors for parathyroid hormone and parathyroid hormone-related peptide in Jansen's metaphyseal chondrodysplasia. N Engl J Med 1996;335:708–714.
118. Coley BL. Neoplasms of Bone and Related Conditions. 2nd ed. Paul Hocher Inc., New York, 1960.
119. Collins M, Shenker A. McCune-Albright Syndrome: New Insights. Curr Opin Endocrinol Diabetes 1999;6:119–125.
120. Albright F, Butler AM, Hamstra AJ, Smith R. Syndrome characterized by osteitis fibrosis disseminata, areas of pigmentation and endocrine dysfunction, with precocious puberty in females. N Engl J Med 1937;216:727–746.
121. Weinstein LS, Shenker A, Gejman PV, Merino MJ, Freidman E, Spiegel MA. Activating mutations of the stimulatory G protein in the McCune-Albright syndrome. N Engl J Med 1991;325:1688–1695.
122. Bianco P, Riminucci M, Majolagbe A, Kuznetsov SA, Collins MT, Mankani MH, et al. Mutations of the GNAS1 gene, stromal cell dysfunction, and osteomalacic changes in non-McCune-Albright fibrous dysplasia of bone. J Bone Min Res 2000;15:120–128.
123. Chapurlat RD, Delmas PD, Liens D, Meunier PJ. Long-term effects of intravenous pamidronate in fibrous dysplasia of bone. J Bone Min Res 1997;12(10):1746–1752.
124. Hopwood JJ, Morris CP. The mucopolysaccharidoses. Diagnosis, molecular genetics and treatment. Mol Biol Med 1990;7(5):381–404.
125. Chen SJ, Li YW, Wang TR, Hsu JCY. Bony changes in common mucopolysaccharidoses. Acta Paed Sin 1996;37(3):178–184.
126. Connor JM, Evans DAP. Genetic aspects of fibrodysplasia ossificans progressiva. J Med Genet 1982; 19:35–39.
127. Feldman G, Li M, Martin S, Urbanek M, Urtizberea A, Fardeau M, et al. Fibrodysplasia ossificans progressiva, a heritable disorder of severe heterotopic ossification, maps to human chromosome 4q27-31. Am J Hum Genet 2000;66:128–135.
128. Lucotte G, Bathelier C, Mercier G, Gerard N, Lenoir G, Semonin O, et al. Localization of the gene for fibrodysplasia ossificans progressiva (FOP) to chromosome 17q21-22. Genet Counsel 2000;11(4): 329–334.
129. Connor JM, Evans DAP. Fibrodysplasia ossificans progressiva: the clinical features and natural history of 34 patients. J Bone Joint Surg 1982;64:76–83.
130. Smith R, Athanasou NA, Vipond SE. Fibrodysplasia (myositis) ossificans progressiva: clinicopathological features and natural history. Q J Med 1996;89:445–456.
131. Shafritz AB, Shore EM, Gannon FH, Zasloff MA, Taub R, Muenke M, et al. Overexpression of an osteogenic morphogen in fibrodysplasia ossificans progressiva. N Engl J Med 1996;335:555–561.
132. NIH Consensus Development Panel on Optimal Calcium Intake. Optimal calcium intake. J Am Med Assoc 1994;272:1942–1948.

V GONADAL DEVELOPMENT

11

Transcriptional Development of the Hypothalamic-Pituitary-Gonadal Axis

Sally Radovick, MD, Helen H. Kim, MD, Diane E. J. Stafford, MD, Andrew Wolfe, PhD, and Marjorie Zakaria, MD

CONTENTS

THE HYPOTHALAMUS

GnRH Neuronal Migration and Anatomy

Unlike other hypothalamic neuropeptide-producing cells, GnRH neurons do not arise from the developing basal forebrain. They originate in the olfactory placode in mammals and migrate across the nasal cavity and cribiform plate into the forebrain *(1,2)*. In mice, for example, the GnRH neurons are derived from the neural ectoderm, are born on d 10.5 postcoitus (pc), and begin to express GnRH mRNA and protein between d 10.75 and 11.5 pc. GnRH neurons then migrate across the olfactory cavity to the forebrain between d 12.5 pc and d 16.5 pc *(2,3)*. GnRH neurons migrating across the nasal cavity appear to be guided, in part, by the polysialic acid-rich form of the neural cell adhesion molecule (PSA-NCAM) *(4)* in association with the vomeronasal nerves (VNN). Recent evidence in studies of chick forebrain development has further implicated PSA-NCAM as an important component in GnRH neuronal migration *(5)*. Other investigators have posited that factors such as gamma aminobutyric acid (GABA) *(6,7)*, adhesion-related kinase *(8)*, or peripherin *(9)* might play a role in the guidance of the GnRH neurons. The initial migration to the forebrain follows the vomeronasal and terminal nerves. However, after entering the rostral forebrain, GnRH neurons become disassociated from the caudal branch of the VNN. Therefore, it is unclear what guides them during the remaining portion of their migration to the basal hypothalamus. At this time, it is felt that GnRH neurons are no longer guided by a defined anatomical structure *(10)*. Instead, neuronal migration may trail behind

From: *Contemporary Endocrinology: Developmental Endocrinology: From Research to Clinical Practice*
Edited by: E. A. Eugster and O. H. Pescovitz © Humana Press Inc., Totowa, NJ

as axonal migration to the median eminence and organum vasculosum of the lamina terminalis (OVLT) is occurring. Axonal migration is directed by chemoattractive signals from the medial basal hypothalamus *(11)*. Additional factors that regulate forebrain development, such as Pax-6 *(12)*, Otx-1 and 2 *(13–15)* may also play specific roles in directing GnRH neuronal migration, but further study is needed to identify their mechanism of action.

The lack of migration of GnRH neurons into the forebrain can result in reproductive dysfunction. For example, some cases of hypogonadotropic hypogonadism are due to a deletion of an X-linked gene referred to as Kalig *(16–18)*. This disorder, Kallmann's Syndrome, results in a lack of proper neuronal migration in humans. The Kalig locus contains four fibronectin type III repeats *(19,20)*, a motif associated with adhesion molecules *(21)*. Forms of idiopathic hypogonadotropic hypogonadism not associated with Kallmann's syndrome have been described in humans, but the mechanisms of dysregulation of the GnRH neurons remain unknown *(22,23)*. Certainly, a lack of developmental progression of GnRH neurons due to the absence of proteins important for migration may result in some of these cases of idiopathic hypogonadotropic hypogonadism.

A mouse model exists for a non-Kallmann's-like associated hypogonadotropic hypogonadism. The hpg mouse was identified as reproductively dysfunctional, and contained a large genetic deletion that included much of the GnRH gene *(24)*. Neurons expressing the truncated form of the GnRH gene are still present in the usual locations in the forebrain indicating that migration of the neurons is unaffected by the absence of the GnRH decapeptide in these animals *(25)*. Transplantation of hypothalamic grafts *(26)*, or GnRH-expressing cell lines *(27,28)* into the hypothalami of the hpg mice rescued the phenotypic hypogonadism. This further underscores the central importance of the GnRH neurons as the primary regulators of pituitary gonadotropin secretion.

It should be stressed that it is unclear whether GnRH neurons are merely passively responding to signals in their immediate milieu, or whether local signals trigger changes in gene expression in GnRH neurons that are ultimately responsible for migration, and for changes in cellular morphology or GnRH gene expression. Several studies have shown that there may be important differences in the proteins produced at each developmental stage, for example, that there are as-yet-unidentified receptors or adhesion molecules produced in GnRH neurons between 12.5 and 16.5 d pc that are essential for their migration. There is evidence for this arrangement in another system, the developmental organization of the cerebellum. Normally granule cells migrate along radial glia to their correct location in the cerebellum. In the mutant weaver mouse, the granule cells fail to migrate to their final location in the cerebellum *(29,30)*. Studies in chimeric mice have suggested that the defect in the weaver mouse is intrinsic to the migrating granule cell *(31)*. Evidence for these types of changes during development in GnRH neurons comes from studies looking at differences in gene expression in GN10 vs GT1 GnRH expressing cells *(8,32)*. The former is derived from an olfactory tumor (migratory GnRH neurons), and the latter from an hypothalamic tumor (postmigratory GnRH neurons). These studies identified more than 10 factors differentially expressed in the two cell lines including adhesion related kinase (Ark), an anti-apoptotic factor found in GN10 cells but not GT1 cells *(32)*. Additional evidence comes from a biochemical analysis of GnRH neurons during development showing that the growth and plasticity associated peptide, GAP43, was expressed at much higher levels in neurons within the nasal septum than in neurons that have already migrated into the forebrain *(10)*. Taken together, these studies indicate that there are additional differentiation events that occur following the onset of GnRH gene expression at day 10.75 pc.

In the adult mouse, the vast majority of GnRH containing neurons are located in the hypothalamus at the level of the organum vasculosum of the lamina terminalis (OVLT) and the pre-optic area (POA), but some GnRH neurons have also been localized in the cerebral cortex and the limbic system *(1,33,34)*. In addition, GnRH neurons are scattered within the olfactory bulbs. Therefore, it appears as if GnRH neurons are strewn along the migratory pathway to the basal hypothalamus. It is not clear what signals are responsible for the organization of the microarchitecture of the mammalian GnRH neurons in the basal forebrain, although there is some evidence that there are important functional groupings within the scattered GnRH neurons. For example there are quiescent subpopulations of GnRH neurons activated during various physiological events, such as during the pre-ovulatory surge in female mammals *(35,36)*, that have a specific anatomical arrangement.

Subpopulations of GnRH Neurons

In the hypothalamus, during a variety of physiologic stimuli, GnRH neurons have been shown to be "recruited" into increasing their expression of GnRH *(35–39)*. For example, during the preovulatory GnRH surge in rats, it appears that a normally quiescent population of GnRH neurons is activated *(35,36)*. Although these differences in GnRH neuronal activation may be a result of variations in the afferent inputs to each population of GnRH neurons, the pattern of release of GnRH from the median eminence during the GnRH surge is radically different from that seen during nonsurge periods *(40,41)*, and may reflect profound differences in the physiology of the surge generating, and the nonsurge generating populations of GnRH neurons. The intracellular events required for activation of GnRH neurons during the surge are unknown.

Another instance where GnRH neurons are recruited to produce higher levels of GnRH gene expression is during the period preceding the onset of puberty in the mouse *(39,42)*, and rat *(38)*, perhaps to prepare the neurons for the increased levels of GnRH secretion that occurs during puberty. Increases in GnRH gene expression after the onset of puberty when compared with prepubertal animals have been observed in the hamster *(43)*. Again, it is not clear what factors (neurotransmitters, growth factors, second messengers or transcription factors) are involved in these puberty-related changes in GnRH gene expression, although there is some evidence that the amino acid family of neurotransmitters (GABA *[44,45]* or N-methyl-D-aspartate [NMDA] *[44,46,47]*) may play a role in regulating the initiation of puberty.

The GnRH Gene

The GnRH neurons are particularly difficult to study due both to their low abundance in the brain (about 800 neurons in the mouse *[2]*), and to their diffuse and widely scattered distribution. Despite these obstacles the GnRH gene has been cloned in a number of species *(48–51)*, and has been found to be about 4Kb in length and to contain four exons. The first exon consists of the 5' untranslated region, the second exon encodes the signal sequence of GnRH, the GnRH decapeptide, and the first 11 amino acids of GnRH-associated peptide (GAP), and the last two exons encode the remaining amino acids of GAP as well as the 3' untranslated region. No clear function has been described for GAP, but interestingly, the infertile hpg mouse contains a large deletion of the GnRH gene that, while not including the coding region for the GnRH decapeptide, includes part of the coding region for GAP *(24)*. This suggests that GAP may play a role in GnRH post-translational processing and transport. Low levels of GnRH immunoreactivity have also been localized in the placenta, the gonads, and the mammary glands *(52)*. Interestingly, placental GnRH transcription is initiated from a different promoter initiation site than that used for transcription of hypothalamic GnRH mRNA *(53)*. In addition, the hypothalamic and placental GnRH genes undergo differential RNA splicing, with the first intron being retained in the placental mRNA and removed in the hypothalamic mRNA *(48,53)*. It is unclear what the significance is of the extrahypothalamic expression of GnRH. In the mouse hypothalamus, studies have shown that two differential splicing events can occur. One form of mRNA contains all four exons while the other does not contain the second exon, which encodes the GnRH decapeptide *(54)*. The former splice variant is the dominant form in GN11 cells that are thought to possess a more migratory phenotype *(54)*. Mature GnRH neurons (NLT cells and adult mouse hypothalamus) express mainly GnRH mRNA with all four exons. The factors responsible for this differential splicing are unknown, but clearly a better understanding of the transcription factors that regulate these different splicing events will advance our understanding of both the cell-specific expression and the regulated expression of the hGnRH gene. Surprisingly, despite the efforts of a number of investigators, no mutation of the GnRH gene has been identified in humans.

GnRH Expressing Neuronal Cell Lines

As a means of developing an in vitro model for the study of GnRH neuronal-cell activity, immortalized GnRH-expressing neuronal cell lines have been created by targeted tumorigenesis *(55,56)*. Radovick et al. *(56)* targeted the expression of the simian virus 40 T antigen (SV40-Tag) to the GnRH neurons with 1131 bps of the human GnRH gene 5'-upstream regulatory sequence. One of these transgenic mice developed an olfactory tumor *(56)* from which several GnRH immunoreactive cell lines (NLT, GN10, GN11) were subsequently derived. Both cell lines are able to synthesize and secrete GnRH. However, NLT cells secrete about 10-fold higher levels of GnRH than GN11 cells *(54)*.

Mellon et al. *(55)* developed the GT1 cell lines which were harvested from an hypothalamic tumor and may represent a more mature GnRH neuronal cell line. Indeed, one group has used a polymerase chain reaction (PCR)-based differential-display system to identify genes expressed differentially in olfactory bulb-derived GN11 cells and hypothalamus-derived GT1 cells *(8,32)*. These genes have been hypothesized to produce proteins important for the regulation of migration and for preventing apoptosis. The primary GT-1 cell lines studied have been the GT1-1, GT1-3, and GT1-7 cell lines *(55)*. These cell lines, like the cell lines obtained by Radovick et al. from the olfactory tumor *(56)*, possess significant physiological, electrophysiological, morphological, and molecular differences from each other *(55,57–61)*.

These cell lines have been invaluable for examining intracellular and extracellular regulators of GnRH gene expression. A number of different factors have been shown to regulate GnRH synthesis, including extracellular mediators such as growth factors *(62)*, as well as the steroid hormones including estradiol *(17,63,64)* and glucocorticoids *(65)*.

One method of isolating transcription factors that regulate GnRH gene expression is to identify differentially expressed genes in high GnRH-expressing cell lines (such as the NLT cell line) vs low GnRH-expressing cell lines (such as the GN11 cell line) in these two cell lines that may contribute to their differences in phenotype *(54)*. Wolfe et al. have shown that Brn-2 mRNA is present in NLT cells, but not in GN11 cells *(66)* and may play a role in regulating GnRH gene expression. In addition, Stafford et al. have identified a novel factor, NLT expression factor-1 (NLT-EF1) that is more highly expressed in NLT cells than GN11 cells *(67)*.

Promoter elements of the GnRH gene important for cell-specific expression, or to mediate regulation by various second-messenger pathways are poorly understood at this time. There is some evidence that the Oct-1 POU homeodomain protein may play a role in regulating the rat, mouse, and human GnRH genes *(65)*. Work from the Radovick laboratory has provided evidence that both the POU homeodomain transcription factor Brn-2 *(66)*, and the AP1 complex *(68)* can regulate hGnRH gene expression. A number of other transcription factors, and second-messenger pathways have been implicated in the regulation of the GnRH gene including SCIP *(70)*, Ras/Raf-1 *(62)*, GATA 4 *(70)*, protein kinase C (PKC) *(68,71–73)* and nitric oxide/cGMP *(74)*. These studies, demonstrating the presence of developmental transcription factors in GnRH neurons, have invited speculation that other unidentified factors may be required in the development and migration of GnRH neurons.

THE PITUITARY GONADOTROPES

Transcriptional Development of the Pituitary Gland

The anterior pituitary gland contains six phenotypically distinct cell types. These hormone-secreting cells include gonadotropes that secrete luteinizing hormone (LH) and follicle-stimulating hormone (FSH); thyrotropes that secrete TSH; somatolactotrophs that secrete GH and prolactin; corticotropes that secrete ACTH; and melanotropes that secrete MSH. These pituitary-specific cell lineages develop from a common primordium known as Rathke's pouch. Rathke's pouch forms by invagination of the midline oral ectoderm to form a pouch rudiment that, as a second step, will develop into the definitive pouch. Rathke's pouch makes direct cell-cell contact with the overlying neural ectoderm of the ventral diencephalon that will evaginate from the posterior pituitary gland. Sequential induction signals from the adjacent diencephalon are required to induce Rathke's pouch formation *(75)*. These signals include brain morphogenic protein 4 (BMP4) and fibroblast growth factor 8 (FGF8). BMP4 is required for the formation of the pouch rudiment very early in embryonic development (e8.5) and thus for the initial phase of organ commitment. FGF8 is necessary for activation of the LHX3 (LIM homeobox 3) gene and development of the definitive Rathke's pouch that closes at e10.5 *(75)*. BMP2 signaling from the adjacent mesenchymal cells ventral to Rathke's pouch is involved in positional determination of pituitary cell types *(76)*.

Positional determination of the different pituitary-cell lineages occurs between e10.5 and e12.5 d, and is followed by terminal differentiation of these cell types by e17.5. Early in pituitary organogenesis, cell types are positionally determined in a spatially restricted pattern according to signaling gradients in Rathke's pouch. An opposing ventral-dorsal BMP2 and dorsal-ventral FGF8 gradient serves to determine the fate of precursors cells to form the ventral/medial cell phenotypes including gonadotrophs, thyrotrophs, and somatolactotrophs, and dorsal-cell phenotypes including corticotrophs and melanotrophs *(76)*. The gonadotropes are the most ventrally located cells in the developing pituitary, followed spatially by thyrotrophs. The ventral BMP2 signal selectively induces transcription of GATA2 in the most ventral cells of the developing pituitary gland. These cells are the presumptive precursors of the gonadotrope-cell lineage. Spatial restriction is later lost as the different cell populations are dispersed in the adult pituitary gland.

GATA2 Induction of the Gonadotrope Cell Lineage

GATA2 is a zinc-finger protein that is expressed ventrally in the Rathkes' pouch throughout early pituitary development. In the adult pituitary, expression of GATA2 is colocalized to gonadotropes and thyrotropes, the two most ventrally arising pituitary-cell types. Transgenic mice overexpressing BMP2 under the control of the alpha-GSU promoter (alpha-GSU/BMp2 mice) demonstrate an increased transcriptional induction and dorsal expansion of GATA2 in the pituitary (77). Dorsal expansion is observed as the alpha-GSU promoter targets expression of the transgene to Rathke's pouch and later to gonadotropes and thyrotropes. Other ventrally expressed genes are not induced in the alpha-GSU/BMP2 transgene. On the other hand, overexpression of Shh, another ventrally expressed gene, under the control of alpha-GSU does not affect the amount or spatial distribution of GATA2 expression in the pituitary. These results are consistent with the hypothesis that ventrally expressed BMP2 is responsible for induction of GATA2 expression in the pituitary gland. The highest level of GATA2 expression is localized to the most ventral pituitary cells that are the presumptive gonadotrope precursors.

GATA2 in turn seems to play an important role in induction of the gonadotrope lineage during pituitary development. Studies from transgenic mice with targeted expression of GATA2 to the pituitary under the control of the pit-1 promoter (pit-1/GATA2 mice) indicate loss of the pit-1 dependent cell lineages (thyrotropes and somatolactotrophs) along with dorsal expansion of the gonadotrope-cell lineage expressing alpha-GSU and LH-beta (77). Early activation of GATA2 expression in the dorsal cell-type precursors seems sufficient to induce a gonadotrope fate in these cells as the targeting of GATA2 dorsally inhibits early pit-1 expression. In addition, these mice show evidence of dorsal expansion of transcription factors that are normally expressed ventrally including Isl1 (a ventral lineage marker), and SF-1 (a gonadotrope-specific lineage marker). These results indicate an epistatic relationship of GATA2 and other ventral markers. Examination of the pituitary cells in adult mice indicate that >90% of the cells were gonadotropes, and that all GATA2-expressing cells derived from the transgene coexpressed alpha-GSU (77).

There was no effect on pituitary-cell phenotypes in mice overexpressing Isl1 under the control of the same pit1 promoter indicating that the effect of GATA2 in determining the fate of the gonadotrope precursors is specific (77). This is further confirmed by studies of transgenic mice expressing a dominant negative mutant of GATA2 under the control of the alpha-GSU promoter (77). These mice fail to develop gonadotropes and thyrotropes. Examination of the pituitary gland in these mice indicates an absence of gonadotrope specific markers including LH-beta and SF-1, and a marked reduction in expression of alpha-GSU and the thyrotrope-specific marker TSH-beta.

In summary, there is evidence that BMP2 induces ventral expression of GATA2, and that GATA2 expression is required for the commitment of pituitary cell-type precursors to the gonadotrope lineage.

LIM Homeobox Gene 3 and 4 (lhx3 and lhx4)

Lhx3 is expressed in the pituitary gland throughout development and is important for organ commitment of the Rathke's pouch to become a pituitary gland, and for differentiation and proliferation of pituitary-cell lineages. Lhx3 expression is regulated by FGF8 arising from the ventral diencephalon, and later by BMP2 from the mesenchymal cells ventral to Rathke's pouch. Mice that are homozygous for the lhx3 null mutation (lhx3−/ lhx3−) exhibit a Rathke's pouch rudiment that failed to grow and differentiate with lack of pituitary-specific cell lineages *(78)*. *In situ* hybridization and immunocytochemistry analysis of the Rathke's pouch rudiment of these mice failed to detect transcripts for the alpha-glycoprotein sub-unit (alpha-GSU), thyroid-stimulating hormone beta sub-unit (TSH-beta), growth hormone, and pit-1. LH-positive cells were undetectable by immuno-staining of the pouch rudiment at e18.5. Thus, four anterior pituitary-cell lineages including gonadotrophs were specifically missing in the lhx3−/lhx3− mice. These results suggest that lhx3 is important for determination of cell-type commitment in the developing pituitary.

While lhx3 seems to be important for cell-type differentiation, lhx4 seems to be impor-tant for the proliferation of the differentiated cells. Transgenic mice homozygous for the lhx4 null mutation (lhx4−/lhx4−) exhibit a distinctly hypoplastic anterior pituitary lobe and a reduced number of all five cell lineages including GnRHR+ and LH+ gonadotrope pre-cursors *(79)*. In summary, these results indicate that lhx3 plays an important role in con-trolling pituitary organ and cell-fate commitment, and that lhx4 is required for proliferation of five of the anterior pituitary cell lineage precursors including gonadotropes.

Pituitary Homeobox 1 (Ptx1)

Ptx1 is the earliest in the cascade of transcription factors that are involved in pituitary organogenesis. It is expressed early on in the stomodeum even before the development of Rathke's pouch. Its expression continues throughout pituitary development and orga-nogenesis. In vitro studies indicate that Ptx1 is expressed in all pituitary-cell lineages with the highest level of expression present in alpha-GSU-expressing cells. Ptx1 is the predominant ptx protein expressed in gonadotropes. In vitro experiments indicate that ptx1 expression is essential for expression of the lhx3 transcription factor and for sus-tained expression of the alpha-GSU promoter *(80)*. In addition, synergism between ptx1 and sf1 was observed in gonadotrope cells on the LHbeta- promoter *(80)*. Thus, ptx1 seems to play a role in directing pituitary development and is one of the earliest regulators of pituitary transcription-activating expression of lhx3 and alpha-GSU.

Alpha-Glycoprotein Subunit (Alpha-GSU)

The alpha-GSU is the first hormonal marker of the developing pituitary gland and is expressed on e11.5 in mice, with beta-TSH expression occurring on e14.5, LH on e16.5 and FSH on e17.5 *(81)*. All pituitary cells expressing the ventral marker Isl1 seem to develop into alpha-GSU-expressing cells. Studies from mice with targeted disruption of the alpha-GSU indicate that the alpha-GSU is not required for further differentiation of the gona-dotropes *(82)*. These mice are hypogonadal and hypothyroid, but exhibit a normal number of gonadotropes but dramatic hyperplasia of the thyrotropes in the pituitary. Gonado-tropes stained for both LH-beta and FSH-beta subunits but not for the alpha-GSU indicat-ing that the alpha-GSU is not required for terminal differentiation of the gonadotropes. Mice were functionally hypogonadal as LH and FSH can not be secreted without the alpha-GSU.

Prophet of Pit-1 (Prop-1)

Prop-1 is a paired-like homeodomain transcription factor whose expression is restricted to the anterior pituitary. It is transiently expressed during pituitary development between e10-e14.5. Prop-1, as the name indicates, plays a role in cell-fate determination of the pit-1 cell lineages including the thyrotropes, and somatolactotropes. Interestingly, there is evidence in both mice and humans that prop-1 may also play a role in gonadotrope proliferation and/or maintenance of gonadotrope function. The Ames dwarf mouse has a homozygous mutation of the prop-1 gene resulting in failure of development of the pit-1-dependent cell lineages, and reduced gonadotropin secretion *(83)*. In contradistinction, pit-1 gene mutations in human and mice do not affect gondotropin secretion suggesting that prop-1 and not pit-1 may regulate gonadotrope differentiation and/or function. Several human mutations of Prop-1 result in combined pituitary deficiency of the pit-1 lineages. In addition, some patients have reduced LH and FSH secretion *(84)* or age-related decline in LH and FSH secretion *(85)* resulting in delayed onset of puberty.

Steroidogenic Factor I (SF-1)

SF-1 is an orphan nuclear receptor that is a member of the superfamily of nuclear hormone receptors. No ligand for the SF-1 receptor has been identified to date. SF-1 plays an important role in the regulation of the neuroendocrine reproductive system at all three levels of the axis. Studies from the SF-1 knockout mouse indicate agenesis of the ventro-medial hypothalamic nucleus, impaired gonadotrope function, agenesis of the gonads and adrenals, and male-female sex-reversal of the internal and external genitalia *(92)*.

THE GONAD

Overview

The gonads have two main functions that are critical for reproductive function. First, they are the reservoir of germ cells that are destined to become oocytes in the ovary and spermatocytes in the testes. Secondly, they produce the sex-steroid hormones that regulate sexual differentiation as well as the maturation of these germ cells into functional gametes.

The genetic sex of the embryo (XY vs XX) is established at fertilization and determines whether male gonads (testes) or female gonads (ovaries) will develop. Gonadal development is complex event requiring coordinated signaling between various cell types. Recent studies have identified several transcription factors that are critical for the development of gonads. The mechanisms by which these transcription factors regulate early gonadal development are only beginning to be elucidated.

Development of the Bipotential Gonadal Anlagen

The ovary and the testis arise from common anlagen during embryonic development, and the adult structures contain homologous cell types. The gonadal cells derive from three embryologic precursors: the primordial germ cell, the coelomic epithelium, and the underlying mesenchyme *(87)*. The primordial germ cells differentiate into the male and female gametes. The coelomic epithelial cells give rise to Sertoli cells in the testes and granulosa cells in the ovary. The ovarian theca cells and testicular Leydig cells derive from the mesenchymal cells.

The undifferentiated or bipotential gonad arises from within the developing urogenital system. The development of the urinary and genital systems are closely associated since the kidneys, ureters, adrenal cortex, and reproductive tracts all arise from the intermediate mesoderm. The Wolffian or mesonephric ducts differentiate into the male reproductive system, including the vasa deferentia, seminal vesicles, and epididymis, while the Mullerian or paramesonephric ducts fuse in the midline to form the uterus, upper portion of the vagina, and the fallopian tubes *(87)*.

Although the genetic sex of the embryo is determined at fertilization, early gonadal development occurs identically in male and female embryos. The gonadal or genital ridge, develops as a thickening on the on the ventral aspect of the mesonephros and represent the primitive gonad. The genital ridges can be seen during the fifth wk of human gestation *(87)* and at 10 d pc in the mouse embryo, referred to as embryonic d 10 or E10 *(88)*. The primordial germ cells originate outside the embryo in the yolk sac and migrate into the genital ridges by the sixth wk of human gestation *(87)*.

Gonadal Sex Differentiation

Morphologically, male and female gonads are identical until embryonic d 12 in the mouse *(88)* and 7 wk, gestation in the human embryo *(87)* at which time testicular differentiation begins in embryos bearing Y chromosomes. The hallmark of testis formation is the differentiation of somatic cells into Sertoli cells, which aggregate to form seminiferous tubules *(90)*. The production of Antimullerian Hormone (AMH) by the Sertoli cells induces the regression of Mullerian ducts. Leydig cells begin to synthesize testosterone at approx 8 wk gestation in the human embryo *(89)* and embryonic d 12.5–13 *(88)* in the mouse embryo. Testosterone maintains the Wolffian structures and promotes the development of male internal and external genitalia.

Ovarian development occurs in embryos lacking the Y chromosome. In contrast to the testes, ovaries do not undergo structural differentiation until later in gestation. Ovarian morphology is not identifiable until 10 wk gestation, and the primordial follicles are not seen until 16 wk gestation *(87)*. In the absence of AMH, the Mullerian ducts persist and differentiate into the female reproductive tract, and in the absence of testosterone, the Wolffian structures regress. Although the development of the female phenotype has traditionally been considered the default condition resulting from a lack of testicular hormones in XX individuals, recent evidence suggests that Wnt-4 signaling is essential for development of the Mullerian ducts and suppression of the Wolffian ducts *(90)*.

Transcription Factors Mediating Early Gonadogenesis

Several transcription factors appear to regulate the development of the bipotential gonadal anlagen *(88,91–93)*. Disruption of the genes encoding these transcription factors will result in gonadal agenesis or dysgenesis. Because gonadal development is arrested prior to sexual differentiation, both testicular and ovarian development are impaired. Furthermore, the lack of testicular AMH and androgens results in pseudohermaphroditism, the formation of female internal and external genitalia, in XY individuals.

he precise mechanisms by which these transcription factors interact to direct gonadal development have not yet been elucidated and are the focus of intense study. SF1, WT1, and Lhx1 have been identified as transcription factors with critical roles in the differentiation of the intermediate mesoderm *(88)*. Mutations in the genes encoding SF1, WT1, and Lhx1 are also associated with defective development of other structures that derive from the intermediate mesoderm, such as the kidney or adrenal cortex *(88,91,92)*. Recently, Lhx9 has been identified as a transcription factor that may specifically control gonadal-cell proliferation early in development *(93)*.

SF-1

Steroidogenic factor 1 (SF1) is an orphan receptor for which no clear activating ligand has been found *(86)*. SF1 was first identified as a transcription factor that regulates expression of many genes involved in steroid biosynthesis *(94–97)*. SF-1 is expressed in mouse embryos from the time of gonadal-ridge development *(98)*. With sexual differentiation, the levels of SF-1 transcripts increase in the testes and decrease in the ovaries. In addition to the gonads, SF-1 is present in the hypothalamus, pituitary, and adrenals of mouse embryos *(88,92)*, suggesting that SF-1 may regulate endocrine function at multiple levels.

Studies of SF-1 knockout mice confirmed essential roles of SF-1 on the development of the hypothalamus, pituitary, adrenals, and gonads. Homozygous SF-1 knockout mice lack the ventromedial hypothalamic nucleus *(98,99)*, have impaired gonadotrope function *(98,100)*, and lack adrenal glands and gonads *(101,102)*. In mouse embryos lacking SF-1, the genital ridges develop and are colonized by germ cells, indicating that SF-1 is not necessary for initial development of the gonad *(101,102)*. Without SF-1, however, the gonads degenerate by apoptosis after 11–11.5 d pc *(101)*. As expected with gonadal loss before the production of testicular AMH and testosterone, SF-1 knockout mice also exhibit male to female sex reversal of their internal and external genital tracts.

The human SF-1 gene shares extensive homology with its mouse counterpart *(103,104)* and is expressed in many of the same tissues *(105)*. Recently, a patient bearing a heterozygous missense mutation in the DNA-binding domain of SF-1 has been described *(106)*. The patient presented with primary adrenal failure during the first weeks of life. This individual had a 46 XY karyotype, but was phenotypically female with normal Mullerian structures found on ultrasound. Gonadotropin release was preserved, but testicular development was severely affected. No androgenic response was elicited after human chorionic gonadotropin (hCG) administration.

WT-1

Because mutations in the Wilms' Tumor associated gene (WT1) are associated with Wilms' tumors (childhood kidney tumors of embryonic origin), it was initially described as a tumor-suppressor gene *(107,108)*. WT1 encodes a zinc-finger transcription factor, which shares homology with members of the early growth response (EGR) gene family. Several different protein isoforms are generated by alternative splicing *(109)*, alternative translation start sites *(110)*, and post-translational RNA editing *(111)*. These isoforms differ in their DNA binding *(112)* and may have distinct cellular functions.

Studies in mice indicate that WT1 has a critical role in normal gonadal development *(88,92,113)*. WT1 expression has been demonstrated as early as 9.5 d pc in the intermediate mesoderm, the embryonic layer from which the kidneys and gonads derive *(114)*. Homozygous WT1 knockout mice lack gonads and kidneys *(115)*. Without testicular AMH and androgens, the internal and external genitalia develop along the female pathway. In the developed gonad, WT1 expression is restricted to the granulosa cells of the ovary and the Sertoli cells of the testes *(116,117)*, suggesting that WT1 may have a role in germ-cell maturation.

WT1 mutations also produce three human syndromes, which are all associated with urogenital anomalies: WAGR syndrome, Denys-Drash syndrome, and Fraiser syndrome *(91,92,113)*. Even within a syndrome, the gonadal and reproductive tract defects can vary widely. In general, however, XX individuals often appear normal whereas XY individuals may present with ambiguous genitalia or varying degrees of pseudohermaphroditism.

The WAGR phenotype includes Wilms' tumor, aniridia, genitourinary, and mental retardation. WAGR syndrome reflects the contiguous deletion of several genes, including WT1, on chromosome 11p13, which may account for the syndrome's distinct clinical features *(107,108,118)*. The associated gonadal anomalies, such as cryptorchidism and hypospadias, are usually mild and are found in only a subset of patients with WAGR syndrome *(92)*.

The Denys-Drash syndrome (DDS) consists of developmental anomalies of the gonads and urogenital systems in association with diffuse mesangial sclerosis causing end-stage renal disease early in childhood *(92)*. Because Wilms' tumors are common in Denys-Drash families, point mutations in the zinc-finger (DNA binding) region of WT1 were found in DDS patients *(116)*. DDS is inherited as an autosomal dominant disorder, suggesting that the mutant WT1 protein inhibits the function of normal WT1 in a dominant-negative manner *(119,120)*. A wide range of gonadal abnormalities is associated with DDS, and gonadal dysgenesis occurs in both XX and XY individuals indicating the importance of WT1 in the development of the early bipotential gonads. Pseudohermaphroditism, however, results from lack of testicular hormones and is found only in XY individuals.

Frasier syndrome is also associated with gonadal dysgenesis, male pseudohermaphroditism, and focal glomerular sclerosis. Compared to DDS, the glomerulopathy in Frasier syndrome is less severe, and some renal function may be preserved into adulthood *(92)*. Although patients with Frasier syndrome do not develop Wilms' tumors, mutations in the WT1 gene are responsible for the syndrome *(121)*. Normally, alternative splicing produces WT1 isoforms with or without three amino acids, lysine, threonine, and serine (KTS), between the third and fourth zinc fingers. The WT1 isoforms containing KTS (+KTS) are associated with spliceosomes, suggesting a role in RNA processing *(122)*. In Frasier syndrome, donor splice-site mutations in WT1 selectively interfere with production of the +KTS isoform *(121)*. Perhaps, RNA processing by WT1 is essential for gonadal development, but has no role in Wilms' tumor suppression.

LIM Homeobox Domain Transcription Factors

No human mutations have been described in either Lhx1 or Lhx9, but mouse studies suggest that these two members of the LIM homeobox domain gene family of transcription factors are essential for gonad formation. Lhx1 (Lim1) and Lhx9 are expressed early in the urogenital ridge, by embryonic d 9.5 *(93)*. Mice homozygous for deletions in Lhx1 are reminiscent of the SF1 and WT1 knockout mice: they lack kidneys, and gonadal development is arrested prior to sexual differentiation *(93)*.

In contrast to the other transcription factors involved in early gonadal development, Lhx9 may have a more specific role in formation of the bipotential gonadal anlagen. Mice homozygous for deletions in Lhx9 are viable and had isolated gonadal agenesis without associated adrenal or renal anomalies *(93)*. Both XX and XY mice are phenotypically female, but with atrophic Mullerian structures. The urogenital ridges developed until embryonic d 11.5 with normal migration of the primordial germ cells. Unlike the gonads of the WT1 and SF1 knockout mice, there was no evidence of apoptosis, suggesting that gonadal agenesis reflects a failure of cell proliferation.

Gene Interactions in Early Gonadogenesis

Formation of the bipotential gonad anlagen from the developing urogenital system is a complex event that requires coordinated signals from various cell types. Analyses of patients with gonadal dysgenesis and knockout mice have identified several transcription factors, which appear to have critical roles in the early gonadal development. Recent studies have begun to examine the mechanisms by which these transcription factors interact to direct formation of the gonadal anlagen.

Studies, performed in vitro, suggest that WT1 may form heterodimers with SF1 and augment SF1-dependent activation of downstream genes, such as the AMH promoter (113). Cotransfection of WT1 increases the expression of reporter genes driven by the SF1 promoter, indicating that WT1 may also increase SF1 expression (92). WT1, however, does not appear to be essential for SF1 expression as WT1 knockout mice have detectable SF-1 transcripts in their degenerating gonads (92).

Examination of SF1, WT1, Lhx1, and Lhx9 expression in different knockout mouse models provides insight into the interactions of the genes involved in the development of the bipotential gonad. Compared to wild-type mice at embryonic d 11.5, SF1 transcripts were reduced in the gonadal ridge of Lhx9-deficient mice. In contrast, Lhx9 expression was unchanged in the SF1-deficient mice, suggesting that Lhx9 acts upstream of SF1 in the regulatory pathway leading to the formation of the bipotential gonad (93). The expression of Lhx1 and WT1, on the other hand, may be independent of Lhx9 and SF1. WT1 expression did not differ between Lhx9 deficient and wild-type mice, and *in situ* hybridization demonstrated normal localization of Lhx1 in the gonadal ridge of Lhx9 deficient mice at embryonic d 9.5 (93).

REFERENCES

1. Schwanzel-Fukuda M, Garcia MS, Morrell JI, Pfaff DW. Distribution of luteinizing hormone-releasing hormone in the nervus terminalis and brain of the mouse detected by immunocytochemistry. J Comp Neurol 1987;255(2):231–244.
2. Wray S, Grant P, Gainer H. Evidence that cells expressing luteinizing hormone-releasing hormone mRNA in the mouse are derived from progenitor cells in the olfactory placode. Proc Natl Acad Sci USA 1989;86:8132–8136.
3. Wu TJ, Gibson MJ, Rogers MC, Silverman AJ. New observations on the development of the gonadotropin-releasing hormone system in the mouse. J Neurobiol 1999;33:983–998.
4. Yoshida K, Rutishauser U, Crandall JE, Schwarting GA. Polysialic acid facilitates migration of luteinizing hormone-releasing hormone neurons on vomeronasal axons. J Neurosci 1999;19:794–801.
5. Murakami S, Seki T, Rutishauser U, Arai Y. Enzymatic removal of polysialic acid from neural cell adhesion molecule perturbs the migration route of luteinizing hormone-releasing hormone neurons in the developing chick forebrain. J Comp Neurol 2000;420(2):171–181.
6. Tobet SA, Chickering TW, King JC, Stopa EG, Kim K, Kuo-Leblank V, Schwarting GA. Expression of gamma-aminobutyric acid and gonadotropin-releasing hormone during neuronal migration through the olfactory system. Endocrinology 1996;137:5415–5420.
7. Fueshko SM, Key S, Wray S. GABA inhibits migration of luteinizing hormone-releasing hormone neurons in embryonic olfactory explants. J Neurosci 1998;18:2560–2569.
8. Fang Z, Xiong X, James A, Gordon DF, Wierman ME. Identification of novel factors that regulate GnRH gene expression and neuronal migration. Endocrinology 1998;139:3654–3657.
9. Wray S, Key S, Qualls R, Fueshko SM. A subset of peripherin positive olfactory axons delineates the luteinizing hormone releasing hormone neuronal migratory pathway in developing mouse. Dev Biol 1994;166:349–354.
10. Livne I, Gibson MJ, Silverman AJ. Biochemical differentiation and intercellular interactions of migratory gonadotropin-releasing hormone (GnRH) cells in the mouse. Dev Biol 1993;159:643–656.
11. Rogers MC, Silverman AJ, Gibson MJ. Gonadotropin-releasing hormone axons target the median eminence: in vitro evidence for diffusible chemoattractive signals from the mediobasal hypothalamus. Endocrinology 1997;138:3956–3966.
12. Dellovade TL, Pfaff DW, Schwanzel-Fukuda M. The gonadotropin-releasing hormone system does not develop in Small-Eye (Sey) mouse phenotype Brain. Res Dev Brain Res 1998;107:233–240.

13. Acampora D, Mazan S, Tuorto F, Avantaggiato V, Tremblay JJ, Lazzaro D, et al. Transient dwarfism and hypogonadism in mice lacking Otx1 reveal prepubescent stage-specific control of pituitary levels of GH, FSH and LH. Development 1998;125:1229–1239.

14. Ang SL, Jin O, Rhinn M, Daigle N, Stevenson L, Rossant J. A targeted mouse Otx2 mutation leads to severe defects in gastrulation and formation of axial mesoderm and to deletion of rostral brain. Development 1996;122:243–252.

15. Simeone A. Otx1 and Otx2 in the development and evolution of the mammalian brain. EMBO J 1998; 17:6790–6798.

16. Franco B, Guioli S, Pragliola A, Incerti B, Bardoni B, Tonlorenzi R, et al. A gene deleted in Kallmann's syndrome shares homology with neural cell adhesion and axonal path-finding molecules. Nature 1998; 353:529–536.

17. Wierman ME, Kepa JK, Sun W, Gordon DF, Wood WM. Estrogen negatively regulates rat gonadotropin releasing hormone (rGnRH) promoter activity in transfected placental cells. Mol Cell Endorinol 1992;86:1–10.

18. Schwanzel-Fukuda M, Bick D, Pfaff DW. Luteinizing hormone-releasing hormone (LHRH)-expressing cells do not migrate normally in an inherited hypogonadal (Kallmann) syndrome. Mol Brain Res 1989;6:311–326.

19. Legouis R, Cohen-Salmon M, Del Castillo I, Petit C. Isolation and characterization of the gene responsible for the X chromosome-linked Kallmann syndrome. Biomed Pharmacother 1994;48:241–246.

20. Legouis R, Hardelin J-P, Levilliers J, Claverie J-M, Compain S, Wunderie V, et al. The candidate gene for the X-linked Kallmann syndrome encodes a protein related to adhesion molocules. Cell 1995; 423–435.

21. Yokosaki Y, Matsuura N, Higashiyama S, Murakami I, Obara M, Yamakido M, et al. Identification of the ligand binding site for the integrin alpha9 beta1 in the third fibronectin type III repeat of tenascin-C. J Biol Chem 1998;273:11,423–11,428.

22. Quinton R, Hasan W, Grant W, Thrasivoulou C, Quiney RE, Besser GM, Bouloux PM. Gonadotropin-releasing hormone immunoreactivity in the nasal epithelia of adults with Kallmann's syndrome and isolated hypogonadotropic hypogonadism and in the early midtrimester human fetus. J Clin Endocrinol Metab 1997;82:309–314.

23. Waldstreicher J, Seminara SB, Jameson JL, Geyer A, Nachtigall LB, Boepple PA, et al. The genetic and clinical heterogeneity of gonadotropin-releasing hormone deficiency in the human. J Clin Endocrinol Metab 1996;81:4388–4395.

24. Mason AJ, Hayflick JS, Zoeller RT, Young WS, Phillips HS, Nikolics K, Seeburg PH. A deletion truncating the gonadotropin-releasing hormone gene is responsible for hypogonadism in the hpg mouse. Science 1986;234:1366–1371.

25. Livne I, Gibson MJ, Silverman AJ. Gonadotropin-releasing hormone (GnRH) neurons in the hypogonadal mouse elaborate normal projections despite their biosynthetic deficiency. Neurosci Lett 1993; 151:229–233.

26. Rogers MC, Silverman AJ, Gibson MJ. Preoptic area grafts implanted in mammillary bodies of hypogonadal mice: patterns of GnRH neuronal projections. Exp Neurol 1998;151:265–272.

27. Kokoris GJ, Lam NY, Ferin M, Silverman AJ, Gibson MJ. Transplanted gonadotropin-releasing hormone neurons promote pulsatile luteinizing hormone secretion in congenitally hypogonadal (hpg) male mice. Neuroendocrinology 1988;48:45–52.

28. Silverman AJ, Roberts JL, Dong KW, Miller GM, Gibson MJ. Intrahypothalamic injection of a cell line secreting gonadotropin-releasing hormone results in cellular differentiation and reversal of hypogonadism in mutant mice. Proc Natl Acad Sci USA 1992;89:10,668–10,672.

29. Rakic P, Sidman RL. Sequence of developmental abnormalities leading to granule cell deficit in cerebellar cortex of weaver mutant mice. J Comp Neurol 1973;15:103–132.

30. Rakic P, Sidman RL. Weaver mutant mouse cerebellum: defective neuronal migration secondary to abnormality of Bergmann glia. Proc Natl Acad Sci USA 1973;70:240–244.

31. Goldowitz D, Mullen RJ. Granule cell as a site of gene action in the weaver mouse cerebellum: evidence from heterozygous mutant chimeras. J Neurosci 1982;2:1474–1485.

32. Allen MP, Zeng C, Schneider K, Xiong X, Meintzer MK, Bellosta P, et al. Growth arrest-specific gene 6 (Gas6)/adhesion related kinase (Ark) signaling promotes gonadotropin-releasing hormone neuronal survival via extracellular signal-regulated kinase (ERK) and Akt. Mol Endocrinol 1999;13:191–201.

33. Barry J, Hoffman GE, Wray S. LHRH-containing systems. In: Björklund A, Hökfelt T, eds. Handbook of Chemical Anatomy. Vol. 4: GABA and Neuropeptides in the CNS, part 1. Elsevier Science Publishers B.V., Amsterdam, 1996, pp. 166–215.

34. King JC, Tobet SA, Snavely FL, Arimura AA. LHRH imminopositive cells and their projections to the median eminence and organum vasculosum of the lamina teminalis. J Comp Neurol 1982;209:287–300.

35. Hiatt ES, Brunetta PG, Seiler GR, Barney SA, Selles WD, Wooledge KH, King JC. Subgroups of luteinizing hormone-releasing hormone perikary defined by computer analysis in the basal forebrain of intact female rats. Endocrinology 1992;13(2):1030–1043.

36. Porkka-Heiskanen T, Urban JH, Turek FW, Levine JE. Gene expression in a subpopulation of luteinizing hormone- releasing hormone (LHRH) neurons prior to the preovuluatory gonadotropin surge. J Neurosci 1994;14(9):5548–5558.

37. Dutlow CM, Rachman J, Jacobs TW, Millar RP. Prepubertal increases in gonadotropin-releasing hormone mRNA, gonadotropin-releasing hormone precursor, and subsequent maturation of precurso processing in male rats. J Clin Invest 1992;90:2496–2501.

38. Gore AC. Diurnal rhythmicity of gonadotropin-releasing hormone gene expression in the rat. Neuroendocrinology 1998;68:257–263.

39. Gore AC, Roberts JL, Gibson MJ. Mechanisms for the regulation of gonadotropin-releasing hormone gene expression in the developing mouse. Endocrinology 1999;140(5):2280–2287.

40. Levine JE, Ramirez VD. Luteinizing hormone-releasing hormone release during the rat estrous cycle and after ovariectomy, as estimated with push-pull cannulae. Endocrinology 1982;111:1439–1448.

41. Moenter SM, Caraty A, Locatelli A, Karsch FJ. Pattern of gonadotropin-releasing hormone (GnRH) secretion leading up to ovulation in the ewe: existence of a preovulatory GnRH surge. Endocrinology 1991;129(3):1175–1182.

42. Wolfe AM, Wray S, Westphal H, Radovick S. Cell-specific expression of the human gonadotropin-releasing hormone gene in transgenic animals. J Biol Chem 1995;271:20,018–20,023.

43. Parfitt DB, Thompson RC, Richardson HN, Romeo RD, Sisk CL. GnRH mRNA increases with puberty in the male syrian hamster brain. J Neuroendocrinol 1999;11:621–627.

44. Terasawa E, Luchansky LL, Kasuya E, Nyberg CL. An increase in lutamate release follows a decrease in gamma aminobutyric acid and the pubertal increase in luteinizing hormone releasing hormone release in the female rhesus monkeys. J Neuroendocrinol 1999;11:275–282.

45. Mitsushima D, Hei DL, Terasawa E. Gamma-aminobutyric acid is an inhibitory neurotransmitter restricting the release of luteinizing hormone-releasing hormone before the onset of puberty. Proc Natl Acad Sci USA 1994;91:395–399.

46. Zamorano PL, Mahesh VB, De Sevilla L, Brann DW. Excitatory amino acid receptors and puberty. Steroids 1994;63:268–270.

47. Gore AC, Wu TJ, Rosenberg JJ, Roberts JL. Gonadotropin-releasing hormone and NMDA receptor gene expression and colocalization change during puberty in female rats. J Neurosci 1996;16:5281–5289.

48. Radovick S, Wondisford FE, Nakayama Y, Yamada M, Cutler GB Jr, Weintraub BD. Isolation and characterization of the human gonadotropin- releasing hormone gene in the hypothalamus and placenta. Mol Endorinol 1990;4:476–480.

49. Bond CT, Hayflick JS, Seeburg PH, Adelman JP. The rat gonadotropin-releasing hormone: SH locus: structure and hypothalamic expression, Mol Endocrinol 1989;3(8):1257–1262.

50. Hayflick JS, Adelman JP, Seeburg PH. The complete nucleotide sequence of the human gonadotropin-releasing hormone gene. Nucleic Acid Res 1989;17(15):6403–6404.

51. Kepa JK, Wang C, Neeley CI, Raynolds MV, Gordon DF, Wood WM, Wierman ME. Structure of the rat gonadotropin-releasing hormone (rGnRH) gene promoter and functional analysis in hypothalamic cells. Nucleic Acid Res 1992;20(6):1393–1399.

52. Seeburg PH, Mason AJ, Stewart TA, Nikolics K. The mammalian GnRH gene and its pivotal role in reproduction. Rec Prog Horm Res 1987;41:69–98.

53. Dong K-W, Yu K-L, Roberts JL. Identification of a major up-stream transcription start site for the human progonadotropin-releasing hormone gene used in reproductive tissues and cell lines. Mol Endocrinol 1993;7:1654–1666.

54. Zhen S, Dunn IC, Wray S, Liu Y, Chappell PE, Levine JE, Radovick S. An alternative gonadotropin-releasing hormone (GnRH) RNA splicing product found in cultured GnRH neurons and mouse hypothalamus. J Biol Chem 1997;272:12,620–12,625.

55. Mellon PL, Windle JJ, Goldsmith PC, Padula CA, Roberts JL, Weiner RI. Immortalization of hypothalamic GnRH neurons by genetically targeted tumorigenesis. Neuron 1990;5:1–10.

56. Radovick S, Wray S, Lee E, Nicols DK, Nakayama Y, Weintraub BD, et al. Migratory arrest of gonadotropin-releasing hormone neurons in transgenic mice. Proc Natl Acad Sci USA 1991;88:3402–3406.

57. Bosma MM. Ion channel properties and episodic activity in isolated immortalized gonadotropin-releasing hormone (GnRH) neurons. J Membr Biol 1993;136:85–96.

58. Martinez dLE, Choi AL, Weiner RI. Generation and synchronization of gonadotropin-releasing hormone (GnRH) pulses: intrinsic properties of the GT1-1 GnRH neuronal cell line. Proc Natl Acad Sci USA 1992;89:1852–1855.

59. Poletti A, Melcangi RC, Negri-Cesi P, Maggi R, Martini L. Steroid binding and metabolism in the luteinizing hormone-releasing hormone-producing neuronal cell line GT1-1. Endocrinology 1994; 135(6):2623–2628.

60. Weiner RI, Martinez DLE. Pulsatile release of gonadotrophin releasing hormone (GnRH) is an intrinsic property of GT1 GnRH neuronal cell lines. Hum Reprod 1993;8(Suppl);2:13–17.

61. Wetsel WC, Mellon PL, Weiner RI, Negro-Vilar A. Metabolism of pro-luteinizing hormone-releasing hormone in immortalized hypothalamic neurons. Endocrinology 1991;129:1584–1595.

62. Zhen S, Zakaria M, Wolfe A, Radovick S. Regulation of gonadotropin-releasing hormone (GnRH) gene expression by insulin-like growth factor I in a cultured GnRH-expressing neuronal cell line. Mol Endocrinol 1997;11:1145–1155.

63. Radovick S, Ticknor CM, Nakayama Y, Notides AC, Rahman A, Weintraub BD, et al. Evidence for direct estrogen regulation of the human gonadotropin-releasing hormone gene. J Clin Invest 1991;88: 1649–1655.

64. Radovick S, Wondisford FE, Wray S, Ticknor C, Nakayama Y, Cutler GB Jr, et al. Characterization expression and estradiol regulation of lthe GnRH gene. In: Crowley WF Jr, Conn PM, eds. Modes of Action of GnRH and GnRH Analogs Springer-Verlag, New York, 1993, pp. 85–105.

65. Chandran UR, Attardi B, Friedman R, Zheng Z, Roberts JL, DeFranco DB. Glucocorticoid repression of the mouse gonadotropin-releasing hormone gene is mediated by promoter elements that are recognized by heteromeric complexes containing glucocorticoid receptor. J Biol Chem 1996;271:20,412–20,420.

66. Wolfe A, Kim HH, Tobet S, Staffor DEJ, Radovick S. Identification of a discreet promoter region of the human GnRH gene that is sufficient for directing neuron-specific expression: a role for PDU Homeodomain Transcription Factors. Mol Endocrinol, in press.

67. Stafford D, Wolfe A, Radovick S. Endocrinology Meeting Abstracts 80th Annual Meeting, 1998, Abstract #OR5-4.

68. Zakaria M, Dunn IC, Zhen S, Su E, Smith E, Patriquin E, Radovick S. Phorbol ester regulation of the gonadotropin-releasing hormone (GnRH) gene in GnRH-secreting cell lines: a molecular basis for species differences. Mol Endocrinol 1996;10:1282–1291.

69. Wierman ME, Xiong X, Kepa JK, Spaulding AJ, Jacobsen BM, Fang Z, et al. Repression of gonadotropin-releasing hormone promoter activity by the POU homeodomain transcription factor SCIP/Oct-6/Tst-1: a regulatory mechanism of phenotype expression? Mol Cell Biol 1997;17:1652–1665.

70. Lawson MA, Whyte DB, Mellon PL. GATA factors are essential for activity of the neuron-specific enhancer of the gonadotropin-releasing hormone gene. Mol Cell Biol 1996;16:3596–3605.

71. Bruder JM, Krebs WD, Nett TM, Wierman ME. Phorbol ester activation of the protein kinase C pathway inhibits gonadotropin-releasing hormone gene expression. Endocrinology 1992;13:2552–2558.

72. Eraly SA, Mellon PL. Regulation of gonadotropin-releasing hormone transcription by protein kinase C is mediated by evolutionarily conserved promoter-proximal elements. Mol Endocrinol 1995;9:848–859.

73. Wetsel WC, Eraly SA, Whyte DB, Mellon PL. Regulation of gonadotropin-releasing hormone by protein kinase-A and -C in immortalized hypothalamic neurons. Endocrinology 1993;132:2360–2370.

74. Belsham DD, Evangelou A, Roy D, Duc VL, Brown TJ. Regulation of gonadotropin-releasing hormone (GnRH) gene expression by 5alpha-dihydrotestosterone in GnRH-secreting GT1-7 hypothalamic neurons. Endocrinology 1998;139:1108–1114.

75. Takuma N, Sheng HZ, Furuta Y, Ward JM, Sharma K, Hogan BLM, et al. Formation of rathke's pouch rewquires dual induction from the diencephalon. Development 1998;125:4835–4840.

76. Treier M, Gleiberman AS, O'Connell SM, Szeto DP, McMahon JA, McMahon AP, Rosenfeld MG. Multistep signaling requirement for pituitary organogenesis in vivo. Genes Dev 1998;12:1691–1704.

77. Dasen JS, O'Connell SM, Flynn SE, Treier M, Geliberman AS, Szeto DP, et al. Reciprocal Interactions of PIT1 and GATA2 mediate signaling gradient-induced determination of pituitary cell types. Cell 1999;97:587–598.

78. Sheng HZ, Zhadanov AB, Mosinger B, Fuji T, Bertuzzi S, Grinberg A, et al. Specification of pituitary cell lineages by the LIM homeobox gene lhx3. Science 1996;272:1004–1007.

79. Sheng HZ, Moriyama K, Yamashita T, Li H, Potter SS, Mahon KA, Westphal K. Multistep control of pituitary organogenesis. Science 1997;278:1809–1812.

80. Tremblay JJ, Lanctot C, Drouin J. The pan-pituitary activator of transcription, ptx1 (pitltary homeobox 1), acts in synergy with SF-1 and Pit1 and as an upstream regulator of the Lim–homeodomain gene Lim3/lhx3. Mol Endocrinol 1998;12(3):428–441.

81. Japon MA, Rubinstein M, Low MJ. In situ hybridization analysis of anterior pituitary hormone gene expression during fetal mouse development. J Histochem Cytochem 1994;42:1117–1125.

82. Kendall SS, Samuelson LC, Saunders TL, Wood RI, Camper SA. Targeted disruption of the pituitary glycoprotein hormone a-subunit produces hypogonadla and hypothyroid mice. Genes Dev 1995;9: 2007–2019.

83. Sornson MW, Wu W, Dasen JS, Flynn SE, Norman DJ, O'Connell SM, et al. Pituitary lineage determination by the prophet of pit-1 homeodomain factor defective in Ames dwarfism. Nature 1996;384: 327–333.

84. Wu W. Mutations in Prop1 cause familial combined pituitary hormone deficiency. Nat Genet 1998;18: 147–149.

85. Fluck C, Deladoey J, Rutishauser K, Able A, Marti U, Wu W, Mullis PE. Phenotypic variability in familial combined pituitary hormone deficiency caused by a PROP1 gene mutation resulting in the substitution of arg-cys at codon 120 (R120C). JCEM 1998;83:3727–3734.

86. Parker KL. The roles of steroidogenic factor 1 in endocrine development and function. Mol Cell Endocrinol 1998;145(1-2):15–20.

87. Moore KL. The urogenital system. In: Schmitt W, ed. The Developing Human: Clinically Oriented Embryology, 6th ed. WB Saunders, Philadelphia, PA, 1988, pp. 303–348.

88. Swain A, Lovell-Badge R. Mammalian sex determination: a molecular drama. Genes Dev 1999;13: 755–767.

89. Josso N. Sexual differentiation. In: Adashi EY, Rock JA, Rosenwaks Z, eds. Reproductive Endocrinology, Surgery, and Technology. Lippincott-Raven Publishers, Philadelphia, PA, 1996, pp. 59–74.

90. Vainio S, Heikkila M, Kispert A, Chin N, McMahon AP. Female development in mammals is regulated by Wnt-4 signaling. Nature 1999;397:405–409.

91. Hiort O, Holterhaus P-M. The molecular basis of male sexual differentiation. Eur J Endocrinol 2000; 142:101–110.

92. Parker KL, Schedl A, Schimmer BP. Gene interactions in gonadal development. Annu Rev Physiol 1999;61:417–433.

93. Birk OS, Casiano DE, Wassif CA, Cogliati T, Zhao L, Zhao Y, et al. The LIM homeobox gene, LHx9 is essential for mouse gonad formation. Nature 2000;403:909–913.

94. Honda SI, Morohashi KI, Nomura M, Takeya H, Kitajima M, Omura T. AdBP regulating steroidogenic p-450 gene is a member of steroid hormone receptor superfamily. J Biol Chem 1993;268:7494–7502.

95. Lala DS, Rice DA, Parker KL. Steroidogenic factor 1, a key regulator of steroidogenic enzyme expression, is the mouse homolog of fushi tarazu factor 1. Mol Endocrinol 1992;6:1249–1258.

96. Morohashi K, Honda S, Inomata Y, Handa H, Omura T. A common trans-acting factor, Ad4-binding protein, to the promoters of steroidogenic P-450s. J Biol Chem 1992;267:17,913–17,919.

97. Morohashi K, Zanger UM, Honda S, Hara M, Waterman MR, Omura T. Activation of CYP11A and CYP11B gene promoters by the steroidogenic cell-specific transcription factor, Ad4BP. Mol Endocrinol 1993;7:1196–1204.

98. Ikeda Y, Luo X, Abbud R, Nilson JH, Parker KL. The nuclear receptor steroidogenic factor 1 is essential for the formation of the ventromedial hypothalamic nucleus. Mol Endocrinol 1995;9:478–486.

99. Shinoda K, Lei H, Yoshii H, Nomura M, Nagano M, Shiba H, et al. Developmental defects of the ventromedial hypothalamic nucleus and pituitary gonadotrophe in the FTz-F1 disrupted mice. Dev Dyn 1995;204:22–29.

100. Ingraham HA, Lala DS, Ikeda Y, Luo X, Shen WH, Nachtigal MW, et al. The nuclear receptor steroidogenic factor 1 acts at multiple levels of the reproductive axis. Genes Dev 1994;8:2302–2312.

101. Luo X, Ikeda Y, Parker KL. A cell-specific nuclear receptor is essential for adrenal and gonadal development and for male sexual differentiation. Cell 1994;77:481–490.

102. Sadovsky Y, Crawford PA, Woodson KG, Polish JA, Clements MA, Tourtellotte LM, et al. Mice deficient in the orphan receptor steroidogenic factor 1 lack adrenal glands and gonads, but express P450 side chain cleavage enzyme in the placenta and have normal embryonic serum levels of corticosteroids. Proc Natl Acad Sci USA 1995;92:10,939–10,943.

103. Oba K, Yanase T, Nomura M, Morohashi K, Takayanagi R, Nawata H. Structural characterization of human Ad4BP (SF-1) gene. Biochem Biophys Res Commun 1996;226:261–267.

104. Wong M, Ramayya MS, Chrousos GP, Driggers PH, Parker KL. Cloning and sequence analysis of the human gene encoding steroidogenic factor 1. J Mol Endocrinol 1996;17:139–147.

105. Ramayya MS, Zhou J, Kino T, Segars JH, Bondy CA, Chrousos GP. Steroidogenic factor 1 messenger ribonucleic acid expression in steroidogenic and nonsteroidogenic human tissues; Northern blot and in situ hybridization studies. J Clin Endocrinol Metab 1997;82:1799–1806.

106. Achermann JC, Ito M, Hindmarsh PC, Jameson JL. A mutation in the gene encoding steroidogenic factor 1 causes XY sex reversal and adrenal failure in humans. Nature Genet 1999;22:125–126.

107. Call KM, Glaser T, Ito CY, Buckler AJ, Pelletier J, Haber DA, et al. Isolation and characterization of a zinc finger polypeptide gene at the human chromosome 11 Wilms' tumor locus. Cell 1990;60:509–520.

108. Gessler M, Poustka A, Cavenee W, Neve RL, Orkin SH, Bruns GA. Homozygous deletion in Wilms tumours of a zinc-finger gene identified by chromosome jumping. Nature 1990;343:774–778.

109. Haber DA, Sohn RL, Buckler AJ, Pelletier J, Call KM, Housman DE. Alternative splicing and genomic structure of the Wilms' tumor gene WT1. Proc Natl Acad Sci USA 1991;88:9618–9622.

110. Bruening W, Pelletier J. A non-AUG translation initiation event generates novel WT1 isoforms. J Biol Chem 1996;271:8646–8654.

111. Sharma PM, Bowman M, Madden S, Rauscher FJ, Sukumar S. RNA editing in the Wilms' tumor susceptibility gene, WT1. Genes Dev 1994;8:720–731.

112. Bickmore WA, Oghene K, Little MH, Seawright A, van Heyningen V, Hastie ND. Modulation of DNA binding specificity by alternative splicing of the Wilms' tumor WT1 gene transcript. Science 1992;257:235–237.

113. Natchigal MW, Hirokawa Y, Enyeart-VanHouten DL, Flanagan JN, Hammer GD, Ingraham HA. Wilms' Tumor 1 and Dax-1 modulate the orphan nuclear receptor SF-1 in sex-specific gene expression. Cell 1998;93:445–454.

114. Pritchard-Jones E, Fleming S, Davidson D, Bickmore W, Porteouse D, Gosden C, et al. The candidate Wilms' tumor gene is involved in genitourinary development. Nature 1990;346:194–197.

115. Kreidberg JA, Sariola H, Loring JM, Maeda M, Pelletier J, Housman D, Jaenisch R. WT-1 is required for early kidney development. Cell 1993;74:679–691.

116. Pellitier J, Schalling M, Buckler AJ, Rogers A, Haber DA, Housman DE. Expression of the Wilm's tumor gene WT1 in the murine urogenital system. Genes Dev 1991a;5:135–1356.

117. Sharma PM, Yang X, Bowman M, Roberts V, Sukumar S. Molecular cloning of rat Wilms' tumor complementary DNA and a study of messenger RNA expression in the urogenital system and the brain. Cancer Res 1992;52:6407–6412.

118. Haber DA, Buckler AJ, Glaser T, Call KM, Pelletier J, Sohn RL, et al. An internal deletion within an 11p13 zinc finger gene contributes to thet developmeont of Wilms' tumor. Cell 1990;61:1257–1269.

119. Hastie ND. Dominant negative mutations in the Wilms' timor (WT1) gene cause Denys-drash syndrome: proof that a tumour-suppressor gene plays a crucial role in normal genitourinary development. Hum Mol Genet 1993;1:293–295.

120. Little MH, Williamson KA, Mannens M, Kelsey A, Gosden C, Hastie ND, Vanbeyningen V. Evidence that WT1 mutations in Denys-Drash sundrom patients may act in a dominat negative fashion. Jum Mol Genet 1993;2:259–264.

121. Barbaux S, Niaudet P, Gubler MC, Grunfeld JP, Jaubert F, Kuttenn F, et al. Donor splice-site mutations in WT1 are responsible for Frasier syndrome. Nat Genet 1997;17:467–470.

122. Larsson SH, Charlieu JP, Miyagawa K, Engelkamp D, Rassoulzadegan M, Ross A, et al. Subnuclear localization of WT1 in splicing or transcription factor domians is regulated by alternative splicing. Cell 1995;81:391–401.

12 Sexual Differentiation

Tamara S. Hannon, MD
and John S. Fuqua, MD

INTRODUCTION

Sexual differentiation is a complex process, and many new developments have arisen over the past few years. In addition, our clinical approach to patients with intersex disorders is currently undergoing significant changes. In this chapter, we will first review the embryology of sexual differentiation, with an emphasis on the genetic control of various aspects of ontogeny. Much of what has been learned about sexual differentiation comes from studies of the rodent. How closely this represents analogous processes in humans is not known. We will then discuss abnormal sexual differentiation, emphasizing that at each step of embryology, there is a corresponding pathological condition. Finally, we will review the diagnosis of intersex disorders and recent progress in the management of affected patients.

NORMAL SEXUAL DIFFERENTIATION

Establishment of Chromosomal Sex

The process of sex determination begins at fertilization, with the ovum normally carrying an X chromosome, and the sperm normally carrying either an X or a Y chromosome. However, meiosis, the process of forming a haploid gamete from a diploid germ cell, must take place normally in order for the establishment of chromosomal sex to occur normally. Disorders of meiosis such as nondisjunction may lead to abnormal sex chromosome number in developing embryos. In addition, loss of sex chromosomes very early in embryonic development may result in mosaicism and lead to anomalies of sex differentiation. This is discussed further below.

From: *Contemporary Endocrinology: Developmental Endocrinology: From Research to Clinical Practice*
Edited by: E. A. Eugster and O. H. Pescovitz © Humana Press Inc., Totowa, NJ

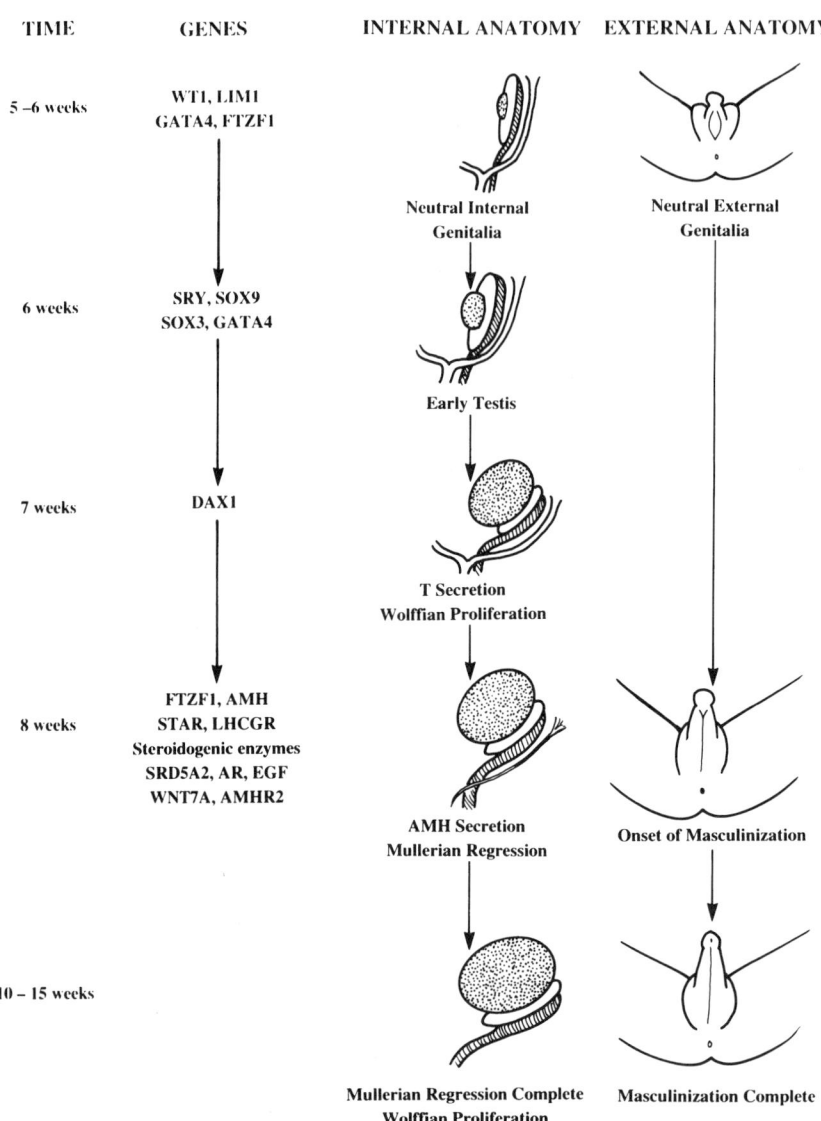

Fig. 1. Timeline of male sexual development, with gestational age, genes thought to be important at various stages, and internal and external anatomy. Internally, the urogenital ridge is flanked by the Wolffian duct and the Müllerian duct. Following testis differentiation, the Müllerian duct involutes and the Wolffian duct develops into the epididymis, vas deferens, and seminal vesicle under the influences of anti-Müllerian hormone and testosterone. Externally, the genital tubercle lies immediately anterior to the urethral folds and the labioscrotal folds. Under the influence of dihydrotestosterone, the genital tubercle enlarges into the penis, and the urethral and labioscrotal folds fuse to form the urethra and scrotum.

Embryology and Genetic Regulation of the Gonadal Ridge

EMBRYOLOGY

At approx 5 wk of gestation in the human embryo, the mesonephros or primitive kidney appears as an outgrowth of the dorsal mesenchyme (1). On the ventromedial surface of each mesonephros, the gonadal ridge appears at about the same time (Fig. 1). The

Table 1
Genes Involved in Sexual Differentiation

Gene	Chromosomal location	Gene product	Location of expression
WT1	11p13	Zn finger transcription factor	Urogenital ridge
LIM1	11p12-p13	Transcription factor	Urogenital ridge
FTZF1	9q33	SF1, Orphan nuclear receptor	Gonads, adrenals, hypothalamus
GATA4	8p22-p23.1	Zn finger transcription factor	Bipotential gonads
SRY	Yp11.3	Transcription factor	Sertoli cells
SOX9	17q24.3-q25.1	Transcription factor	Sertoli cells, cartilage
DAX1	Xp21	Nuclear hormone receptor	Gonads, adrenals, hypothalamus
WNT4	1p35	Secreted glycoprotein	Developing ovary
DMRT1	9p24.3	DNA binding protein	Testis
MTM1	Xq28	Tyrosine phosphatase	Testis, skeletal muscle
XH2	Xq13.3	DNA helicase	Widespread
AMH	19p13.3	TGF-β family of cytokines	Sertoli cells
LHCGR	2p16-p21	G-protein coupled receptor	Leydig cells
STAR	8p11.2	Cholesterol transport protein	Leydig cells, adrenal
HSD17B3	9q22	Steroidogenic enzyme	Leydig cells
SRD5A2	2p23	Steroidogenic enzyme	External genitalia
AR	Xq11-q12	Nuclear hormone receptor	Androgen-responsive tissues
EGF	4q25	Epidermal growth factor	Androgen-responsive tissues
AMHR2	12q13	Membrane hormone receptor	Mullerian ducts
WNT7A	3p25	Secreted glycoprotein	Mullerian ducts
HOXA	7p14.2-p15	Transcription factors	Mullerian ducts

gonadal ridge is morphologically undifferentiated and appears identical in both XX and XY embryos, hence it is frequently termed the bipotential or indifferent gonad. The combination of the mesonephros and gonadal ridge is called the urogenital ridge (1). Germ cells arise from the wall of the yolk sac, migrate along the dorsal mesentery, then move laterally toward the undifferentiated gonad, arriving at 5–6 wk gestation (1,2). At this point, the development of the bipotential gonad is complete.

Genetic Regulation

WT1. Our understanding of the genetic mechanisms regulating differentiation of the urogenital and gonadal ridges has expanded remarkably over the past decade. One of the first genes discovered to be involved in urogenital ridge development was the Wilms tumor-suppressor gene, WT1 (Table 1). mRNAs from WT1 have been detected in the mesonephros and genital ridge of early human embryos by *in situ* hybridization (3). In mice, targeted disruption of the homologous gene leads to renal agenesis and arrest of gonadal development at the gonadal ridge stage (4). In humans with WT1 mutations, gonadal differentiation disorders are always found in association with renal anomalies. This association has been taken as evidence of an early involvement in urogenital ridge morphogenesis (5). In addition, WT1 mutation interrupts both testicular development in XY individuals and ovarian development in XX individuals, hence the assumption that the primary defect occurs at the bipotential gonad stage (6). However, the precise action of the WT1 gene product and its interaction with other genes involved in early differentiation are not known.

LIM1. More recently, the LIM1 gene has been implicated in gonadal-ridge differentiation *(7)* (Table 1). The mRNA of its mouse homolog has been detected in gonadal mesoderm and nephrogenic cords in mouse embryos *(8)*. Targeted disruption of the gene in mice produces offspring lacking gonads, kidneys, and head structures *(9)*. No mutations of this gene have been detected in humans *(7)*.

FTZF1. The FTZF1 gene and its product, steroidogenic factor-1 (SF1), play a major role in sexual differentiation (Table 1). SF1 performs numerous functions related to sexual differentiation in a tightly controlled and tissue-specific manner *(7)*. Its role begins at the urogenital ridge stage. *In situ* hybridization studies in the mouse have shown the presence of Ftz-F1 mRNA in the urogenital ridge. Expression was also found in the bipotential gonad *(10)*. Gene knockout studies resulted in mice that lacked gonads, adrenal glands, and the ventromedial hypothalamic nuclei, important in the production of hormones regulating gonadal function *(10)*. The absence of both testes and ovaries in these mice is further evidence of a role in early gonadal development *(11)*. Additional actions of SF1 are reviewed below.

GATA4. Recent evidence suggests that the GATA4 gene may also play a role in early gonadal differentiation (Table 1). This gene belongs to the GATA family of genes, members of which play roles in the differentiation of a variety of cells and organs *(12)*. The GATA-4 gene is expressed in mouse embryos at 11.5 d post coitus (pc) in the gonadal ridge, localized in the somatic cells of the gonads, with no expression in germ cells *(12)*.

Embryology and Genetic Regulation of the Testis

Embryology

The earliest morphologic changes specific to the testis occur at about 6 wk of gestation *(11)* (Fig. 1). At this time, the coelomic epithelium invades the gonadal mesenchyme to form cords of cells called the primitive sex cords *(1)*. Germ cells are incorporated into these cords, having recently migrated into the gonad from the yolk-sac membrane. Simultaneously, Sertoli cells begin to differentiate within the primitive sex cords, initially in the central portion of the gonad and then spreading in a wave-like fashion toward the periphery *(13)*. The Sertoli cells cluster around the germ cells as the primitive sex cords lengthen and develop into the seminiferous tubules. The appearance of Sertoli cells is generally recognized to be the first sign that the gonad will become a testis *(14)*. In addition, Sertoli cells are thought to have an inductive effect on surrounding cells, promoting their differentiation into other cell lineages important in testis structures *(15)*. Approximately 1 wk after Sertoli cells appear, Leydig cells differentiate from the mesenchyme between the primitive sex cords *(16)* and become functional soon after their appearance. As development progresses, the epithelium covering the testis thickens into a dense collagenous layer called the tunica albuginea.

Genetic Regulation

SRY. The genetic signal that initiates the conversion of the bipotential gonad into a testis was the object of a long series of studies, culminating in the identification of the SRY gene (Table 1). The SRY gene is located on the Y chromosome at p11.3. SRY expression occurs in the precursors of Sertoli cells *(17)*. The SRY protein contains a central DNA binding domain that is highly conserved among mammals, called the HMG box. The protein binds to DNA in a sequence-specific manner. In addition, it also binds nonspecifically to hairpin secondary structures of DNA. The precise relationship of the SRY protein to other factors controlling sex determination is not well-known. SRY protein binds to the promotors of the AMH gene and the P450arom gene in vitro *(18)*. This potential inter-action would suggest a control mechanism for Müllerian duct involution (*see* p. 268). However, conflicting evidence exists for an interaction in vivo, hence the significance of this binding is uncertain *(7)*. It is also thought that SRY may potentiate SF1 transcrip-tion, increasing SF1's effect on the synthesis of steroidogenic enzymes *(11)*. It has been postulated that SRY functions as an inhibitory factor, repressing the action of a down-stream gene controlling testis determination. This downstream gene may itself be a repres-sor of testis determination; that is, SRY may repress a repressor. In this scenario, the presence of SRY would allow testis determination to proceed, but in the absence of SRY, testis determination would be blocked *(19)*. The identity of this putative downstream repressor is unknown, but may be DAX1 *(20)* or a gene related to SRY known as SOX3 *(21)*.

SOX9. Another member of the SOX group of genes (SRY-like, HMG box genes) that plays a part in early testis differentiation is SOX9 *(7)* (Table 1). Although it is expressed in the urogenital ridge prior to SRY in mice, the expression is increased as testis determi-nation proceeds and becomes confined to Sertoli cells. Because expression is extinguished if the bipotential gonad becomes an ovary, a role for SOX9 in Sertoli cell differentiation is postulated *(15)*. The interaction of SOX9 with other genes important in the developing testis is unclear. It is postulated that SRY may upregulate SOX9 expression in the gonad, promoting Sertoli cell differentiation and subsequent induction of other testis cell lines *(15)*. However, although it is an appealing hypothesis, there is no evidence at present for SRY regulation of SOX9. It has also been proposed that another SOX gene, SOX3, may be a negative regulator of SOX9 expression, and that SRY binding may relieve the inhib-itory effect of SOX3 *(21)*. Again, evidence supporting this theory is lacking.

GATA4. The GATA4 gene, the homolog of which has its earliest expression in the gonadal ridge in mice, is thought to have an ongoing role as testis differentiation pro-ceeds. This gene is expressed in Sertoli cells and, like SOX9, its expression continues in the testis while being suppressed in the developing ovary. In addition, GATA4 has been shown to activate the promotor of the AMH gene in heterologous cells *(12)*.

Embryology and Genetic Regulation of the Ovary

EMBRYOLOGY

In the absence of testis determination, ovarian determination normally occurs (Fig. 2). The earliest sign that the bipotential gonad will become an ovary occurs at approx 7 wk gestation, when cells from the coelomic epithelium of the gonad invade the underlying mesenchyme to form the cortical cords *(1)*. Germ cells become incorporated into these cords and enter prophase I of meiosis at approx 10 wk gestation *(2)*. The cortical cords sub-sequently break up into clusters of cells surrounding each germ cell. These cells secrete a lamina propria and, along with the germ cells, form the ovarian follicles. This process begins in the medullary portion of the gonad and spreads outward toward the epithelium. The precursors of the follicular cells are of the same lineage as the Sertoli cells of the testis *(22)*. Ovarian hilar cells subsequently arise between 12 and 20 wk gestation *(13)*.

GENETIC REGULATION

DAX1. Our understanding of the genetic regulation of ovarian differentiation remains relatively primitive at this time. Although several genes are recognized to participate in

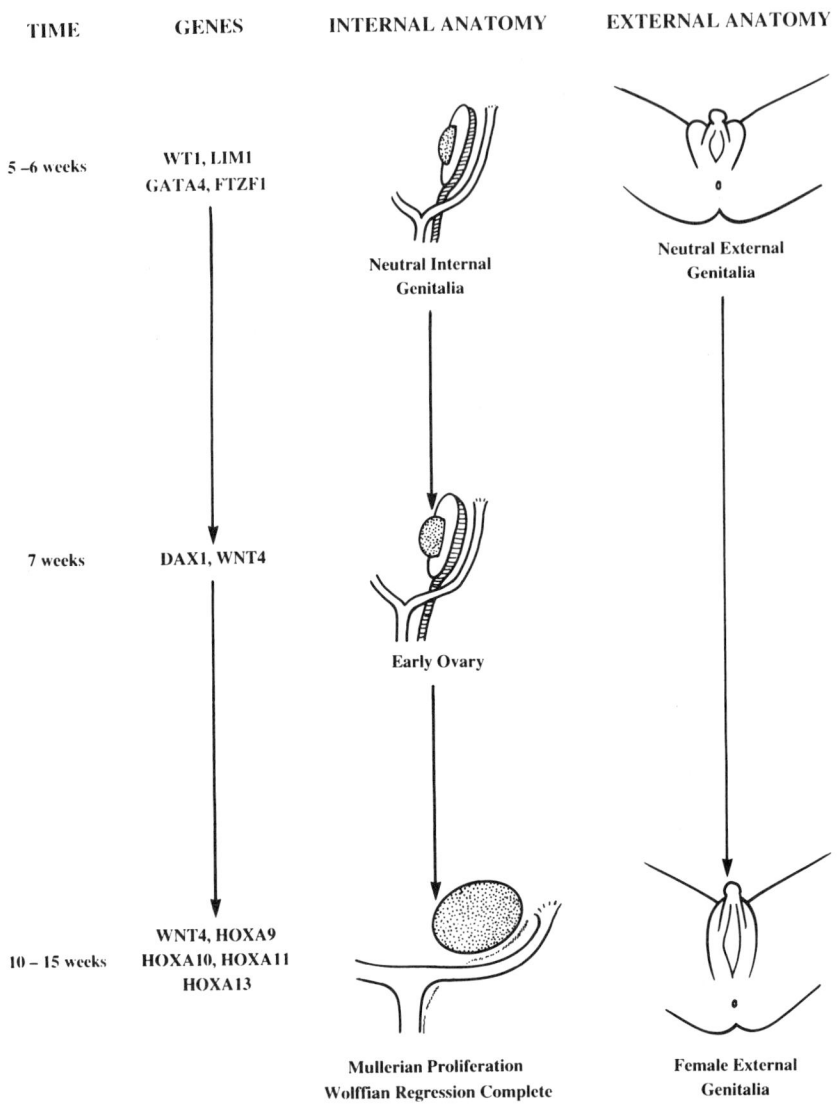

Fig. 2. Timeline of female sexual development, with gestational age, genes thought to be important at various stages, and internal and external anatomy. Internally, the urogenital ridge is flanked by the Wolffian duct and the Müllerian duct. These structures eventually develop into the ovary, Fallopian tubes, uterus and posterior one-third of the vagina in the absence of anti-Müllerian hormone and testosterone. Externally, the genital tubercle lies immediately anterior to the urethral folds and the labioscrotal folds. These structures develop into the normal female genitalia in the absence of androgen.

testis differentiation, only two candidates are felt to be involved in ovarian differentiation. The first of these, the DAX1 gene, is felt to be an "antitestis" gene, whose presence is important in the promotion of ovarian development *(23)* (Table 1). Its homolog in mice is present in gonadal ridge tissue, rapidly disappears if testis determination occurs, but continues if ovarian differentiation proceeds *(20)*. In humans, XY individuals carrying 2 active copies of this gene due to a duplication of the X chromosome have dysgenetic testes. Loss of the DAX1 gene through mutation in XY subjects does not interfere with testis formation, but does lead to hypoplasia of the adrenal glands. This indicates the effects of gene dosage, whereby the presence of zero or one copy of the gene allows testis differentiation to progress, but two copies prevent such differentiation from occurring.

The regulation of DAX1 transcription has been the subject of intense research. It is thought that SF1 may regulate DAX1 expression in a positive fashion, based on the presence of SF1 binding sites in the DAX1 promotor and stimulation of DAX1 expression by SF1 in cultured cell lines *(23)*. In addition, DAX1 may autoregulate, perhaps by inhibition of SF1 stimulation *(24)*. The precise actions of the DAX1 protein also have yet to be fully elucidated. It appears to recognize and bind to hairpin loops of DNA, similar to the nonspecific binding properties of SRY *(24)*. DAX1 seems to be a potent transcriptional repressor of a number of systems, including the actions of SF1 and the synergy of SF1 and WT1 *(23)*. In addition, a number of investigators have theorized that SRY may work in concert with DAX1 in testis determination, either by directly repressing DAX1 transcription and allowing subsequent expression of downstream genes or by competing directly with DAX1 for binding sites in the promotors of downstream genes *(7)*. There is little evidence for these proposals, however. Obviously, much more information needs to be obtained before the full process can be understood.

WNT4. The second candidate gene for ovarian differentiation is WNT4 (Table 1). The WNT family of genes is important in several developmental contexts, particularly in patterning and cell-cell communication *(25)*. In the mouse, Wnt4 appears to be important in ovarian differentiation. This gene appears to inhibit the differentiation of Leydig cells in the developing gonad, hence suppressing androgen biosynthesis. Wnt4 deficient female mice produce inappropriate amounts of testosterone from their ovaries, resulting in masculinization *(26)*.

Other Genes Involved in Gonadal Differentiation

Several other genes have been proposed to participate in gonadal development, but the nature of their actions is unknown *(7)* (Table 1). A locus at the telomeric end of chromosome 9p has long been recognized to be important due to the presence of gonadal dysgenesis in XY subjects with terminal 9p deletions *(27)*. A gene called DMRT1 has been localized to this region. The homologs of DMRT1 in *Caenhorhabditis elegans* and *Drosophila* are known to be involved in sex differentiation, although no mutations of this gene in mammals have been described *(28)*. Other relevant genes are thought to be present on chromosomes 10q and 18p, as deletions of these regions lead to abnormal testis development *(29,30)*. Two other X chromosomal genes, MTM1 and XH2, have also been implicated in testis development, although their molecular actions are not known *(7)*.

Endocrinology of the Testis

AMH SECRETION

As discussed earlier, the earliest morphologic evidence of testis determination is the appearance of Sertoli cells. The Sertoli cells produce the first hormone secreted by the testes, anti-Müllerian hormone (AMH, also called Müllerian inhibiting substance), beginning at 7 wk gestation *(31)*. AMH subsequently acts to disrupt development of the Müllerian ducts (*see* next page). Unlike other hormonal products of the fetal testis, AMH secretion does not appear to be regulated by trophic hormones.

TESTOSTERONE SECRETION

At 8 wk of gestation, approx 1 wk after AMH secretion begins, the fetal testis starts to produce testosterone. Leydig cells require stimulation by hCG to proliferate, differentiate, and produce testosterone in appropriate amounts. The effects of hCG are mediated via the luteinizing hormone/chorionic gonadotropin (LH/CG) receptor on the Leydig cell surface. Pituitary LH is not initially required for testosterone production, and indeed, it is not secreted from the pituitary until 11.5 wk gestation *(32)*. Stimulation of this receptor causes an increase in the transport of cholesterol from the outer to the inner mitochondrial membrane, the rate-limiting step in steroid biosynthesis mediated by the steroidogenic acute regulatory protein (StAR) *(33)*. Inside the mitochondria, the first of a series of enzymatic steps resulting in testosterone synthesis occurs, with subsequent steps taking place in the endoplasmic reticulum. Enzymes important in this pathway include p450scc (side chain cleavage enzyme), 3-β-hydroxysteroid dehydrogenase/$\Delta 5 \rightarrow \Delta 4$ isomerase, P450 c17 (17α-hydroxylase/c17-20 lyase), and 17-β-hydroxysteroid dehydrogenase. Testosterone is then secreted by the Leydig cell and subsequently diffuses into target cells. In the target cells, it may act directly or be enzymatically converted by 5-α-reductase to the more potent androgen, dihydrotestosterone.

The aromatase enzyme is present in fetal testes, but is of unclear significance. Aromatase activity has been detected in the fetal ovary as well, although its importance is not known *(11)*. Aromatase activity is also present in the placenta, serving the important role of protecting XX fetuses from the masculinizing effects of placentally transferred maternal androgens.

Genetic Control of Hormone Production

Many of the enzymes required for sex-hormone production are also required for glucocorticoid and mineralocorticoid production. The genetics of these enzymes will be discussed in the chapter on congenital adrenal hyperplasia. However, some pertinent genes will be discussed here.

AMH

Although not a steroid hormone, AMH plays an important role in male sex differentiation as discussed above (Table 1). The AMH gene is highly conserved across species, particularly in the C-terminal region, which becomes the bioactive portion after proteolytic cleavage *(34)*. The genetic regulation of the AMH gene has not been fully determined. SF1 can bind to the AMH promotor and is thought to influence its expression *(31)*. As AMH is produced in a sex-specific manner and is the earliest secreted product of the testis, the role of SRY in its regulation has been investigated. Although SRY has been shown to bind the AMH promotor *(18)*, it is still not known whether SRY regulates AMH expression. There is also a consensus binding site for the GATA family of transcription factors, but it is not known if GATA4 plays a role in AMH regulation *(35)*.

LHCGR

The gene for the LH/CG receptor is termed LHCGR (Table 1). The protein is a member of the G-protein-coupled superfamily of receptors. As with other such receptors, ligand binding induces a conformational change, eventually allowing release of activated G-protein and subsequent signal transduction.

STAR

The StAR protein controls the rate-limiting step of steroidogenesis, the transfer of cholesterol across the mitochondrial membrane, as mentioned earlier (Table 1). In the absence of StAR protein, steroidogenesis can proceed at a slow rate, with accumulation of cholesterol esters within the steroidogenic cell and subsequent disruption of function *(36)*. Hence, testosterone cannot be produced in normal amounts in the absence of StAR activity. The STAR gene promotor contains a binding site for SF1, and targeted disruption of the FTZF1 gene in mice also produces a lack of STAR expression *(10)*. In contrast, DAX1 appears to be a repressor of STAR gene transcription, acting by binding to hairpin DNA structures in the STAR promotor. It has been postulated that SF1 and DAX1 may have direct protein-protein interactions affecting target genes *(37)*.

FTZF1

SF1 has effects at other levels of steroidogenesis, independent of its effect on the StAR protein. SF1 was first discovered in its role as a transcription factor controlling the activity of the P450 steroid hydroxylases *(38)*. The genes for the enzymes thus far identified as responsive to SF1 all share common regulatory sequences in their promotors. Their promotors have been individually shown to be responsive to binding of these sequences by SF1 *(38)*.

HSD17B3

The final step in biosynthesis of testosterone in the testis is mediated by the enzyme 17-β-hydroxysteroid dehydrogenase. This enzyme exits in five known isoforms *(39)*, with the type 3 isoform controlling the conversion of androstenedione to testosterone in the endoplasmic reticulum of the Leydig cell.

Embryology of the Internal Ducts and External Genitalia

By about 6 wk of gestation, the embryo possesses two sets of ducts, precursors of the male and female internal ducts (Figs. 1, 2). Both sets form initially, regardless of the karyotype of the embryo and the ultimate fate of the bipotential gonads. The Wolffian ducts, precursors of the male system, originate as the excretory ducts of the mesonephros at about 4 wk gestation. They are located lateral to the urogenital ridge and pass caudally. Caudal to the mesonephros, they course medially, then run parallel to each other to reach the urogenital sinus *(13)*. The Müllerian ducts, precursors of the female system, initially form at approx 6 wk of gestation as invaginations of the coelomic epithelium lateral to the Wolffian ducts. These invaginations proceed caudally and medially, becoming closely apposed to the Wolffian ducts. They cross over the Wolffian ducts and meet in the midline to form the uterine canal, which progresses caudally to reach the urogenital sinus, with the Wolffian ducts lying on either side. It is thought that along the distal two-thirds of their course, the Müllerian ducts actually arise from the epithelium of the Wolffian ducts, as the two are enclosed in a common basement membrane *(40)*.

In the XY fetus (Fig. 1), testis determination subsequently occurs, and AMH secretion begins at 7 wk gestation. In the presence of AMH, the Müllerian ducts involute. The timing of this is critical, as the ducts become insensitive to the effects of AMH after 8 wk of gestation *(41)*. Müllerian duct regression correlates with the peak levels of AMH produced *(42)*, and is essentially complete by 10 wk gestation.

In the presence of testosterone, produced from the fetal testis starting at 8 wk gestation, the Wolffian ducts proliferate. Testosterone effects mainly occur in the vicinity of the gonad. Some investigators postulate that testosterone is secreted into the Wolffian duct, which allows it to be concentrated there, promoting its action *(43)*. Under the influence of androgen, the Wolffian duct differentiates into the epididymis, vas deferens, and seminal vesicles.

In the XX fetus (Fig. 2), no testosterone or AMH is produced early in gestation. The Wolffian ducts regress if they are not exposed to androgen by 10 wk of gestation. In the absence of AMH exposure early in gestation, the Müllerian ducts proliferate. It should be noted that the fetal ovary does produce AMH, although its production does not begin until after the period of AMH sensitivity has passed. The function of AMH in the female fetus is not known. The superior parts of the Müllerian ducts eventually differentiate into the Fallopian tube, while the uterine canal differentiates into the uterus, cervix, and upper one-third of the vagina. At the junction of the Müllerian duct with the urogenital sinus, there is a thickening and proliferation of epithelium called the sinovaginal bulb. This tissue elongates and canalizes to form the lower two-thirds of the vagina *(1,40)*.

Analogous to the bipotential gonads, the external genitalia of an XY embryo prior to 8 wk of gestation cannot be distinguished from those of an XX embryo (Figs. 1, 2). Bilateral ridges of tissue form lateral to the urogenital membrane and are known as the urethral folds. These folds meet anteriorly to form a swelling called the genital tubercle. A secondary set of folds develops lateral to the urethral folds, called the labioscrotal folds. Under the influence of androgen, beginning by 8 wk gestation, the genital tubercle elongates to form the phallus. The urethral folds begin to fuse, starting posteriorly and moving anteriorly along the ventral surface of the phallus to form the penile urethra (Fig. 1). The labioscrotal folds increase in size and fuse in the midline to form the scrotum. The differentiation of the external genitalia in the male is complete by 12–13 wk gestation *(13)*. If androgen secretion is delayed past this time, development of the external genitalia cannot be completed, even in the face of normal androgen levels *(13)*. Masculinization of the external genitalia in XY fetuses occurs under the influence of the androgen dihydrotestosterone (DHT), formed from testosterone by the enzyme 5-α-reductase. As discussed earlier, DHT is more potent than testosterone and allows masculinization to occur early in gestation, while testosterone levels are still low.

In the XX embryo (Fig. 2), few changes occur in the appearance of the external genitalia after 6 wk gestation. The genital tubercle enlarges slightly to form the clitoris, while the urethral folds form the labia minora and the labioscrotal folds develop into the labia majora.

Genes Important in the Differentiation of Internal Ducts and External Genitalia

SRD5A2

The gene SRD5A2 encodes for the enzyme 5-α-reductase type 2, responsible for the synthesis of dihydrotestosterone. Mutation of the type 2 isoenzyme may inhibit the synthesis of DHT and impair masculinization of the external genitalia in XY fetuses *(44)*.

ANDROGEN RECEPTOR (AR)

The final link in the chain of events leading to male sex development is the interaction of androgen, either testosterone or DHT, with the androgen receptor. The gene for this receptor (Table 1) is expressed by 9 wk gestation in equal amounts in XX and XY fetuses *(45)*. The AR protein is located in the cytoplasm, but it is translocated to the nucleus upon ligand binding *(46)*. There, it binds to specific DNA sequences of its target genes. A large number of genes are androgen-responsive, some being induced and others repressed *(47)*. In general, morphologic changes caused by androgen action are mediated by the subepithelial mesenchyme, which subsequently involves the overlying epithelium in the differentiation process. The downstream genetic mediators of morphogenesis are not known *(47)*.

EGF

It has been recognized that binding of androgen to the AR is not sufficient by itself to promote male development *(48)*. Epidermal growth factor appears to be an enhancer of AR-mediated transcriptional activity, potentiating the effects of testosterone and DHT *(49)*.

AMHR2

In order for AMH to exert its effects, it must also interact with a receptor. Members of the TGF-β family of transcription factors generally use two receptors for signal transduction. Type 2 receptors are the primary forms which bind ligand, but type 1 receptors are required for signal transduction to occur *(50)*. The gene for the type 2 AMH receptor, AMHR2 has been isolated; however, the gene for a type 1 AMH receptor has not yet been identified *(31)*.

WNT4 AND WNT7A

As discussed earlier in this chapter, the WNT family of genes appears to be involved in sexual differentiation. The Wnt4 gene in mice is required for normal growth of the Müllerian ducts in both male and female animals, based on the study of gene knockout models *(26)*. Another member of the WNT family, Wnt7a, is also required for normal Müllerian duct formation in mice *(51)*. Wnt7a gene expression influences the synthesis of the type 2 AMH receptor in periductal mesenchyme. Wnt7a appears to be expressed in Müllerian duct epithelium, but then signals the mesenchyme to express the AMH receptor *(51)*. Mice lacking the Wnt7a gene have persistence of Müllerian duct structures. No mutations of this gene in humans have been reported yet.

HOXA GENE CLUSTER

Recently, a role in sexual differentiation for the HOX family of genes has been discovered. These genes are responsible for the differentiation of structures along a spatial axis. In vertebrates, there are four clusters of these genes. Within a cluster, the spatial expression of the genes corresponds to the genetic order along the chromosome, with the most 3' gene being the most anteriorly expressed. Each gene product gives its region of expression its own identity by controlling the expression of downstream genes *(52)*. The "A" cluster, consisting of 8 genes, has a role in Müllerian duct development, with HOXA9, HOXA10, HOXA11, and HOXA13 controlling the differentiation of the Fallopian tubes, uterus, cervix, and posterior vagina. The regulation of these genes and the mechanisms controlling their spatial expression are not known *(52)*. Mutation of the HOXA13 gene has been described in humans with abnormalities of Müllerian duct differentiation *(53)*.

ABNORMAL SEXUAL DIFFERENTIATION

Normal sexual differentiation as described earlier requires a multitude of embryologic and physiologic actions to occur in the fetus. Any abnormality of this sequence can lead to abnormal sexual differentiation with overmasculinization of XX individuals or undermasculinization of XY individuals (Table 2). These abnormalities are described in the following sections.

Table 2

Etiologies of Intersex Disorders

I.   Disorders of gonadal differentiation and sex-chromosome abnormalities
     A. Gonadal dysgenesis
          1. 46,XY complete gonadal dysgenesis
          2. 46,XY partial gonadal dysgenesis
          3. 46,XX gonadal dysgenesis
     B. XX maleness
     C. True hermaphroditism
     D. 45,X/46,XY mosaicism
II. Overmasculinization of 46,XX infants
     A. Virilizing congenital adrenal hyperplasia
          1. 21α-hydroxylase deficiency
          2. 11β-hydroxylase deficiency
          3. 3β-hydroxysteroid dehydrogenase deficiency
     B. Maternal androgen exposure
     C. Fetal aromatase deficiency
III. Undermasculinization of 46,XY infants
     A. Abnormal testicular function
          1. Leydig-cell hypoplasia
          2. Defects in testosterone biosynthesis
               a. Feminizing congenital adrenal hyperplasia
                    i.   StAR deficiency (lipoid adrenal hyperplasia
                    ii. 3β-hydroxysteroid dehydrogenase deficiency
                    iii. 17α-hydroxylase/17,20 lyase deficiency
               b. 17β-hydroxysteroid dehydrogenase deficiency
     B. 5α-reductase deficiency
     C. Androgen insensitivity syndrome
          1. Complete androgen insensitivity syndrome
          2. Partial androgen insensitivity syndrome
IV. Other abnormalities of sexual differentiation
     A. Micropenis
     B. Cryptorchidism
     C. Hypospadias
     D. Testicular regression syndrome
     E. Syndromes of multiple congenital anomalies
     F. Persistent Mullerian duct syndrome

Disorders of Gonadal
Differentiation and Sex Chromosome Abnormalities

Gonadal dysgenesis refers to defective embryonic gonadal development and differentiation. There are varying classes of abnormality, often described as complete, incomplete (partial), and mixed gonadal dysgenesis. The etiologies of these disorders are likely related to mutations in various genes playing roles in the control of gonadal differentiation including SRY, SF-1, WT1, DAX-1, SOX9, and others as yet unidentified *(54,55)*. Mosaic karyotypes, such as 45,XO/46,XY, also are associated with defects in gonadal differentiation. Other conditions with abnormal karyotypes, such as Turner syndrome (45,X) and Klinefelter syndrome (47,XXY), are well known to have abnormal germ-cell function and will not be discussed in this chapter.

GONADAL DYSGENESIS

Complete gonadal dysgenesis describes individuals with 46,XY or 46,XX karyotypes and undifferentiated gonadal tissue. In 46,XY complete gonadal dysgenesis there is defective testis determination in the presence of a 46,XY karyotype. This leads to streak gonads without germ cells, persistence of Müllerian structures, absence of Wolffian structures, and female external genitalia (54). 46,XX gonadal dysgenesis can occur if ovarian development does not proceed normally and is also characterized by streak gonads and normal internal and external female genitalia (13). Although these girls have streak gonads, much the same as those with Turner syndrome, they generally lack the phenotypic features of Turner syndrome, such as short stature, pterygium coli, cubitus valgus, and so on. The etiology of 46,XY gonadal dysgenesis has been attributed to mutations in SRY and specific SRY-related genes (56). However, this only explains a minority of the cases, leading to the assumption that mutations in other genes may result in this condition as well (57). The etiology of 46,XX gonadal dysgenesis is unknown, but may be due to mutations in genes related to ovarian maintenance. One possible candidate gene reported by Aittomaki et al. is the follicle-stimulating hormone (FSH) receptor gene, mutations of which were found in cases of 46,XX ovarian dysgenesis (58). Clinical presentation of 46,XY and 46,XX complete gonadal dysgenesis is usually that of normal female genitalia, delayed puberty with poorly developed secondary sex characteristics, and primary amenorrhea (54). Gonadal tumors occur in approx 25–30% of patients with 46,XY gonadal dysgenesis, and arrangements should be made for the removal of gonadal tissue when the diagnosis is made (59). Neoplasia occurs more frequently in dysgenetic gonadal tissue containing Y-bearing cell lines. Treatment with estrogen replacement may be instituted to achieve secondary female sex characteristics in both conditions.

46,XY incomplete (or partial) gonadal dysgenesis is defined by incomplete testis determination with varying degrees of dysgenesis (54). Histologically, the seminiferous tubules are poorly formed and sparsely distributed, with areas of wavy, ovarian-like stroma. The tunica albuginea is frequently thin and poorly developed. There is impairment of both Sertoli and Leydig cell function. Patients usually present with ambiguous genitalia at birth and have a mixture of Wolffian and Müllerian duct structures due to deficient testosterone and anti-Müllerian hormone production (54). Abnormal gonadal differentiation in these individuals and in those with complete gonadal dysgenesis has been ascribed to various gene mutations, but clearly there are unidentified genes involved in this complex process. As outlined previously, these patients have a significant risk of gonadal neoplasia, and early gonadectomy or placement of testes in the scrotum where they may be periodically examined is recommended.

45,X/46,XY KARYOTYPE

45,X/46,XY mosaic karyotypes occur when there is loss of the Y chromosome in one cell line during mitosis. This is usually caused by nondisjunction and is most likely to occur if the Y chromosome is abnormal (54). Gonadal dysgenesis may result, as may true hermaphroditism. The term "mixed gonadal dysgenesis" is used to refer to individuals with a dysgenetic gonad on one side with a normal testis present on the other. 45,X/46,XY individuals may have male, female, or ambiguous genitalia depending on the degree of testis differentiation. However, in a series reported by Chang et al., 95% of 92 prenatally diagnosed patients with 45,X/46,XY mosaicism had normal male genitalia (60). It may be necessary to analyze the chromosomes in gonadal tissue to make the diagnosis, because mosaicism may not exist in all tissues *(13)*. This patient population also carries an increased risk of gonadal tumors, and prophylactic gonadectomy is recommended *(59)*.

TRUE HERMAPHRODITISM

True hermaphroditism occurs in individuals carrying both testicular tissue with seminiferous tubules and ovarian tissue with ovarian follicles. Patients may have a 46,XY, 46,XX, or mosaic karyotype. There may be bilateral ovotestes or various combinations of ovaries, testes, and ovotestes positioned anywhere from the abdomen to the labioscrotum. The most common combination is an ovary and an ovotestis. In a review of 228 cases, 46,XX was the most common karyotype (70.6%), chromosomal mosaicism was the second most common karyotype (20.2%), and 7% had a 46,XY karyotype *(61)*. Genitalia are almost always ambiguous in this patient population. Ovarian tissue and female sex organs can function normally, as pregnancies have occurred; however, seminiferous tubules are often atrophic and spermatogenesis is extremely rare. The etiology of true hermaphroditism is unknown. Cases of XX maleness and 46,XX true hermaphroditism are reported to coexist in the same kindred, implying a genetic mechanism that excludes the role of the Y chromosome in these patients, who were SRY-negative *(62,63)*. Most likely, true hermaphroditism is a genetically heterogeneous condition. Diagnosis is made by biopsy of the gonads and examination of external and internal genitalia. Gonadal tumors occur in approx 10% of patients with 46,XY or 46,XX/46,XY true hermaphroditism and less frequently (4%) in those with 46,XX karyotypes *(59)*.

OTHER CAUSES OF XX MALENESS

46,XX maleness is a condition in which testicular tissue develops in the presence of a 46,XX karyotype. Sometimes called 46,XX sex reversal, this is a genetically heterogeneous condition *(64)*. While some individuals have Y-chromosome sequences translocated to the X chromosome, this is not consistently found in this population *(64)*. It is not known why testis determination occurs in the absence of the SRY gene. Cases of familial XX maleness and 46,XX true hermaphroditism have been shown to coexist in the same pedigree, which suggests there is a shared genetic defect in the two conditions *(62,63)*. Kuhnle et al. *(62)* reported a family in which 46,XX true hermaphroditism and 46,XX maleness coexisted and which exhibited maternal as well as paternal transmission, suggesting the possibility that both autosomal dominant and X-linked dominant inheritance may occur. Clinical presentation is variable, with most having normal male genitalia, but 10–15% exhibiting some form of genital ambiguity or hypospadias *(65)*. Patients with translocated Y sequences may present similarly to patients with Klinefelter syndrome (47,XXY karyotype) *(65)*. Those patients lacking Y chromosomal material have been reported to have more variable presentations, ranging from normal male phenotype to ambiguous genitalia with minimal testicular development and Leydig and Sertoli cell dysfunction *(64)*.

Disorders Causing Masculinization of 46,XX Infants

CONGENITAL ADRENAL HYPERPLASIA

Congenital adrenal hyperplasia (CAH) accounts for the majority of cases of masculinization of 46,XX infants. CAH is caused by a group of autosomal recessive disorders of adrenal steroidogenesis in which there is deficient activity of one of the enzymes necessary for the production of cortisol. Cortisol deficiency causes increased levels of ACTH via lack of the negative feedback to the hypothalamus and pituitary, leading to adrenal hyperplasia and overproduction of adrenal androgens. Virilizing CAH may be caused by 21-hydroxylase deficiency, 11-β-hydroxylase deficiency, or 3-β-hydroxysteroid dehydrogenase deficiency.

21-Hydroxylase Deficiency. 21-hydroxylase deficiency (21-OHD) accounts for more than 90% of CAH and is the most important diagnosis to consider in an intersex infant. Based on newborn screening studies, the classical form of the disease occurs in 1/10,000–1/15,000 live births *(66)*. The clinical presentation of 21-OHD is dependent on the form of disease. In the classical form there is masculinization at birth, with or without salt-wasting. The salt-wasting form accounts for 75% of classic 21-OHD, while the simple-virilizing form accounts for approx 25% of cases *(67)*.

Diagnosis of 21-OH deficiency is supported by increased baseline and ACTH stimulated 17-OH-progesterone and increased serum androgens. Prenatal diagnosis is available via molecular analysis of the CYP21 gene and has been used in conjunction with prenatal dexamethasone treatment of mothers carrying CAH affected fetuses *(68)*. Prenatal treatment has been shown to be efficacious in reducing masculinization of affected females as compared with CAH-affected sisters *(68)*. However, prenatal treatment remains controversial, as ill-desired side effects often occur in the mother and potential long-term risks to the fetus have not been completely established *(68)*.

11β-Hydroxylase Deficiency. 11β-hydroxylase deficiency (11βHD) accounts for about 5% of cases of CAH. Although salt asting may occur in the newborn period, it is less common than in 21OHD. In later infancy and childhood, hypertension may occur due to accumulation of 11-deoxycorticosterone (DOC) and its metabolites *(69)*. The diagnosis is supported by increased baseline and ACTH-stimulated 11-deoxycortisol, DOC, and serum androgens.

3-β-Hydroxysteroid Dehydrogenase Deficiency. 3-β-hydroxysteroid dehydrogenase deficiency (3βHSDD) is the least common form of CAH. Clinical presentation in affected females is usually that of mild masculinization (mild clitoromegaly) secondary to accumulation of DHEA and its peripheral conversion to testosterone via the type I 3βHSD enzyme, with salt-wasting *(70)*. Diagnosis of 3βHSDD is supported by increased ACTH-stimulated Δ_5 steroids (pregnenolone, 17-OH pregnenolone, DHEA).

Exposure to Maternal Androgens

Masculinization of female external genitalia has occurred after exposure to endogenous or ingested maternal androgens during pregnancy *(71,72)*. This may occur due to ingestion of androgenic progestational compounds, maternal androgen-secreting tumors, or maternal congenital adrenal hyperplasia (CAH). Many women with CAH have given birth to normal female infants despite adrenal androgen excess, which is attributed to the protective effect of placental aromatization of androgens to estrogens. However, placental aromatase activity may be insufficient to prevent virilization in all cases, as was reported recently by Zacharin *(73)*.

Aromatase Deficiency

P450arom, which catalyzes the conversion of androgens to estrogens, is found in multiple tissues such as the placenta, gonads, brain, liver, breast, skin, and adipose tissue *(70)*. Aromatase deficiency may lead to an accumulation of maternal and fetal androgens, such as DHEA, which are then converted to androstenedione and testosterone by placental 3βHSD and 17βHSD enzymes. Virilization of both the infant and the mother is usually seen in this extremely rare condition. Furthermore, gonadotropin and androgen levels (testosterone and androstenedione) are elevated while estrogen levels are very low or undetectable. Affected females later develop multicystic ovaries because of elevated gonadotropins and androgens, while affected males have normal sexual maturation. Both sexes have delayed bone maturation, unfused epiphysis, and very tall adult stature *(74)*.

Disorders Causing Under-Masculinization of 46,XY Infants

ABNORMAL TESTICULAR FUNCTION

Leydig Cell Hypoplasia. First described by Berthezene et al. *(75)* Leydig cell hypoplasia is a condition in which there is unresponsiveness to luteinizing hormone (LH) and human chorionic gonadotropin (hCG) secondary to an abnormal LH/CG receptor *(76)*. This results in insufficient production of testosterone and incomplete or absent differentiation of male external genitalia. Multiple loss-of-function mutations of the LH/CG receptor gene have been reported *(77)* that are inherited in an autosomal recessive fashion *(78)*. Patients with Leydig cell hypoplasia have 46,XY karyotypes with phenotypes varying from that of normal female external genitalia to hypospadias and undescended testes *(76)*. Müllerian structures are not present. Testes are undescended, with normal seminiferous tubules but without mature Leydig cells. Secondary sexual characteristics do not develop at puberty. Levels of testosterone and its biochemical precursors are low or undetectable, LH levels are elevated, and there is no steroid hormone response to hCG stimulation testing *(76)*. Therapy needs to be tailored to the individual, as less severe forms may respond to testosterone administration.

Abnormal Androgen Biosynthesis. Deficiencies of enzymes involved in the biosynthesis of testosterone from cholesterol, including StAR, 17α-hydroxylase/17,20-lyase, 3β-hydroxysteroid dehydrogenase (3β-HSD), and 17β-hydroxysteroid dehydrogenase (17β-HSD), are all associated with abnormal differentiation of male genitalia. Furthermore, 5α-reductase deficiency impairs the conversion of testosterone to dihydrotestosterone, leading to undermasculinization of the external male genitalia and genital ambiguity.

StAR Protein Deficiency. StAR facilitates the movement of cholesterol to the inner mitochondrial membrane, and multiple STAR gene mutations have been identified. Clinically, patients with lipoid CAH present between one day and 6 mo of age regardless of chromosomal sex with hyponatremia, hyperkalemia (salt-wasting crisis), and female external genitalia *(79)*. Other clinical and laboratory features include: hypergonadotropic hypogonadism, low serum cortisol and other steroids, high ACTH leading to hyperpigmentation, high plasma renin, and adrenal hyperplasia with foamy cholesterol ester deposits in adrenal cells *(79)*. There is a correlation between the severity of the gene mutation and the age of clinical presentation (salt-wasting), as some mutations may allow residual StAR activity *(79)*.

Cytochrome P450c17 (17α-hydroxylase/17,20 lyase) Deficiency. Cytochrome P450c17 provides two enzymatic functions, 17α-hydroxylase and 17,20-lyase activities *(80)*. P450c17 is encoded by the gene CYP17. Mutations of this gene impair steroid formation in the adrenals and gonads, leading to male pseudohermaphroditism and CAH *(81)*. The 17α-hydroxylase and 17,20-lyase reactions are differentially regulated, and both enzymatic activities may be deficient, or 17,20-lyase alone may be deficient. In isolated 17,20-lyase deficiency, 17α-hydroxylation is relatively unaffected, but 17,20-lyase activity is severely diminished due to gene mutations selectively abolishing 17,20-lyase activity.

Complete deficiency of cytochrome P45017 results in inadequate cortisol and androgen synthesis. Cortisol deficiency then leads to increased secretion of ACTH and accumulation of DOC and corticosterone. Elevated levels of DOC result in hypertension and suppression of the renin-angiotensin system *(81)*. In isolated 17,20-lyase deficiency, cortisol synthesis is normal, but androgen synthesis is deficient. Both forms of this disorder result in female or ambiguous appearing genitalia *(13)*.

3β-Hydroxysteroid Dehydrogenase Deficiency. Complete absence of 3βHSD results in aldosterone, cortisol, and testosterone deficiency. The clinical manifestations of 3βHSD deficiency in XY infants vary from female external genitalia with salt-wasting crises if there is complete deficiency to ambiguous genitalia without salt-wasting if there is partial deficiency *(13)*. The diagnosis is supported by elevated levels of Δ5, 3-β-hydroxysteroids.

17-β-Hydroxysteroid Dehydrogenase-3 Deficiency. 17β-hydroxysteroid dehydrogenase-type 3 (17βHSD-3) is responsible for the conversion of androstenedione to testosterone in the testis. Mutations in the gene for the type 3 isozyme, cause undermasculinization of male genitalia due to inadequate testosterone levels in utero *(82)*.

The clinical presentation of affected XY infants is that of genital ambiguity, often with palpable inguinal gonads, Wolffian structures, and female external genitalia with a blind-ending vagina. Often there is virilization at puberty, which may be due either to increased conversion of androstenedione to testosterone by 17βHSD isozymes other than type 3 or to incomplete deficiency of the 17βHSD type 3 isozyme *(83)*. In some cultures, a male-gender role is then adopted at the time of puberty *(84)*. The diagnosis is suggested by an increased androstenedione/testosterone ratio and elevated LH level. hCG stimulation testing may be useful for diagnosis in the newborn and prepubertal age groups, but is not as helpful in adults. Treatment is determined by the sex of rearing. Patients raised as male may require surgical modification of the genitalia as well as testosterone replacement and possible excision of gynecomastia at the time of puberty. Those raised as female will ultimately require removal of the testes to prevent further virilization. The timing of these operations is controversial, as discussed on page 284.

5α-REDUCTASE DEFICIENCY

5α-Reductase deficiency impairs the conversion of testosterone to DHT, the more potent androgen, leading to undermasculinization of the external male genitalia. Mutations in the gene, SRD5A2, are responsible for the phenotypic findings caused by 5α-reductase deficiency *(85)*. Large kindreds of affected individuals have been reported *(85)*, and there is some evidence of mutational hot spots within the gene causing identical mutations in individuals with different ethnic backgrounds *(86)*.

The clinical presentation of 5α-reductase deficiency in infancy is one of ambiguous or female-appearing external genitalia. Affected infants have normal wolffian structures and abnormal external genitalia, as differentiation of the external genitalia is dependent upon the conversion of testosterone to DHT. Genitalia often consist of a clitoris-like phallus, bifid scrotum, perineal hypospadias, and cryptorchidism. Pubertal virilization occurs, hypothesized to be due to the actions of testosterone at puberty. In cultures where this is socially acceptable, there is often reversal of the gender role during puberty *(87)*. Furthermore, there have been reported cases of fertility *(88)*.

Laboratory data indicating this diagnosis include normal to increased testosterone and LH levels, low levels of DHT, an increased ratio of testosterone to DHT before or after hCG administration, and a demonstrable decrease in 5α-reductase activity in cultured fibroblasts from genital skin *(89)*.

Male sex assignment has been recommended in this patient population *(89)*, with therapy including surgical reconstruction and supplemental androgen treatment. Of course, this is best decided on a case-by-case basis.

ANDROGEN RECEPTOR INSENSITIVITY

Androgen insensitivity syndrome (AIS) occurs because abnormalities of the AR result in complete or partial insensitivity to androgens (testosterone and dihydrotestosterone) and abnormal male sexual differentiation. A wide variety of gene defects may occur, and over 300 specific mutations have been described *(90)*. These mutations may cause complete or partial AIS depending on the location of the mutation within the gene and the resulting function of the receptor.

Wolffian structures and the external genitalia cannot form properly in AIS. Adult patients with complete AIS have a female body habitus, normal feminine breast development, absent or scant axillary and pubic hair, female appearing external genitalia with a blind-ending vagina, and testes which are intra-abdominal or found along the inguinal canal *(13)*. As the testes produce normal amounts of anti-Müllerian hormone, Müllerian structures are not usually found. Unless there is a family history of AIS, discordant prenatal sex chromosome analysis, or palpable testes or inguinal masses in infancy, the diagnosis is usually not made until the postpubertal period, when the patient presents with primary amenorrhea. In contrast, partial AIS may present with a variety of phenotypes. A classification system for partial AIS has been developed consisting of seven grades ranging from normal male phenotype (grade I) to normal female phenotype without pubic or axillary hair (grade VII) *(91)*. At puberty, increased androgen levels may lead to some maturation of the genitalia, anabolic growth, and spermatogenesis in individuals with partial AIS; however, the degree of virilization at puberty is variable *(47)*.

Laboratory investigations in individuals with AIS reveal normal testosterone and LH in prepubertal patients *(91)*. AMH levels are high in these patients, and the use of AMH levels is helpful in diagnosis *(92)*. During and after puberty, the absence of a normally functioning AR leads to increased LH, increased testosterone, and increased aromatization of testosterone to estradiol *(91)*. Binding assays may be performed on cultured fibroblasts from genital skin; however, general mutation screening strategies are replacing these *(93)*.

Individuals with complete AIS are reared as girls and should have gonadectomies in order to reduce the risk of gonadal tumors *(94)*. The timing of gonadectomy is controversial, however. If the gonads are removed before puberty, hormonal therapy to initiate and maintain puberty must be instituted. Another option is to remove the gonads after puberty has begun, allowing for spontaneous breast development. Following gonadectomy, estrogen replacement will be required *(94)*. This option is acceptable because the incidence of gonadal tumors in AIS patients is very low before puberty, and there may be psychological benefits from spontaneous puberty *(13)*. Those infants with partial AIS pose more treatment dilemmas *(94)*, as their response to androgens at puberty cannot be accurately predicted and the effects of prenatal androgen exposure on the brain are uncertain. If the male sex of rearing is contemplated, a short course of testosterone may be useful to determine the responsiveness of the genitalia *(94)*. Testicular tumors may also occur more frequently in individuals with partial AIS, making close follow-up necessary *(95)*.

Other Abnormalities of Sexual Differentiation

MICROPENIS

Micropenis is present when the penis is normally formed, but when fully stretched, measures 2.5 SD below the mean for age (<2.5 cm at birth for a term infant) *(13,96)*. Micropenis must be distinguished from a buried penis in which the penis is of normal size, but is hidden in the suprapubic fat pad. The etiology of micropenis may be hypogonadotropic hypogonadism due to pituitary or hypothalamic disorders or may be due to growth hormone deficiency (GHD), primary testicular deficiency, partial androgen insensitivity, or other unknown causes *(13)*. Levels of gonadotropins and testosterone, the testicular response to hCG stimulation testing, and evaluation of anterior pituitary function may be helpful in defining the etiology. Short courses of testosterone therapy in infancy and childhood may help to attain a normal penile size *(97)*.

CRYPTORCHIDISM

Cryptorchidism occurs when there is failure of testicular descent, bilaterally or unilaterally. The testis is joined to the area of the inguinal canal by a collection of mesenchymal tissue called the gubernaculum. Testicular descent occurs with migration of the gubernaculum and testis toward the bottom of the scrotum. The first stage of testicular descent, which involves swelling of the gubernaculum and testicular descent to the inguinal region, is hypothesized to be controlled by MIS *(98)*. The descent of the testis from the internal inguinal ring to the scrotum appears to be androgen-dependent *(98)*. The pathogenesis of cryptorchidism may be related to abnormalities of the hypothalamic-pituitary-testicular axis, defects in androgen synthesis, androgen insensitivity, or anatomical defects.

HYPOSPADIAS

Hypospadias is incomplete fusion of the penile urethra and is reported to occur in approx 4–8 of 1000 male births, although the true incidence is unknown *(99)*. Hypospadias can be classified as primary (glandular), secondary (penile), or tertiary (perineoscrotal). Tertiary hypospadias is often associated with abnormalities of sexual differentiation; however, primary hypospadias is generally an isolated anomaly. It is recommended that all infants with severe hypospadias undergo a thorough diagnostic evaluation, as many of these patients will have an identifiable etiology *(100)*.

TESTICULAR REGRESSION SYNDROME

The etiology of testicular regression syndrome is unknown. Occurring in 46,XY individuals, there is apparent loss of testicular tissue and cessation of testicular function sometime during or after the embryologic period of male sexual differentiation. Differentiation of the genital ducts, urogenital sinus, and external male genitalia is variable and depends on when testicular function ceases; thus, individuals affected with this disorder have variable phenotypes *(96)*. Invariably, however, they are found to have absent or rudimentary testes. Affected individuals have increased gonadotropin levels secondary to lack of testosterone. AMH levels are useful in determining presence of testicular tissue, as AMH levels are very low in the absence of testes *(92)*.

PERSISTENT MÜLLERIAN DUCT SYNDROME

Persistent Müllerian duct syndrome (PMDS) occurs in 46, XY individuals due to the lack of production or action of anti-Müllerian hormone (AMH). The etiology is a defect of either the AMH gene or the AMH receptor gene, and inheritance is sex-limited autosomal recessive *(101)*. Affected individuals have normally masculinized genitalia, well-developed but undescended testes, normal male genital ducts, and persistence of Müllerian structures *(101)*. With AMH gene defects, there are low serum AMH levels; conversely, with receptor defects, AMH levels are increased *(101)*. These patients do not have obvious phenotypic features and are detected in infancy when undergoing surgical repair of an inguinal hernia or undescended testes. As adults, they may have infertility due to surgical trauma incurred during removal of the Müllerian structures.

SYNDROMES AND MULTIPLE CONGENITAL ANOMALIES

There are several known syndromes of multiple congenital anomalies that are associated with ambiguous genitalia or abnormal sexual differentiation. This section is not meant to be all-inclusive, but to briefly outline some of these anomalies.

Midline anomalies can be associated with abnormal sexual differentiation. Kallman syndrome is the most frequent cause of isolated hypogonadotrophic hypogonadism and is associated with cryptorchidism, small phallus, anosmia, and other midline anomalies *(102)*.

Renal and genital anomalies often are related. Denys-Drash syndrome, caused by a mutation in the Wilm's tumor-suppressor gene (WT1), is associated with XY gonadal dysgenesis and genital ambiguity, progressive renal failure, and Wilm's tumor *(103)*. Also caused by a mutation in WT1, Frasier syndrome is associated with XY karyotype, streak gonads, female external genitalia, progressive glomerulopathy, and gonadoblastoma *(104)*. Interestingly, Wilm's tumor is not a feature of Frasier syndrome. Smith-Lemli-Opitz syndrome is characterized by mental retardation, hypotonia, facial dysmorphisms, limb anomalies including syndactyly, and upper and lower genitourinary tract anomalies including hypospadias, cleft scrotum, and cryptorchidism *(105)*. Syndromes of multiple congenital anomalies that feature renal anomalies, such as VACTERL *(106)* and CHARGE *(107)* syndromes, are also associated with abnormal sexual differentiation.

Robinow syndrome is associated with facial dysmorphism, short stature, and skeletal and genital anomalies *(108)*. The genital anomalies in Robinow syndrome include small phallus or hypoplastic clitoris and cryptorchidism.

EVALUATION

The evaluation of an infant with abnormal sexual differentiation or ambiguous genitalia is an endocrinologic emergency (Fig. 3). The initial contact with the family must be established in a timely, yet sensitive and confidential manner. The complex medical work-up required for diagnosis must be well-coordinated with appropriate consultation including endocrinology, urology, genetics, neonatology, and social work/clergy/patient support quickly initiated.

History

The family and pregnancy histories should be obtained as soon as possible. Family history of other intersex conditions, deaths in early infancy, or infertility may be of significance. Pregnancy history of exposures (drugs, chemicals, or androgens) or of virilization during pregnancy is important to establish.

Physical Examination

A careful and objective physical examination must be performed (Fig. 4) and should include the following observations. The general appearance of the infant (level of con-

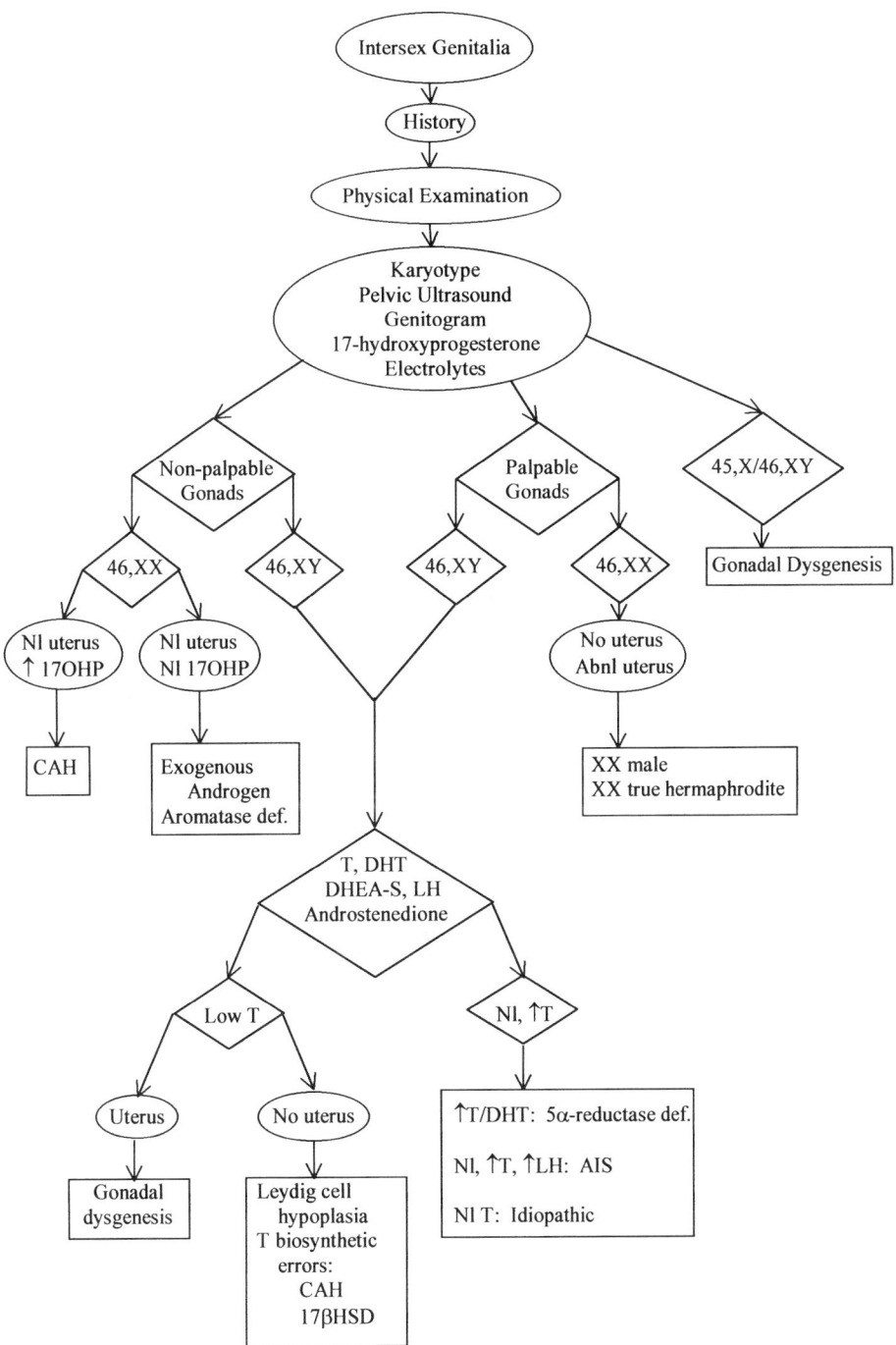

Fig. 3. Algorithm for the evaluation and diagnosis of intersex disorders in children. Nl, normal; Abnl, abnormal; ↑, increased; 17OHP, 17-hydroxyprogesterone; CAH, congenital adrenal hyperplasia; def, deficiency; T, testosterone; DHT, dihydrotestosterone; DHEA-S, dehydroepiandrosterone sulfate; LH, luteinizing hormone; 17βHSD, 17-β-hydroxysteroid dehydrogenase deficiency.

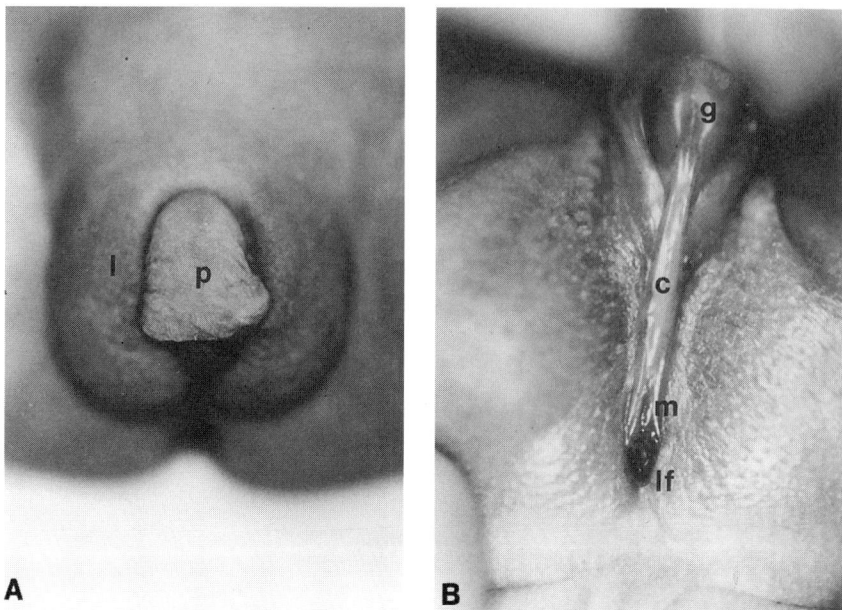

Fig. 4. (**A**) Genitalia of a term infant born with partially masculinized genitalia due to a 45,X/46,XY karyotype and subsequent gonadal dysgenesis. l, labioscrotal fold with mild rugation and pigmentation; p, phallus measuring 2.3 cm in length. (**B**) Same patient as in (A), with phallus lifted to reveal underlying structures. g, glans of phallus; c, chordee; m, urethral meatus; lf, posterior labial fusion partially obscuring a vaginal orifice.

sciousness, perfusion) should be noted. Dysmorphic features or evidence of other anomalies should be noted. Midline structures, face, thorax, abdomen, limbs, anus, and spine should be carefully inspected. The abdomen should be carefully palpated for masses. The presence or absence of palpable gonads in the scrotum or inguinal canal is of utmost importance to note, as this will help to direct the laboratory evaluation. The genitalia should be examined in a careful, objective manner, with specific attention to phallic size and structure, location of the urethral meatus, presence of a vaginal orifice or posterior labial fusion (defined as a ratio of the distance from anus to fourchette/anus to base of clitoris >0.5) *(109)*, presence of rugation of the labioscrotal folds, and the placement of the anus. It is important to note whether the genitalia are symmetrical.

Studies

Imaging studies are very helpful in evaluating the internal genital structures and the kidneys. A pelvic ultrasound should be obtained in an urgent manner in a patient undergoing work-up for ambiguous genitalia and awaiting sex assignment. A genitogram is often useful in evaluating the urethra and the presence of structures such as a urogenital sinus or vagina. These imaging studies will help to document the presence of a uterus or other Müllerian structures, the lack of which indicates AMH secretion from testicular tissue.

Laboratory studies should include a rapid karyotype (fluorescent Y study), which should be obtained and sent to a reliable laboratory as soon as possible. Electrolytes are important to obtain after 24 h of life, looking for salt-wasting as evidence of adrenal insufficiency. 17-hydroxyprogesterone is always indicated in the case of genital ambiguity, as 21-hydroxylase deficiency is the most frequent cause of this condition. If gonads are palpable, the infant is likely to have a 46,XY karyotype, and additional adrenal and testicular hormones including dehydroepiandrosterone, androstenedione, testosterone, and dihydrotestosterone are indicated for diagnosis. ACTH stimulation testing is useful if adrenal hormone levels are borderline or nondiagnostic *(109)*. Other useful diagnostic studies include measurement of gonadotropin levels, AMH, and AR studies. AMH levels can be used to indicate the presence of testes and Sertoli-cell function and are becoming more available as a useful diagnostic tool *(92)*. hCG stimulation testing is useful to evaluate Leydig-cell function and 5α-reductase activity *(109)*. When the aforementioned evaluation fails to indicate a diagnosis, gonadal dysgenesis and true hermaphroditism should be considered. These two diagnoses are dependent on histologic examination of gonadal tissue, hence surgical exploration may be necessary.

ISSUES IN THE MANAGEMENT OF INTERSEX CONDITIONS

Gonadal Tumors

It has long been noted that individuals with intersex disorders are at risk for the development of gonadal tumors. However, this risk appears to be largely confined to patients with gonadal dysgenesis who carry a Y chromosome-bearing cell line. Intersex individuals born without Y chromosome material appear to have no increased risk of gonadal tumors *(59)*. Likewise, patients who have abnormalities of sex differentiation without gonadal dysgenesis (Table 2) appear to have a low rate of gonadal tumor development, approximating that of patients with cryptorchidism. In contrast, it is estimated that the prevalence of gonadal tumors in individuals with a 46,XY karyotype and gonadal dysgenesis is at least 30%, while the risk for 45,X/46,XY patients is 15–20% *(59)*. The most common gonadal tumors are gonadoblastoma and dysgerminoma.

Gonadoblastomas occur almost exclusively in dysgenetic gonads, with only 4% arising in normal gonads. They occur most commonly in the second decade of life, after the onset of puberty, although gonadoblastoma has been reported in infants as young as 15 mo of age *(110)*. Histologically, the tumor contains nests of germ cells mixed with cells from the Sertoli-granulosa-cell lineage. Surrounding these nests, Leydig-cell derivatives may be found in some cases. These tumors may be functional, secreting both testosterone and estrogens. An individual suspected to have 46,XY gonadal dysgenesis who develops signs of sex-hormone secretion should be evaluated for the presence of gonadal tumor.

The etiology of gonadoblastoma is not known. Studies of patients with 45,X/46,XY mosaicism suggest that the tumor arises predominately in cells carrying a Y chromosome *(111)*. A locus on the Y chromosome called GBY (GonadoBlastoma locus on the Y), has been postulated to confer the increased tumor risk *(112)*, although a gene has not yet been isolated.

Dysgerminomas are thought to arise from pre-existing gonadoblastomas. These tumors consist of germ-cell elements alone and are considered malignant. They have a tendency to metastasize, and have a disease-free survival rate of 80% *(113)*. Teratoma, embryonal carcinoma, choriocarcinoma, and endodermal sinus tumor also occur in dysgenetic gonads, making up approx 10% of gonadal tumors *(96)*.

Because of the high risk of gonadoblastoma and malignant degeneration into dysgerminomas, it is usually recommended that dysgenetic gonadal tissue be removed from patients with a Y chromosome-bearing cell line *(59,95)*. This surgery is recommended at the time of diagnosis. In patients assigned a male gender, gonadectomy may not be necessary if the dysgenetic testes are placed in the scrotum. Intrascrotal gonads may be easily palpated, and tumors may be clinically detected at an early stage. Nevertheless, biopsy of the gonad at the time of diagnosis and again at the time of puberty has been recommended in order to detect carcinoma *in situ*, which may precede clinical tumor development *(114)*.

Sex Assignment

In the area of gender assignment, there are several issues that are important to review: the provision of appropriate information to parents and patients, criteria for making gender assignments, and surgical management of the genitalia.

In order to reinforce the assigned gender, it was recommended in the past that individuals with intersex disorders not be informed about their conditions. They may have been told nothing at all or the information may have been presented in a misleading manner. For example, a 46,XY individual with dysgenetic testes who was raised as a female might be told that the gonads needed to be removed because "they were not normal ovaries." However, it is usually impossible to hide information fully from an inquisitive patient, who will often discover the details of the condition. Creating an atmosphere of secrecy in response to a patient's questioning can undermine the trust that is required for any relationship to succeed, be it parent and child or physician and patient. Arguments for hiding patients' diagnoses from them have even appeared recently in the literature *(115)*. However, the current consensus among ethicists is that deception of this sort is unethical *(116)*. There is no ideal time at which to discuss the child's condition with him or her. When it is discussed, it should be at the appropriate developmental level. Formal psychological counselling is recommended for all such patients and their families *(117)*.

Assigning a gender to a child with an intersex disorder is one of the most difficult decisions to be made in Pediatric Endocrinology. Several goals should be considered, such as potential for fertility, future sexual function, and perhaps most importantly, selection of a gender which ultimately will most closely match the preference of the individual patient.

It is important to make a distinction between gender identity and gender role. Gender role refers to actions and statements made by an individual that would indicate gender. Gender identity refers to the experience of one's self as male or female *(118)*. The determinants of gender identity are not fully known. Although it has been taught in the past that gender identity was plastic at birth and was predominantly influenced by parental and societal factors, many now believe that early exposure to sex steroids plays a predominant role, primarily in utero but also possibly in the early postnatal period *(116,119,120)*. Although not directly applicable to humans, a significant amount of evidence from animal models has accumulated that relates prenatal androgen exposure to behavioral variables *(119)*. There are also studies of human exposure to abnormal amounts of androgens in utero *(121)*, but this evidence generally deals with gender role rather than gender identity *(119)*.

There have been three reported cases of hormonally normal XY infants who were reassigned to the female gender in infancy after traumatic loss of the penis *(120,122,123)*. In two of these cases, the individuals subsequently decided to change back to the male gender during adolescence, suggesting that early exposure to androgens influenced their gender identity. There are several series of patients with 5-α-reductase deficiency and 17-β-hydroxysteroid dehydrogenase deficiency in which individuals who were initially assigned to the female gender later changed to male following puberty *(124,125)*. Presumably, these patients also had significant in utero androgen exposure, although less than that of the XY infants with penile trauma. However, cultural influences may have played a large part in these individuals' decisions, as there may have been a significant societal benefit to being male. No such series from developed countries have been published. In addition, although studies of patients with male pseudohermaphroditism from a wide variety of causes have shown that the majority of individuals remain in their assigned gender, a significant number elect to switch *(119)*.

Given the potential effects of prenatal androgen exposure on the establishment of gender identity, how can a gender assignment be made that will match the patient's identified gender following puberty? Unfortunately, there is presently no way to determine how significant this androgen effect will be in a given individual. In the absence of a marker for this effect, the extent of masculinization of the genitalia may be used as a surrogate measure, but evidence supporting this is lacking. Studies to provide such evidence are in progress. The masculinizing effects of androgen on the brain are discussed further in Chapter 13. In any case, careful psychological counseling is important for both the patient and the family, an aspect of care that is frequently omitted *(117)*.

Fertility may be possible for intersex individuals, depending on the specific condition. Obviously, if the treatment involves removal of the gonads, fertility is also sacrificed. However, fertility may be problematic in other situations as well. While women with CAH are generally fertile, the frequency of childbearing does appear to be reduced, particularly among those with the salt-wasting variety of CAH *(126)*. In addition, those intersex infants with testicular tissue assigned to the male gender may require removal of Müllerian duct remnants, potentially disrupting the anastomoses of the vas deferens with the urethra. In many cases of gonadal dysgenesis, all cell lines may be deficient, including Sertoli cells, Leydig cells, and germ cells. In other cases of XY intersex patients, there may be insufficient local concentrations of testosterone to support spermatogenesis in the testes. Regardless of the karyotype, if an adequate uterus is present, pregnancy following in vitro fertilization using a donor egg may be possible.

Satisfactory future sexual function is also a goal when making a gender assignment. In the past, it was the policy in many centers to raise an infant as female if the phallus was less than an arbitrary length, usually 2.5–3.0 SD below the mean *(13,127)*. Recent evidence indicates that males born with micropenis who are treated in infancy and childhood with supplemental testosterone have normal-sized penises in adulthood, many being sexually active and all having male gender identity and normal psychosocial behavior *(97)*. It is not known if these results can be extrapolated to intersex infants. However, even in untreated males with micropenis, sexual function has been reported to be adequate *(128, 129)*. Sexual function in females has focused on the vagina and the ability to have heterosexual intercourse. There are various techniques used to create a vagina or to enlarge an existing vaginal pouch, each with its own advantages *(116)*. However, the function of the clitoris is also important, and some groups advocate not surgically modifying it to achieve a more typical appearance, as surgery may interfere with clitoral sensitivity *(130)*.

In addition to the aforementioned general goals, a number of other factors should be considered in a decision regarding gender assignment.

The karyotype by itself has little impact on the decision regarding gender. However, individuals carrying a 45,X cell line may tend to be shorter than those without a 45,X line. With all else being equal, this may provide some support for the female gender, as it is generally easier in modern society for a female to be short than for a male to be short *(13)*.

Anatomic considerations include the phallic size as discussed previously, the position of the urethral meatus, and the presence of a utriculo-vaginal pouch. An infant assigned as male whose urethral meatus is located on the perineum will require more significant surgery than those with a more distal location, with a higher rate of complications such as fistula formation or stenosis. However, improvements in surgical techniques now allow many of these procedures to be performed successfully as single-stage operations *(131)*. Alternatively, the presence of a large utriculo-vaginal pouch allows easier construction of a vagina in an infant raised as female *(116)* but increases the likelihood of infertility in an infant with testes raised as male *(13)*.

CONCLUSION

Our knowledge of the basic science of sexual differentiation is rapidly expanding. In order to understand the implications of this new knowledge and to apply it clinically, the embryology of the genital system should be understood. Although there is a large number of well-described abnormalities of sexual differentiation, this number will certainly increase in the future, as previously idiopathic conditions become associated with defects of the newly discovered genes. On a broader level, although changes in our treatment of individuals with these conditions have recently occurred, more studies aimed at directing gender assignment and surgical treatment are desperately needed.

REFERENCES

1. Langman J. Urogenital System. Medical Embryology. Williams & Wilkins, Baltimore, MD, 1981, pp. 234–267.
2. Jirasek J. Morphogenesis of the genital system in the human. In: Blandau R, Bergsma D, eds. Morphogenesis and Malformation of the Genital System. Alan Liss, New York, 1977, pp. 13–40.
3. Pritchard-Jones K, Fleming S, Davidson D, et al. The candidate Wilms' tumour gene is involved in genitourinary development. Nature 1990;346:194–197.
4. Kreidberg JA, Sariola H, Loring JM, et al. WT-1 is required for early kidney development. Cell 1993; 74:679–691.
5. Clarkson PA, Davies HR, Williams DM, Chaudhary R, Hughes IA, Patterson MN. Mutational screening of the Wilms's tumour gene, WT1, in males with genital abnormalities. J Med Genet 1993;30:767–772.
6. Little M, Wells C. A clinical overview of WT1 gene mutations. Hum Mutat 1997;9:209–225.
7. Lim HN, Hawkins JR. Genetic control of gonadal differentiation. Baillieres Clin Endocrinol Metab 1998;12:1–16.
8. Barnes JD, Crosby JL, Jones CM, Wright CV, Hogan BL. Embryonic expression of Lim-1, the mouse homolog of Xenopus Xlim-1, suggests a role in lateral mesoderm differentiation and neurogenesis. Dev Biol 1994;161:168–178.
9. Shawlot W, Behringer RR. Requirement for Lim1 in head-organizer function. Nature 1995;374:425–430.
10. Caron KM, Clark BJ, Ikeda Y, Parker KL. Steroidogenic factor 1 acts at all levels of the reproductive axis. Steroids 1997;62:53–56.
11. Migeon CJ, Wisniewski AB. Sexual differentiation: from genes to gender. Horm Res 1998;50:245–251.
12. Viger RS, Mertineit C, Trasler JM, Nemer M. Transcription factor GATA-4 is expressed in a sexually dimorphic pattern during mouse gonadal development and is a potent activator of the Müllerian inhibiting substance promoter. Development 1998;125:2665–2675.
13. Migeon CJ, Berkovitz GD, Brown TR. Sexual differentiation and ambiguity. In: Kappy MS, Blizzard RE, Migeon CJ, eds. Wilkins The Diagnosis and Treatment of Endocrine Disorders in Childhood and Adolescence. Charles C. Thomas, Springfield, IL, 1994, pp. 573–715.
14. Styne D. The testis: disorders of sexual differentiation and puberty. In: Sperling M, ed. Pediatric Endocrinology. WB Saunders Company, Philadelphia, PA, 1996, pp. 423–476.

15. Morais da Silva S, Hacker A, Harley V, Goodfellow P, Swain A, Lovell-Badge R. Sox9 expression during gonadal development implies a conserved role for the gene in testis differentiation in mammals and birds. Nat Genet 1996;14:62–68.

16. Migeon CJ, Berkovitz GD, Brown TR. Sexual differentiation and ambiguity. In: Kappy MS, Blizzard RE, Migeon CJ, eds. Wilkins the Diagnosis and Treatment of Endocrine Disorders in Childhood and Adolescence. Charles C. Thomas, Springfield, IL, 1994, p. 586.

17. Palmer SJ, Burgoyne PS. In situ analysis of fetal, prepuberal and adult XX–XY chimaeric mouse testes: Sertoli cells are predominantly, but not exclusively, XY. Development 1991;112:265–268.

18. Haqq CM, King CY, Donahoe PK, Weiss MA. SRY recognizes conserved DNA sites in sex-specific promoters. Proc Natl Acad Sci USA 1993;90:1097–1101.

19. McElreavey K, Vilain E, Abbas N, Herskowitz I, Fellous M. A regulatory cascade hypothesis for mammalian sex determination: SRY represses a negative regulator of male development. Proc Natl Acad Sci USA 1993;90:3368–3372.

20. Swain A, Zanaria E, Hacker A, Lovell-Badge R, Camerino G. Mouse Dax1 expression is consistent with a role in sex determination as well as in adrenal and hypothalamus function. Nat Genet 1996;12:404–409.

21. Graves JA. Two uses for old SOX [news; comment]. Nat Genet 1997;16:114–115.

22. Burgoyne PS, Buehr M, McLaren A. XY follicle cells in ovaries of XX–XY female mouse chimaeras. Development 1988;104:683–688.

23. Goodfellow PN, Camerino G. DAX-1, an 'antitestis' gene. Cell Mol Life Sci 1999;55:857–863.

24. Zazopoulos E, Lalli E, Stocco DM, Sassone-Corsi P. DNA binding and transcriptional repression by DAX-1 blocks steroidogenesis. Nature 1997;390:311–315.

25. Miller C, Pavlova A, Sassoon DA. Differential expression patterns of Wnt genes in the murine female reproductive tract during development and the estrous cycle. Mech Dev 1998;76:91–99.

26. Vainio S, Heikkila M, Kispert A, Chin N, McMahon AP. Female development in mammals is regulated by Wnt-4 signalling. Nature 1999;397:405–409.

27. Bennett CP, Docherty Z, Robb SA, Ramani P, Hawkins JR, Grant D. Deletion 9p and sex reversal. J Med Genet 1993;30:518–520.

28. Raymond CS, Shamu CE, Shen MM, et al. Evidence for evolutionary conservation of sex-determining genes. Nature 1998;391:691–695.

29. Wilkie AO, Campbell FM, Daubeney P, et al. Complete and partial XY sex reversal associated with terminal deletion of 10q: report of 2 cases and literature review. Am J Med Genet 1993;46:597–600.

30. Telvi L, Bernheim A, Ion A, Fouquet F, Le Bouc Y, Chaussain JL. Gonadal dysgenesis in del (18p) syndrome. Am J Med Genet 1995;57:598–600.

31. Rey R, Picard JY. Embryology and endocrinology of genital development. Baillieres Clin Endocrinol Metab 1998;12:17–33.

32. Thliveris JA, Currie RW. Observations on the hypothalamo-hypophyseal portal vasculature in the developing human fetus. Am J Anat 1980;157:441–444.

33. Kallen CB, Arakane F, Christenson LK, Watari H, Devoto L, Strauss JF III. Unveiling the mechanism of action and regulation of the steroidogenic acute regulatory protein. Mol Cell Endocrinol 1998;145:39–45.

34. Lee MM, Donahoe PK. Müllerian inhibiting substance: a gonadal hormone with multiple functions. Endocr Rev 1993;14:152–164.

35. Lane AH, Donahoe PK. New insights into Müllerian inhibiting substance and its mechanism of action. J Endocrinol 1998;158:1–6.

36. Bose HS, Sugawara T, Strauss JF III, Miller WL. The pathophysiology and genetics of congenital lipoid adrenal hyperplasia. International Congenital Lipoid Adrenal Hyperplasia Consortium. N Engl J Med 1996;335:1870–1878.

37. Swain A, Narvaez V, Burgoyne P, Camerino G, Lovell-Badge R. Dax1 antagonizes Sry action in mammalian sex determination. Nature 1998;391:761–767.

38. Parker KL, Schimmer BP. Steroidogenic factor 1: a key determinant of endocrine development and function. Endocr Rev 1997;18:361–377.

39. Andersson S, Moghrabi N. Physiology and molecular genetics of 17 beta-hydroxysteroid dehydrogenases. Steroids 1997;62:143–147.

40. Ludwig KS. The Mayer-Rokitansky-Kuster syndrome. An analysis of its morphology and embryology. Part II: Embryology. Arch Gynecol Obstet 1998;262:27–42.

41. Taguchi O, Cunha GR, Lawrence WD, Robboy SJ. Timing and irreversibility of Müllerian duct inhibition in the embryonic reproductive tract of the human male. Dev Biol 1984;106:394–398.

42. Rey R, al-Attar L, Louis F, et al. Testicular dysgenesis does not affect expression of anti-Müllerian hormone by Sertoli cells in premeiotic seminiferous tubules. Am J Pathol 1996;148:1689–1698.

43. Tong SY, Hutson JM, Watts LM. Does testosterone diffuse down the wolffian duct during sexual differentiation? J Urol 1996;155:2057–2059.

44. Thigpen AE, Davis DL, Milatovich A, et al. Molecular genetics of steroid 5 alpha-reductase 2 deficiency. J Clin Invest 1992;90:799–809.

45. Kalloo NB, Gearhart JP, Barrack ER. Sexually dimorphic expression of estrogen receptors, but not of androgen receptors in human fetal external genitalia. J Clin Endocrinol Metab 1993;77:692–698.

46. Georget V, Lobaccaro JM, Terouanne B, Mangeat P, Nicolas JC, Sultan C. Trafficking of the androgen receptor in living cells with fused green fluorescent protein-androgen receptor. Mol Cell Endocrinol 1997;129:17–26.

47. Hiort O, Holterhus PM, Nitsche EM. Physiology and pathophysiology of androgen action. Baillieres Clin Endocrinol Metab 1998;12:115–132.

48. Gupta C, Chandorkar A, Nguyen AP. Activation of androgen receptor in epidermal growth factor modulation of fetal mouse sexual differentiation. Mol Cell Endocrinol 1996;123:89–95.

49. Gupta C. Modulation of androgen receptor (AR)-mediated transcriptional activity by EGF in the developing mouse reproductive tract primary cells. Mol Cell Endocrinol 1999;152:169–178.

50. Massague J. TGFbeta signaling: receptors, transducers, and Mad proteins. Cell 1996;85:947–950.

51. Parr BA, McMahon AP. Sexually dimorphic development of the mammalian reproductive tract requires Wnt-7a. Nature 1998;395:707–710.

52. Taylor HS, Vanden Heuvel GB, Igarashi P. A conserved Hox axis in the mouse and human female reproductive system: late establishment and persistent adult expression of the Hoxa cluster genes. Biol Reprod 1997;57:1338–1345.

53. Mortlock DP, Innis JW. Mutation of HOXA13 in hand-foot-genital syndrome. Nat Genet 1997;15:179–180.

54. Berkovitz GD, Seeherunvong T. Abnormalities of gonadal differentiation. Bailliere's Clin Enocrinol Metab 1998;12:133–142.

55. Lim HN, Hawkins JR. Genetic control of gonadal differentiation. Baillierre's Clin Endocrinol Metab 1998;12:1–15.

56. Lim HN, Freestone SH, Romero D, Kwok C, Hughes IA, Hawkins JR. Candidate genes in complete and partial XY sex reversal: mutation analysis of SRY, SRY-related genes and FTZ-F1. Mol Cell Endocrinol 1998;140:51–58.

57. Scherer G, Held M, Erdel M, et al. Three novel SRY mutations in XY gonadal dysgenesis and the enigma of XY gonadal dysgenesis cases without SRY mutations. Cytogenet Cell Genet 1998;80:188–192.

58. Aittomaki K, Lucena JL, Pakarinen P, et al. Mutation in the follicle-stimulating hormone receptor gene causes hereditary hypergonadotropic ovarian failure. Cell 1995;82:959–968.

59. Verp MS, Simpson JL. Abnormal sexual differentiation and neoplasia. Cancer Genet Cytogenet 1987; 25:191–218.

60. Chang HJ, Clark RD, HB. The phenotype of 45,X/46,XY mosaicism: an analysis of 92 prenatally diagnosed cases. Am J Human Genet 1990;46:156–167.

61. Krob G, Braun A, Kuhnle U. True hermaphroditism: geographical distribution, clinical findings, chromosomes and gonadal histology. Eur J Pediatr 1994;153:2–10.

62. Kuhnle U, Schwarz HP, Lohrs U, Stengel-Ruthkowski S, Cleve H, Braun A. Familial true hermaphroditism: paternal and maternal transmission of true hermaphroditism (46,XX) and XX maleness in the absence of Y-chromosomal sequences. Human Genet 1993;92:571–576.

63. Slaney SF, Chalmer IJ, Affara NA, Chitty LS. An autosomal or X linked mutation results in true hermaphrodites and 46,XX males in the same family. J Med Genet 1998;35:17–22.

64. Fechner PY, Marcantonio SM, Jaswaney V, et al. The role of the sex-determining region Y gene in the etiology of 46.XX maleness. J Clin Endocrinol Metab 1993;76:690–695.

65. de la Chapelle A. Analytic review: nature and origin of males with XX sex chromosomes. Am J Human Genet 1972;24:71–105.

66. Speiser PW, White PC. Congenital adrenal hyperplasia due to steroid 21-hydroxylase deficiency. Clin Endocrinol 1998;49:411–417.

67. Pang S, Clark A. Congenital adrenal hyperplasia due to 21-hydroxylase deficiency: newborn screening and its relationship to the diagnosis and treatment of the disorder. Screening 1993;2:105.

68. Mercado AB, Wilson RC, Cheng KC, Wei JQ, New MI. Prenatal treatment and diagnosis of congenital adrenal hyperplasia. J Clin Endocrinol Metab 1995;80:2014–2020.

69. White PC, Curnow KM, Pascoe I. Disorders of steroid 11 beta-hydroxylase isozymes. Endocr Rev 1994;15:421–438.

70. Hughes IA. The masculinized female and investigation of abnormal sexual development. Bailliere's Clin Endocrinol Metab 1998;12:157–171.

71. Kirk JM, Perry L, Shand W, Kirk BR, Besser G, Savage M. Female pseudohermaphroditism due to a maternal adreno-cortical tumour. J Clin Endocrinol Metab 1990;70:1280–1284.

72. Grumbach MM, Ducharme JR. The effects of androgens on fetal sexual development. Fertil Steril 1960;11:157–180.

73. Zacharin M. Fertility and its complications in a patient with salt losing congenital adrenal hyperplasia. J Pediatr Endocrinol Metab 1999;12:89–94.

74. MacGillivray MH, Morishima A, Conte F, Grumbach M, Smith EP. Pediatric endocrinology update: an overview. The essential roles of estrogens in pubertal growth, epiphyseal fusion and bone turnover: lessons from mutations in the genes for aromatase and the estrogen receptor. Horm Res 1998;49:2–8.

75. Berthezene F, Forest MG, Grimaud JA, Claustrat B, Mornex R. Leydig-cell agenesis: a cause of male pseudohermaphroditism. N Engl J Med 1976;295:969–972.

76. Chan W. Molecular genetic, biochemical, and clinical implications of gonadotropin receptor mutations. Mol Genet Metab 1998;63:75–84.

77. Laue LL, Wu SM, Kudo M, et al. Compound heterozygous mutations of the luteinizing hormone receptor gene in Leydig cell hypoplasia. Mol Endocrinol 1996;10:987–997.

78. Saldanha PH, Arnhold IJP, Mendonca BB, Bloisse W, Toledo SPA. A clinico-genetic investigation of Leydig cell hypoplasia. Am J Med Genet 1987;26:337–344.

79. Miller WL, Strauss III JF. Molecular pathology and mechanism of action of the steroidogenic acute regulatory protein, StAR. J Steroid Biochem Mol Biol 1999;69:131–141.

80. Miller WL. Early steps in androgen biosynthesis: from cholesterol to DHEA. Bailliere's Clin Endocrinol Metab 1998;12:67–81.

81. Yanase T, Simpson ER, Waterman MR. 17α-hydroxylase/17,20-lyase deficiency from clinical investigation to molecular definition. Endocr Rev 1991;12:91–107.

82. Andersson S, Geissler WM, Wu L, et al. Molecular genetics and pathophysiology of 17 beta hydroxysteroid dehydrogenase 3 deficiency. J Clin Endocrinol Metab 1996;81:130–136.

83. Andersson S, Russell DW, Wilson JD. 17β-hydroxysteroid dehydrogenase 3 deficiency. Trends Endocrinol Metab 1996;7:121–126.

84. Eckstein B, Cohen S, Farkas A, Rosler A. The nature of the defect in familial male pseudohermaphroditism in Arabs of Gaza. J Clin Endocrinol Metab 1989;68:477–485.

85. Andersson S, Berman DM, Jenkins EP, Russell DW. Deletion of steroid 5α-reductase 2 gene in male pseudohermaphroditism. Nature 1991;354:159–161.

86. Canto P, Vilchis F, Chavez B, et al. Mutations of the 5 alpha-reductase type 2 gene in eight Mexican patients from six different pedigrees with 5 alpha-reductase-2 deficiency. Clin Endocrinol (Oxf) 1997; 46:155–160.

87. Herdt GH, Davidson J. The Sambia "turnim-man": sociocultural and clinical aspects of gender formation in male pseudohermaphrodites with 5-alpha-reductase deficiency in Papua New Guinea. Arch Sex Behav 1988;17:33–56.

88. Katz MD, Kligman I, Cai LQ, et al. Paternity by intrauterine insemination with sperm from a man with 5alpha-reductase-2 deficiency. N Engl J Med 1997;336:994–997.

89. Zhu YS, Katz MD, Imperato-McGinley J. Natural potent androgens: lessons from human genetic models. Bailliere's Clin Endocrinol Metab 1998;12:83–113.

90. Gottlieb B, Trifiro M, Lumbroso R, Pinsky L. The androgen receptor gene mutations database. Nucleic Acids Res 1997;25:158–162.

91. Quigley CA, De Bellis A, Marschke KB, el-Awady MK, Wilson EM, French FS. Androgen receptor defects: historical, clinical, and molecular perspectives. Endocr Rev 1995;16:271–321.

92. Rey RA, Belville C, Nihoul-Fekete C, et al. Evaluation of gonadal function in 107 intersex patients by means of serum antiMüllerian hormone measurement. J Clin Endocrinol Metab 1999;84:627–631.

93. Marcelli M, Tilley WD, Wilson CM, Griffin JE, Wilson JD, McPhaul MJ. Definition of the human androgen receptor gene structure permits the identification of mutations that cause androgen resistance: premature termination of the receptor protein at amino acid residue 588 causes complete androgen resistance. Mol Endocrinol 1990;4:1105–1116.

94. Wiener JS, Teague JL, Roth DR, Gonzales ET Jr, Lamb DJ. Molecular biology and function of the androgen receptor in genital development. J Urol 1997;157:1377–1386.

 95. Manuel M, Katayama PK, Jones HW Jr. The age of occurrence of gonadal tumors in intersex patients with a Y chromosome. Am J Obstet Gynecol 1976;124:293–300.
 96. Grumbach MM, Conte FA. Disorders of sex differentiation. In: Wilson JD, Foster DW, Kronenberg HM, Larsen PR, eds. Williams Textbook of Endocrinology. WB Saunders, Philadelphia, PA, 1998, pp. 1303–1426.
 97. Bin-Abbas B, Conte FA, Grumbach MM, Kaplan SL. Congenital hypogonadotropic hypogonadism and micropenis: effect of testosterone treatment on adult penile size why sex reversal is not indicated. J Pediatr 1999;134:579–583.
 98. Clarnette TD, Sugita Y, Hutson JM. Genital anomalies in human and animal models reveal the mechanisms and hormones governing testicular descent. Br J Urol 1997;79:99–112.
 99. Paulozzi LJ, Erickson JD, Jackson RJ. Hypospadias trends in two US surveillance systems. Pediatrics 1997;100:831–834.
100. Albers N, Ulrichs C, Gluer S, et al. Etiologic classification of severe hypospadias: implications for prognosis and management [see comments]. J Pediatr 1997;131:386–392.
101. Josso N, Picard JY, Imbeaud S, di Clemente N, Rey R. Clinical aspects and molecular genetics of the persistent Müllerian duct syndrome. Clin Endocrinol (Oxf) 1997;47:137–144.
102. Dissaneevate P, Warne GL, Zacharin MR. Clinical evaluation in isolated hypogonadotrophic hypogonadism (Kallmann syndrome). J Pediatr Endocrinol Metab 1998;11:631–638.
103. Gallo GE, Chemes HE. The association of Wilms' tumor, male pseudohermaphroditism and diffuse glomerular disease (Drash syndrome): report of eight cases with clinical and morphologic findings and review of the literature. Pediatr Pathol 1987;7:175–189.
104. Barbaux S, Niaudet P, Gubler MC, et al. Donor splice-site mutations in WT1 are responsible for Frasier syndrome. Nat Genet 1997;17:467–470.
105. Joseph DB, Uehling DT, Gilbert E, Laxova R. Genitourinary abnormalities associated with the Smith-Lemli-Opitz syndrome. J Urol 1987;137:719–721.
106. Schuler L, Salzano FM. Patterns in multimalformed babies and the question of the relationship between sirenomelia and VACTERL. Am J Med Genet 1994;49:29–35.
107. Ragan DC, Casale AJ, Rink RC, Cain MP, Weaver DD. Genitourinary anomalies in the CHARGE association. J Urol 1999;161:622–625.
108. Schorderet DF, Dahoun S, Defrance I, Nussle D, Morris MA. Robinow syndrome in two siblings from consanguineous parents. Eur J Pediatr 1992;151:586–589.
109. Anhalt H, Neely EK, Hintz RL. Ambiguous genitalia. Pediatr Rev 1996;17:213–220.
110. Olsen MM, Caldamone AA, Jackson CL, Zinn A. Gonadoblastoma in infancy: indications for early gonadectomy in 46XY gonadal dysgenesis. J Pediatr Surg 1988;23:270–271.
111. Iezzoni JC, Von Kap-Herr C, Golden WL, Gaffey MJ. Gonadoblastomas in 45,X/46,XY mosaicism: analysis of Y chromosome distribution by fluorescence in situ hybridization. Am J Clin Pathol 1997; 108:197–201.
112. Page DC. Hypothesis: a Y-chromosomal gene causes gonadoblastoma in dysgenetic gonads. Development 1987;101:151–155.
113. Casey AC, Bhodauria S, Shapter A, Nieberg R, Berek JS, Farias-Eisner R. Dysgerminoma: the role of conservative surgery. Gynecol Oncol 1996;63:352–357.
114. Muller J, Skakkebaek NE. Testicular carcinoma in situ in children with the androgen insensitivity (testicular feminisation) syndrome. BMJ (Clin Res Ed) 1984;288:1419–1420.
115. Natarajan A. Medical ethics and truth telling in the case of androgen insensitivity syndrome. CMAJ 1996;154:568–570.
116. Schober JM. Long-term outcomes and changing attitudes to intersexuality. BJU Int 1999;83(Suppl) 3:39–50.
117. Diamond M, Sigmundson HK. Management of intersexuality. Guidelines for dealing with persons with ambiguous genitalia. Arch Pediatr Adolesc Med 1997;151:1046–1050.
118. Money J. Hormones, hormonal anomalies, and psychologic health care. In: Kappy M, Blizzard R, Migeon C, eds. Wilkins the Diagnosis and Treatment of Endocrine Disorders in Childhood and Adolescence. Charles C. Thomas, Springfield, IL, 1994, pp. 1141–1178.
119. Meyer-Bahlburg HF. Gender assignment and reassignment in 46,XY pseudohermaphroditism and related conditions. J Clin Endocrinol Metab 1999;84:3455–3458.
120. Diamond M, Sigmundson HK. Sex reassignment at birth. Long-term review and clinical implications [see comments]. Arch Pediatr Adolesc Med 1997;151:298–304.

121. Berenbaum SA. Effects of early androgens on sex-typed activities and interests in adolescents with congenital adrenal hyperplasia. Horm Behav 1999;35:102–110.

122. Bradley SJ, Oliver GD, Chernick AB, Zucker KJ. Experiment of nurture: ablatio penis at 2 months, sex reassignment at 7 months, and a psychosexual follow-up in young adulthood. Pediatrics 1998;102:e9.

123. Dittmann RW. Ambiguous genitalia, gender-identity problems, and sex reassignment. J Sex Marital Ther 1998;24:255–271.

124. Imperato-McGinley J, Guerrero L, Gautier T, Peterson RE. Steroid 5alpha-reductase deficiency in man: an inherited form of male pseudohermaphroditism. Science 1974;186:1213–1215.

125. Rosler A, Kohn G. Male pseudohermaphroditism due to 17 beta-hydroxysteroid dehydrogenase deficiency: studies on the natural history of the defect and effect of androgens on gender role. J Steroid Biochem 1983;19:663–674.

126. Mulaikal RM, Migeon CJ, Rock JA. Fertility rates in female patients with congenital adrenal hyperplasia due to 21-hydroxylase deficiency. N Engl J Med 1987;316:178–182.

127. Newman K, Randolph J, Anderson K. The surgical management of infants and children with ambiguous genitalia. Lessons learned from 25 years. Ann Surg 1992;215:644–653.

128. van Seters AP, Slob AK. Mutually gratifying heterosexual relationship with micropenis of husband. J Sex Marital Ther 1988;14:98–107.

129. Reilly JM, Woodhouse CR. Small penis and the male sexual role. J Urol 1989;142:569–571; discussion 572.

130. Diamond M. Pediatric management of ambiguous and traumatized genitalia. J Urol 1999;162:1021–1028.

131. Glassberg KI. Gender assignment and the pediatric urologist [editorial; comment]. J Urol 1999;161:1308–1310.

13 Prenatal Androgens and Sexual Differentiation of Behavior

Sheri A. Berenbaum, PhD

INTRODUCTION

There is now little doubt that sex-steroid hormones affect human behavioral sexual differentiation, much as they affect physical sexual differentiation. The ubiquity, magnitude, and complexity of the behavioral effects of these hormones have important implications for the management of children with endocrine conditions. This chapter provides a discussion of this topic, including the evidence for the behavioral effects of sex-steroid hormones present during early development periods, the significance of this evidence for current controversies in pediatric medicine regarding the best treatment for children with intersex conditions, and speculations about the mechanisms mediating the behavioral effects of sex steroid hormones.

Much of the rationale for studying hormonal influences on human behavior comes from studies in nonhuman mammals showing that gonadal hormones exert powerful influences on sex-typed behavior, paralleling their effects on physical characteristics. Behavioral variations associated with early hormones have been demonstrated in many ways in other mammalian species, including experimental manipulation of hormones and examination of subtle naturally occurring hormonal variations related to intrauterine position *(1–5)*.

From: *Contemporary Endocrinology: Developmental Endocrinology: From Research to Clinical Practice*
Edited by: E. A. Eugster and O. H. Pescovitz © Humana Press Inc., Totowa, NJ

EVIDENCE FOR ANDROGEN
EFFECTS ON HUMAN BEHAVIOR

The evidence for human behavioral effects of sex-steroid hormones comes primarily from individuals with intersex conditions, in whom there is discordance among aspects of sexual differentiation. The behavior of intersex individuals has been of interest for a long time, and early reports about these individuals have played a role in their treatment (e.g., ref. 6). There is increasing recognition, however, of the limitations of early reports, especially with respect to sample bias (of particular concern is loss of subjects with unusual histories); the objectivity, reliability, and validity of the measures used; the comparison groups; and statistical power for detecting differences between intersex and comparison individuals. Therefore, most of the compelling evidence about behavioral effects of sex hormones comes from contemporary studies of intersex individuals using good methodology. In recent years, there have also been studies of normal participants with typical variations in prenatal hormones, providing important converging evidence for studies in clinical populations (for other reviews, *see* refs. *7,8*).

The most commonly studied intersex condition is congenital adrenal hyperplasia due to 21-hydroxylase deficiency (CAH). CAH is relatively common (occurring in about 1 in 10,000–15,000 live births and accounting for most cases of intersexuality) and relatively uncomplicated. Not surprisingly, then, most of the evidence regarding behavioral effects of sex-steroid hormones comes from studies of individuals with CAH. There are numerous case reports, but few systematic studies, of individuals with other intersex conditions. Therefore, studies in CAH will be the focus of this chapter, with systematic data from other forms of intersexuality discussed when they are available.

Individuals with CAH provide a unique opportunity to examine the behavioral effects of early androgens. The inability to synthesize cortisol (caused by a mutation in the gene coding 21-OH) results in production of high levels of adrenal androgens beginning early in gestation and continuing throughout gestation; once a diagnosis is made, usually in the early neonatal period, patients with CAH are treated with corticosteroids, which normalize androgen levels (for reviews, *see* ref. *9,10*). Thus, individuals with CAH are exposed to high levels of masculinizing hormones in the prenatal and perinatal periods, but relatively normal levels postnatally with good treatment. If sexual differentiation of human behavior is affected by androgen levels present during sensitive periods of development (as it is in other species), then females with CAH should be behaviorally "masculinized" and "defeminized," that is, compared to control females, they should behave more like males and less like females. And they do in some, but not all, ways. Finding that females with CAH are not uniformly masculinized and defeminized means that they can provide important information about the ways in which androgens are involved in sexual differentiation of behavior. It is not surprising to find that androgen has differential effects on different aspects of behavior, given that sex-typed behavior is multidimensional *(11)*.

Play Behavior and Activities

Early androgens appear to have big effects on childhood play behavior and associated interests *(12–15)*. Girls with CAH spend considerably more time playing with boys' toys than do their unaffected sisters. This difference is apparent when the girls are directly observed playing, when they are asked about their favorite activities, and when their parents are asked about the girls' activities. The sex-atypical interests of girls with CAH continue into adolescence, as manifested in the girls' reports of their activities and career interests, and their parents' reports of their activities (16). These sex-atypical preferences characterize not just the group of CAH girls, but most individuals within the group; this is most apparent when activities are assessed with multiple measures to increase reliability of individual differences. In both childhood and adolescence, there is very little overlap between girls with CAH and unaffected girls in their scores on composite measures of activities (13,16). Given continuities in interests found in typical males and females (17), it is reasonable to expect adult females with CAH to have male-typical leisure interests and occupations, but this awaits confirmation.

Gender Identity

Moderate levels of androgens characteristic of females with CAH do not masculinize all aspects of sex-typed behavior. Almost all females with CAH have female-typical gender identity, with little evidence of gender dysphoria either in childhood or adulthood (15,18–20). A very small minority of females with CAH are unhappy living as females or live successfully as males, and this number is greater than would be expected among typical women (18,21). Many, but not all, of those who live as males were not diagnosed until later in childhood. It is unclear what differentiates females with CAH with male gender identity from the vast majority with female gender identity, but it is likely that both continuing postnatal androgenization and rearing environment play a role.

It is important to consider the data from females with CAH in the context of data from individuals with other intersex conditions, most of them associated with much higher androgen levels than typical of females with CAH. Unfortunately, much of those data come from case reports, which can be difficult to interpret because rigorous methods are not always used, follow-up is often selective, and intersex children vary considerably in their degree of early hormone exposure and consistency of rearing sex (20).

One case has played a key role in refocusing attention on determinants of gender identity (22,23). This was a boy with male-typical prenatal and neonatal development whose penis was ablated after a mishandled circumcision and who was subsequently reassigned and reared female. Contrary to early reports, the child never adjusted to the female assignment, despite having no knowledge of his early history. Sex reassignment was requested and the individual is now reported to live successfully and happily as a man. Because this individual is a normal genetic male who was exposed to male-typical hormones in prenatal and early neonatal life, this case lends credence to the view that gender identity is determined by early hormones acting on the developing brain, and argues against the view that rearing sex is the main determinant of gender identity (23).

This conclusion must be considered in light of other details of this case and other cases. The individual described earlier (23) was reared unequivocally as a boy at least until age 7 mo when the accident occurred, and perhaps longer, because the final decision about female reassignment was not made until his second year, and surgery was not completed until age 21 mo. Further, another case of ablatio penis had a very different outcome: after an accident at age 2 mo, this second child was reassigned female at 7 mo, and has reportedly adapted well to this identity. As an adult, she shows no evidence of gender dysphoria, although she has a male-typical occupation and a bisexual orientation (24).

The evidence from males with micropenis also suggests variations in outcome, and it is currently unclear what differentiates those with good vs poor outcome when they are reared as males or as females. Nevertheless, it does seem clear that males with micropenis can develop male gender identity and experience normal heterosexual activities, especially with testosterone treatment to increase penile size *(25,26)*.

Ongoing studies on boys with cloacal exstrophy who are reared as girls should help to provide systematic evidence regarding malleability of gender identity. These boys have a malformed or absent penis, but normal testes; they are usually reassigned as girls because of concerns about adjustment problems associated with inadequate male genitalia. Preliminary reports from an ongoing systematic study *(27)* indicate that more than half of these children identify as boys, consistent with their male-typical prenatal androgen exposure and not with their female-typical rearing. Interestingly, however, some of these children do identify as girls, so it will be important to determine what differentiates children with male identity from those with female identity.

Thus, there is not a simple association between degree of prenatal hormone exposure and gender identity. It appears that moderate levels of androgen present during prenatal development are necessary, but are not sufficient, to masculinize gender identity. It also appears that sex-typical genitalia are neither necessary nor sufficient for sex-typical gender identity. It is unclear what factors modify influences of prenatal androgens on gender identity, but they probably include rearing sex and continuing postnatal androgenization. There is an urgent need for systematic studies of gender identity in children with ambiguous genitalia, especially children with XY karyotype and reduced prenatal androgen levels.

Sexual Orientation

Early studies of sex steroid-hormone influences on sexual orientation assessed in females with CAH are difficult to interpret because of methodological limitations. Two recent studies with good methodology suggest that women with CAH have less heterosexual experience, but not more homosexual experience, than do unaffected women *(19, 28)*. This may reflect consequences of the disease and its treatment, rather than prenatal androgens, including poorer body image, reduced sexual sensitivity, and discomfort with intercourse because of reconstructive genital surgery. These possibilities are rendered less likely in light of evidence regarding sexual arousal and fantasy. Compared to their unaffected sisters, women with CAH express more sexual interest in women and less sexual interest in men, although the majority of women with CAH appear to have heterosexual interests, and the others bisexual, not exclusively homosexual, interests *(19)*. For example, on a lifetime global rating of sexual orientation in fantasy, among women with CAH, 66% were classified as exclusively heterosexual, 27% as bisexual, and 7% had no sexual fantasies; 100% of controls were classified as exclusively heterosexual *(19)*. It is possible that these numbers underestimate the incidence of homosexual interest in women with CAH, because of underreporting or sample bias (women with homosexual interests might be less likely to participate or to reveal those interests than would women with heterosexual interests), so it is important to conduct additional studies in samples where biases are minimized. There is also a need to conduct systematic studies of sexual behavior in individuals with other intersex conditions.

Other Social Behaviors

There is suggestive evidence that prenatal androgens affect other social behaviors that show sex differences, including maternal behavior and aggression. Compared to unaffected females (unaffected sisters or other controls), girls and women with CAH have less interest in babies and in having their own children *(15,29,30)*. This is not likely to reflect a psychological response to the disease, such as reduced fertility, because women with Turner syndrome (who are completely infertile) do not show reduced interest in babies *(6)*, nor do males with CAH *(30)*.

Evidence from two sources suggest that early masculinizing hormones increase aggression later in life. Females (aged 6–17 yr) exposed to androgenizing progestins in utero because of maternal ingestion to prevent miscarriage were more likely than their unexposed sisters to report that they would use physical aggression in hypothetical conflict situations *(31)*. Females with CAH also appear to be more likely than unaffected female relatives to report that they would use aggression, but the difference emerges most clearly in adolescents and adults, not in children *(15,32)*. This apparent developmental effect needs to be replicated in a longitudinal study, and future studies also need to consider the multidimensionality of aggression (e.g., unprovoked aggression vs response to frustration).

Cognitive Abilities

Early androgens also appear to play a role in aspects of cognition. Sex differences are not found in general intelligence, but rather in the pattern of cognitive abilities. Males, on average, outperform females on measures of spatial, mechanical, and mathematical abilities, whereas females, on average, outperform males on measures of verbal fluency, verbal memory, emotional perception, and perceptual speed *(33)*. There are several pieces of evidence to suggest that the sex differences in at least some of these abilities are influenced by prenatal androgens acting to organize the brain early in development. Females with CAH have been reported to have higher spatial ability than their unaffected female relatives *(34,35)* and males with low early androgen levels (due to idiopathic hypogonadotropic hypogonadism, IHH) to have lower spatial ability than controls *(36)*. Although it is unclear exactly at what age androgen levels begin to decline in males with IHH, three pieces of evidence suggest that the reduced spatial ability results from reduced androgens early in development: spatial ability has been reported to correlate with testicular volume and not to improve with androgen replacement in males with IHH, and not to be reduced in males with acquired (late-onset) hypogonadism *(36)*.

There is very little information about the effects of early hormones on other aspects of cognitive abilities. It will be interesting to study, for example, whether females with CAH have lower (more male-typical) verbal memory than unaffected females. These studies will be challenging to do, however, because sex differences in these abilities are smaller than those in spatial ability, so that large samples will be necessary to detect any effects of early hormones.

Failures to Find Evidence
of Behavioral Effects of Early Androgens

Not all studies of individuals with CAH or other endocrine conditions have shown behavioral effects of prenatal androgens, but it is important to remember that the absence of significant hormone-behavior associations in a single study does not mean that those associations do not exist in the population. There are a variety of methodological criteria that must be met in order to conclude with confidence that there are no associations in the population. Studies failing to find differences related to early hormone exposure generally did not include large enough samples to provide sufficient power to detect hypothesized differences, and used measures with limited reliability and validity (particularly measures that did not show sex differences in the age ranges studied).

RULING OUT ALTERNATIVE EXPLANATIONS

The evidence reviewed above from intersex individuals strongly suggests that early androgens affect a variety of aspects of human sex-typical behavior, confirming experimental studies in other species. It appears that this masculinization results directly from the effects of excess androgens on the developing brain in utero. But, intersex and typical individuals differ in several ways besides prenatal androgen exposure, and it is important to examine how these factors contribute to the behavioral differences.

Social Influences

Many intersex individuals have genitalia that look different from those of typical individuals, and it is possible that this physical difference elicits different responses from other individuals, which in turn cause the behavioral differences. For example, differences between females with CAH and unaffected females might result from differential treatment by parents in response to the virilized genitalia of girls with CAH *(37)*. Evidence suggests that this is not likely. Parents report that they do not treat girls with CAH differently than they treat their unaffected daughters, but, of course, parents' reports may not necessarily reflect their behavior *(12,15)*. Two pieces of evidence from studies from androgenized female rhesus macaques also suggest that maternal responses to genitalia do not account for masculinized behavior *(38)*. Female offspring exposed to androgens late in gestation had normal external genitalia, but were behaviorally masculinized in several ways, including rough play. Mothers' behavior, particularly inspection of offspring genitalia, was not associated with either the amount or kind of offspring masculine behavior shown to peers.

More compelling data are provided by a Swedish study in which girls with CAH and control girls were observed playing with sex-typed toys alone and with a parent (usually the mother) *(39)*. As expected, when alone, girls with CAH played more with boys' toys than did control girls. When the girls played with a parent, the difference between girls with CAH and control girls was reduced, not increased, suggesting that parents actually discourage rather than encourage sex-atypical play.

Data from other intersex conditions also weaken the argument for the primacy of social influences on differences between intersex and typical individuals. Males with IHH have lower spatial ability than controls, but their external genitalia are not obviously different. A meaningful number of males with endocrine disorders or traumatic injuries resulting in small or absent penis and subsequent female sex assignment still have male gender identity, despite female-appearing genitalia and female-typical socialization.

Further, data from studies involving normal participants with typical variations in prenatal hormones and normal external genitalia provide important converging evidence for studies in clinical populations in showing prenatal androgens to be associated with some aspects of sex-typed behavior. Females thought to be exposed to high-average levels of testosterone by virtue of sharing a uterine environment with a male co-twin appear to show some behavioral masculinization: compared to females with a female co-twin, they have higher spatial ability *(40)*, higher sensation-seeking *(41)*, and a male-typical pattern of auditory function *(42)*, although they do not play more with boys' toys *(43)*. Seven-yr-old girls who had high levels of testosterone in utero (assessed in amniotic fluid at 14–16 wk of gestation) had faster mental rotation (an aspect of spatial ability) than girls who had low levels of prenatal testosterone *(44)*.

Postnatal Androgens

Some causes of intersexuality are associated with atypical hormones in postnatal life also, so it is possible that some behavioral changes reflect postnatal rather than prenatal hormones. Evidence also suggests that this is unlikely. Behavior in females with CAH has been found to relate to indicators of prenatal androgen excess, such as degree of 21-OH deficiency reflected in genetic mutation *(45)* and severity of illness *(14,46)*, and not to indicators of postnatal androgen excess, such as advanced bone age or hormones measured close in time to behavioral assessment *(46)*. In fact, females with CAH are likely to have subnormal androgens *(46,47)*. Evidence from other conditions also argues against the primacy of postnatal androgens. Reduced spatial ability is found only in males with IHH, and not in males with acquired hypogonadism *(36)*. Chromosomal males with cloacal exstrophy who are castrated in the perinatal period, and thus exposed to androgens only in the prenatal period, are masculinized in gender identity and aspects of gender role *(27)*.

Other Disease Characteristics

Intersex individuals often have abnormalities besides sex-atypical androgens, but, again, it is unlikely that these factors are responsible for the behavioral changes. The other hormones that are abnormal in CAH, such as progesterone and corticosteroids, have smaller and less consistent behavioral effects than androgen, and may actually prevent masculinization *(48)*. Behavioral similarities between CAH and control males make it unlikely that behavioral changes in CAH females reflect general disease characteristics or other hormonal abnormalities *(12,13,16,30,32)*.

Consistency of Evidence

Although these other factors, such as socialization in girls with CAH or postnatal androgens, might account for some findings, they cannot account for all findings. The most parsimonious explanation of the data involves the organizing action of prenatal androgen on the developing brain. Further, the findings are consistent with theoretical expectations and with studies in other species where hormones have been directly manipulated *(1–3,5)*. Importantly, differences between intersex and typical individuals are found only on measures that show sex differences and thus would be reasonably expected to be sensitive to effects of early hormones.

WHAT ACCOUNTS FOR VARIATIONS?

An interesting question concerns the variation in effects of prenatal androgens across behaviors and across individuals with the same cause of intersexuality. With respect to variations across behavior, for example, it is important to consider findings from females with CAH that gender identity is less affected by prenatal androgens than is childhood toy play. With respect to variations across individuals with the same condition, for example, it is important to consider findings that some boys with cloacal exstrophy successfully adjust to a female sex assignment, whereas others do not, or findings that some women with CAH show sexual arousal to other women, but most report completely heterosexual arousal.

Table 1
Behavioral Differences Between Females
with CAH and Control Females Compared to Sex Differences[a]

	Sex difference	CAH vs control females
Childhood play and activities	3.3	1.5
Adolescent activities	2.4	1.3
Playmate preference	3.6	0.8
Sexual orientation	5.9	0.8
Interest in babies	1.0	0.7
Aggression	1.4	1.1
Spatial ability	1.0	0.7

Data from refs. *(13,16,19,30,32,35,94)*.
[a]Differences are expressed in standard deviation units, *d (49)*.

Comparing Androgen Effects Across Behaviors

Before evaluating possible reasons for apparent varying effects of androgen, it would be useful to quantify the effects. Comparison of effects across behaviors is complicated by measurement variations, that is, different behaviors are measured with differing reliability and validity. A solution to this problem is to evaluate the difference between intersex and typical individuals in relation to the sex difference. Behavioral differences between typical males and females result from a variety of factors; differences between individuals exposed to sex-atypical and sex-typical androgen levels approximate the proportion of the behavioral sex difference that reflects a sex difference in early androgen levels.

Variations in androgen effects across behaviors can be assessed with data from females with CAH. Table 1 shows the size of each behavioral difference between females with CAH and comparison females compared to the size of the sex difference on that behavior. Differences are expressed in standard deviation units, *d (49)*. It is preferable to calculate both the sex difference and CAH-control female difference in the same sample, but that is not always possible, particularly with regard to behaviors that show large sex differences (such as sex of sexual partner and gender identity). In the latter case, estimates of sex differences were obtained from other studies. Figure 1 shows the ratio of the CAH-control female difference to the sex difference; this is interpreted as the proportion of the sex difference that is due to the effect of early androgen. This analysis suggests that moderate androgens characteristic of females with CAH have larger effects on aspects of gender-role behavior and cognition than on gender identity and sex of partners (as playmates and as targets of sexual arousal). Possible reasons for these differences are considered below.

Behavioral Issues

Multidimensionality of Sex-Typed Behavior

It is clear from developmental studies in typical children that there are many aspects of sex-typed behavior and that they develop at different rates and correlate with different criteria *(11)*. Some behaviors show little overlap between typical males and females (e.g., sex of identification, sex of sex partner), whereas others show only moderate-sized differences and substantial overlap between the sexes (e.g., verbal memory). The size of the

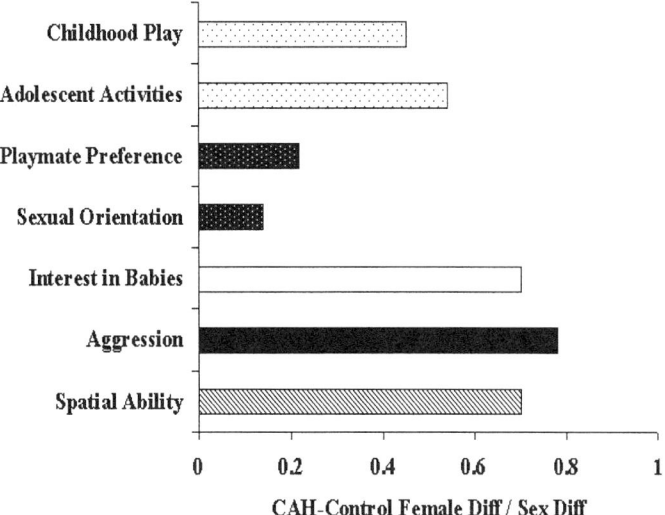

Fig. 1. Proportion of behavioral sex difference attributed to effects of prenatal androgens, measured as ratio of difference between females with CAH and control females to sex difference.

population sex difference and the within-sex variability thus set a limit on the size of androgen effects and the likely variation within groups of intersex individuals. The big differences seen in activities and interests between girls with CAH and unaffected girls probably reflects the very large differences in these behaviors between typical boys and girls. In this context, it is compelling that the moderate levels of androgens that are characteristic of females with CAH have such a small effect on gender identity, given the fact that gender identity shows almost no overlap between typical males and females.

MEASUREMENT

Some of the variation can be explained by method variance. Most behaviors are assessed with a single measure with imperfect reliability, but individual differences are best captured by multiple measures *(50)*. This is easily overlooked, but dramatically illustrated with data on childhood play and activities in girls with CAH. On a single observational measure, girls with CAH spend more time than control girls playing with boys' toys, but there is considerable variation within both groups of girls and overlap between the groups. In this single session, some girls with CAH play a lot with boys' toys and some do not play with these toys at all, whereas a few unaffected girls play a considerable amount with boys' toys *(12)*. But, measuring toy play with multiple measures (observations and reports) on more than one occasion substantially reduces the variance among both groups of girls, so that there is little overlap among the groups *(13)*. Although within-group variations in some behaviors will likely be reduced with more reliable measurement, some variations probably reflect other factors.

Characteristics of Hormone Exposure

TIMING OF EXPOSURE

It is likely that behaviors are differentially affected by the amount and levels of hormones present during different sensitive periods. The early prenatal period has been generally thought to be the crucial time for organizational effects of hormones on brain development and later behavior, but studies in nonhuman mammals suggest that other periods may be important too. In primates, for example, there appear to be several distinct sensitive periods for androgen effects on behavior, with different behaviors masculinized by exposure early vs late in gestation *(38)*: female rhesus macaques exposed to androgen early in gestation (and thus with virilized genitalia) show increased mounting behavior, reduced mother-grooming, and delayed puberty onset, whereas those exposed late in gestation (with no genital virilization) show increased rough play.

DOSE

The relation between hormone dose and behavioral masculinization does not appear to be the same for all behaviors and it is not always linear. This is clear from experimental studies in nonhuman mammals and suggested by findings from intersex individuals described earlier. Moderate departures from sex-typical androgen levels appear to affect some behaviors more than others. Moderate changes in androgens affect spatial ability in females with CAH and males with IHH (enhancing and reducing spatial ability, respectively). Moderate increases in androgens in females with CAH also masculinize or defeminize some aspects of gender-role behavior (toy play, adolescent activities, interest in babies) more than others (playmate preferences). Nevertheless, a moderate dose of androgen alone is insufficient for the development of male gender identity: the vast majority of females with CAH have female-typical gender identity. Although a high dose of androgen is likely to masculinize gender identity, it may not be sufficient to do so, given variations in gender identity seen in males with normal or slightly reduced male-typical androgens, such as cloacal exstrophy, ablatio penis, and micropenis.

SPECIFIC HORMONES AND THEIR INTERACTIONS

Masculinizing hormones come in many forms, and each affects different aspects of physical and behavioral sexual differentiation. For example, dihydrotestosterone is responsible for differentiation of the external genitalia *(51)*; in monkeys, dihydrotestosterone and testosterone propionate have different effects on learning *(52)*. Different forms of androgen have different potency; for example, dihydrotestosterone is more effective than testosterone in masculinizing the external genitalia, and both are more potent that dihydroepiandrostenedione. In some species, masculine-typical development results from estradiol metabolized from androgen in the brain, although aromatized estrogens do not appear to play a role in masculinizing the human brain and behavior *(53)*. For example, women exposed to high prenatal levels of estrogens only, because of complete androgen insensitivity syndrome or exposure to diethystilbestrol (DES), appear to have female-typical behavior *(54–57)*, except perhaps for increased homosexuality in women exposed to DES *(58)*.

The effects of specific hormones may be modified by other hormones *(5)*, and some discrepancies across intersex conditions may be explained by differences in ovarian hormones such as progesterone and estrogen. Progesterone, for example, can act as an antiandrogen in female rodents, providing protection against the masculinizing effects of androgen *(48,59)*, and may function similarly in human females *(60,61)*. There is also increasing recognition of the importance of ovarian estrogens in feminization (feminization is no longer considered to be a completely passive process). For example, depriving female rats of ovarian estrogens results in reduced sexual behavior and decreased activity. Interestingly, the sensitive periods for the behavioral effects of ovarian estrogens may be later than those for androgens *(62)*. If ovarian hormones play an active role in sexual differentiation, a given amount of androgen may have different effects in males and females. This may explain why sexual orientation and gender identity are less masculinized in females with CAH than in individuals with other intersex conditions. In this context, it is interesting to consider behavior in females with Turner syndrome who have low or absent estrogens. Their female-typical gender identity and sex-typed behavior *(63)* would seem to argue that estrogens are not necessary for female-typical behavior, but some of the cognitive deficits found in females with Turner syndrome, especially in memory, have been interpreted to reflect brain dysfunction secondary to low estrogen *(64,65).* It is important to remember, however, that Turner syndrome involves major genetic and physical abnormalities, so it is difficult to ascribe behavioral changes to estrogens alone.

SENSITIVITY TO HORMONES

Behavioral effects of hormones likely are modified by genetic variations in hormone-receptor sensitivity. Mutations in the human androgen receptor gene cause androgen resistance to varying degrees, with phenotypic abnormalities in men ranging from complete insensitivity to androgen and thus female differentiation to men with infertility and minor undervirilization *(66).* These receptor variations have not yet been studied with respect to behavioral consequences, but such effects are likely, given mouse studies showing genotype-dependent behavioral effects of early exposure to testosterone (increased aggression in one strain but not another) *(67).* Variations in hormone sensitivity might account for some findings described earlier, for example, that some females with CAH have homosexual interests, or that some 46XY males with cloacal exstrophy adjust well to a female sex assignment and develop female gender identity. In the case of CAH, these variations might be in the androgen receptor or in the glucocorticoid receptor (affecting the individual's ability to use relatively low levels of endogenous corticosteroids or in responding to treatment).

Early hormones may modify an individual's later sensitivity to those hormones. For example, the response to exogenous testosterone in adult gerbils depends on their early exposure *(4).* If this occurs in people, then it might explain differences among individuals with the same intersex condition but different postnatal hormone histories. A given amount of postnatal androgen might have a greater behavioral effect on an individual with exposure to high prenatal levels than one with exposure to only moderate levels. For example, 46XY individuals with cloacal exstrophy reared as females but reassigned as males and receiving testosterone replacement might be more behaviorally masculinized than 46XX individuals with CAH reared as males with continuing postnatal androgenization, because of greater sensitivity to the postnatal androgens induced by exposure to higher prenatal androgens.

OTHER CONTRIBUTORS TO SEXUAL DIFFERENTIATION

Some variations across conditions may reflect nonhormonal influences on sexual differentiation, particularly effects of the sex chromosomes. For example, differences between females with CAH and males with cloacal exstrophy may reflect not just differences in the amount of androgen exposure but the fact that the latter have the SRY gene.

Environmental Modification

There is evidence from other species that behavioral effects of hormones can be modified by the social and physical environment, and this malleability is likely to be more pronounced in human beings than in other species *(68)*. It will be very important to study in a systematic fashion the environments of children with intersex conditions, to determine how rearing environment modifies effects of prenatal androgens. It is important to remember, however, that the social environment is probably not independent of the person, that is, individuals are responded to and actively select their environments in part based on their predispositions, including those that are affected by prenatal androgens. For example, girls with CAH almost certainly have a home environment that contains more toy vehicles and construction sets than girls without CAH. It is more likely that this environment was shaped by the child (through requests for toys and differential play with toys received as gifts) than it was imposed on her.

MECHANISMS FOR BEHAVIORAL EFFECTS OF HORMONES

Some of the most interesting and important questions about the behavioral effects of early androgens concern the mechanisms that underlie these effects *(69)*. Androgens undoubtedly affect behavior directly by changing brain regions subserving specific behaviors, but they also likely have their behavioral effects in indirect ways. There are currently no human data to reveal what mediates hormone-behavior associations, but studies in other species and from other areas of research in people suggest some possibilities that might be subjected to empirical test. The following section is speculative and intended to stimulate discussion of possible mechanisms.

Neural Mechanisms

There is considerable interest in documenting sex differences in the human brain, and in determining how these brain differences underlie behavioral sex differences, and how they are affected by sex-steroid hormones. This work follows logically from studies in other species, in which a substantial number of brain sex differences have been described and related to behavior and to exposure to sex-steroid hormones *(1–3,5)*. For example, sex differences in spatial learning in rats may be mediated by early androgen effects on the developing hippocampus *(70,71)*. In other species, gonadal hormones have been shown to affect neuronal size, survival, and outgrowth, synapse number and organization, dendritic branching patterns, gross nuclear volume, cortical thickness, and neurotransmitter systems.

A variety of sex differences have been reported in human brain structure and function (for review, *see* ref. *72*). In terms of structure, for example, the splenium of the corpus callosum has been reported to be wider and more bulbous in females than in males *(73)*, the relative size of the language areas has been reported to be larger in females than in males *(74)*, and females have been reported to have greater neuronal density than do males in regions of the temporal lobe known to subserve language functions *(75)*. Functional sex differences have been observed with brain-imaging techniques while subjects are performing simple cognitive tasks. For example, during the processing of rhymes, females have been reported to activate both left and right inferior frontal gyrus regions, whereas males activate only the left *(76)*.

The results of studies of both structural and functional sex differences are very exciting, and have encouraged investigators to examine these differences in individuals with atypical early hormones, such as females with CAH (e.g., refs. *77,78*). But, for several reasons, it is important to be cautious about studies of sex differences and hormone effects on brain structure and function. First, it has proven difficult to replicate results. This may reflect statistical issues associated with the methods and samples typically used in imaging studies. On the one hand, many regions are examined in imaging studies and it is likely that some will show sex differences in a given sample simply as a result of sampling fluctuation and multiple comparisons. On the other hand, nonreplications may result from low statistical power: even moderate to large differences require larger samples than is usually feasible in imaging studies. Second, brain sex differences have not been specifically found to relate to behavioral sex differences. For example, sex differences in cortical activation while subjects solve a rhyming task do not translate into sex differences in performance. This may partly reflect the fact that tasks used in imaging studies are very simple, so there is little variation across participants. But this is not the complete explanation, because this problem is not unique to human studies; in rodents, destruction of regions that show sex differences and sensitivity to early androgens often has no behavioral effect. Third, very little is known about the brain regions that subserve many of the human behaviors that show sex differences and sensitivity to early hormones. For example, although there is good evidence that spatial abilities involve frontal and parietal structures (and thus these regions might differ in females with CAH and controls), it is unclear what brain regions might underlie childhood toy play and adolescent activities.

Behavioral Mechanisms

The search for the neural substrates mediating the behavioral effects of androgens might be enhanced by better analysis of behavioral or psychological mechanisms associated with androgens. For example, hormones may affect "higher-order" behaviors through effects on basic perceptual or sensory processes *(79)*. It is intriguing to speculate that androgen effects on toy play might be mediated by affective properties of moving stimuli associated with limbic structures. Of course, such speculations await empirical test.

Environmental Interactions

Hormones may affect behavior by changing the way in which the individual interacts with the environment (physical and social environment). Studies in rodents reveal that hormones affect not only the behavior of the organism but others' responses to the individual, including grooming by the mother and attraction of peers (e.g., ref. *4*). There are currently no studies of this possibility in people, but it is easy to speculate that early androgen exposure in girls with CAH might create an affective bias for moving stimuli, which is then reinforced by the environment, through selection by the child and provision by the parents of transportation and action toys. This familiarity and comfort with machines and action might then lead the girls to use computers, which in turn might foster their spatial skills. Of course, this speculation also awaits empirical assessment.

RESOLVING CONTROVERSIES IN THE TREATMENT OF CHILDREN WITH AMBIGUOUS GENITALIA

Questions about the relative contributions of hormones and the social environment have recently assumed critical importance in pediatric medicine with new data casting doubt on two key tenets that have guided the treatment of children with intersex conditions (e.g., refs. *23,80*). The first tenet, derived from the early work of Money, is that children are "psychosexually neutral" at birth, with gender identity determined solely by sex of rearing and not by genes or hormones *(81,82)*. (Money's emphasis on the relative primacy of the social environment applied primarily to gender identity. He did argue for the importance of early androgens for other aspects of behavior, e.g., ref. *6*). This has generally resulted in female sex assignment, because it is easier to reconstruct female than male external genitalia. Gender identity is considered to be fixed by the end of the second year of life, so any change in sex assignment after the age of two (which might be considered in cases with delayed diagnoses) is not usually considered because it is assumed to cause psychological disturbance. The second tenet guiding treatment of intersex individuals is that genital anatomy must be concordant with assigned sex. "Normal" sex-typical genitalia are deemed to be necessary both for the individual's self-image and for acceptance by others, and thus for satisfactory gender identity and psychological adjustment.

These tenets have guided medical treatment of newborns with ambiguous genitalia (e.g., ref. *83–86*), although changes are occurring *(87,88)*. The birth of a child with abnormalities of the genitalia is still considered a "social emergency" and early sex assignment is encouraged. One recent change has been the recognition that prenatal androgens may affect the brain and behavior, so gender identity cannot be assumed to depend solely on rearing sex *(87)*. In order to maximize female-typical development, children receive early genital surgery and their parents are instructed to provide unwavering female-typical socialization. If diagnosis is delayed after age two, sex reassignment is rarely considered, because of assumed psychological harm.

Recent challenges to this treatment have emphasized the lack of empirical support of the key tenets or their application *(22,23,89)*. Much of the evidence cited to support the current treatment derives from case reports of individuals who may not be representative or completely described. Recent evidence suggests the need to consider modifications in treatment and some, but not all, of these are being incorporated into practice *(87)*.

First, with respect to the notion of psychosexual neutrality, as noted earlier, gender identity does not appear to be completely malleable. In particular, 46XY individuals with at least moderate androgen exposure may do better as males than as females. Second, with respect to late sex reassignment, there are no systematic studies of its psychological consequences. In some cases, late sex reassignment may actually ameliorate psychological distress in individuals assigned as females who later experienced severe gender dysphoria *(22,23,27)*. Of course, these cases may not be representative. Third, with respect to the importance of early genital surgery, there is no evidence that gender identity and psychological adjustment require sex-typical genitalia. In females with CAH, psychological adjustment appears unrelated or only weakly related to the degree of genital virilization or the age at which genital surgery is performed *(90)*, and the small minority who have male-typical gender identity are not necessarily those with the most masculinized genitalia *(18,21)*. It is also worth repeating data showing that gender identity can be clearly and unequivocally established even in the absence of sex-typical genitals and sometimes in the presence of genitalia of the nonidentified sex, as in boys with clocal exstrophy or ablatio penis reared as females but self-identified as males. But, before declaring a moratorium on early genital reconstructive surgery, we should remember that there are no systematic studies of long-term outcome in children with sex-atypical genitalia who did not receive such surgery. Fourth, the costs of surgery have been noted by intersex individuals whose sexual response has been compromised *(28,91–93)*.

It is important that policy regarding the medical treatment of children with ambiguous genitalia be reexamined in light of empirical evidence. It is just as important that changes to current policy be based on empirical evidence. Consider, for example, the recommendation that females with CAH and severe genital masculinization be reared as males *(80)*. The recommendation is based on an assumption not currently supported by data, that there is a simple linear relation between genital virilization and brain masculinization. With specific respect to gender identity in females with CAH, most live successfully and happily as females, and the small minority who are unhappy as females or who live as males include those with only moderate genital masculinization *(18,21)*. Further, hormones do not affect all behaviors—and therefore the brain—uniformly, so it is unclear how to define "brain masculinization."

There is an urgent need for systematic data to assess the adequacy of the current treatment for children with ambiguous genitalia, as well as for the likely benefit of suggested changes to that treatment. This includes assessment of psychological outcome in different causes of intersexuality, examining gender identity in relation to initial sex assignment, and consequences of surgical interventions for gender identity, sexual function, and overall psychological adjustment. Treatment is also likely to be enhanced by further understanding of the specific ways that behaviors are influenced by prenatal androgens acting directly on the brain and through the social environment.

SUMMARY AND CONCLUSIONS

There is now little question that human behavioral sexual differentiation parallels, at least in part, physical sexual differentiation. Aspects of sex-typed behavior in childhood and adulthood are affected by hormones that were present very early in development, confirming findings in other mammalian species. Nevertheless, these effects are not simple and uniform across all behaviors. This causes difficulties in prediction, for example, from degree of genital ambiguity to gender identity, or from play behavior to sexual orientation. Many questions remain about the extent, nature, and mechanisms of hormonal influences on human behavior. It is encouraging to know that this is an active area of current investigation and that answers to these questions are likely to be found in the near future. These answers should result in improved treatment for children with intersex conditions.

ACKNOWLEDGMENTS

Preparation of this chapter and my own research reported here were supported by National Institutes of Health grant HD19644. I thank the following people for their contributions to my research: Kristina Korman Bryk provided outstanding research assisstance, including coordination of the project, and data collection, processing, and management; Drs. Stephen Duck, Deborah Edidin, Orville Green, David Klein, Ora Pescovitz, Gail Richards, Julio Santiago, Bernard Silverman, and David Wyatt generously provided access to their patients and answered medical questions; Elizabeth Snyder, Lori Alegnani, Kathleen Bechtold, Jackie Ewing, Kim Ketterling, Robyn Reed, and George Vineyard assisted in data collection and/or processing; Dr. Stephen Duck examined medical records and provided ratings on androgen excess and disease characteristics. I am particularly grateful to the families who have participated in my studies.

REFERENCES

1. Arnold AP, Gorski RA. Gonadal steroid induction of structural sex differences in the central nervous system. Ann Rev Neurosci 1984;7:413–442.
2. Becker JB, Breedlove SM, Crews D, eds. Behavioral Endocrinology. MIT Press, Cambridge, MA, 1992.
3. Breedlove SM. Sexual differentiation of the human nervous system. Ann Rev Psych 1994;45:389–418.
4. Clark MM, Galef BG. Effects of intrauterine position on the behavior and genital morphology of litter-bearing rodents. Dev Neuropsych 1998;14:197–211.
5. Goy RW, McEwen BS. Sexual Differentiation of the Brain. Oxford University Press, London, 1980.
6. Money J, Ehrhardt AA. Man and Woman, Boy and Girl. Johns Hopkins University Press, Baltimore, MD, 1972.
7. Collaer ML, Hines M. Human behavioral sex differences: a role for gonadal hormones during early development? Psych Bull 1995;118:55–107.
8. Hampson E, Kimura D. Sex differences and hormonal influences on cognitive function in humans. In: Becker JB, Breedlove SM, Crews D, eds. Behavioral Endocrinology. MIT Press, Cambridge, MA, 1992, pp. 357–398.
9. Hannon T, Fuqua J. Sexual differentiation. In: Eugster E, Pescovitz OH, eds. Developmental Endocrinology: From Research to Clinical Practice. Humana Press, Totowa, NJ, 2002, pp. 261–292.
10. Pang S. Congenital adrenal hyperplasia. Endo Metab Clin NA 1997;26:853–891.
11. Ruble DN, Martin CL. Gender development. In: Damon W, series ed., Eisenberg N, vol ed., Handbook of Child Psychology: vol 3. Social, Emotional, and Personality Development, 5th ed. Wiley, New York, 1998, pp. 933–1016.
12. Berenbaum SA, Hines M. Early androgens are related to childhood sex-typed toy preferences. Psych Sci 1992;3:203–206.
13. Berenbaum SA, Snyder E. Early hormonal influences on childhood sex-typed activity and playmate preference: implications for the development of sexual orientation. Dev Psych 1995;31:31–42.
14. Dittmann RW, Kappes MH, Kappes ME, Borger D, Stegner H, Willig RH, Wallis H. Congenital adrenal hyperplasia I: gender-related behaviors and attitudes in female patients and their sisters. Psychoneuroendocrinology 1990;15:401–420.
15. Ehrhardt AA, Baker SW. Fetal androgens, human central nervous system differentiation, and behavior sex differences. In: Friedman RC, Richart RR, Vande Weile RL, eds. Sex Differences in Behavior. Wiley, New York, 1974, pp. 33–51.
16. Berenbaum SA. Effects of early androgens on sex-typed activities and interests in adolescents with congenital adrenal hyperplasia. Horm Behav 1999;35:102–110.
17. Swanson JL. Stability and change in vocational interests. In: Savickas ML, Spokane AR, eds. Vocational Interests: Meaning, Measurement, and Counseling Use. Davies-Black Publishers, Palo Alto, CA, 1999, pp. 135–158.
18. Berenbaum SA, Bailey JM. Prenatal androgens and gender identity: evidence from girls with congenital adrenal hyperplasia, tomboys, and typical girls. Submitted.
19. Zucker KJ, Bradley SJ, Oliver G, Blake J, Fleming S, Hood J. Psychosexual development of women with congenital adrenal hyperplasia. Horm Behav 1996;30:300–318.
20. Zucker KJ. Intersexuality and gender identity differentiation. Ann Rev Sex Res 1999;10:1–69.
21. Meyer-Bahlburg HFL, Gruen RS, New MI, Bell JJ, Morishima A, Shimshi M, et al. Gender change from female to male in classical congenital adrenal hyperplasia. Horm Behav 1996;30:319–332.
22. Colapinto J. As Nature Made Him: The Boy Who Was Raised As a Girl. Harper Collins, New York, 2000.
23. Diamond M, Sigmundson HK. Sex reassignment at birth. Arch Pediatr Adolesc Med 1997;151:298–304.
24. Bradley SJ, Oliver GD, Chernick AB, Zucker KJ. Experiment of nurture: ablatio penis at 2 months, sex reassignment at 7 months, and a psychosexual follow-up in young adulthood. Pediatrics (electronic version) 1998; 102:e9. www.pediatrics.org/cgi/content/full/102/1/e9.
25. Bin-Abbas, B, Conte FA, Grumbach MM, Kaplan SL. Congenital hypogonadotropic hypogonadism and micropenis: effect of testosterone treatment on adult penile size. Why sex reversal is not indicated. J Pediatr 1999 May;134(5):579–583.
26. Reilly JM, Woodhouse CR. Small penis and the male sexual role. J Urol 1989;142:569–571.
27. Reiner W. Outcomes in gender assignment: cloacal exstrophy. In: Grumbach M, Chair. "Neonatal Management of Genital Ambiguity." Symposium presented at the meeting of the Lawson Wilkins Pediatric Endocrine Society, Boston, MA, May 2000.

28. Mulaikal RM, Migeon CJ, Rock JA. Fertility rates in female patients with congenital adrenal hyperplasia due to 21-hydroxylase deficiency. N Engl J Med 1987;316:178–182.
29. Helleday J, Edman G, Ritzen EM, Siwers B. Personality characteristics and platelet MAO activity in women with congenital adrenal hyperplasia (CAH). Psychoneuroendocrinology 1993;18:343–354.
30. Leveroni C, Berenbaum SA. Early androgen effects on interest in infants: evidence from children with congenital adrenal hyperplasia. Dev Neuropsych 1998;14:321–340.
31. Reinisch JM. Prenatal exposure to synthetic progestins increases potential for aggression in humans. Science 1981;211:1171–1173.
32. Berenbaum SA, Resnick SM. Early androgen effects on aggression in children and adults with congenital adrenal hyperplasia. Psychoneuroendocrinology 1997;22:505–515.
33. Halpern DF. Sex Differences in Cognitive Abilities, 3rd ed. Lawrence Erlbaum Associates, Mahwah, NJ, 2000.
34. Hampson E, Rovet JF, Altmann, D. Spatial reasoning in children with congenital adrenal hyperplasia due to 21-hydroxylase deficiency. Dev Neuropsychol 1998;14:299–320.
35. Resnick SM, Berenbaum SA, Gottesman II, Bouchard TJ. Early hormonal influences on cognitive functioning in congenital adrenal hyperplasia. Dev Psychol 1986;22:191–198.
36. Hier DB, Crowley WF. Spatial ability in androgen-deficient men. N Engl J Med 1982;306:1202–1205.
37. Quadagno DM, Briscoe R, Quadagno JS. Effects of perinatal gonadal hormones on selected nonsexual behavior patterns: a critical assessment of the nonhuman and human literature. Psychol Bull 1977;84: 62–80.
38. Goy RW, Bercovitch FB, McBrair MC. Behavioral masculinization is independent of genital masculinization in prenatally androgenized female rhesus macaques. Horm Behav 1988;22:552–571.
39. Servin A. Sex Differences in Children's Play Behavior: A Biological Construction of Gender? Comprehensive Summaries of Uppsala Dissertations from the Faculty of Social Sciences, Acta Universitatis Upsaliensis, Uppsala, Sweden, 1999.
40. Cole-Harding S, Morstad AL, Wilson JR. Spatial ability in members of opposite-sex twin pairs. [Abstract]. Behav Genet 1988;18:710.
41. Resnick SM, Gottesman II, McGue M. Sensation seeking in opposite-sex twins: an effect of prenatal hormones? Behav Genet 1993;23:323–329.
42. McFadden DM. A masculinizing effect on the auditory systems of human females having male co-twins. Proc Nat Acad Sci USA 1993;90, 11,900–11,904.
43. Henderson BA, Berenbaum SA Sex-typed play in opposite-sex twins. Dev Psychobiol 1997;31:115–123.
44. Grimshaw GM, Sitarenios G, Finegan JK. Mental rotation at 7 years: relations with prenatal testosterone levels and spatial play experience. Brain Cog 1995;29:85–100.
45. Nordenstrom A, Servin A, Larsson A, Bohlin G. Psychological follow up of children with congenital adrenal hyperplasia. In: Berenbaum SA, Chair. "Neuropsychological Follow-Up of Neonatal Screening." Symposium conducted at the 4th meeting of the International Society for Neonatal Screening, Stockholm, Sweden, June 1999.
46. Berenbaum SA, Duck SC, Bryk K. Behavioral effects of prenatal vs. postnatal androgen excess in children with 21-hydroxylase-deficient congenital adrenal hyperplasia. J Clin Endocrinol Metab 2000;85: 727–733.
47. Helleday J, Siwers B, Ritzen EM, Carlstrom K. Subnormal androgen and elevated progesterone levels in women treated for congenital virilizing 21-hydroxylase deficiency. J Clin Endo Metab 1993;76:933–936.
48. Hull EM, Franz JR, Snyder AM, Nishita JK. Perinatal progesterone and learning, social and reproductive behavior in rats. Physiol Behav 1980;24:251–256.
49. Cohen J. Statistical Power Analysis for the Behavioral Sciences, 2nd ed. Lawrence Erlbaum Associates, Hillsdale, NJ, 1988.
50. Epstein S. The stability of behavior: II. Implications for psychological research. Am Psychol 1980;35: 790–806.
51. Siiteri PK, Wilson JD. Testosterone formation and metabolism during male sexual differentiation in the human embryo. J Clin Endocrinol Metab 1974;38:113–125.
52. Bachevalier J, Hagger C. Sex differences in the development of learning abilities in primates. Psychoneuroendocrinology 1991;16:177–188.
53. Grumbach MM, Auchus RJ. Estrogen: consequences and implications of human mutations in synthesis and action. J Clin Endocrinol Metab 1999;84:4677–4694.
54. Hines M, Sandberg EC. Sexual differentiation of cognitive abilities in women exposed to diethylstilbestrol (DES) prenatally. Horm Behav 1996;30:354–363.

55. Hines M, Shipley C. Prenatal exposure to diethylstilbestrol (DES) and the development of sexually dimorphic cognitive abilities and cerebral lateralization. Dev Psychol 1984;20:81–94.

56. Imperato-McGinley J, Pichardo M, Gautier T, Voyer D, Bryden MP. Cognitive abilities in androgen-insensitive subjects: comparison with control males and females from the same kindred. Clin Endocrinol 1991;34:341–347.

57. Lish JD, Meyer-Bahlburg HFL, Ehrhardt AA, Travis BG, Veridiano NP. Prenatal exposure to diethylstilbestrol (DES): childhood play behavior and adult gender-role behavior in women. Arch Sex Behav 1992;21:423–441.

58. Meyer-Bahlburg HFL, Ehrhardt AA, Rosen LR, Gruen RS, Veridiano NP, Vann FH, Neuwalder HF. Prenatal estrogens and the development of homosexual orientation. Dev Psychol 1995;31:12–21.

59. Shapiro BH, Goldman AS, Bongiovanni AM, Marino JM. Neonatal progesterone and feminine sexual development. Nature 1976;264:795–796.

60. Ehrhardt AA, Meyer-Bahlburg HFL. Effects of prenatal sex hormones on gender-related behavior. Science 1981;211:1312–1318.

61. Ehrhardt AA, Meyer-Bahlburg HFL, Feldman JF, Ince SE. Sex-dimorphic behavior in childhood subsequent to prenatal exposure to exogenous progestogens and estrogens. Arch Sex Behav 1984;13:457–477.

62. Fitch RH, Denenberg VH. A role for ovarian hormones in sexual differentiation of the brain. Behav Brain Sci 1998;21:311–327.

63. McCauley E. Psychosocial aspects of the Turner syndrome. In: Bender BG, Berch DB, eds. Sex Chromosome Abnormalities and Behavior: Psychological Studies. AAAS/Westview Press, Boulder, CO, 1990, pp. 78–99.

64. Buchanan L, Pavlovic J, Rovet J. A reexamination of the visuospatial deficit in Turner syndrome: contributions of working memory. Dev Neuropsychol 1998;14:341–367.

65. Ross J, Zinn A, McCauley E. Neurodevelopmental and psychosocial aspects of Turner syndrome. Mental Retardation Dev Disabilities Res Rev 2000;6:135–141.

66. McPhaul MJ, Marcelli M, Zoppi S, Griffin JE, Wilson JD. Genetic basis of endocrine disease 4. The spectrum of mutations in the androgen receptor gene that causes androgen resistance. J Clin Endocrinol Metab 1993;76:17–23.

67. Michard-Vanhee C. Aggressive behavior induced in female mice by an early single injection of testosterone is genotype dependent. Behav Genet 1988;18:1–12.

68. Wallen K. Nature needs nurture: the interaction of hormonal and social influences on the development of behavioral sex differences in rhesus monkeys. Horm Behav 1996;30:364–378.

69. Berenbaum SA. How hormones affect behavioral and neural development: introduction to the special issue on "Gonadal Hormones and Sex Differences in Behavior." Dev Neuropsychol 1998;14:175–196.

70. Juraska JM. Sex differences in cognitive regions of the rat brain. Psychoneuroendocrinology 1991;16:105–119.

71. Roof RL, Havens MD. Testosterone improves maze performance and induces development of a male hippocampus in females. Brain Res 1992;572:310–313.

72. Resnick SM, Maki PM. Sex differences in regional brain structure and function. In: Kaplan PW, ed. The Neurology of Women. Demos Vermande, New York, 1999, pp. 3–10.

73. de Lacoste-Utamsing C, Holloway RL. Sexual dimorphism in the corpus callosum. Science 1982;216:1431–1432.

74. Harasty J, Double KL, Halliday GM, Kril J, McRitchie DA. Language-associated cortical regions are proportionally larger in the female brain. Arch Neurol 1997;54:171–176.

75. Witelson SF, Glezer II, Kigar DL. Women have greater density of neurons in posterior temporal cortex. J Neurosci 1995;15:3418–3428.

76. Shaywitz BA, Shaywitz SE, Pugh KR, Constable RT, Skudlarski P, Fulbright RK, et al. Sex differences in the functional organization of the brain for language. Nature 1995;373:607–609.

77. Merke D. Personal communication, May 2000.

78. Plante E, Boliek C, Binkiewicz A, Erly WK. Elevated androgen, brain development and language/learning disabilities in children with congenital adrenal hyperplasia. Dev Med Child Neurol 1996;38:423–437.

79. McFadden DM. Sex differences in the auditory system. Dev Neuropsychol 1998;14:261–298.

80. Diamond M, Sigmundson HK. Management of intersexuality. Arch Pediatr Adolesc Med 1997;151:1046–1050.

81. Meyer-Bahlburg HFL. 1998 Gender assignment in intersexuality. J Psych Human Sexuality 102:1–21.

82. Money J, Hampson JG, Hampson JL. Hermaphroditism: recommendations concerning assignment of sex, change of sex, and psychologic management. Bull Johns Hopkins Hosp 1955;97:284–300.

83. Donahoe PK, Schnitzer JJ. Evaluation of the infant who has ambiguous genitalia, and principles of operative management. Semin Ped Surg 1996;5:30–40.

84. Grumbach MM, Conte F. Disorders of sex differentiation. In: Wilson JW, Foster DW, eds. Williams Textbook of Endocrinology, 9th ed. WB Saunders, Philadelphia, PA, 1998, pp. 1400–1405.

85. Hendren WH. Surgical approach to intersex problems. Semin Ped Surg 1998;7:8–18.

86. Pinsky L, Erickson RP, Schimke RN. Genetic Disorders of Human Sexual Development. Oxford University Press, New York, 1999.

87. American Academy of Pediatrics. Evaluation of the newborn with developmental anomalies of the external genitalia. Pediatrics 2000;106:138–142.

88. Grumbach M, Chair. "Neonatal Management of Genital Ambiguity." Symposium presented at the meeting of the Lawson Wilkins Pediatric Endocrine Society, Boston, MA, May 2000.

89. Kessler S. Lessons From the Intersexed. Rutgers University Press, New Brunswick, NJ, 1998.

90. Berenbaum SA, Duck SC, Bryk K, Resnick SM. Psychological adjustment in children and adults with congenital adrenal hyperplasia. Poster presented at the joint meeting of the Pediatric Academic Societies and American Academy of Pediatrics, Boston, MA, May 2000.

91. Chase C. Letter: re-measurement of evoked potentials during feminizing genitoplasty: techniques and application. J Urol 1996;156:1139–1140.

92. Intersex Society of North America. Web page. www.isna.org.

93. Slijper FME, van der Kamp HJ, Brandenburg H, de Muinck Keizer-Schrama SMPF, Drop SLS, Molenaar JC. Evaluation of psychosexual development of young women with congenital adrenal hyperplasia: a pilot study. J Sex Educ Ther 1992;18:200–207.

94. Bailey, JM. Unpublished data, 2000.

14 Normal and Precocious Puberty

Joan DiMartino-Nardi, MD

CONTENTS

INTRODUCTION

Puberty refers to the achievement of reproductive maturity. It is a period of acceleration in linear growth, increase in muscle mass, and changes in ovarian and testicular function *(1)*. The initial evaluation of the young child with early sexual development is to distinguish true central precocious puberty with activation of the hypothalamic/pituitary/gonadal axis from peripheral or gonadotropin-independent precocious puberty so that specific treatment can be initiated. The decision to treat medically the child with central precocious puberty requires an understanding of the variable progression of puberty. Hence, the evaluation of the child with central precocious puberty should identify those children who might benefit by treatment with long-acting analogs of Gonadotropin Releasing Hormone (GnRHa) to halt their pubertal progression.

NORMAL PUBERTY

Clinical Features

NORMAL AGE OF ONSET

Pubertal onset occurs in 95% of girls between the ages of 8–13 yr with a mean age of 11 yr *(2)*. In boys the pubertal onset is between 9–14 yr with a mean of 11.5 yr *(2)*. The pubertal changes for both sexes have been staged according to Marshall and Tanner *(3,4)*.

TANNER STAGING

In girls, the development of the breast bud (thelarche) and the enlargement of the areola, are the result of increased estradiol production from the ovary. Other estrogen effects include the development of the female fat distribution, uterine and genital maturation

From: *Contemporary Endocrinology: Developmental Endocrinology: From Research to Clinical Practice*
Edited by: E. A. Eugster and O. H. Pescovitz © Humana Press Inc., Totowa, NJ

with modifications of the vulva—including growth of the labia minora and change of color of the vaginal mucosa—and menstruation *(5)*. The duration of breast development spans approx 2–3.5 yr *(2)*.

Sexual hair development (pubarche) results from androgens derived from the adrenals (adrenarche) and gonads (gonadarche). Other androgen induced effects include the development of axillary hair and odor, seborrhea, and acne. Generally, thelarche precedes pubarche. However, pubarche may occasionally precede thelarche. Menarche, the first menstrual period, occurs at a mean age of 12.8 yr in North America and generally occurs 2.3 yr after the onset of breast development, but there is considerable variation *(6)*. Menarche generally occurs during Tanner stages IV–V. Frequently, girls have irregular menses without ovulation for 1–2 yr after menarche.

In boys, the first evidence of puberty is an increase in testicular volume to more than 3 mL using the elliptical models developed by Zachmann and Prader *(7)*. Progressive genital enlargement spans 3–5 yr and is the result of increasing testosterone production from the testes and androgens from the adrenals. The period is characterized by an increase in the size of the penis, erections, sexual hair development, increase in muscle mass, acne, seborrhea, and a decrease in body fat *(8)*. Gynecomastia (breast development) occurs in approx two-thirds of boys during normal puberty *(9)*. Regression of breast tissue generally occurs when puberty is complete.

GROWTH

In girls, the pubertal growth spurt occurs during the earlier Tanner stages. After menarche, growth is variable with an average increase in height of 4–6 cm. In boys, the pubertal growth spurt occurs during the later stages of puberty. In both sexes, the pubertal growth spurt is due to the combined effect of growth hormone and sex steroids *(10)*. In both boys and girls, estrogen, rather than testosterone, stimulates growth hormone (GH) secretion such that basal serum (GH) and its response to specific stimulation tests increase during puberty *(11,12)*. Twenty-four hour GH production is increased, and this is an amplitude modulated phenomenon as the number of pulses remains unchanged *(13)*. Also, the increase in the mean 24-hr GH concentrations corresponds to the increase in height velocity of North American males *(14)*. Estrogen has an important role in the maturation of the epiphyseal growth plate and the advancement of the bone age. The importance of estrogen in epiphyseal maturation has been supported by the delayed epiphyseal maturation reported in the estrogen-insensitive male and in aromatase-deficient males and females *(15,16)*. Furthermore, in either sex, estrogen is crucial for the accumulation of calcium in bones and the attainment of a normal bone mineral density (BMD) *(17)*.

Hormonal Features

The physical changes described are the results of two generally simultaneous processes: gonadarche, activation of the hypothalamic/pituitary/gonadal axis; and, adrenarche, activation of the hypothalamic/pituitary/adrenal axis.

GONADARCHE

The increase in the pulsatile release of gonadotropin-releasing hormone (GnRH) from the hypothalamus results in an increase in the amplitude and frequency of follicle-stimulating hormone (FSH) and luteinizing hormone (LH) released from the pituitary gland *(18,19)*. Initially, FSH and LH pulses increase primarily at night, followed by an increase in both daytime and nighttime gonadotropin release *(20,21)*. LH stimulates increased testosterone production from the Leydig cells of the testes; FSH stimulates the maturation of spermatogonia *(9)*. In girls, both FSH and LH are necessary for sex-hormone production and FSH affects maturation of the ova *(18)*.

The presence of gonadarche can be confirmed with the GnRH stimulation test and the leuprolide stimulation test *(22,23)*. In either test, the gonadotropin response is diminished in the prepubertal child. As puberty progresses, the incremental rise of FSH and LH increases. The LH response to an exogenous dose of GnRH and leuprolide is more indicative of pubertal maturation than is the FSH response.

Adrenarche

Adrenarche refers to the rise of adrenal androgen production from the zona reticularis *(24)*. This contributes to the development of sexual hair growth as well as certain skin changes including acne and oily skin. The control of adrenarche is poorly understood. Adrenarche begins about the same time as the preadolescent rise in body mass index (BMI) *(25)*, the gradual increase in plasma insulin, and the increase in insulin-like growth factor (IGF-1) serum levels *(26)*. Nutritional status, measurable in the form of a change in BMI (and not BMI alone) is an important physiological regulator of adrenarche *(27)*.

Normal Variants

Premature Thelarche

Premature thelarche refers to the early appearance of breast tissue usually in toddler girls. Modest overfunction of the pituitary-ovarian axis has been implicated *(28)*. Basal levels of FSH can be increased and there is often an exaggerated FSH response to GnRH stimulation. Basal and GnRH stimulated LH levels are low. Slight elevations of estradiol can occur.

Typically, the areola is not estrogenized in appearance, i.e., the diameter is approx 1 cm and it is not hyperpigmented. The urogenital mucosa is prepubertal in appearance, or there may be modest estrogenization. Growth and bone-age maturation are normal. Ovarian ultrasound may detect microcysts *(29)*. Follow-up should be performed to confirm the nonprogressive nature of this condition and that growth and development remain normal.

Premature Adrenarche

Premature adrenarche refers to the early maturation of the zona reticularis in girls before the age of 8 yr and in boys before the age of 9 yr *(24)*. Adrenocorticotropin (ACTH)-stimulated androgens and levels of dehydroepiandrosterone sulfate are within the range seen in children in the early pubertal stages (Tanner II–III). The modest hyperandrogenism causes the early appearance of pubic and axillary hair, axillary odor, mild oily skin, and acne. Virilization (i.e., change in body habitus, clitoromegaly, and hirsutism) does not occur. Growth and bone-age maturation remain normal.

Premature Adrenarche and Polycystic Ovarian Syndrome (PCOS)

Recently, premature adrenarche has been proposed to be a risk factor for polycystic ovary syndrome (PCOS) and insulin resistance *(30)*. In contrast to the modest hyperandrogenism described in children with premature adrenarche, approx one-third of the 72 prepubertal African-American and Carribbean Hispanic girls with premature adrenarche evaluated had ACTH-stimulated androgens (particularly 17-hydroxypregnenolone) that were more than 2 standard deviations (SD) above the mean for normal girls who were in the Tanner II–III stages of puberty *(31)*. Furthermore, approx half of the prepubertal minority girls evaluated had acanthosis nigricans and reduced insulin sensitivity when tested with the frequently sampled intravenous glucose tolerance test. Those girls who were more insulin resistant were heavier, had higher ACTH stimulated androgens, and had a strong family history of diabetes. In a study performed by Ibanez et al., 45% of 35 adolescent girls with a history of premature adrenarche had clinical and hormonal findings consistent with functional ovarian hyperandrogenism when evaluated with the leuprolide challenge test *(32)*. Hence, in certain girls, premature adrenarche may be an early clinical feature of PCOS and insulin resistance.

PRECOCIOUS PUBERTY

Until recently, in the US, a child was considered to have precocious sexual development when the secondary sex characertistics appeared before the age of 8 yr in girls and before the age of 9 yr in boys. In 1997, Herman-Giddens reported the pubertal staging of more than 17,00 girls between 3 and 12 yr of age *(33)*. The examinations were from the Pediatric Research in Office Settings network. Breasts and pubic hair were reported to occur significantly earlier especially in African-American girls. In this 1997 study, stage 2 of breast and pubic hair development occurred approx 1 yr earlier in white girls and 2 yr earlier in African-American girls than previous studies had shown. The Herman-Giddens report did not include endocrine testing or follow-up data to confirm that these girls had truly progressive puberty nor did the report include information regarding the rate of pubertal progression in these young children. Based on this report, the Drug and Therapeutics and Executive Committees of the Lawson Wilkins Pediatric Endocrine Society have recommended new guidelines for the age at which early sexual development be considered precocious *(34)*. The Lawson Wilkins Pediatric Endocrine Society has proposed that girls with either breast development or pubic hair should be evaluated if these occur before age 7 in white girls and before age 6 in African-American girls. Boys with signs of puberty younger than 9 yr should be evaluated. However, these recommendations have not been uniformly accepted by Pediatric Endocrinologists and many still adhere to the previous guidelines (girls should be evaluated if puberty occurs before the age of 8 yr; boys, before the age of 9 yr). Important is that the evaluation of the child with early puberty should be individualized. The child with early puberty should be followed carefully to confirm that psychological or behavioral issues do not arise, that the child's growth and development progress normally, and that the child's bone age does not mature too rapidly and possibly result in a short adult stature.

The initial evaluation of the child with early sexual development is to assess whether the early pubertal development is the result of the early activation of the hypothalamic/pituitary/gonadal axis (central or gonadotropin-dependent precocious puberty) or is the result of increased sex-steroid production from either the gonads or adrenals independent of gonadotropin release (peripheral or gonadotropin-independent precocious puberty). The GnRH stimulation test is sometimes useful in distinguishing between the two subsets.

Central or Gonadotropin-Dependent Precocious Puberty

DEFINITION

Central precocious puberty refers to the early activation of the hypothalamic/pituitary/gonadal/axis. In the classical situation, children with CPP have elevated basal levels of

Table 1
Differential Diagnosis of Gonadotropin-Dependent (Central) Precocious Puberty

• Idiopathic
• CNS abnormalities: surgery, trauma, post-infection (meningitis abscess, granulomatous
  disease, encephalitis), postchemotherapy, postirradiation, arachnoid or ventricular cyst, suprasellar cyst, inflammatory disorders, septo-optic dysplasia, tumors (LH-secreting adenoma,
  astrocytoma, optic glioma, [neurofibromatosis] craniopharyngioma, dysgerminoma, ganglio-
  neuroma, ependymoma, hypothalamic hamartoma, teratoma, pinealoma), hydrocephalus,
  empty sella syndrome, tuberous sclerosis, epilepsy
• Secondary to chronic exposure to sex steroids (also referred to as combined precocious
  puberty): congenital adrenal hyperplasia, McCune-Albright syndrome, ovarian cysts,
  familial gonadotropin-independent precocious puberty
• Misc. conditions:
  Boys with Russell-Silver syndrome
  Hypothyroidism
  Prader-Willi syndrome

LH and FSH and a rise of gonadotropins in response to a bolus dose of GnRH or leuprolide
as seen in the normal pubertal child.

DIFFERENTIAL

The majority of girls with early sexual development have central precocious puberty.
In these children, imaging of the pituitary by magnetic resonance imaging (MRI) with
gadolinium contrast is performed to rule out a space-occupying lesion within the hypothalamus or the pituitary. The conditions known to be associated with central precocious
puberty are listed in Table 1.

More commonly, a specific etiology of the sexual precocity is not identified, and the
diagnosis of idiopathic central precocious puberty is made. Ninety-five percent of girls
have idiopathic precocious puberty whereas more than 50% of boys have an identifiable
lesion *(35)*. Essentially, any central nervous system (CNS) pathology can be associated with
true precocious puberty. Precocious puberty has also been described in association with
Russell-Silver syndrome, Prader-Willi syndrome, and severe hypothyroidism, although
the precise etiology is not known.

A hypothalamic hamartoma is a benign hyperplasia of nervous tissue having a normal
histological appearance and frequently presenting as a pedunculated mass at the base of the
brain *(35)*. Most of these tumors contain ectopic GnRH-secreting neurons that function
independently of the normal hypothalamic/pituitary axis. Ectopic GnRH in the hypothalamic hamartoma produces premature activation of pulsatile GnRH release. Recently, transforming growth factor-alpha (TGF-α) mRNA was identified in the tumors of two girls
with hypothalamic hamartomas *(36)*. Neither tumor had neurons producing GnRH. Hence,
peptides such as TGF-α may hasten the onset of puberty.

Precocious puberty can be characterized by an increase in growth velocity, acceleration
of bone maturation, early epiphyseal fusion, and, in certain cases, short adult stature *(37–
39)*. Therefore, an important part of the evaluation of the precocious child is to determine
whether the child is at risk for short stature. Short stature, with a height below the 5th percentile, can occur in 10–30% of girls with untreated central precocious puberty. The mean
adult height in untreated girls with idiopathic precocious puberty has been reported to be

short (150.9–155.3 cm m) *(37–41)*. However, 29 of the 89 girls reported achieved an adult height greater than five feet. The mean adult height of untreated boys with precocious puberty ranges from 149.8–159.6 cm *(38,39,41)*. In addition, mild, slowly progressive variants of precocious puberty have been reported. Fontoura described girls with central precocious puberty and moderate estrogen activity in whom bone-age advancement was less than 2 yr above chronologic age at the time of evaluation *(42)*. Initially the height prediction was normal and did not deteriorate after 2 yr of follow-up without therapy. Kreiter also described a group of girls with precocious puberty who had a normal mean height prediction of 165.4 cm, which did not deteriorate after 2 yr of observation *(43)*.

Recently, the final height and near final heights for 27 untreated children with precocious puberty were reported to be 161.4 ± 7.7 cm (32th percentile) and 165 cm (59th percentile), respectively *(44)*. Ninety percent of the girls achieved a height of more than 153 cm (3rd percentile). Only 10% were shorter than 150 cm. Final height significantly correlated with the initial height prediction (using the method of Bayley-Pinneau) and with the degree of height age advancement (Fig. 1) *(44)*. Although final height correlated very well with the Bayley Pinneau height prediction, this method overestimated the final height by 4.2 +/– 4.4 cm. As this study did not include a large cohort of girls whose sexual precocity occurred before the age of 5 yr, the Bayley-Pinneau method of height prediction for these younger girls should be interpreted with caution.

In that same study, the mean interval between the onset of breast development and menarche was 4.9 +/– 2.4 yr. This indicates that many of these girls had the more slowly progressive variant of precocious puberty, which has a less detrimental effect on adult height and does not warrant therapy. However, three girls with a normal height prediction at the time of their initial evaluation ultimately had a height of less than 150 cm. This underscores that careful follow-up is necessary to ensure that sexual maturation remains slowly progressive and that there is no deterioration of the height prediction.

Palmert also reported the initial presentation and long-term follow-up of 20 untreated patients with slowly progressive puberty *(45)*. These girls reached their genetic targets for final height (mean final height of 165.5 +/– 2.2 cm; mean genetic target height 164.0 +/– 1.1 cm). The average age of menarche was 11.0 +/– 0.4 yr. Hence, slowly progressive puberty in young girls does not warrant therapy with GnRH analog.

TRANSIENT SEXUAL PRECOCIOUS PUBERTY

Transient central precocious puberty has also been described in which the clinical symptoms wax and wane *(46)*. Hence, for the early pubertal child, follow-up with confirmation of its progressive nature should occur before therapy is initiated.

Peripheral or Gonadotropin Independent Precocious Puberty

DEFINITION

Peripheral precocious puberty refers to the production of sex steroids from the gonads or adrenal glands without activation of the hypothalamic/pituitary/gonadal axis. Basal gonadotropins are low, and there is a negligible rise of gonadotropins in response to GnRH testing.

DIFFERENTIAL

The conditions associated with peripheral precocious puberty are listed in Table 2. Familial gonadotropin-independent precocious puberty refers to an autosomal dominant

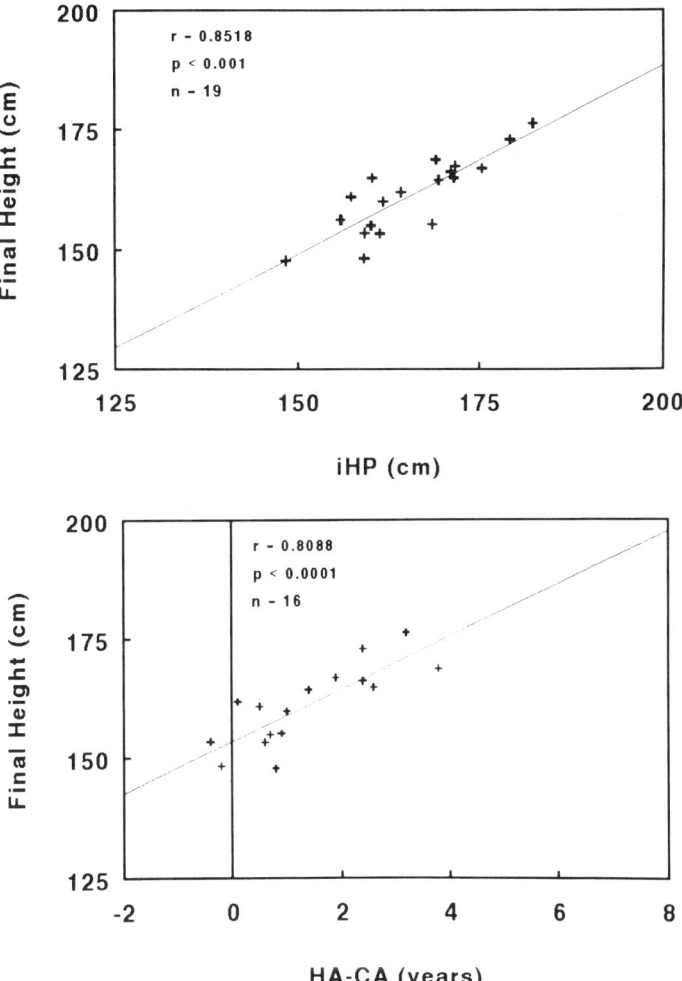

Fig. 1. Final height significantly correlated with initial HP (*iHP*) ($r = 0.85; p < 0.001$) and with degree of height age advancement ($HA - CA$) ($r = 0.8; p < 0.001$). Adapted with permission from ref. *(91)*.

mutation in the LH receptor, resulting in its constitutive activation and the resultant autonomous production of testosterone independent of LH release *(47)*. Males generally exhibit penile enlargement and bilateral testicular enlargement by the age of 4 yr *(48)*. Gonadotropin levels are prepubertal. The chronic production of testosterone in boys can result in the secondary activation of the hypothalamic/pituitary/gonadal axis with result-ant central preococious puberty as well.

The McCune-Albright syndrome is a form of peripheral precocious puberty character-ized by the classic triad of precocious puberty, polyostotic fibrous dysplasia, and café au lait spots *(49)*. Additional endocrine abnormalities may include hyperthyroidism, GH excess, and Cushing's disease. This condition is caused by an activating mutation in the gene encoding the stimulatory subunit of the G protein, causing autonomous activation of G-protein stimulated cAMP formation and resulting in episodic excessive sex-steroid production *(49)*. The sporadic formation of ovarian cysts leads to transient excessive ele-vations of serum estradiol, the early development of breasts, and vaginal bleeding. As in

Table 2
Differential Diagnosis
of Gonadotropin-Independent (Peripheral or Pseudo) Precocious Puberty

---

- Familial Gonadotropin-Independent Precocious Puberty
- McCune-Albright syndrome
- Congenital adrenal hyperplasia
- Adrenal lesion (adenoma, carcinoma)
- Ovarian lesion (granulosa cell, granulosa-theca cell, cystadenoma, gonadoblastoma, lipoid)
- Leydig-cell tumor, teratoma
- Human chorionic gonadotropin (hCG) producing lesion: (choriocarcinoma, chorioepithelioma, dysgerminoma, hepatoblastoma, teratoma, hepatoma)

---

males with familial gonadotropin-independent precocious puberty, girls with this condition can have secondary central precocious puberty as well.

The term adrenal hyperplasia refers to the histologic change that occurs in the adrenal gland as a result of the deficiency of one of the several enzymes necessary for steroid biosynthesis *(50)*. Cortisol is the most important of the glucocorticoids made by the adrenal gland and its synthesis is regulated by pituitary ACTH. In the enzymatic defects of cortisol biosynthesis deficient production of cortisol is associated with a compensatory rise in ACTH and the accumulation of steroids proximal to the enzymatic defect. These precursors are shunted to the androgen pathways and hyperandrogenism results. The three autosomal resessive disorders that cause cortisol deficiency and hyperandrogenism include 21-hydroxylase deficiency, 11-hydroxylase deficiency, and 3β-hydroxysteroid dehygenase deficiency. Symptoms of the disorder depend on which classes of steroids are deficient and which are overproduced. For example, in the severe salt-wasting form of 21-hydroxylase deficiency, both the cortisol and mineralocorticoid synthesis are interrupted and androgens are overproduced. In the genetic female, the prenatal exposure to high androgens in the first trimester causes genital ambiguity and children of either sex will develop salt-wasting symptoms generally within the first 3 mo of life. However, in the simple virilizing form of 21-hydroxylase deficiency, cortisol, but not mineralocorticoid biosynthesis is interrupted, the genetic male will not be born with genital ambiguity, the genetic female will be born with genital ambiguity, and salt-wasting symptoms do not occur. Delay in diagnosis or inadequate treatment in either case will result in postnatal virilization with progressive clitoral and phallic enlargement, early development of axillary and pubic hair, axillary hair and odor, acne, increased growth velocity with crossing of a percentile growth channels, advanced bone age, precocious puberty, and ultimately short stature. Young women inadequately treated may develop PCOS. The nonclassic late onset form of 21-hydroxylase deficiency has clinical variability and can present at any age with symptoms of hyperandrogenism. Because the enzymatic defect is milder than the congenital form, affected girls do not have general ambiguity. The clinical symptoms include premature pubic and axillary hair growth, premature axillary odor, acne, increased growth velocity, advanced bone age, hirsutism, male pattern baldness in young women, and PCOS. In both the nonclassic and the classic forms of adrenal hyperplasia, the diagnosis can be confirmed by finding an elevated basal 17-hydroxyprogesterone and in response to a bolus dose of ACTH. However, in the milder enzymatic defects, basal 17-hydroxyprogesterone may not be elevated.

Like the 21-hydroxylase deficiency, the 11β-hydroxylase enzyme can also present with the more severe congenital syndrome characterized by sexual ambiguity in affected females, and, similarly, inadequate therapy can result in early virilization. In addition, the accumulation of deoxycorticosterone (a weak mineralocorticoid) will eventually lead to low renin hypertension. Milder forms of 11-β hydroxylase deficiency have been described and present similar to the late-onset form of 21-hydroxylase deficiency. The diagnosis is made by finding an elevated 11-hydroxycortisol in the basal state that is stimulated by ACTH and suppressed by dexamethasone.

The deficiency of the 3-β hydroxysteroid dehydrogenase enzyme also present with a severe form with ambiguity in both sexes in the salt-wasting crisis in the neonatal period *(51)*. However, milder forms have also been described similar to 21-hydroxylase deficiency and 11-hydroxylase deficiency. Molecular genetic studies have identified defects in the gene encoding this enzyme only in those patients whose precursor hormones, 17-hydroxypregnenolone and dehydroepiandosterone, are markedly elevated to approx 8 standard deviations (SD) above the mean of normal of normal individuals *(52)*.

Virilization of girls (sexual hair growth, oily skin, acne, clitoromegaly, and hirsutism) can occur in association with a virilizing adrenal or ovarian neoplasm. Virilization of boys can occur with a testicular tumor (Leydig-cell tumor, teratoma) or an human chorionic gonadotropin (hCG)-producing tumor, which stimulates testosterone production by the Leydig cells.

Combined Precocious Puberty

Combined precocious puberty refers to activation of the hypothalamic/pituitary/gonadal axis that occurs after the long-standing sex-steroid exposure of peripheral precocious puberty. This can be seen with congenital adrenal hyperplasia, the McCune-Albright syndrome, and familial gonadotropin-independent precocious puberty.

EVALUATION OF THE SEXUALLY PRECOCIOUS CHILD

History

The evaluation of the child with early sexual development includes a complete history with particular attention to symptoms suggestive of CNS pathology (headache, vomiting, visual disturbances, etc.). A family history should include the pubertal history and heights of parents and other family members.

Physical Examination

The physical examination should include height, weight, and careful Tanner staging of pubertal development. In boys, testicular size should be measured using the Prader orchidometer. Bilateral or unilateral testicular enlargement can be seen with testicular tumors or with adrenal rest tissue associated with adrenal hyperplasia.

Psychological Assessment

In the young child, difficulty coping with tall stature and advancing pubertal development may present with behavioral changes *(53–55)*. The dyssynchrony between physical appearance and chronological age may predispose certain children to stress, abuse, and early pregnancy. Psychologic counseling may be helpful for the parents and child to decrease the fears they may have regarding the early sexual development.

Laboratory Evaluation

The laboratory evaluation involves direct measurement of basal sex steroids (testosterone and estradiol) and gonadotropins (FSH, LH). Human chorionic gonadotropin (hCG) should be measured in boys (to evaluate for a possible hCG-producing lesion). Thyroid-function tests and adrenal androgen levels should also be obtained. A GnRH stimulation test is useful to confirm the activation of the hypothalamic/pituitary/gonadal axis. GnRH (100 mcg bolus) is administered intravenously with FSH and LH measured at 0, 20, 40, and 60 min *(22)*. Alternatively in the leuprolide stimulation test, leuprolide (20 mcg/kg) is administered subcutaneously and gonadotropins are measured 0, 1, 2, 3, 4, 6, and 24 h; serum estradiol (in girls) or testosterone (in boys) are obtained at baseline, 6 and 24 h *(23)*. Interpretation of the gonadotropin response requires a knowledge of the prepubertal and pubertal levels for the particular assay utilized. An ACTH stimulation test (adrenal steroids measured before and 60 min after an intravenous bolus of ACTH 0.25 mg) and dexamethasone suppression test (adrenal steroids measured before and after dexamethasone 20 mcg/kg/d or 2 mg/d for 2 d) should be performed if adrenal pathology is suspected.

Radiographic Evaluation

For those children with central precocious puberty, an MRI of the pituitary gland with gadolinium should be performed to rule out a CNS lesion. An adrenal computed tomography (CT) scan, MRI, or adrenal/pelvic ultrasound should be performed if the GnRH test is consistent with peripheral precocious puberty. A bone age should be obtained so that a height prediction can be made *(44)*.

THERAPY

Central Precocious Puberty

INDICATIONS

When precocious puberty is not idiopathic, treatment should be directed towards the etiology. In central precocious puberty, the goal of therapy is to halt pubertal progression in order to avoid psychosocial and behavioral problems and to improve adult height in those children at risk for short stature. The Bayley-Pinneau method of height prediction can be used to identify those patients at risk for short stature who might benefit from therapy *(44)*.

GnRH ANALOG THERAPY

Long-acting analogs of GnRH (GnRHa) are now considered the treatment of choice for select children with gonadotropin-dependent precocious puberty. After an initial activation of the hypothalamic/pituitary/gonadal axis, they cause reversible suppression of gonadotropins and a decline in gonadal sex-steroids levels *(56)*. Clinically in girls, menses cease and breast development regresses after several months of therapy. In boys, testicular size also gradually decreases. Sexual hair growth in both sexes continues to progress slowly as GnRH analogs do not suppress adrenarche *(557)*. The rate of linear growth and bone-age advancement decreases and ultimately, the adult height is improved. GnRH testing is used periodically to confirm suppression of the hypothalamic/pituitary/gonadal axis. Urinary gonadotropin determinations are not reliable for assessing gonadotropin suppression *(58)*. GnRH analogs are not effective for the treatment of gonadotropin-independent precocious puberty such as McCune-Albright syndrome or familial gonadotropin-independent precocious puberty unless it is complicated by secondary central precocious puberty.

GnRH Therapy: Long-Term Follow-Up

Gonadal Function. The menstrual function of girls after treatment with GnRH analogs has been studied by several groups. Jay et al. reported the menstrual function of 46 girls with central precocious puberty who had been treated with GnRH for at least 2 yr *(59)*. Menses occurred on the average of 1.2 ± 0.8 yr post-therapy (range 0.1–4.3 yr). Menstrual cycles of 25–35 d duration were reported to occur in 41% of the girls in the first yr postmenarche and 65% of the girls studied 3 or more yr postmenarche. Ovulation was demonstrated in 50% of the girls studied within 1yr of menarche and in 90% of the girls studied 2 yr or more postmenarche, similar to documented patterns for normal adolescents. Fertility after GnRHa has not been assessed as yet. However, pregnancies have been reported to occur in young adolescents who had completed therapy with GnRHa *(59)*.

Feuillan compared the reproductive axis after discontinuation of GnRH therapy in girls with hypothalamic hamartoma and idiopathic precocious puberty to that of normal perimenarcheal girls *(60)*. By 1 yr after discontinuation of therapy, gonadotropins and estradiol were in the pubertal range in both groups of girls. However, the ratio of peak LH/FSH in response to a bolus of GnRH was less than that observed in the normal controls. The mean age of menarche in the patients was comparable to that in normal girls, and, seven patients demonstrated fertility. Those girls with hypothalamic hamartomas had a higher incidence of oligomenorrhea. The mean ovarian volume as determined by ultrasound was greater in the girls with hamartomas than in the girls with idiopathic precocious puberty, but by 4–5 yr after therapy, ovarian volume in both groups of treated girls was higher than the normals. Baseline and stimulated gonadotropin levels were not consistent with PCOS. Continued follow-up is necessary to determine whether these girls will develop PCOS. Of note is that both groups of treated girls had a BMI that was greater than normal prior to and during therapy. It is not clear whether the observed increase in ovarian volume is due to the therapy itself or is in some way related to their obesity, as is functional ovarian hyperandrogenism.

In contrast, Baek Johnson from Denmark reported the ultrasound findings in 33 girls with idiopathic precocious puberty *(61)*. Although precocious girls had a higher mean ovarian volume prior to therapy than normal prepubertal girls, GnRHa therapy resulted in a reduction in mean ovarian volume similar to that of prepubertal girls. After discontinuation of therapy, ovarian volume remained in the normal range. None of the girls' ovaries had a polycystic appearance during or after treatment with GnRH analogs.

Bone Mineral Density. Puberty is characterized by major changes in BMD. Neely measured BMD in treated girls with precocious puberty using dual-energy X-ray absorptometry *(62)*. Prior to treatment, BMD was elevated for age and concordant for the advanced skeletal age. During therapy, BMD SD scores for age and skeletal age did not change. These findings have been substantiated by Boot, who noted that mean spinal BMD SDS and total body BMD SDS did not change substantially after 2 yr of GnRHa analog therapy *(63)*.

Obesity. There has been concern that children with central precocious puberty are prone to the development of obesity. This question was recently addressed in the report of Palmert et al., who analyzed several parameters of obesity (including skinfold thickness, percent body fat by dual-energy X-ray absorptiometry and BMI) in a large cohort of treated children with precocious puberty *(45)*. Girls and boys with precocious puberty had a mean BMI SD score that was increased prior to the initiation with therapy. The children remained obese and GnRHa therapy had little impact on weight or weight gain.

Height. GnRHa therapy causes a decrease in growth velocity that results from a decrease in the amplitude of nocturnal GH peaks without affecting GH pulse frequency *(64)*. Changes in IGF-1 levels are variable *(65)*. The combined effects of the decrease in growth velocity as well as a decrease in the rate of bone-age maturation results in an increase in the child's height prediction. Several long-term studies report a significant increase in the mean adult height of GnRHa-treated patients *(66–80)*. The reported mean adult heights of treated girls are very variable and range from 154.7–164.9 cm with a height gain of approx 2–5.2 cm when the final height is compared to the initial height prediction made at the time of diagnosis. However, because the Bayley Pinneau method of height prediction tends to overestimate the final height in girls with precocious puberty, the height gains with therapy are probably underestimated *(44)* (*see* Fig. 1). There is sparse information available regarding the adult height of boys treated with GnRH analogs. Mean adult heights of treated boys range from 168–184 cm which constitute a 6.3–9.9 cm gain in adult height compared to the initial height prediction made at the time of diagnosis *(75,76)*. The tremendous variability of the impact of treatment on adult height reflects several factors including genetic potential, the age of initiation of puberty, the degree of bone-age advancement at the time of diagnosis, and the timing of initiation of therapy. In the 1994 review by Kletter and Kelch, the adult heights of GnRHa-treated girls was assessed according to the age of the child when sexual precocity was diagnosed and evaluated *(79)*. In that review, the adult heights of 17 treated children with precocious puberty diagnosed before 6 yr of age was compared to the heights of 10 untreated children of the same age. The adult heights of the treated children was 160.4 ± 1.8 cm in comparison to the untreated children who achieved an adult height of 153.9 ± 3.8 cm. The heights of the 114 treated children who were more than 6 yr of age at the time of evaluation, were not significantly different than the height of the 54 untreated children of the same age (157.5 cm and 157 cm, respectively). Hence, the treatment of children who were diagnosed and treated before the age of 6 yr, resulted in a significant improvement in adult height.

Brauner reserved GnRHa therapy for those girls with a poor height prediction less than 155 cm and did not treat those girls with a height prediction greater than 155 cm *(80)*. The group who received therapy achieved a mean adult height that was 6.5 cm greater than their initial height prediction. In the untreated children, the adult height was similar to the predicted height at the initial evaluation.

GnRH Analogs and GH Therapy

Growth Hormone Deficiency. In general, adult heights tend to be below the target heights in both boys and girls. Furthermore, in certain children, GnRHa therapy results in a marked decline in growth velocity below normal. Standard provocative testing should be performed to evaluate for coexistent growth hormone deficiency (GHD). GH therapy in these children can improve their growth velocity and height prediction *(81)*. Information regarding final height in those children treated with combination therapy is limited.

Growth Hormone Sufficiency. The observations that GH decreases during GnRHa therapy for precocious puberty combined with the poor growth velocity and poor height prediction in certain children despite GnRHa therapy have prompted the theory that perhaps improved growth could be achieved by combination GH and GnRHa therapy. GH therapy has also been extended to precocious pubertal children treated with GnRHa whose height prediction is impaired but who are not GH deficient by standard testing *(66, 68,82,83)*. In these children, combination therapy can result in an improved growth velocity and predicted adult height. Pasquino et al. administered combination GH and GnRHa therapy for 2–4 yr to 10 of 20 girls with central precocious puberty until adult height was achieved *(84)*. Patients treated with GH plus GnRHa showed an adult height significantly higher than pretreatment predicted adult height with a mean gain of 7.9 +/− 1.1 cm. Patients treated with GnRHa only achieved an adult height of only 1.6 +/− 1.2 cm greater than their initial height prediction. Furthermore, those children treated with combination therapy did not develop ovarian cysts.

Therefore, although certain children may benefit from combination therapy, the amount of benefit reaped by combination therapy is not clear. Of potential concern is the report by Bridges, that those girls treated with combination therapy developed very large ovaries during therapy and had an increased prevalence of ovaries with a polycystic appearance *(85)*.

Gonadotropin-Independent Preococious Puberty

Therapy for gonadotropin-independent precocious puberty should be directed toward the etiology. Tumors are treated both surgically and with chemotherapy. In familial gonadotropin-independent precocious puberty (testotoxicosis), inhibitors of androgen biosynthesis (ketoconazole), anti-androgens (flutamide, spironolactone), and inhibitors of androgen to estrogen conversion (testolactone) are being investigated *(86)*.

The treatment the enzymatic defects of steroidogenesis dependent on whether or not there is isolated glucocorticoid and/or mineralocorticoid deficiency. For those patients with isolated glucocorticoid deficiency, a dose of hydrocortisone of 10–25 mg/m^2/d may be necessary in order to maintain normal growth and development and a normal rate of bone-age advancement *(50)*. The salt-wasting patients generally require the salt-retaining steroid 9α-fludrocortisone acetate. This is sometimes useful for those simple virilizers who tend to have elevated plasma renin activity. Although the introduction of steroid radioimmunoassay methods has facilitated management of these children, growth and development may not be optimal. Hence, currently studies are underway to determine if the addition of androgen-receptor blockers will improve growth *(87)*. Preliminary data suggest that flutamide and testolactone can be used with a reduced dose of hydrocortisone in patients with adrenal hyperplasia *(88)*.

Treatment of McCune-Albright syndrome has not been optimal. Testolactone (an aromatase inhibitor) has been used but has variable success due to problems both with efficacy and compliance *(89)*. Tamoxifen (a nonsteroidal antiestrogen with both potent antiestrogenic and weakly estrogenic properties) has been used in a limited number of children and has been found to be beneficial in halting pubertal progression and improving adult height predictions in girls with this condition *(90)*. Large-scale studies need to be done to confirm the effectiveness and safety of this therapy.

SUMMARY

For the child who has early sexual development, the initial evaluation should be directed toward identification of the specific etiology so that appropriate treatment can be provided. For those children with central puberty, therapy with long-acting analogs is effective in halting pubertal progression, improving adult height, and promoting the psychosocial adjustment of the child and family. There is a wide spectrum of clincial progression of the early sexual development ranging from the nonprogressive forms to the more rapidly progressive variants. Hence, not all children with sexual precocity require GnRH analog-suppressive therapy. For those children whose families opt not to choose treatment because the height prediction is acceptable and the early development is not interfering with their psychosocial adjustment, careful follow-up of growth and development should continue.

REFERENCES

1. Wilkins, L. The diagnosis and treatment of endocrine disorders in childhood and adolescence. Charles C. Thomas, Springfield, IL, 1968, p. 250.
2. Lee PA. Normal ages of pubertal events among American males and females. J Adolesc Health Care 1980;1:26–29.
3. Marshall WA, Tanner JM. Variations in pattern of pubertal changes in girls. Arch Dis Child 1969;44:291–303.
4. Marshall WA, Tanner JM. Variations in pattern of pubertal changes in boys. Arch Dis Child 1970;45:13–23.
5. DeRidder CM, Thijssen JHH, Bruning PF, Van Den Brande JL, Zonderland ML, Erich WBM. Body fat mass, body fat distribution, and pubertal development: a longitudinal study of physical and hormonal sexual maturation of girls. J Clin Endocrinol Metab 1992;75:442–446.
6. Kaplan SL, Grumbach MM. Clinical Review 14: pathophysiology and treatment of sexual precocity. J Clin Endocrinol Metab 1990;71:785–789.
7. Zachmann M, Prader A, Kind HP, Hafliger H, Budliger H. Testicular volume during adolescence: cross-sectional and longitudinal studies. Helv Paediatr Acta 1974;29:61–72.
8. Forbes GB, Porta CR, Herr BE, Griggs RC. Sequence of changes in body composition induced by testosterone and reversal of changes after drug is stopped. JAMA 1992;267–399.
9. Nielson CT, Skakkabak NE, Darling JA, et al. Longitudinal study of testosterone and luteinizing hormone (LH) in relation to supermarche, pubic hair, height and sitting height in normal boys. Acta Endocrinol (Copenh) 1986;279(Suppl):98–106.
10. Attie KM, Ramirez RR, Conte FA, Kaplan SL, Grumbach MM. The pubertal growth spurt in eight patients with true precocious puberty and growth hormone deficiency: evidence for a direct role of sex steroids. J Clin Endocrinol Metab 1990;71:975–983.
11. Gelato MC, Malozowski S, Caruso-Nicolett M, et al. Growth hormone (GH) responses to GH-releasing hormone during pubertal development in normal boys and girls: comparison to idiopathic short stature and GH deficiency. J Clin Endocrinol Metab 1986;63:174–179.
12. Zadik Z, Chalew SA, Kowarski A. Assessment of growth hormone secretion in normal stature children using 24-hour integrated concentration of GH and pharmacological stimulation. J Clin Endocrinol Metab 1990;71:932–936.
13. Mauras N, Blizzard RM, Link, Johnson ML, Rogol AD, Veldhuis JD. Augmentation of GH secretion during puberty: evidence for a pulse amplitude-modulated phenomenon. J Clin Endo Metab 1987;64:596–601.
14. Martha PM J, Rogol AD, Veldhuis JD, Kerrigan JR, Goodman DW, Blizzard RM. Alterations in the pulsatile properties of circulating GH concentrations during puberty in boys. J Clin Endocrinol Metab 1989;69:563–570.
15. Federman DD. Life without estrogen. N Engl J Med 1994;331:1088–1089.
16. Smith EP, Boyd J, Frank GR, et al. Estrogen resistance caused by a mutation in the estrogen-receptor gene in a man. N Engl J Med 1994;331:1056–1061.
17. Bachrach LK. Bone mineralization in childhood and adolescence. Curr Opin Pediatr 1993;5:467–473.
18. Knobil E. The neuroendocrine control of the menstrual cycle. Recent Prog Horm Res 1980;36:53–88.
19. Lee PA. Pubertal neuroendocrine maturation: early differentiation and stages of development. Adolesc Pediatr Gynecol 1988;1:3–12.
20. Burr IM, Sizonenko PC, Kaplan SL, Grumbach MM. Hormonal changes in puberty. I. Correlation of serum lutenizing hormone and follicle stimulating hormone with stages of puberty, testicular size, and bone age in normal boys. Pediatr Res 1970;4:25–35.
21. Sizonenko PC, Burr IM, Kaplan SL, Grumbach MM. Hormonal changes in puberty. II. Correlation of serum luteinizing hormone and follicle stimulating with stages of puberty and bone age in normal girls. Pediatr Res 1970;4:36–45.

22. Reiter EO, Kaplan SL, Conte FA. Responsivity of pituitary gonadotropes to luteinizing hormone-releasing factor in idiopathic precocious puberty, precocious thelarche, precocious adrenarche and in patients treated with medroxy-progesterone acetate. Pediatr Res 1975;9:111–116.

23. Garibaldi LR, Aceto T Jr, Weber C, Pang S. The relationship between luteinizing hormone and estradiol secretion in female precocious puberty: evaluation by sensitive gonadotropin assays and the leuprolide stimulation test. J Clin Endocrinol Metab 1993;76:851–856.

24. Saenger P, Reiter EO. Editorial: premature adrenarche: a normal variant of puberty? J Clin Endocrinol Metab 1992;74:236–238.

25. Rolland-Cachera MF. Body composition during adolescence: methods, limitations and determinants. Horm Res 1993;39(Suppl 3):25–40.

26. Smith CP, Dunger DB, Williams AJK, et al. Relationship between insulin, insulin-like growth factor I, and dehydroepiandrosterone sulfate concentrations during childhood, puberty, and adult life. J Clin Endocrinol Metab 1989;68:932–937.

27. Remer T, Manz F. Role of nutritional status in the regulation of adrenarche. J Clin Endocrinol Metab 1999;84:3936–3944.

28. Pescovitz OH, Hench KD, Barnes KM, Loriaux DL, Cutler GB Jr. Premature thelarche and central precocious puberty: the relationship between clinical presentation and the gonadotropin response to luteinizing hormone-releasing hormone. J Clin Endocrinol Metab 1988;67:474–479.

29. Salardi S, Orsini LF, Cacciari E, Partesotti S, Brondelli L, Cicognani A, et al. Pelvic ultrasonography in girls with precocious puberty, congenital adrenal hyperplasia, obesity, or hirsutism. J Pediatr 1988; 112:880–887.

30. DiMartino-Nardi J. Premature adrenarche: findings in prepubertal African-American and Caribbean-Hispanic girls. Acta Paediatr 1999;433(Suppl):67–72.

31. Vuguin P, Linder B, Rosenfeld RG, Saenger P, DiMartino-Nardi J. The roles of insulin sensitivity, insulin-like growth factor I (IGF-I), and IGF-binding protein-1 and -3 in the hyperandrogenism of African-American and Caribbean Hispanic girls with premature adrenarche. J Clin Endocrinol Metab 1999;84:2037–2042.

32. Ibanez L, Potau N, Virdis R, et al. Postpubertal outcome in girls diagnosed of premature pubarche during childhood. Increased frequency of functional ovarian hyperandrogenism. J Clin Endocrinol Metab 1993;76:1599–1603.

33. Herman-Giddens ME, Slora EJ, Wasserman RC, et al. Secondary sexula characteristics and menses in young girls seen in office practice: a study from the pediatric research in office settings network. Pediatrics 1997;99:505–512.

34. Kaplowitz PB, Oberfield SE, and the Drug and Therapeutics and Executive Committees of the Lawson Wilkins Pediatric Endocrine Society. Reexamination of the age limit for defining when puberty is precocious in girls in the United States: implications for evaluation and treatment. Pediatrics 1999; 104(4):936–941.

35. Judge DM, Kulin HE, Page R, Santen R, Trapukdi S. Hypothalamic hamartoma: a source of luteinizing-hormone release factor in precocious puberty. N Engl J Med 1977;296:7–10.

36. Jung H, et al. Some hypothalamic hamartomas contain transforming growth factor alpha, a puberty-inducing growth factor, but not luteinizing hormone-releasing hormone neurons. J Clin Endocrinol Metab 1999;84:4695–4701.

37. Thamdrup E. Precocious Sexual Developmental: A Clinical Study of 100 Children. Charles C. Thomas, Springfield, IL, 1961, p. 237.

38. Sigurjonsdottir TJ, Hayles AB. Precocious puberty: a report of 96 cases. Am J Dis Child 1968;115: 309–321.

39. Werder EA, Mueset G, Zachmann M, et al. Treatment of precocious puberty with cyproterone acetate. Pediatr Res 1974;8:248–256.

40. Lee PA. Medroxyprogesterone therapy for sexual precocity in girls. Am J Dis Child 1981;135:443–445.

41. Murram D, Dewhurst J, Grant DB. Precocious puberty: a follow-up study. Arch Dis Child 1984;59: 77–78.

42. Fontoura M, Brauner R, Prevot C, Rappoport R. Precocious puberty in girls: early diagnosis of a slowly progressing variant. Arch Dis Childhood 1989;64:1170–1176.

43. Kreiter M, Burstein S, Rosenfield RL, Moll GW, Cara JF, Yousefzadeh DK, et al. Preserving adult height potential in girls with idiopathic true precocious puberty. J Pediatr 1990;117:364–370.

44. Bar A, Linder B, Sobel EH, Saenger P, DiMartino-Nardi J. The Bayley-Pinneau method for height prediction in girls with central precocious puberty: correlation with adult height. J Pediatr 1995;126:955–958.

45. Palmert MR, Mansfield MJ, Crowley WF Jr, Crigler JF Jr, Crawford JD, Boepple PA. Is obesity an outcome of gonadotropin-releasing hormone agonist administration? Analysis of growth and body composition in 110 patients with central precocious puberty. J Clin Endocrinol Metab 1999;84:4480–4488.

46. Schwarz HP, Tschaeppeler H, Zuppinger K. Case Report: Unsustained central sexual precocity in four girls. Am J Med Sci 1990;290:260–264.

47. Shenker A, Laue L, Kosugi S, et al. A constitutively activating mutation of the luteinizing hormone receptor in familial male precocious puberty. Nature 1993;365:652–654.

48. Egli CA, Rosenthal SM, Grumbach MM, et al. Pituitary gonadotropin-independent male-limited autosomal dominant sexual precocity in nine generations: familial testotoxicosis. J Pediatr 1985;106:33–40.

49. Weinstein LS, Shenker A, Gejman PV, et al. Activating mutations of the stimulatory G protein in the McCune-Albright syndrome. N Engl J Med 1991;325:1688–1695.

50. New MI, Ghizzoni L, Speiser PW. Update on congenital adrenal hyperplasia. In: Lifshitz F, ed. Pediatric Endocrinology. Marcel Dekker, New York, NY, 1996.

51. Pang S. The molecular and clinical spectrum of 3-β hydroxysteroid dehydrogenase deficiency disorder. Trends Endocrinol Metab 1998;9:82–86.

52. Chang YT, Zhang L, Alkaddour HS, Mason JI, Lin K, Yang X, et al. Absence of molecular defect in the type II 3β-hydroxysteroid dehydrogenase (3β-HSD) gene in premature pubarche children and hirsute female patients with moderately decreased adrenal 3β-HSD activity. Pediatr Res 1995;37:820–824.

53. Money Y, Clopper RR Jr. Psychosocial and psychosexual aspects of errors of pubertal onset and development. Hum Biol 1974;46:173–181.

54. Sonis WA, Comite F, Blue J, et al. Behavior problems and social competence in girls with true precocious puberty. J Pediatr 1985;106:156–160.

55. Ehrhardt AA, Meyer-Bahlburg HFL, Bell JJ, et al. Idiopathic precocious puberty in girls: psychiatric follow-up in adolescence. J Am Acad Child Psychiatry 1984;23:23–33.

56. Crowley WF, Comite F, Vale W, Rivier J, Loriaux DL, Cutler GB Jr. Therapeutic use of pituitary desensitization with a long-acting LHRH agonist: a potential new treatment for idiopathic precocious puberty. J Clin Endocrinol Metab 1981;52:370–372.

57. Wierman ME, Beardswork DE, Crawford JD, et al. Adrenarche and skeletal maturation during luteinizing hormone releasing-hormone analogue suppression of gonadarche. J Clin Invest 1986;77:121–126.

58. Witchel SF, Baens-Bailon RG, Lee PA. Treatment of central precocious puberty: comparison of urinary gonadotropin excretion and gonadotropin-releasing hormone (GnRH) stimulation tests in monitoring GnRH analog therapy. J Clin Endocrinol Metab 1996;81:1353–1356.

59. Jay N, Mansfield MJ, Blizzard RM, Crowley WF Jr, Shoenfeld D, Rhubin L, Boepple PA. Ovulation and Menstrual function of adolescent girls with central precocious puberty after therapy with gonadotropin-releasing hormone agonists. J Clin Endocrinol Metab 1992;75:890–894.

60. Feuillan PP, Jones JV, Barnes K, Oerter-Klein K, Culter GB Jr. Reproductive axis after discontinuation of gonadotropin-releasing hormone analog treatment of girls with precocious puberty: long term follow-up comparing girls with hypothalamic hamartoma to those with idiopathic precocious puberty. J Clin Endocrinol Metab 1999;84:44–49.

61. Baek Jenson AM, Brocks V, Holm K, Laursen EM, Miller J. Central precocious puberty in girls: internal genitalia before, during, and after treatment with long-acting gonadotropin-releasing hormone analogues. J Pediatr 1998;132:105–108.

62. Neely EK, Bachrach LK, Hintz RL, Habiby RL, Slemenda CW, Feezle L, Pescovitz OH. Bone mineral density during treatment of central precocious puberty. J Pediatr 1995;127:819–822.

63. Boot AM, De Munick Keizer-Schrama SMPF, Pols HAP, Krenning EP, Drop SLS. Bone mineral density and body composition before and during treatment with gonadotropin-releasing hormone agonist in children with central precocious and early puberty. J Clin Endocrinol Metab 1998;83:370–373.

64. DiMartino-Nardi J, Wu R, Varner R, Wong WLT, Saenger P. The Effect of luteinizing hormone-releasing hormone analog for precocious puberty on growth hormone (GH) and GH-binding protein. J Clin Endocrinol Metab 1994;78:664–668.

65. Harris DA, Van Vliet G, Egli CA, et al. Somatomedin-C in normal puberty and in true precocious puberty before and after treatment with a potent luteinizing hormone-releasing hormone agonist. J Clin Endocrinol Metab 1985;61:152–159.

66. Saggese G, Pasquino AM, Bertelloni S, et al. Effect of combined treatment with gonadotropin releasing hormone analogue and growth hormone in patients with central precocious puberty who had subnormal growth velocity and impaired height prognosis. Acta Paediatr 1995;84:299–304.

67. Kreiter M, Burstein S, Rosenfield RL, et al. Preserving adult height potential in girls with idiopathic true precocious puberty. J Pediatr 1990;117:364–370.

68. Tató L, Saggese G, Cavallo L, et al. Use of combined Gn-RH agonist and hGH therapy for better attaining the goals in precocious puberty treatment. Horm Res 1995;44:49–54.

69. Bertelloni S, Baroncelli GI, Sorrentino MC, Perri G, Saggese G. Effect of central precocious puberty and gonadotropin-releasing hormone analogue treatment on peak bone mass and final height in females. Eur J Pediatr 1998;157:363–367.

70. Kauli R, Galatzer A, Kornreich L, Lazar L, Pertzelan A, Laron A. Final height of girls with central precocious puberty, untreated versus treated with cyproterone acetate or GnRH analogue: a comparative study with re-evaluation of predictions by the Bayley-Pinneau method. Horm Res 1997;47:54–61.

71. Oerter KE, Manasco PK, Barnes KM, Jones J, Hill S, Cutler GB Jr. Effects of luteinizing hormone-releasing hormone agonist on final height in luteinizing hormone-releasing hormone-dependent precocious puberty. Acta Pediatr 1993;388(Suppl):62–68.

72. Paul D, Conte FA, Grumbach MM, Kaplan SL. Long term effect of gonadotropin-releasing hormone agonist therapy on final and near final height in 26 children with true precocious puberty treated at a median age of less than 5 years. J Clin Endocrinol Metab 1995;80:546–551.

73. Galluzzi F, Salti R, Bindi G, Pasquini E, La Cauza C. Adult height comparison between boys and girls with precocious puberty after long-term gonadotropin-releasing hormone analogue therapy. Acta Pediatr 1998;87:521–527.

74. Brauner R, Adan L, Malandry F, Zantleifer D. Adult height in girls with idiopathic true precocious puberty. J Clin Endocrinol Metab 1994;79:415–420.

75. Oerter K, Manasco P, Barnes KM, Jones J, Hill S. Cutler G. Adult height in precocious puberty after long-term treatment with Deslorelin. J Clin Endocrinol Metab 1991;73:1235–1240.

76. Oostdijk W, Drop SLS, Odink RJH, Hummelink R, Partsch CJ, Sippel WG. Long-term results with a slow-release gonadotropin-releasing hormone agonist in central precocious puberty. Acta Paediatr Scan 1991;372(Suppl):39–45.

77. Boepple PA, Crowley WF Jr. Growth, final height, and reproductive function following GnRH agonist-induced pituitary-gonadal suppression in central precocious puberty [Abstract 6A]. Proceedings of the 75th Annual Meeting of the Endocrine Society, 1993, p. 10.

78. Cacciari E, Cassio A, Balsamo A, Colli C, Cicognani A, Pirazzoli P, et al. Long-term follow-up and final height in girls with central precocious puberty treated with luteinizing hormone-releasing hormone analogue nasal spray. Arch Pediatr Adolesc Med 1994;148:1194–1199.

79. Kletter GB, Kelch R. Effects of gonadotropin-releasing hormone analog therapy on adult stature in precocious puberty. J Clin Endocrinol Metab 1994;79:331–334.

80. Brauner R, Adam L, Malandry F, Zantleifer D. Adult height in girls with idiopathic true precocious puberty. J Clin Endocrinol Metab 1994;79:415–420.

81. Cara JF. Kreiter ML. Rosenfield RL. Height prognosis of children with true precocious puberty and growth hormone deficiency: effect of combination therapy with gonadotropin releasing hormone agonist and growth hormone. J Peds 1992;120:709–715.

82. Oostdijk W, Drop SLS, Odink RJH, HDmmelink R, Partsch CJ, Sippell WG. Long-term results with a slow-release gonadotropin-releasing hormone agonist in central precocious puberty. Acta Paediatr Scand 1991;372(Suppl):39–45.

83. Pasquino AM, Municchi G, Pucarelli I, Segni M, Mancini MA, Troiani S. Combined treatment with gonadotropin-releasing hormone analogue and growth hormone in central precocious puberty. J Clin Endocrinol Metab 1996;81:948–951.

84. Pasquino AM, Pucarelli I, Segni M, Matruzola M, Cerrone F. Adult height in girls with central precocious puberty treated with gonadotropin-releasing hormone analogues and growth hormone. J Clin Endocrinol Metab 1999;84:449–452.

85. Bridges NA, Cooke A, Healy MJR, Hindmarsh PC, Brook CGD. Ovaries in sexual precocity. Clin Endocrinol 1995;42:135–140.

86. Holland FJ, Fishman L, Bailey JD, et al. Ketoconazole in the management of precocious puberty not responsive to LHRH-analogue therapy. N Engl J Med 1985;312:1023–1028.

87. Laue L, Merke DP, Jones JV, Barnes KM, Hill S, Cutler GB Jr. A preliminary study of flutamide, testolactone and reduced hydrocortisone dose in the treatment of congenital adrenal hyperplasia. J Clin Endocrinol Metab 1996;81:3535–3539.

88. Merke DP, Keil MF, Jones JV, Fields J, Hill S, Cutler GB Jr. Flutamide, testolactone, and reduced hydrocortisone dose maintain normal growth velocity and bone maturation despite elevated androgen levels in children with congenital adrenal hyperplasia. J Clin Endocrinol Metab 2000;85:1114–1120.

89. Forster CM, Pescovitz DH, Comite F, et al. Testolactone treatment of precocious puberty in McCune-Albright syndrome. Acta Endocrinol (Copenh) 1985;109:254–257.

90. Eugster EA, Shankar R, Feezle LK, Pescovitz OH. Tamoxifen treatment of progressive precocious puberty in a patient with McCune Albright. Pediatr Endocrinol Metab 1999;12:681–686.

91. Bar A, Linder B, Sobel EH, Saenger P, DiMartino-Nardi J. Bayley-Pinneau method of height prediction in girls with central precocious puberty: correlation with adult height. J Pediatr 1995;126:955–958.

15 Delayed Puberty

Steven G. Waguespack, MD
and Ora Hirsch Pescovitz, MD

CONTENTS

INTRODUCTION

The onset of puberty marks the beginning of an intriguing period of growth and development. The hypothalamic-pituitary-gonadal (HPG) axis, once quiescent in childhood, reawakens to promote the sexual maturation, changes in body composition, and alterations in psyche that accompany the attainment of fertility. Puberty is heralded by the pulsatile secretion of gonadotropin releasing hormone (GnRH) from the hypothalamus, which in turn activates the pituitary release of luteinizing hormone (LH) and follicle-stimulating hormone (FSH). This sequence results in gonadal maturation, increasing levels of sex steroids, and the physical changes that mark the pubertal process. Fortunately, this course of events most often transpires without disruption. However, in some children, the onset or progression of puberty does not occur as expected (Table 1).

Based on older population studies, delayed puberty can be defined as the lack of breast development in a girl at the age of 13 yr or a testicular volume less than 4 mL in a boy who has reached the age of 14. The term pubertal delay also encompasses the absence of menarche by 16 yr of age or a prolonged tempo of pubertal progression, greater than 5 yr from pubertal onset to completion. These conventional definitions are recognized as imperfect and may not apply to all populations, but they do serve as a good guide to the clinician. However, given the fact that the normal age of pubertal onset in girls is under review *(1)*, the accepted definitions of delayed puberty may warrant reconsideration as well.

From: *Contemporary Endocrinology: Developmental Endocrinology: From Research to Clinical Practice*
Edited by: E. A. Eugster and O. H. Pescovitz © Humana Press Inc., Totowa, NJ

Table 1
Differential Diagnosis of Delayed Puberty

Constitutional delay of growth and development	Hypergonadotropic Hypogonadism
Hypogonadotropic Hypogonadism	Congenital Disorders
Isolated Gonadotropin Deficiency	Turner syndrome
Kallmann syndrome (KAL mutation)	Klinefelter syndrome
Idiopathic hypogonadotropic hypogonadism	46,XX Gonadal dysgenesis
Partial gonadotropin deficiency/fertile	Disorders of sexual differentiation
eunuch syndrome	5α-reductase deficiency
GnRH receptor gene mutations	Biosynthetic defects
LH and FSHβ subunit mutations	StAR deficiency (congenital lipoid
Adrenal Hypoplasia Congenita	adrenal hyperplasia)
(DAX-1 mutations)	CYP17 deficiency
Leptin deficiency/Leptin receptor mutations	17α-hydroxylase deficiency
Developmental abnormalities	(females have pubertal delay)
Empty sella	17,20-lyase deficiency
Septo-optic dysplasia (de Morsier syndrome)	3β-hydroxysteroid dehydrogenase def.
Holoprosencephaly	17β-hydroxysteroid dehydrogenase
Congenital Syndromes	deficiency
(May also have primary hypogonadism)	Androgen insensitivity syndromes
Prader-Willi syndrome	Complete androgen resistance
Laurence-Moon syndrome	(Testicular feminization)
Bardet-Biedl syndrome	Partial androgen resistance
Hypopituitarism of any cause	(Reifenstein syndrome)
Trauma, irradiation, infection, hypophysitis	XY gonadal dysgenesis
Multiple Pituitary Hormone Deficiencies	(Swyer syndrome)
(PROP1 mutations)	Testicular regression syndrome
Space occupying lesions	Leydig cell hypoplasia/LH receptor defects
Vascular lesions	Vanishing testes/testicular regression
Craniopharyngioma	syndrome
Germinoma	Resistant Ovary syndrome/LH and
Pituitary macroadenoma	FSH receptor gene mutations
Granulomatous disease	Aromatase (CYP 19) deficiency
Langerhans cell histiocytosis	Metabolic disorders
Functional Gonadotropin Deficiency	Galactosemia
Chronic disease	Carbohydrate-deficient glycoprotein
Strenuous exercise	syndrome type 1
Malnutrition/weight loss	Nephropathic cystinosis
Eating disorders	Other congenital syndromes
Severe obesity	Myotonic dystrophy
Endocrinopathies	Noonan syndrome
Hypothyroidism	Trisomy 21
Hyperprolactinemia	Ataxia-telangiectasia syndrome
Cushing disease	Leopard syndrome
Isolated growth hormone deficiency	Acquired disorders
Poorly controlled diabetes mellitus	Irradiation
	Cytotoxic therapy, e.g., alkylating agents
	Infection (mumps, coxsackie, TB)
	Gonadal injury/cryptorchidism
	Autoimmune disorders

Adapted with permission from ref. *(117).*

CONSTITUTIONAL DELAY:
A VARIANT OF NORMAL PUBERTY

By far, the majority of children with pubertal delay will ultimately prove to have constitutional delay of puberty (CDP), a transient lag in the maturation of the HPG axis that is a variant of normal development. Although it may occur as an isolated finding, CDP is more commonly associated with short stature (constitutional delay of growth and puberty or CDGP). In fact, many of these children come to medical attention initially due to height concerns, not pubertal delay. Constitutional delay most often presents in boys, and this may reflect the natural genetic and physiologic differences between boys and girls. On the other hand, boys are more likely to be teased and socially isolated due to their delay in pubertal development, particularly if they also have concomitant short stature. Thus, the perceived failure to live up to societal expectations may be the underlying reason why more boys than girls present for evaluation.

The typical adolescent with CDP presents when his relative small stature and delayed sexual development become apparent as the majority of his peers enter puberty. Generally, the child's growth velocity has been normal for his age, although there may be a subnormal growth velocity during the protracted phase of prepubertal growth deceleration commonly seen in CDP. The child's family history is frequently positive for similar developmental patterns, and physical exam and laboratory testing are normal. Adrenarche and gonadarche are similarly delayed. There is an invariable delay in bone age, which usually correlates with the child's height age. The onset of puberty most often occurs in parallel with the bone age, typically occurring before the bone age is 13 yr. Children with CDGP are expected to attain a normal adult stature, but it is unclear whether or not these children truly achieve their genetic potential. Many studies demonstrate that final adult height is not significantly different from midparental height, whereas others suggest that target height is not achieved (2–4).

The exact etiology of CDP is unclear. Transient growth hormone deficiency (GHD), relative to the chronological age, is well-described in children with constitutional delay. This is most likely a secondary effect of low sex steroid levels, as secretion of GH usually normalizes after both sex-steroid priming and/or the onset of puberty (5,6). Therefore, a primary GH defect is not implicated as the etiology of CDP. However, it is possible that this relative "GH deficiency" may play a contributing role, as low insulin-like growth factor (IGF-1) levels do impair the gonadal response to gonadotropins (7). Given its familial predilection, CDP may have a specific genetic origin. The finding of transient hypogonadotropic hypogonadism and GHD in mice that lack the pituitary transcription factor Otx1 may prove to be a good animal model of CDGP (8). However, until more research is done, the genetic basis for constitutional delay in humans remains elusive.

HYPOGONADOTROPIC HYPOGONADISM

Pathologic pubertal delay may be caused by ineffective gonadotropin production that occurs as a result of hypothalamic and/or pituitary dysfunction. Regardless of etiology, the term most commonly used to describe this circumstance is hypogonadotropic hypogonadism (HH). HH is due either to a congenital defect in LH or FSH production, or it results from an acquired problem in gonadotropin secretion, which may be permanent or transient in nature. Clinical entities will be discussed first, followed by a summary of the molecular genetic aspects of these conditions.

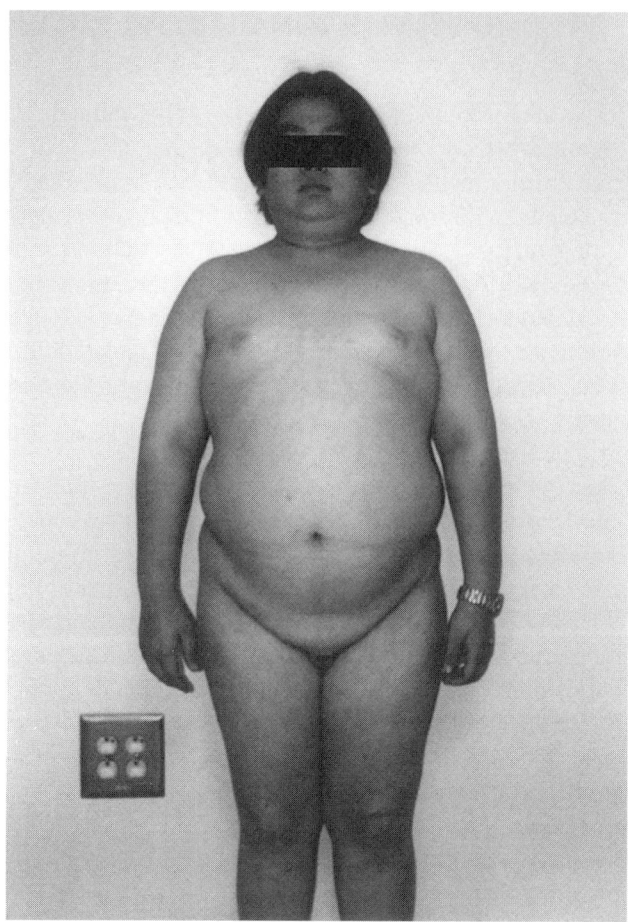

Fig. 1. Nineteen-yr-old male with hypogonadotropic hypogonadism as part of a syndrome of multiple anterior pituitary hormone deficiencies. Height was 148 cm and bone age was 14 yr at the time of presentation. LH was 0.3 mIU/mL, FSH was 1.0 mIU/mL, and total testosterone was 6 ng/dl. Central hypothyroidism and growth hormone deficiency were also present; adrenal insufficiency was not. MRI was normal except for the presence of a small pituitary gland. Adapted with permission from ref. *117.*

Defective gonadotropin secretion may be isolated, or it may be a component of multiple anterior pituitary-hormone deficiencies or hypothalamic dysfunction. Essentially any event or factor that results in hypopituitarism can cause HH (Fig. 1). Although pubertal delay may be the presenting complaint, it is more common for these children to develop symptoms of associated endocrine deficiencies, e.g., growth failure, prior to the expected age of puberty. Multiple pituitary hormone deficiencies can occur in association with head trauma, central nervous system (CNS) infection, and cranial irradiation, as well as with congenital developmental or anatomic defects such as septo-optic dysplasia (de Morsier syndrome), holoprosencephaly, or primary empty sella. HH may also be caused by CNS lesions that disrupt the hypothalamic-pituitary axis. Most commonly encountered in this setting is craniopharyngioma, a congenital tumor originating from Rathke's pouch (Fig. 2). Germinomas, pituitary macroadenomas, granulomatous disease (e.g., sarcoidosis, tuberculosis [TB], and Langerhans cell histiocytosis are other rare entities to consider.

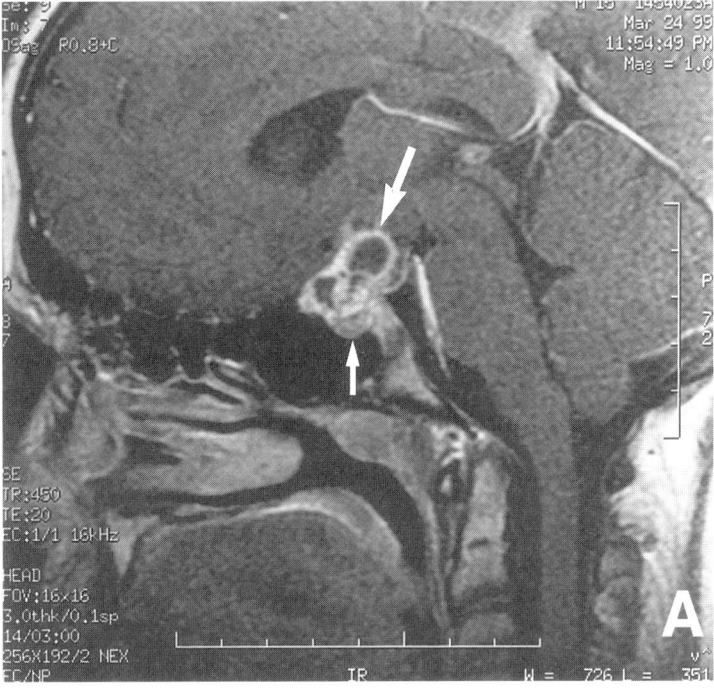

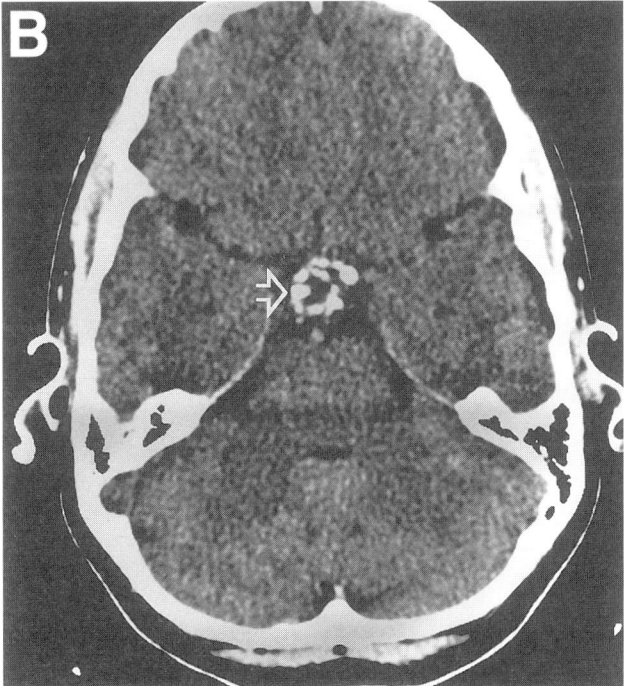

Fig. 2. Craniopharyngioma. (**A**) A 15-yr-old boy presented with short stature and delayed puberty. Hypogonadotropic hypogonadism was diagnosed, in addition to growth hormone and thyroid hormone deficiencies. MRI revealed a cystic, 2.5 cm suprasellar mass (large arrow) with intrasellar extension. Note the normal pituitary gland within the sella turcica (small arrow). Pathologic evaluation confirmed the diagnosis of craniopharyngioma. (**B**) Characteristic appearance of craniopharyngioma on CT. Note the scattered calcifications (open arrow) in the suprasellar mass.

Isolated Gonadotropin Deficiency

Unlike the aforementioned problems, gonadotropin deficiency without associated anterior pituitary-hormone deficiencies may not be diagnosed until adolescence when delayed puberty is the sole complaint. It is most often due to a congenital defect in GnRH, and most cases of GnRH deficiency appear to be sporadic in nature, without a specific genetic defect identified *(9)*. Within this category are a spectrum of disorders that ranges from a complete lack of gonadotropin production to varying degrees of partial LH and FSH deficiencies. Therefore, the clinical phenotype of individuals affected by isolated HH is heterogeneous and may range from the most severe form, in which there is complete sexual infantilism, to the mildest end of the spectrum, in which pubertal delay occurs with an otherwise normal pubertal sequence *(10)*.

Kallmann syndrome (KS) is the best characterized of these conditions and is used to describe isolated gonadotropin deficiency in association with anosmia or hyposmia. This is in contrast to idiopathic hypogonadotropic hypogonadism (IHH), a term that specifies isolated gonadotropin deficiency in the absence of a known defect in olfaction. KS is a clinically heterogeneous disorder, and cases occur sporadically or are inherited in an autosomal dominant, autosomal recessive, or X-linked fashion. The specific genetic defect has been discovered in X-linked KS and is due to mutations of the KAL gene, located at Xp22.3. Despite being an uncommon cause of familial KS *(9)*, the KAL gene offers significant insight into heritable GnRH deficiency *(see* below).

HH may be difficult to distinguish from CDGP, except for the fact that children with HH often have normal stature, in contrast to the short stature commonly seen in constitutional delay. The history and physical exam may be entirely normal except for pubertal delay, eunuchoid body proportions (arm span 5 cm or more greater than height; upper-to-lower body segment ratio < 0.9), and an altered sense of smell that may not be identified unless formal testing is undertaken. Individuals with KS may have other associated midline defects such as cleft lip and/or palate as well as neurological abnormalities, including cerebellar ataxia and sensorineural hearing loss. Furthermore, boys with X-linked KS may have synkinesis *(11)*, or mirror movements, as well as unilateral renal agenesis *(12)*.

The fertile eunuch syndrome has been used traditionally to describe a clinical phenotype that results from incomplete GnRH deficiency. As implied by the name, these men have eunuchoid body proportions. Since GnRH secretion is only partially impaired, the testes are pubertal and produce enough testosterone to cause varying degrees of virilization. Despite incomplete virilization and low systemic levels of testosterone, intratesticular concentrations are sufficient to support spermatogenesis and testicular growth *(13)*. Therefore, these men may achieve fertility with the use of exogenous testosterone or human chorionic gonadotropin (hCG) alone *(14)*.

Congenital Syndromes

There are several well-described syndromes in which hypogonadotropic hypogonadism is prevalent. Prader-Willi syndrome (PWS) is a disorder of genomic imprinting, a process by which certain genes are programmed during gametogenesis to be either activated or inactivated, depending on the parent of origin. In PWS, there is a defect on chromosome 15 at the 15q11-q13 locus that causes the paternally derived genes in this location not to be expressed *(15)*. In contrast, similar defects at this locus in the genes of maternal origin cause a clinically distinct syndrome, the Angelman syndrome. In PWS, 70% of

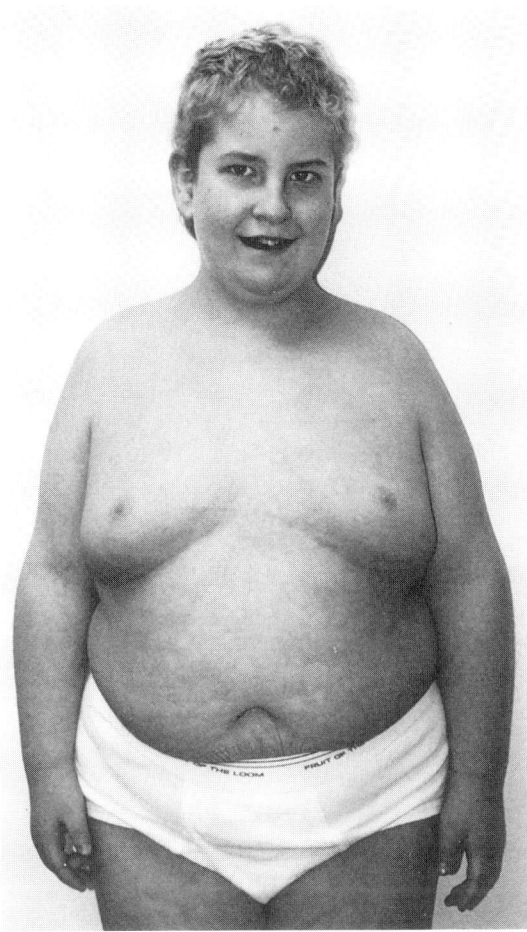

Fig. 3. Eleven-yr-old boy with classic features of Prader-Willi syndrome. Note the characteristic obesity, small hands, and typical facies: prominent forehead, bitemporal narrowing, almond-shaped eyes, strabismus, thin upper lip, and submental adiposity. On exam, genital hypoplasia is also apparent.

cases are due to an interstitial deletion of chromosome 15. Most of the remaining cases result either from maternal uniparental disomy (both chromosomes 15 are inherited from the mother) or from mutations in the imprinting process itself *(16)*. Diagnosis is possible using standard fluorescent *in situ* hybridization (FISH) or by methylation-specific polymerase chain reaction (PCR).

PWS is characterized by infantile hypotonia and associated poor suck during the neonatal period. These children are not typically born large for gestational age and may initially have failure to thrive secondary to their feeding difficulties *(15)*. Obesity becomes a central part of the syndrome in early childhood, as insatiable hunger, hyperphagia, and extreme food-seeking behaviors ensue. Behavioral problems and mental deficiency are universal. Children with PWS have a distinct appearance, with characteristic facies, central obesity, short stature, and small hands and feet (Fig. 3). Although not uniformly present, hypogonadism is prevalent and is manifested by hypoplastic external genitalia and delayed puberty, both in boys and girls. As expected, menarche in girls with PWS is often delayed or absent altogether, and ovulation frequently does not occur. Cryptorchidism is common in males and, if uncorrected, may occasionally give rise to elevated gonadotropins *(17)*. However, in most cases, the hypogonadism that occurs is secondary to hypothalamic dysfunction. Short stature is also a common feature of PWS and is most likely secondary to growth hormone deficiency *(18)*.

Often described under one eponym, the Laurence-Moon and Bardet-Biedl syndromes are felt to be distinct clinical entities. Similar to PWS, both are characterized by hypogonadism and hypogenitalism, particularly in males. In addition, retinitis pigmentosa, varying degrees of mental deficiency, and autosomal recessive inheritance are features of both. Spastic paraparesis predominates in the Laurence-Moon syndrome, whereas obesity, dystrophic extremities (polydactyly, syndactyly), and renal abnormalities are found in children with the Bardet-Biedl syndrome. Although once thought to have only HH as the cause of pubertal delay, recent reports have refuted this long-held assumption *(19,20)*.

Functional Hypogonadotropic Hypogonadism

The onset and progression of puberty is dependent not only on genetic factors, but also on the overall health and well-being of the individual. Any chronic systemic disease can adversely affect normal gonadotropin secretion and cause pubertal delay *(21)*. The exact pathophysiology is often multifactorial and, in many cases, unknown. Confounding factors in children with chronic disease often include inadequate nutrition or exposure to medications that can have profound effects on growth and development. Fortunately, the HH encountered in the context of chronic disease is often transient. With adequate treatment and optimization of nutrition, most children will ultimately enter puberty without the need for intervention. Well-known disorders that are associated with delayed puberty include: gastrointestinal disease, namely inflammatory bowel disease and celiac disease; chronic lung disease, such as cystic fibrosis and severe asthma; renal disease, including chronic renal failure and renal tubular acidosis; and hemoglobinopathies, such as sickle-cell disease and β-thalassemia major.

A subnormal amount of body fat, as seen in malnutrition and anorexia nervosa, is linked to delayed pubertal development *(22,23)*. Similarly, girls who engage in vigorous exercise may develop HH. In female athletes and dancers, puberty and menarche are frequently delayed and hypothalamic amenorrhea persists after menarche, particularly in those girls who begin their training before the onset of menses *(24)*. An equivalent clinical syndrome has not been definitively identified in male athletes *(13)*.

Although rare, HH can also be caused by an underlying endocrinopathy. Both hypothyroidism and hyperprolactinemia, either due to a prolactinoma or as a medication side effect, disrupt normal gonadotropin secretion. Hyperprolactinemia, however, is an infrequent etiology for pubertal delay and is more commonly associated with galactorrhea and/or secondary amenorrhea. Although not the typical presentation, Cushing disease has presented only as isolated pubertal arrest and growth failure *(25)*. In untreated children with isolated GHD, pubertal development is often delayed in accordance with the degree of bone-age delay. The use of exogenous GH typically initiates normal pubertal development. It is still being debated whether or not GH may actually accelerate the tempo of pubertal progression in these children *(26)*. Finally, very poorly controlled type 1 diabetes mellitus, as in any chronic disease, can also be associated with delayed puberty.

Table 2
Important Genes in Human Hypogonadotropic Hypogonadism (HH)

Gene	Chromosome location	Clinical phenotype of gene mutation
KAL	Xp22.3	Kallmann Syndrome: HH and anosmia/hyposmia
		Renal agenesis, synkinesis, midline defects possible
DAX1	Xp21	In males, adrenal hypoplasia congenita (AHC):
		primary adrenal insufficiency and HH
		In females: pubertal delay or HH
PROP1	5q	Multiple anterior pituitary hormone deficiencies, including HH
HESX1	3p21	Familial septo-optic dysplasia; HH
GnRH receptor	4q21.2	Hypogonadotropic hypogonadism, various degrees of severity.
		HH possible, but unconfirmed
LHβ subunit	19q13.3	Male with pubertal delay
		Elevated immunoreactive LH, but low bioactive LH
		Normal FSH, low testosterone
FSHβ subunit	11p13	Females with pubertal delay (one male with delayed puberty)
		Low FSH, elevated LH, low sex steroid levels
Leptin	7q31.3	Obesity, hyperphagia
(ob, Lep^{ob})		HH
Leptin receptor	1p31	Obesity, hyperphagia, abnormal GH and TSH secretion
(db, $Lepr^{db}$)		HH

Molecular Insights into Hypogonadotropic Hypogonadism

Medical progress has permitted novel and remarkable insights into the molecular and genetic basis of many disease processes. This union of basic science research and clinical medicine has opened the door to a new world of scientific understanding. Currently, there are several genes implicated in varying syndromes of hypogonadotropic hypogonadism: KAL, DAX1, PROP1, and HESX1 (Table 2). In addition, the discovery of leptin has permitted new research into its possible role in the regulation of the pubertal process.

KAL: X-Linked Kallman Syndrome

The genetic understanding of KS began with the observation that KS can be inherited as part of a "contiguous gene syndrome" that includes short stature, mental retardation, X-linked ichthyosis (steroid sulfatase deficiency), and chondrodysplasia punctata. These associated entities were known to occur with large deletions of the pseudoautosomal region of the X chromosome. Thereafter, the putative KS gene was localized to Xp22.3, adjacent to the steroid sulfatase gene *(27)*. Through positional cloning, the responsible gene was ultimately isolated in 1991 and was found to encode a protein (anosmin) that appears to function as an adhesion molecule *(28,29)*. The KAL protein plays a vital role in normal embryonic nerve migration by providing a scaffold for GnRH-producing neurons and olfactory neurons to migrate from the olfactory placode to their final destination *(30)*. Defects in the KAL protein, therefore, cause the clinical phenotype of hypogonadotropic hypogonadism and anosmia/hyposmia (secondary to a lack of GnRH-producing neurons in the hypothalamus and failure of normal development of the olfactory bulbs and tracts, respectively). Subsequent to the discovery of the KAL gene, deletions and point mutations have been described in male patients with KS confirming its causative role in the X-linked form of the syndrome. Interestingly, the study of the KAL gene in chickens has shown that it is also expressed in nonolfactory tissues, such as cerebellum, meso- and metanephros, and facial mesenchyme *(10,30)*. This wider expression of the KAL gene may provide an explanation for the associated anomalies encountered in X-linked KS.

DAX-1: X-Linked Adrenal Hypoplasia Congenita

Adrenal hypoplasia congenita (AHC) is a rare genetic disorder that is inherited either in an X-linked or autosomal recessive fashion. In the X-linked type, there is a failure of adrenocortical development. As expected, the typical presentation is one of acute primary adrenal insufficiency in either infancy or childhood. In adolescence, these boys fail to enter puberty due to HH, which appears to be a result of defects both at the level of the hypothalamus and the pituitary *(31)*. Interestingly, the pubertal hypogonadism in these patients may actually represent a postnatal regression of HPG function, as evidenced by the demonstration of a normal minipuberty of infancy in children with AHC *(32,33)*.

As with KS, the genetic understanding of X-linked AHC began with the study of patients with contiguous gene-deletion syndromes including AHC, glycerol kinase deficiency, and Duchenne muscular dystrophy *(10,33)*. This ultimately led to the isolation of the gene (DAX1) on the short arm of the X chromosome at Xp21. Mutations in this gene were subsequently implicated in both adrenal insufficiency and hypogonadotropic hypogonadism *(34)*. Furthermore, mutations in DAX1 have been found to affect the reproductive axis at multiple levels. Similar to the *Ahch* (DAX1) knockout mouse, affected males may have an intrinsic defect in spermatogenesis that is unresponsive to gonadotropin therapy *(35,36)*.

DAX1 (dosage-sensitive sex-reversal AHC critical region on human X chromosome, gene 1) encodes a protein that is a member of the nuclear hormone-receptor superfamily *(37)*. The DAX1 protein is unique in that it has a DNA-binding domain, in contrast to the zinc fingers characteristic of other nuclear hormone receptors, and it is an orphan receptor with no identified ligand. The regulation of DAX1 is not well-understood, but it appears to have significant interactions with another co-expressed orphan nuclear hormone receptor, steroidogenic factor 1 (SF1) *(10,38)*.

The clinical presentations of DAX1 mutations may be markedly heterogeneous *(10,33, 38)*. Although typically diagnosed in childhood, adrenal insufficiency occurred at age 28 in one adult male with a DAX1 mutation; he also had incomplete pubertal development and partial gonadotropin deficiency *(36)*. Recently, female members of affected families have also been identified with various phenotypic expressions of DAX1 gene mutations. In one case, a woman with isolated HH was found to have a homozygous mutation, which was presumed secondary to a spontaneous gene conversion (the nonreciprocal transfer of DNA from one parental allele to the other) *(39)*. In another family, women with a heterozygous mutation in the DAX1 gene manifested only pubertal delay *(35)*.

PROP1 and HESX1: Important Pituitary Transcription-Factor Genes

The discovery of the PIT1 homeobox protein in 1988 began an era of research and insight into the various transcription-factor genes that direct the ordered embryonic development of the anterior pituitary gland *(40)*. As can be expected, the discovery of mutations in these vital genes has identified the molecular basis for some cases of HH in the context of multiple anterior pituitary-hormone deficiencies.

The name PROP1 (Prophet of PIT1) is derived from the fact that the PROP1 gene product precedes PIT1 in the developmental cascade. In fact, PROP1 is absolutely required for the normal expression of PIT1 *(40)*. PROP1 gene mutations were initially identified in the Ames dwarf (*df/df*) mouse *(41)*. Subsequently, humans with familial combined pituitary-hormone deficiency were found to have inactivating mutations in the PROP1 gene *(42)*. To date, at least 7 mutations have been identified, all of which are inherited in an autosomal recessive fashion *(40)*. The hormonal phenotype of an individual with a PROP1 mutation includes gonadotropin deficiency, in addition to deficiencies in GH, thyrotropin, and prolactin. Interestingly, it also appears that persons with PROP1 gene mutations can ultimately develop ACTH deficiency. In a study of one large family with the common 301-302delAG mutation, adrenal insufficiency was detected in 83% of the affected members who were over the age of 43 yr *(43)*.

HESX1("homeobox gene expressed in embryonic stem cells") and RPX ("Rathke's pouch homeobox") are names given to the same pituitary transcription factor that antedates PROP1 and that plays a major role in anterior pituitary and optic-nerve development *(40)*. The phenotype of the HESX1 null mutant mouse is reminiscent of the human syndrome of septo-optic dysplasia (SOD or De Morsier syndrome), in which varying degrees of pituitary deficiency are associated with optic-nerve hypoplasia and midline neurodevelopmental anomalies, namely absent septum pellucidum and/or agenesis of the corpus callosum *(44)*. However, mutations in the HESX1 gene have only been identified in humans in the very rare setting of familial septo-optic dysplasia *(44)*. Therefore, although HESX1 plays an obvious role in anterior pituitary development, it does not appear to relate to the typical presentation of septo-optic dysplasia, and its role in hypogonadotropic hypogonadism remains unclear. Whether or not it will ultimately be implicated in human cases of multiple pituitary-hormone deficiencies remains to be seen.

GnRH Receptor and Gonadotropin Gene Mutations: Discrete Causes of HH

Mutations in the GnRH gene have only been described in the *hpg/hpg* mouse and have yet to be identified in humans with IHH. On the other hand, mutations in the GnRH receptor gene have been discovered and offer another etiology for the autosomal recessive inheritance of IHH *(45–47)*. Similar to other hormone receptors, the GnRH receptor is a G protein-coupled receptor with seven transmembrane domains. When mutated, the GnRH receptor loses function and becomes resistant to exogenous GnRH. This loss of function ranges from partial inactivation to a total loss of function that results in complete HH *(47)*. The latter case has been identified in individuals with homozygous mutations of the GnRH receptor gene, whereas the cases with a less severe phenotype have compound heterozygous mutations.

Defects in the genes encoding for the β-subunits of LH and FSH have also been described *(30)*. There has been one case of an identified LHβ mutation, in which a 17-yr-old boy presented with delayed puberty, an elevated LH, normal FSH, and decreased testosterone *(48)*. Despite the increased levels of immunoreactive LH, the bioactivity of the LH molecule was markedly diminished due to a lack of binding to the LH receptor. Mutations in the FSHβ gene have also been characterized in two women with delayed puberty who had decreased immunoreactive and bioactive FSH and elevated LH levels *(49,50)*. One woman was homozygous for the specific mutation, whereas the other was a compound heterozygote. It is presumed that the identified mutations prevent efficient combination of the α and β subunits to form intact FSH *(50)*. Although not expected to cause pubertal delay in men, a homozygous FSHβ gene mutation has also been reported in an 18-yr-old male who presented with pubertal delay and a similar biochemical profile *(51)*.

LEPTIN: A ROLE IN HYPOGONADOTROPIC HYPOGONADISM?

The discovery of the *ob* (*Lep^{ob}*) gene and its peptide product leptin has allowed a new understanding of other factors that may be regulating the pubertal process. Leptin is an adipocyte-derived hormone that signals the adequacy of adipose tissue energy stores to the hypothalamus via a specific leptin receptor encoded for by the *db* (*Lepr^{db}*) gene. It thus has significant effects on food intake, metabolism, and energy expenditure *(52)*. Furthermore, studies of the leptin deficient mouse have clearly shown an impact of leptin on neuroendocrine and reproductive function. In the *ob/ob* mouse, puberty is delayed and fertility is impaired via a mechanism of hypogonadotropic hypogonadism. With leptin administration, fertility is restored *(53,54)*. Furthermore, in young prepubertal mice, exogenous leptin administration advances the pubertal process and attainment of fertility *(55,56)*.

The exact role of leptin in human reproductive physiology is not as clear. It is possible that leptin acts only as a permissive factor, signaling the brain that the body's nutritional status and metabolic reserves are adequate for fertility *(57)*. However, in studies of patients with leptin or leptin-receptor mutations, there is concrete evidence that leptin does play an active role in the initiation of puberty. Despite being obese with adequate nutritional stores, individuals with these genetic defects have HH and pubertal delay *(58,59)*. Although no adult with leptin deficiency has been treated with leptin to prove a reversal of the hypogonadism, a 9-yr-old girl with a leptin mutation was treated for 12 mo *(60)*. In this case, the girl was prepubertal, despite having a bone age of 12.5 yr. At the end of therapy, the nocturnal secretion of gonadotropins was consistent with early puberty. Although difficult to confirm that the onset of pulsatile gonadotropin secretion was a direct effect of leptin therapy, the data are suggestive of a role of leptin in the onset of puberty. More research is obviously needed into this fascinating topic.

HYPERGONADOTROPIC HYPOGONADISM

Hypergonadotropic hypogonadism, also known as primary gonadal failure, describes the state in which there are increased levels of gonadotropins in response to inadequate gonadal sex-steroid production. Most frequently due to a chromosomal disorder, the spectrum of hypergonadotropic hypogonadism also encompasses a variety of distinct clinical entities that are unique to each sex.

Chromosomal Disorders

Turner syndrome (Ullrich-Turner syndrome; gonadal dysgenesis) is the term used to describe those women with a distinct clinical phenotype resulting from an incomplete complement of X chromosomes. It occurs with a frequency of 1 in 1500–2500 live-born girls and is most commonly secondary to the complete absence of one of the X chromosomes (45,XO) *(61,62)*. It may also result from partial deletions of an X chromosome or chromosomal mosaicism, in which at least one cell line is 45,XO. Rarely, there may be smaller deletions of the long arm of the X chromosome that result only in primary gonadal failure without the associated features of the syndrome *(63)*.

Resulting from variations in the underlying genotype as well as the severity of fetal lymphedema, there is significant clinical heterogeneity in the phenotype of girls with Turner syndrome. Universally, short stature is prominent and is most likely due to haploinsufficiency of the SHOX (short stature homeobox-containing) gene, which is located in the pseudoautosomal region of the sex chromosomes *(64)*. Other clinical features include prominent rotated ears, high arched palate, webbed neck, low posterior hairline, broad chest with the appearance of widely spaced nipples, increased carrying angle (cubitus valgus), short metacarpals, hypoplastic hyperconvex nails, and congenital lymphedema of the hands and feet (Fig. 4). Otitis media is frequent in childhood secondary to a disturbed relationship of the middle ear to the Eustachian tube *(62)*. Congenital heart disease occurs in approx 25% of cases, with bicuspid aortic valve and aortic coarctation being most common *(65)*. Renal anomalies and autoimmune thyroid disease are also frequent findings, occurring in over one-third of girls *(62)*.

Turner syndrome is characterized by streak gonads and primary gonadal failure in the majority of cases. This gonadal dysgenesis occurs prenatally or early in childhood as a result of a presumed acceleration of oocyte loss with a concomitant increase of stromal fibrosis *(62)*. These processes are not universal, however, and some women with Turner syndrome, particularly those with chromosomal mosaicism or partial X deletions, may have normal pubertal development and even achieve fertility. In fact, as demonstrated in one study, up to 16% of girls may have spontaneous puberty, including menarche *(66)*. Girls with Turner syndrome and primary ovarian failure have markedly elevated levels of gonadotropins that occur in a biphasic pattern, both in infancy to early childhood and after the age of 10 yr *(67)*. Therefore, if measured at these ages, elevated levels of LH and FSH serve as helpful markers of impaired gonadal function. Furthermore, pelvic ultrasonography to assess ovarian size and appearance may also serve as a prognostic indicator of future pubertal development *(68)*.

The observation of individuals with a Turner syndrome phenotype but normal karyotype ultimately led to the description of the Noonan syndrome *(69)*. Noonan syndrome, often aberrantly referred to as male Turner syndrome, is not a sex-chromosome disorder but an autosomal disorder that occurs in both males and females. It occurs sporadically or is inherited in an autosomal dominant fashion, and it has been linked to chromosome 12 *(70)*. Characteristic features include short stature, hypertelorism, low-set ears, webbed neck, chest deformity (pectus excavatum), and cardiac anomalies (namely pulmonic stenosis). Delayed puberty occurs in both sexes. Fertility is preserved in females, but males have a high incidence of cryptorchidism, which appears to be the main factor in the high infertility rate seen in men with Noonan syndrome *(71)*.

Another chromosomal disorder that causes primary gonadal failure and hypergonadotropic hypogonadism is the Klinefelter syndrome. The most frequent etiology of male hypogonadism, affecting 1 in 500–1000 males *(72)*, Klinefelter syndrome most commonly results from the presence of an additional X chromosome (47,XXY). Similar to Turner syndrome, however, Klinefelter syndrome can also result from a variety of sex-chromosome aberrancies (e.g., 48,XXXY; 48,XXYY; 49,XXXXY; and mosaic genotypes) which cause diverse phenotypes. Currently grouped under the unifying title of Klinefelter syndrome, these other genotypes may be distinct syndromes worthy of separate consideration *(73)*.

Individuals with Klinefelter syndrome tend to be tall with eunuchoid body proportions. There is an increased frequency of behavioral problems and learning disabilities. Microphallus may be present and primary gonadal failure results from fibrosis and hyalinization of the seminiferous tubules, a process that begins prepubertally. As a result, the testes are typically small and firm in consistency. Despite this testicular abnormality, Leydig-cell function is often preserved, and testosterone production is frequently sufficient to induce

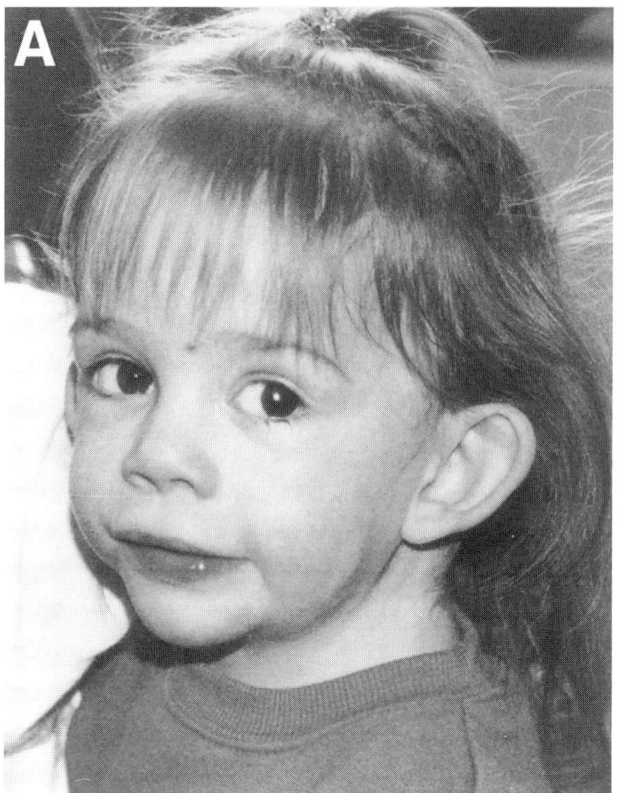

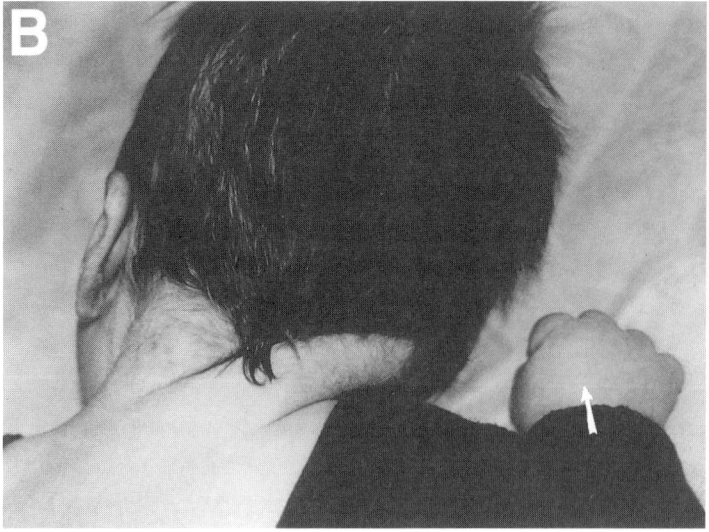

Fig. 4. Turner syndrome. (**A**) Classic facial features of Turner syndrome include epicanthal folds, prominent rotated ears, and downward and outward slant of the palpebral fissures. Note also the webbed neck and low posterior hairline. (**B**) Some features are obvious at birth, as in this child with redundant nuchal skin, a low posterior hairline, and lymphedema of the extremities (arrow).

varying degrees of virilization. Therefore, these boys often enter puberty normally but may not complete pubertal development as expected. Infertility is the norm, although rare cases of successful recovery of spermatozoa and in vitro fertilization have been reported *(74)*. Gynecomastia is present in up to 60% of affected individuals and is secondary to an abnormal estradiol/testosterone ratio *(72)*. In addition, men with Klinefelter syndrome have an increased risk of malignancy, particularly mediastinal germ-cell tumors and breast carcinoma *(75,76)*.

Rare Congenital Causes of Hypergonadotropic Hypogonadism

There are a variety of other infrequent congenital defects that result in primary gonadal failure and hypergonadotropic hypogonadism. In females, delayed puberty and primary amenorrhea may be the presenting signs of the resistant ovary syndrome, a poorly understood disorder in which affected individuals are found to have elevated gonadotropin levels and small ovaries with intact primordial follicles *(77)*. This disorder is most likely secondary to defects at the level of the gonadotropin receptors. In fact, inactivating mutations in both the FSH and LH receptor genes have been described *(78–81)*. Genetic males with mutations in the LH receptor gene are undervirilized and typically have a female phenotype, whereas genetic females present with amenorrhea despite normal pubertal progression *(78,80)*. As expected, inactivating mutations in the FSH receptor cause amenorrhea in females; in males, however, there is not a distinct phenotype, but there is variable suppression of spermatogenesis *(78,81)*. Females with *CYP17* gene mutations (congenital adrenal hyperplasia secondary to 17α-hydroxylase deficiency) also develop hypergonadotropic hypogonadism due to defective gonadal estradiol production *(82)*.

Genetic males with disorders of sexual differentiation (a.k.a. male pseudohermaphroditism) may present with pubertal delay, although the typical clinical presentation is one of genital ambiguity. Rare conditions in this category include the androgen insensitivity syndromes *(83)*, defects in androgen biosynthesis, inactivating LH receptor mutations, 5α-reductase deficiency, and 46,XY pure gonadal dysgenesis. For example, pubertal delay and/or primary amenorrhea may be the presenting complaint in 46,XY individuals who are phenotypic females, as seen in the complete androgen insensitivity syndrome and complete 46,XY gonadal dysgenesis.

The terms vanishing testes syndrome and testicular regression syndrome describe the clinical phenotype of a 46,XY male who is born without palpable testes. In this condition, there is a presumed in utero insult to the testes, but this entity may also be part of the spectrum of 46,XY gonadal dysgenesis *(84)*. If testicular loss occurs late in gestation, after sexual differentiation is complete, the child is born with anorchia but otherwise normal male external genitalia. However, if it happens at an earlier, critical stage of development, varying degrees of genital ambiguity may result.

Aromatase deficiency and estrogen resistance are rare entities that adversely affect the pubertal process. Mutations in the aromatase gene (CYP19) have been identified in both males and females *(85)*, and estrogen resistance due to a disruptive mutation of the estrogen-receptor gene has been isolated in a single male patient *(86)*. Girls with aromatase deficiency have pubertal delay, whereas boys have normal sexual maturation, both with aromatase deficiency and estrogen resistance. The consequence of these defects in estrogen synthesis and action is most noticeable in skeletal growth and maturation. In these disorders, there is no pubertal growth spurt, and affected individuals have delayed bone ages, unfused epiphyses, tall stature, and continued growth into adulthood *(85)*. Bone mineral density (BMD) is invariably decreased despite high levels of androgens. Improved bone mass and epiphyseal fusion have been demonstrated after estrogen therapy in a man with aromatase deficiency *(87)*. These findings support the notion that estrogen is primarily responsible for pubertal growth, bone mineral accretion, and epiphyseal fusion.

Acquired Gonadal Failure

Acquired bilateral gonadal failure is an uncommon cause of delayed puberty, and when it occurs, gonadotropin levels are markedly elevated. Testicular or ovarian failure can result from any insult to the gonads that is sufficient enough to diminish sex steroid production from both gonads. In boys, trauma, cryptorchidism, and testicular torsion are possible etiologies, as is infection with the mumps or coxsackie viruses. In both sexes, the treatment of childhood malignancies, including gonadectomy, chemotherapy with alkylating agents and pelvic irradiation, may lead to primary gonadal failure. Furthermore, the gonads can be affected by autoimmune disease, which may be isolated to the gonad, as seen in autoimmune-mediated premature ovarian failure, or associated with other endocrinopathies, as found in the autoimmune polyglandular syndromes. Hypergonadotropic hypogonadism also occurs over time in certain metabolic diseases, including galactosemia *(88)* and carbohydrate-deficient glycoprotein syndrome type 1 *(89)* in girls and, in boys, nephropathic cystinosis *(90)*.

PRIMARY AMENORRHEA

There is a unique subset of females who present only with primary amenorrhea despite an apparently normal pubertal progression. Separate consideration of these individuals is warranted, as the approach to diagnosis in these cases is often quite distinct from the typical assessment of a girl with delayed breast development. Common etiologies for this clinical scenario include pregnancy, premature ovarian failure, or acquired hypothalamic/pituitary disease after puberty has begun *(91)*. An imperforate hymen or other outflow tract obstruction, such as vaginal septae, may be present and is suggested by a history of cyclic abdominal pain. Developmental abnormalities of the genital tract, such as Mullerian agenesis (Rokitansky-Kuster-Hauser syndrome) *(92)*, should also be considered. A complete pelvic exam to confirm normal vaginal anatomy and the presence of a cervix is clearly warranted in all cases of primary amenorrhea.

Females with the syndrome of complete androgen insensitivity (testicular feminization) *(83)* usually present with primary amenorrhea during adolescence, although the diagnosis may be made in infancy or childhood if the testes descend to give rise to an inguinal hernia or inquiral masses. They have normal, often enhanced, breast development secondary to the aromatization of testosterone, which is elevated due to the underlying androgen resistance. Given the normal testicular production of anti-Mullerian hormone during fetal development, the Mullerian structures are absent and the distal vagina ends as a blind pouch. External genitalia are typically normal, and these children have absent or scant axillary and pubic hair. Karyotype will reveal that the patient is a genetic male (46,XY), and the testes will be located anywhere from the abdominal cavity to the labia. Despite being genetically male, these children have a normal female sexual identity, although psychological counseling may be required in some cases. Therapy should include estrogen replacement, vaginal dilatation as required to allow for intercourse, and gonadectomy, as the testes have a higher risk of malignant transformation.

DIAGNOSIS

The diagnosis of delayed puberty can be a challenge, but with a thoughtful and systematic approach, the clinician will often find an etiology for the pubertal delay. The main goal in the care of these children is to distinguish the benign normal variant of development, i.e., constitutional delay of puberty, from a permanent form of hypogonadism, which will require a precise diagnosis and lifelong hormone replacement. Fortunately, an involved costly investigation is not initially warranted in most children with delayed puberty. Instead, continued observation with accurate growth-velocity assessment and well-documented physical exams may be sufficient. However, if there are concerning features of the presenting history or exam that indicate an underlying pathologic diagnosis, if growth velocity is much less than expected for bone age, or if further growth and development do not occur as anticipated, it is necessary to pursue a more complete evaluation.

Similar to any problem encountered in clinical practice, the initial history and physical exam form the foundation of the investigation. Particular emphasis is given to the child's past medical history, previous growth patterns, and growth velocity over the previous 4–6 mo, if available. A thorough review of systems must be undertaken; questioning for symptoms of chronic disease, searching for symptoms of an intracranial process, and asking about the sense of smell are vital. A detailed family history is essential; the presence of family members with similar developmental patterns may support a diagnosis of constitutional delay. In addition, parental heights and the calculated target height are important adjuncts to the investigation. On physical exam, one should search for stigmata of the various congenital syndromes associated with delayed puberty as well as for subtle evidence of chronic disease, such as clubbing. The exam must incorporate accurate Tanner staging and precise anthropometric measurements (weight, height obtained with a stadiometer, upper/lower body segment ratio, and arm span). The presence of pubic hair should not reassure the clinician that puberty has been attained, since adrenarche alone could explain this milestone. For example, some pubertal disorders, e.g., Turner syndrome and Klinefelter syndrome, may present with normal pubic hair development despite the failure of gonadal maturation.

A bone age (radiograph of the left wrist and hand) should be obtained in all cases. It is an invaluable tool that not only assists with diagnosis, but also provides information regarding the potential for continued growth. Reasonable laboratory tests include a basic chemistry profile, urinalysis, complete blood cell count, and sedimentation rate to assess for the presence of occult renal or gastrointestinal (GI) disease. Thyroid function tests are typically assessed, specifically in those children with growth arrest. IGF-1 and IGFBP-3 levels should be considered if there is significant short stature or subnormal growth velocity, keeping in mind that these values are often low for chronologic age (although appropriate for bone age) in children with constitutional delay *(93)*. A karyotype should be ordered in all girls and boys with elevated gonadotropins or phenotypic features suggestive of a chromosomal disorder. Finally, magnetic resonance imaging (MRI) of the brain and pituitary gland should be obtained in those individuals suspected of having permanent HH as well as those patients with visual field defects or symptoms of increased intracranial pressure. Children with diabetes insipidus or late onset of growth failure would also warrant CNS imaging.

Gonadotropin levels are usually obtained, particularly in the older child who presents with pubertal delay. Measurements of LH and FSH are very helpful when elevated, for they prove primary gonadal failure or end-organ resistance. When they are normal or low, however, the diagnostic challenge remains the differentiation of adolescents with constitutional delay from those with true gonadotropin deficiency, as both groups usually have prepubertal gonadotropin levels. Of course, the findings of micropenis, anosmia, or the stigmata of a particular syndrome may lead one to suspect true HH. However, despite the advances in endocrine testing, there has been no one test that has unequivocally differentiated these disorders (94).

Many tests have been utilized previously in an attempt to distinguish constitutional delay from isolated gonadotropin deficiency, including the measurement of adrenal androgens, testosterone levels after hCG stimulation, and the prolactin response to stimulation by TRH, metoclopramide, domperidone, and chlorpromazine (95). However, each of these tests, as well as the use of random and GnRH-stimulated gonadotropin levels, has limitations. Specifically, there is often considerable overlap in the observed responses of the two groups that precludes definitive diagnosis, although the advent of the ultrasensitive chemiluminometric assays for LH may ultimately permit a more reliable distinction. Other investigations that have been used to delineate the two groups include: frequent nocturnal sampling of LH (96), gonadotropin levels after stimulation with pulsatile GnRH (97) or GnRH analogs (96,98), random early morning testosterone levels (99), urinary excretion of gonadotropins (100), and the free α-subunit response to GnRH (101,102). Unfortunately, many of these tests are either too costly or have yet to be validated for routine clinical use.

Finally, most boys with CDP have evidence of testicular growth after a short course of testosterone therapy (103). Exogenous sex steroids should not substantially increase testicular size. Therefore, it is believed that testicular enlargement represents endogenous puberty that has started secondary to "priming" of the HPG axis by exogenous testosterone. Consequently, many clinicians use a course of testosterone not only as treatment, but also as a diagnostic tool in distinguishing CDP from true gonadotropin deficiency.

MANAGEMENT

The management of delayed puberty is closely linked to its underlying etiology. In cases of transient HH in which the causative factor(s) can be determined, simply treating the underlying problem should result in the attainment or the completion of puberty. However, independent of etiology, any case of pubertal delay can always be treated through the use of exogenous sex steroids to induce and maintain the secondary sexual characteristics.

Constitutional Delay

Since theirs is a functional disorder that invariably resolves over time, children with constitutional delay of growth and puberty do not require specific medical intervention. In many cases, emotional support and reassurance, including pointing out the early signs of puberty that may have been overlooked, are often all that is needed. However, these children are subject to ridicule by their classmates and are often presumed to be younger than their chronologic age. This may lead to significant psychological repercussions for the child who is seen as "different" from his or her peers. Thus, poor self-esteem, social isolation, and prolonged parental dependence are not uncommon in this setting. In addition, studies have shown that pubertal delay may have adverse effects on bone accretion, with diminished peak bone mass and possible osteopenia in adulthood (104). For these reasons, as well as for the diagnostic benefit discussed above, it is appropriate to consider a brief (3–6 mo) course of sex steroids in children with CDGP in order to promote short-term growth and pubertal development. The short-term use of testosterone or estrogen is a safe mode of therapy with few side effects, except for the normal signs of puberty. Studies have clearly shown the benefit of treatment on emotional well-being and physical development. Furthermore, previous concerns about significant advancement of bone age with resultant negative effects on final adult height are unfounded *(105)*. Most children will respond to one course of therapy, but a minority may require a second course. If more than two courses are required, the diagnosis of CDGP should be reconsidered.

Constitutional delay can also be treated with the oral derivatives of testosterone: methyltestosterone, fluoxymesterone, and oxandrolone. However, these 17α-alkylated androgens do carry the risk of hepatotoxicity, cholestasis, and liver tumors, which makes their use less frequent. Oxandrolone is the best-studied and most frequently used anabolic steroid for CDGP. Despite its androgenic action, oxandrolone is generally not sufficient in inducing virilization, and its utility in constitutional delay has been its ability to accelerate linear growth. Therefore, oxandrolone in a dose of 2.5–5 mg/d is a safe alternative (in both males and females) that does not significantly advance bone age or compromise final adult height *(106,107)*. Finally, GH therapy is not indicated in the adolescent with isolated constitutional delay because available data suggest that there is no benefit on final height *(6)*.

Permanent Hypogonadism

Unlike those individuals with CDP, children with permanent hypogonadism absolutely require intervention for the induction and maintenance of the secondary sexual characteristics and for the preservation of BMD. If the diagnosis is previously established, treatment should begin at the approximate age when puberty is anticipated to occur and when appropriate for the psychosocial milieu. Testosterone or estrogen is initially administered in a fashion that attempts to mimic the natural rise of these hormone levels. The timing of pubertal entrance, however, must be considered carefully in those children receiving concomitant therapy with GH. In this setting, the benefit of sex steroids on bone accretion and feminization or masculinization must be weighed against its possible adverse effects on epiphyseal fusion and final adult height.

Testosterone is the mainstay of treatment for boys with hypogonadism (Table 3), and it is most frequently administered as one of its long-acting esters, testosterone cypionate or testosterone enanthate. Testosterone undecanoate is another testosterone ester that is available for use outside of the United States. It has recently been studied for intramuscular use *(108)*, but is most commonly taken as a pill 2–4 times/d. Although good for androgen replacement in adult men, it may not be the first choice in adolescents, given its variable oral absorption *(109)*. Additional testosterone therapies available to the clinician include subcutaneous pellets *(110)*, transdermal patches *(111)*, and the newly approved topical gel *(112)*. However, exact dosing for pubertal induction with these modes of testosterone delivery has not been firmly established, and their role is much greater in maintenance therapy.

Estrogen is available in several forms for the treatment of girls with hypogonadism (Table 3). In the United States, the most commonly used preparations for pubertal induction are the esterified or conjugated estrogens. Alternatively, escalating doses of unconjugated ethinyl estradiol may be prescribed. Once breakthrough bleeding occurs, or by the second year of estrogen therapy, a progestational agent is added to the hormonal regimen, either

Table 3
Hormonal Treatment in Delayed Puberty

Treatment	Induction of Puberty	Maintenance Dose
MALES		
Testosterone enanthate or Testosterone cypionate	50 mg IM Q mo, titrated every 3–6 mo	150–200 mg IM Q 2–3 wk
Testosterone undecanoate	40 mg PO QD, titrated based on response	Up to 240 mg/d
Transdermal testosterone A) Androderm® (2.5 mg; 5 mg) B) Testoderm® (4 mg; 6 mg) C) Testoderm® TTS (5 mg)	Exact dosing unknown	4–6 mg/d A) 5 mg QHS (back, upper arms, abdomen, or thighs) B) 4 mg or 6 mg QHS (scrotal skin) C) 5 mg QHS (back, arms, or upper buttocks)
Testosterone pellets	8–10 mg/kg q 6 mo *(110)*	600–1200 mg subcutaneously every 4–6 mo
Testosterone gel (AndroGel™)	Unknown	5–10 mg/d
FEMALES		
Conjugated estrogens (Premarin®) or Esterified estrogens (Estratab®, Menest™)	0.3 mg PO QD, titrated every 3–6 mo	0.6–1.25 mg PO QD
Ethinyl estradiol	2–5 mcg PO QD, titrated every 3–6 mo	20–35 mcg PO QD
Transdermal 17β-estradiol, various products	Exact dosing unknown	0.05–0.1 mg/d
Estrogen/progesterone combinations, various oral and transdermal preparations	Not used	Product dependent

Adapted with permission from ref. *(117)*.

separately or as part of an oral contraceptive pill. Progestagens protect against endometrial hyperplasia and its attendant risk of adenocarcinoma. Estrogen and estrogen/progesterone combinations are also available via various transdermal patches, which have the advantage of no first-pass metabolism through the liver. Although transdermal therapy with 17β-estradiol has been used to induce puberty in girls with Turner syndrome *(113)*, its use is most valuable in maintenance therapy once attainment of secondary sexual characteristics is complete.

Other therapeutic options in the treatment of children with permanent HH address both the hypogonadism as well as the infertility encountered in these patients. The use of exogenous pulsatile GnRH via a pump can be used in the induction of puberty *(114)*, but it is an inconvenient and expensive means of achieving a goal that has other options. On the other hand, GnRH therapy is an excellent choice for those patients with HH who desire fertility *(13,115)*. The gonadotropins, hCG and either recombinant FSH or human menopausal gonadotropin (hMG), have also been successfully used to induce puberty and spermatogenesis *(13,116)*. Although hCG therapy has the added benefit of stimulating testicular growth, the need for parenteral administration every other day often precludes the routine use of these hormones in pubertal induction.

CONCLUSION

Delayed puberty can result from a multitude of etiologies, including defects at the level of the hypothalamus/pituitary (HH) or ineffective gonadal sex-steroid production (hypergonadotropic hypogonadism). Fortunately, the diagnosis is frequently made with a patient, conscientious approach to the affected child. Furthermore, regardless of cause, pubertal delay can easily be treated, the result of which is best appreciated in the face of the child who now feels like a member of his or her peer group. Although our knowledge of the many factors involved in normal and aberrant puberty remains in its infancy, we can look forward to the future when further advances in science will promote our understanding of this engaging topic.

REFERENCES

1. Kaplowitz PB, Oberfield SE. Reexamination of the age limit for defining when puberty is precocious in girls in the United States: implications for evaluation and treatment. Drug and Therapeutics and Executive Committees of the Lawson Wilkins Pediatric Endocrine Society. Pediatrics 1999;104:936–941.
2. Rensonnet C, Kanen F, Coremans C, Ernould C, Albert A, Bourguignon JP. Pubertal growth as a determinant of adult height in boys with constitutional delay of growth and puberty. Horm Res 1999; 51:223–229.
3. Arrigo T, Cisternino M, Luca De F, et al. Final height outcome in both untreated and testosterone-treated boys with constitutional delay of growth and puberty. J Pediatr Endocrinol Metab 1996;9: 511–517.
4. LaFranchi S, Hanna CE, Mandel SH. Constitutional delay of growth: expected versus final adult height. Pediatrics 1991;87:82–87.
5. Adan L, Souberbielle JC, Brauner R. Management of the short stature due to pubertal delay in boys. J Clin Endocrinol Metab 1994;78:478–482.
6. Ferrandez Longas A, Mayayo E, Valle A, Soria J, Labarta JI. Constitutional delay in growth and puberty: a comparison of final height achieved between treated and untreated children. J Pediatr Endocrinol Metab 1996;9(Suppl 3):345–357.
7. Cara JF, Rosenfield RL. Insulin-like growth factor I and insulin potentiate luteinizing hormone-induced androgen synthesis by rat ovarian thecal-interstitial cells. Endocrinology 1988;123:733–739.
8. Acampora D, Mazan S, Tuorto F, et al. Transient dwarfism and hypogonadism in mice lacking Otx1 reveal prepubescent stage-specific control of pituitary levels of GH, FSH and LH. Development 1998; 125:1229–1239.
9. Waldstreicher J, Seminara SB, Jameson JL, et al. The genetic and clinical heterogeneity of gonadotropin-releasing hormone deficiency in the human. J Clin Endocrinol Metab 1996;81:4388–4395.
10. Seminara SB, Hayes FJ, Crowley WF Jr. Gonadotropin-releasing hormone deficiency in the human (idiopathic hypogonadotropic hypogonadism and Kallmann's syndrome): pathophysiological and genetic considerations. Endocr Rev 1998;19:521–539.
11. Conrad B, Kriebel J, Hetzel WD. Hereditary bimanual synkinesis combined with hypogonadotropic hypogonadism and anosmia in four brothers. J Neurol 1978;218:263–274.
12. Kirk JM, Grant DB, Besser GM, et al. Unilateral renal aplasia in X-linked Kallmann's syndrome. Clin Genet 1994;46:260–262.
13. Hayes FJ, Seminara SB, Crowley WF Jr. Hypogonadotropic hypogonadism. Endocrinol Metab Clin North Am 1998;27:739–763, vii.
14. Smals AG, Kloppenborg PW, van Haelst UJ, Lequin R, Benraad TJ. Fertile eunuch syndrome versus classic hypogonadotrophic hypogonadism. Acta Endocrinol (Copenh) 1978;87:389–399.

15. Cassidy SB, Schwartz S. Prader-Willi and Angelman syndromes. Disorders of genomic imprinting. Medicine (Baltimore) 1998;77:140–151.

16. Nicholls RD, Saitoh S, Horsthemke B. Imprinting in Prader-Willi and Angelman syndromes. Trends Genet 1998;14:194–200.

17. Muller J. Hypogonadism and endocrine metabolic disorders in Prader-Willi syndrome. Acta Paediatr Suppl 1997;423:58–59.

18. Thacker MJ, Hainline B, St. Dennis-Feezle L, Johnson NB, Pescovitz OH. Growth failure in Prader-Willi syndrome is secondary to growth hormone deficiency. Horm Res 1998;49:216–220.

19. Green JS, Parfrey PS, Harnett JD, et al. The cardinal manifestations of Bardet-Biedl syndrome, a form of Laurence-Moon-Biedl syndrome. N Engl J Med 1989;321:1002–1009.

20. Whitaker MD, Scheithauer BW, Kovacs KT, Randall RV, Campbell RJ, Okazaki H. The pituitary gland in the Laurence-Moon syndrome. Mayo Clin Proc 1987;62:216–222.

21. Rosen DS. Pubertal growth and sexual maturation for adolescents with chronic illness or disability. Pediatrician 1991;18:105–120.

22. Pugliese MT, Lifshitz F, Grad G, Fort P, Marks-Katz M. Fear of obesity. A cause of short stature and delayed puberty. N Engl J Med 1983;309:513–518.

23. Frisch RE. The right weight: body fat, menarche and ovulation. Baillieres Clin Obstet Gynaecol 1990; 4:419–439.

24. Frisch RE, Gotz-Welbergen AV, McArthur JW, et al. Delayed menarche and amenorrhea of college athletes in relation to age of onset of training. JAMA 1981;246:1559–1563.

25. Zadik Z, Cooper M, Chen M, Stern N. Cushing's disease presenting as pubertal arrest. J Pediatr Endocrinol 1993;6:201–204.

26. Darendeliler F, Hindmarsh PC, Preece MA, Cox L, Brook CG. Growth hormone increases rate of pubertal maturation. Acta Endocrinol (Copenh) 1990;122:414–416.

27. Ballabio A, Bardoni B, Carrozzo R, et al. Contiguous gene syndromes due to deletions in the distal short arm of the human X chromosome. Proc Natl Acad Sci USA 1989;86:10,001–10,005.

28. Franco B, Guioli S, Pragliola A, et al. A gene deleted in Kallmann's syndrome shares homology with neural cell adhesion and axonal path-finding molecules. Nature 1991;353:529–536.

29. Legouis R, Hardelin JP, Levilliers J, et al. The candidate gene for the X-linked Kallmann syndrome encodes a protein related to adhesion molecules. Cell 1991;67:423–435.

30. Layman LC. The molecular basis of human hypogonadotropic hypogonadism. Mol Genet Metab 1999; 68:191–199.

31. Habiby RL, Boepple P, Nachtigall L, Sluss PM, Crowley WF Jr, Jameson JL. Adrenal hypoplasia congenita with hypogonadotropic hypogonadism: evidence that DAX-1 mutations lead to combined hypothalamic and pituitary defects in gonadotropin production. J Clin Invest 1996;98:1055–1062.

32. Takahashi T, Shoji Y, Haraguchi N, Takahashi I, Takada G. Active hypothalamic-pituitary-gonadal axis in an infant with X-linked adrenal hypoplasia congenita. J Pediatr 1997;130:485–488.

33. Peter M, Viemann M, Partsch CJ, Sippell WG. Congenital adrenal hypoplasia: clinical spectrum, experience with hormonal diagnosis, and report on new point mutations of the DAX-1 gene. J Clin Endocrinol Metab 1998;83:2666–2674.

34. Muscatelli F, Strom TM, Walker AP, et al. Mutations in the DAX-1 gene give rise to both X-linked adrenal hypoplasia congenita and hypogonadotropic hypogonadism. Nature 1994;372:672–676.

35. Seminara SB, Achermann JC, Genel M, Jameson JL, Crowley WF Jr. X-linked adrenal hypoplasia congenita: a mutation in DAX1 expands the phenotypic spectrum in males and females. J Clin Endocrinol Metab 1999;84:4501–4509.

36. Tabarin A, Achermann JC, Recan D, et al. A novel mutation in DAX1 causes delayed-onset adrenal insufficiency and incomplete hypogonadotropic hypogonadism. J Clin Invest 2000;105:321–328.

37. Zanaria E, Muscatelli F, Bardoni B, et al. An unusual member of the nuclear hormone receptor superfamily responsible for X-linked adrenal hypoplasia congenita. Nature 1994;372:635–641.

38. Reutens AT, Achermann JC, Ito M, et al. Clinical and functional effects of mutations in the DAX-1 gene in patients with adrenal hypoplasia congenita. J Clin Endocrinol Metab 1999;84:504–511.

39. Merke DP, Tajima T, Baron J, Cutler GB Jr. Hypogonadotropic hypogonadism in a female caused by an X-linked recessive mutation in the DAX1 gene. N Engl J Med 1999;340:1248–1252.

40. Parks JS, Brown MR, Hurley DL, Phelps CJ, Wajnrajch MP. Heritable disorders of pituitary development. J Clin Endocrinol Metab 1999;84:4362–4370.

41. Sornson MW, Wu W, Dasen JS, et al. Pituitary lineage determination by the Prophet of Pit-1 homeodomain factor defective in Ames dwarfism. Nature 1996;384:327–333.

42. Wu W, Cogan JD, Pfaffle RW, et al. Mutations in PROP1 cause familial combined pituitary hormone deficiency. Nat Genet 1998;18:147–149.

43. Pernasetti F, Toledo SP, Vasilyev VV, et al. Impaired adrenocorticotropin-adrenal axis in combined pituitary hormone deficiency caused by a two-base pair deletion (301-302delAG) in the prophet of Pit-1 gene. J Clin Endocrinol Metab 2000;85:390–397.

44. Dattani MT, Martinez-Barbera JP, Thomas PQ, et al. Mutations in the homeobox gene HESX1/Hesx1 associated with septo-optic dysplasia in human and mouse. Nat Genet 1998;19:125–133.

45. de Roux N, Young J, Misrahi M, et al. A family with hypogonadotropic hypogonadism and mutations in the gonadotropin-releasing hormone receptor. N Engl J Med 1997;337:1597–1602.

46. Layman LC, Cohen DP, Jin M, et al. Mutations in gonadotropin-releasing hormone receptor gene cause hypogonadotropic hypogonadism [letter]. Nat Genet 1998;18:14–15.

47. Pralong FP, Gomez F, Castillo E, et al. Complete hypogonadotropic hypogonadism associated with a novel inactivating mutation of the gonadotropin-releasing hormone receptor. J Clin Endocrinol Metab 1999;84:3811–3816.

48. Weiss J, Axelrod L, Whitcomb RW, Harris PE, Crowley WF, Jameson JL. Hypogonadism caused by a single amino acid substitution in the beta subunit of luteinizing hormone. N Engl J Med 1992;326:179–183.

49. Matthews CH, Borgato S, Beck-Peccoz P, et al. Primary amenorrhoea and infertility due to a mutation in the beta-subunit of follicle-stimulating hormone. Nat Genet 1993;5:83–86.

50. Layman LC, Lee EJ, Peak DB, et al. Delayed puberty and hypogonadism caused by mutations in the follicle- stimulating hormone beta-subunit gene. N Engl J Med 1997;337:607–611.

51. Phillip M, Arbelle JE, Segev Y, Parvari R. Male hypogonadism due to a mutation in the gene for the beta-subunit of follicle-stimulating hormone. N Engl J Med 1998;338:1729–1732.

52. Roemmich JN, Rogol AD. Role of leptin during childhood growth and development. Endocrinol Metab Clin North Am 1999;28:749–764, viii.

53. Chehab FF, Lim ME, Lu R. Correction of the sterility defect in homozygous obese female mice by treatment with the human recombinant leptin. Nat Genet 1996;12:318–320.

54. Mounzih K, Lu R, Chehab FF. Leptin treatment rescues the sterility of genetically obese ob/ob males. Endocrinology 1997;138:1190–1193.

55. Ahima RS, Dushay J, Flier SN, Prabakaran D, Flier JS. Leptin accelerates the onset of puberty in normal female mice. J Clin Invest 1997;99:391–395.

56. Chehab FF, Mounzih K, Lu R, Lim ME. Early onset of reproductive function in normal female mice treated with leptin. Science 1997;275:88–90.

57. Kiess W, Reich A, Meyer K, et al. A role for leptin in sexual maturation and puberty? Horm Res 1999; 51(Suppl)S3:55–63.

58. Clement K, Vaisse C, Lahlou N, et al. A mutation in the human leptin receptor gene causes obesity and pituitary dysfunction. Nature 1998;392:398–401.

59. Strobel A, Issad T, Camoin L, Ozata M, Strosberg AD. A leptin missense mutation associated with hypogonadism and morbid obesity [news]. Nat Genet 1998;18:213–215.

60. Farooqi IS, Jebb SA, Langmack G, et al. Effects of recombinant leptin therapy in a child with congenital leptin deficiency. N Engl J Med 1999;341:879–884.

61. Saenger P. Turner's syndrome. N Engl J Med 1996;335:1749–1754.

62. Lippe B. Turner syndrome. Endocrinol Metab Clin North Am 1991;20:121–152.

63. Ponzio G, Chiodo F, Messina M, et al. Non-mosaic isodicentric X-chromosome in a patient with secondary amenorrhea. Clin Genet 1987;32:20–23.

64. Rao E, Weiss B, Fukami M, et al. Pseudoautosomal deletions encompassing a novel homeobox gene cause growth failure in idiopathic short stature and Turner syndrome. Nat Genet 1997;16:54–63.

65. Mazzanti L, Cacciari E. Congenital heart disease in patients with Turner's syndrome. Italian Study Group for Turner Syndrome (ISGTS). J Pediatr 1998;133:688–692.

66. Pasquino AM, Passeri F, Pucarelli I, Segni M, Municchi G. Spontaneous pubertal development in Turner's syndrome. Italian Study Group for Turner's Syndrome. J Clin Endocrinol Metab 1997;82:1810–1813.

67. Conte FA, Grumbach MM, Kaplan SL. A diphasic pattern of gonadotropin secretion in patients with the syndrome of gonadal dysgenesis. J Clin Endocrinol Metab 1975;40:670–674.

68. Matarazzo P, Lala R, Artesani L, Franceshini PG, De Sanctis C. Sonographic appearance of ovaries and gonadotropin secretions as prognostic tools of spontaneous puberty in girls with Turner's syndrome. J Pediatr Endocrinol Metab 1995;8:267–274.

69. Noonan JA. Noonan syndrome. An update and review for the primary pediatrician. Clin Pediatr (Phila) 1994;33:548–555.

70. Jamieson CR, van der Burgt I, Brady AF, et al. Mapping a gene for Noonan syndrome to the long arm of chromosome 12. Nat Genet 1994;8:357–360.

71. Elsawi MM, Pryor JP, Klufio G, Barnes C, Patton MA. Genital tract function in men with Noonan syndrome. J Med Genet 1994;31:468–470.

72. Schwartz ID, Root AW. The Klinefelter syndrome of testicular dysgenesis. Endocrinol Metab Clin North Am 1991;20:153–163.

73. Peet J, Weaver DD, Vance GH. 49,XXXXY: a distinct phenotype. Three new cases and review. J Med Genet 1998;35:420–424.

74. Ron-el R, Friedler S, Strassburger D, Komarovsky D, Schachter M, Raziel A. Birth of a healthy neonate following the intracytoplasmic injection of testicular spermatozoa from a patient with Klinefelter's syndrome. Hum Reprod 1999;14:368–370.

75. Nichols CR, Heerema NA, Palmer C, Loehrer PJ Sr, Williams SD, Einhorn LH. Klinefelter's syndrome associated with mediastinal germ cell neoplasms. J Clin Oncol 1987;5:1290–1294.

76. Hultborn R, Hanson C, Kopf I, Verbiene I, Warnhammar E, Weimarck A. Prevalence of Klinefelter's syndrome in male breast cancer patients. Anticancer Res 1997;17:4293–4297.

77. Conway GS. Clinical manifestations of genetic defects affecting gonadotrophins and their receptors. Clin Endocrinol (Oxf) 1996;45:657–663.

78. Layman LC. Mutations in human gonadotropin genes and their physiologic significance in puberty and reproduction. Fertil Steril 1999;71:201–218.

79. Aittomaki K, Lucena JL, Pakarinen P, et al. Mutation in the follicle-stimulating hormone receptor gene causes hereditary hypergonadotropic ovarian failure. Cell 1995;82:959–968.

80. Latronico AC, Anasti J, Arnhold IJ, et al. Brief report: testicular and ovarian resistance to luteinizing hormone caused by inactivating mutations of the luteinizing hormone-receptor gene. N Engl J Med 1996;334:507–512.

81. Tapanainen JS, Aittomaki K, Min J, Vaskivuo T, Huhtaniemi IT. Men homozygous for an inactivating mutation of the follicle-stimulating hormone (FSH) receptor gene present variable suppression of spermatogenesis and fertility. Nat Genet 1997;15:205–206.

82. Adashi EY, Hennebold JD. Single-gene mutations resulting in reproductive dysfunction in women. N Engl J Med 1999;340:709–718.

83. Quigley CA, De Bellis A, Marschke KB, el-Awady MK, Wilson EM, French FS. Androgen receptor defects: historical, clinical, and molecular perspectives [published erratum appears in Endocr Rev 1995 Aug;16(4):546]. Endocr Rev 1995;16:271–321.

84. Marcantonio SM, Fechner PY, Migeon CJ, Perlman EJ, Berkovitz GD. Embryonic testicular regression sequence: a part of the clinical spectrum of 46,XY gonadal dysgenesis. Am J Med Genet 1994;49:1–5.

85. MacGillivray MH, Morishima A, Conte F, Grumbach M, Smith EP. Pediatric endocrinology update: an overview. The essential roles of estrogens in pubertal growth, epiphyseal fusion and bone turnover: lessons from mutations in the genes for aromatase and the estrogen receptor. Horm Res 1998;49:2–8.

86. Smith EP, Boyd J, Frank GR, et al. Estrogen resistance caused by a mutation in the estrogen-receptor gene in a man [published erratum appears in N Engl J Med 1995 Jan 12;332(2):131]. N Engl J Med 1994;331:1056–1061.

87. Bilezikian JP, Morishima A, Bell J, Grumbach MM. Increased bone mass as a result of estrogen therapy in a man with aromatase deficiency. N Engl J Med 1998;339:599–603.

88. Kaufman FR, Donnell GN, Roe TF, Kogut MD. Gonadal function in patients with galactosaemia. J Inherit Metab Dis 1986;9:140–146.

89. Kristiansson B, Stibler H, Wide L. Gonadal function and glycoprotein hormones in the carbohydrate-deficient glycoprotein (CDG) syndrome. Acta Paediatr 1995;84:655–659.

90. Winkler L, Offner G, Krull F, Brodehl J. Growth and pubertal development in nephropathic cystinosis. Eur J Pediatr 1993;152:244–249.

91. Braverman PK, Sondheimer SJ. Menstrual disorders. Pediatr Rev 1997;18:17–25.

92. Lindenman E, Shepard MK, Pescovitz OH. Mullerian agenesis: an update. Obstet Gynecol 1997;90:307–312.

93. Rosenfield RL. Clinical review 6: diagnosis and management of delayed puberty. J Clin Endocrinol Metab 1990;70:559–562.

94. Styne DM. New aspects in the diagnosis and treatment of pubertal disorders. Pediatr Clin North Am 1997;44:505–529.

95. Shalet SM. Treatment of constitutional delay in growth and puberty (CDGP). Clin Endocrinol (Oxf) 1989;31:81–86.

96. Ehrmann DA, Rosenfield RL, Cuttler L, Burstein S, Cara JF, Levitsky LL. A new test of combined pituitary-testicular function using the gonadotropin-releasing hormone agonist nafarelin in the differentiation of gonadotropin deficiency from delayed puberty: pilot studies. J Clin Endocrinol Metab 1989;69:963–967.

97. Smals AG, Hermus AR, Boers GH, Pieters GF, Benraad TJ, Kloppenborg PW. Predictive value of luteinizing hormone releasing hormone (LHRH) bolus testing before and after 36-hour pulsatile LHRH administration in the differential diagnosis of constitutional delay of puberty and male hypogonadotropic hypogonadism. J Clin Endocrinol Metab 1994;78:602–608.

98. Zamboni G, Antoniazzi F, Tato L. Use of the gonadotropin-releasing hormone agonist triptorelin in the diagnosis of delayed puberty in boys. J Pediatr 1995;126:756–758.

99. Wu FC, Brown DC, Butler GE, Stirling HF, Kelnar CJ. Early morning plasma testosterone is an accurate predictor of imminent pubertal development in prepubertal boys. J Clin Endocrinol Metab 1993;76:26–31.

100. Kulin H, Demers L, Chinchilli V, Martel J, Stevens L. Usefulness of sequential urinary follicle-stimulating hormone and luteinizing hormone measurements in the diagnosis of adolescent hypogonadotropism in males. J Clin Endocrinol Metab 1994;78:1208–1211.

101. Mainieri AS, Viera JG, Elnecave RH. Response of the free alpha-subunit to GnRH distinguishes individuals with 'functional' from those with permanent hypogonadotropic hypogonadism. Horm Res 1998;50:212–216.

102. Lavoie HB, Martin KA, Taylor E, Crowley WF, Hall JE. Exaggerated free alpha-subunit levels during pulsatile gonadotropin-releasing hormone replacement in women with idiopathic hypogonadotropic hypogonadism. J Clin Endocrinol Metab 1998;83:241–247.

103. Kaplowitz PB. Diagnostic value of testosterone therapy in boys with delayed puberty. Am J Dis Child 1989;143:116–120.

104. Finkelstein JS, Neer RM, Biller BM, Crawford JD, Klibanski A. Osteopenia in men with a history of delayed puberty. N Engl J Med 1992;326:600–604.

105. Richman RA, Kirsch LR. Testosterone treatment in adolescent boys with constitutional delay in growth and development. N Engl J Med 1988;319:1563–1567.

106. Stanhope R, Buchanan CR, Fenn GC, Preece MA. Double blind placebo controlled trial of low dose oxandrolone in the treatment of boys with constitutional delay of growth and puberty. Arch Dis Child 1988;63:501–505.

107. Joss EE, Schmidt HA, Zuppinger KA. Oxandrolone in constitutionally delayed growth, a longitudinal study up to final height. J Clin Endocrinol Metab 1989;69:1109–1115.

108. Zhang GY, Gu YQ, Wang XH, Cui YG, Bremner WJ. A pharmacokinetic study of injectable testosterone undecanoate in hypogonadal men. J Androl 1998;19:761–768.

109. Zachmann M. Therapeutic indications for delayed puberty and hypogonadism in adolescent boys. Horm Res 1991;36:141–146.

110. Zacharin MR, Warne GL. Treatment of hypogonadal adolescent boys with long acting subcutaneous testosterone pellets. Arch Dis Child 1997;76:495–499.

111. De Sanctis V, Vullo C, Urso L, et al. Clinical experience using the Androderm testosterone transdermal system in hypogonadal adolescents and young men with beta-thalassemia major. J Pediatr Endocrinol Metab 1998;11:891–900.

112. Wang C, Berman N, Longstreth JA, et al. Pharmacokinetics of transdermal testosterone gel in hypogonadal men: application of gel at one site versus four sites: a General Clinical Research Center Study. J Clin Endocrinol Metab 2000;85:964–969.

113. Illig R, DeCampo C, Lang-Muritano MR, et al. A physiological mode of puberty induction in hypogonadal girls by low dose transdermal 17 beta-oestradiol. Eur J Pediatr 1990;150:86–91.

114. Hoffman AR, Crowley WF Jr. Induction of puberty in men by long-term pulsatile administration of low-dose gonadotropin-releasing hormone. N Engl J Med 1982;307:1237–1241.

115. Blumenfeld Z, Makler A, Frisch L, Brandes JM. Induction of spermatogenesis and fertility in hypogonadotropic azoospermic men by intravenous pulsatile gonadotropin-releasing hormone (GnRH). Gynecol Endocrinol 1988;2:151–164.

116. Barrio R, de Luis D, Alonso M, Lamas A, Moreno JC. Induction of puberty with human chorionic gonadotropin and follicle-stimulating hormone in adolescent males with hypogonadotropic hypogonadism. Fertil Steril 1999;71:244–248.

117. Waguespack S, Walvoord E, Pescovitz O. Precocious and delayed puberty. In: Becker K, Bilezikian J, Bremner W, et al., eds. Principles and Practice of Endocrinology and Metabolism, 3rd ed. Lippincott Williams & Wilkins, Philadelphia, PA, 2000, pp. 893–908.

VI ADRENAL

16 Molecular Development of the Hypothalamic-Pituitary-Adrenal (HPA) Axis

Sophia P. Tsakiri, MD, George P. Chrousos, MD, and Andrew N. Margioris, MD

CONTENTS

DEVELOPMENT OF HYPOTHALAMUS: THE PARAVENTRICULAR NUCLEUS

The human hypothalamus lies ventrally to the thalamus and extends from the rostral part of the optic chiasm to the caudal edge of the mamillary bodies. It originates in the alar plate of diencephalon, its sulcus becoming identifiable by the 5th wk of gestation. The hypothalamus is a highly complex organ coordinating central nervous system (CNS) centers and neuroendocrine, metabolic, autonomic nervous and behavioral functions. A system of nerve fibers and portal vessels connects the hypothalamus to the pituitary. The axon terminals of neurons originating in several hypothalamic nuclei, including the supraoptic,

From: *Contemporary Endocrinology: Developmental Endocrinology: From Research to Clinical Practice*
Edited by: E. A. Eugster and O. H. Pescovitz © Humana Press Inc., Totowa, NJ

the paraventricular, the arcuate, and the ventromedial nucleus, form the median eminence located rostrally to the mamillary bodies. The median eminence communicates with the anterior pituitary via a local portal venous system, which permits the direct hematogenous communication between neurons and endocrine cells. The hypothalamic neurons regulating the function of anterior pituitary corticotrophs are located in the parvocellular part of the paraventricular hypothalamic nucleus. They synthesize the neuropeptides corticotropin-releasing hormone (CRH) and arginine-vasopressin (AVP), which, packaged in secretory vesicles, travel the neural axons and reach the median eminence, where they are placed in specific secretory areas beneath the subplasmalemal actin network ready to be secreted into the portal system.

CRH and AVP regulate the synthesis and secretion of adrenocorticotropin (ACTH) hormone from the corticotroph cells in anterior pituitary. Neuropeptides, neurotransmitters, cytokines, and catecholamines affect CRH and AVP synthesis; axonal transport; and secretion, while glucocorticoids exert negative feedback on the hypothalamus. It should be noted here that the AVP produced by megakaryocytes in the paraventricullar and the supraoptic nuclei does not participate in the regulation of the HPA axis. Indeed, this AVP is under osmotic control and its physiological mission is to regulate water homeostasis. The posterior pituitary is the anatomical equivalent of the median eminence representing the terminals of megakaryocytic axons. Megakaryocyte-derived AVP reaches the posterior pituitary via axonal transport. AVP is released from the posterior pituitary directly into the systemic circulation. CRH transcript and peptide are detectable in the paraventricular nucleus of the fetal rat hypothalamus by d 15 increasing in concentration steadily up to d 20 (term = 21 d). Following a brief period of decline, CRH reaches adult levels by postnatal d 4 *(1)*. Similarly, in the ovine fetus, the CRH transcript in the paraventricular nucleus is detectable by gestational d 60 (term = 147 d) and increases markedly in late gestation, declining during the immediate postpartum period *(2)*. The presence of hypothalamic CRH may not be a good indicator of the maturation of the HPA axis, since it now appears that the pituitary portal system becomes functional later. Thus, in rat fetuses, exogenous CRH stimulates the transcription of the pro-opic-melanocortin (POMC)-gene and the secretion of POMC-derived peptides by d 15 *(3)*, while endogenous CRH begins to play a physiologic role only by d 17. CRH antiserum administration in pregnant rats significantly decreases fetal corticosterone and ACTH production, but not earlier than d 17 of gestation. Similarly, in human fetuses, ACTH secretion responds to exogenous CRH from the 12th wk of gestation *(4)*. However, endogenous CRH released into the portal system begins only by the 16th wk of fetal life, establishing the CRH-control of pituitary corticotrophs at that time. Fetal anterior pituitary ACTH also responds to AVP *(5)*. It is of interest that, in the ovine fetus, AVP-containing neurons in the median eminence appear early in gestation (by the 42nd d of gestation), well before the appearance of CRH-containing neurons. The earlier appearance of AVP relative to CRH suggests a significant role for AVP in the control of ACTH secretion early in gestation. Hypothalamic concentrations of the AVP transcript and the AVP peptide significantly increase in late gestation, remaining elevated in the newborn *(2,6)*. In the early 1980s, the late professor D.T. Krieger and her colleagues found that human placenta is a major source of CRH during pregnancy *(7–10)*. Placental CRH is secreted in both maternal and fetal circulation. The precise role of placental CRH is unknown. It most probably affects the growth of the fetal adrenals and the production of dehydroepiandrosterone (DHEA), which serves as a precursor for placental-derived estrogens. The major role of placental CRH may be local, affecting myometrial tone, thus regulating the length of pregnancy and the initiation of labor. CRH-R1 receptors are present in human myometrium *(11)*.

DEVELOPMENT
OF ANTERIOR PITUITARY CORTICOTROPHS

The anterior pituitary gland or adenohypophysis arises during the 3rd wk of gestation from Rathke's pouch evaginating from the posterior buccopharyngeal membrane. The mature anterior pituitary gland is formed around the 11th wk of gestation. Mesenchymal cells located around Rathke's pouch proliferate forming the gland's capsule. From the 6th wk of gestation, a downward projection of diencephalon, the infundibulum, starts forming the pituitary stalk and the posterior pituitary (neurohypophysis). By the 8th wk of gestation, the two parts of the pituitary are in close contact. As it grows, the adenohypophysis wraps around the neurohypophysis and upwards around the stalk to form the pars tuberalis. The vascular link between the hypothalamus and pituitary consists of a portal system, the capillaries of which start developing within the pituitary by the 8th wk of gestation, maturing by the 12th wk. Tufts of capillaries in the median eminence and infundibulum form the internal and the external plexuses running along the pituitary stalk. These portal vessels open again into a second tuft of vascular sinusoids spread between the cells of the anterior pituitary. The middle and inferior hypophyseal arteries provide blood supply to the stalk and to the posterior pituitary. The venous blood of the pituitary gland drains mainly toward the cavernous sinus. By the 20th wk of gestation, the hypothalamic-pituitary complex is anatomically mature, although complete functional maturation appears to take place in postnatal life.

Regulation of Anterior Pituitary Development

Commitment of the anterior pituitary progenitor cells to specific cell types occurs very early in the development of the gland, most probably prior to the formation of Rathke's pouch. For example, the expression of the gene encoding the alpha-subunit, common to thyroid-stimulating hormone (TSH), luteinizing hormone (LH), and follicle-stimulating hormone (FSH), takes place as early as the 11th embryonic d *(12)*. The development of the anterior pituitary and its differentiation to the five final phenotypes of pituitary cells can be divided into four distinct phases, each regulated by homeobox-gene products acting as specific transcription factors. The first phase is regulated by the Rpx homeobox gene, which promotes the invagination of Rathke's pouch from the oral ectoderm. The second phase is characterized by the activation of genes, such as the BMP4, FGF8 and Lhx3 genes, instrumental in the maturation of Rathke's pouch. The third phase involves the differentiation of anterior pituitary cells, under the regulation of BMP2 and Shh genes, playing opposing roles. Finally, the fourth phase involves the geographical distribution of each anterior pituitary-cell type, which is regulated by such genes as Pax6 homeobox, Shh, and BMP2 *(13–16)*.

The Ptx (Pitx) family of homeobox transcription factors includes the Ptx1, Ptx2, and Ptx3. Ptx1 homeobox transcription factor acts in the pituitary as a master-regulator of transcription. It interacts with cell-specific factors, such as SF-1, Erg-1, Pit-1, and the basic helix-loop-helix (bHLH) hetero-dimer NeuroD1/Pan1 to activate the transcription of multiple downstream target-genes *(17)*. Pituitary-specific transcription factor-1 (Pit-1) interacts with factor GATA-2 to regulate cell-type specific gene transcription *(18)*. Pit-1 gene transcript (Pit-1/GHF-1) is found in all five types of pituitary cells and transactivates the promoter of growth hormone (GH), prolactin, and thyrotropin genes in somatotroph, lactotroph, and thyrotroph cells, respectively. Pit-1 gene mutations cause a combined GH, prolactin (PRL), and TSH deficiency. The Prophet of Pit-1 (Prop-1) transcription factor is expressed early in pituitary-cell development. Prop-1 gene mutations lead to hypogonadism and GH, PRL, and TSH deficiency. Hesx1 gene expression precedes that of Prop-1 and Pit-1; its inactivating mutations lead to panhypopituitarism *(19)*. The E-box element of the POMC promoter is cell-specific for the corticotroph cells and represents the binding site for corticotroph cell-specific HLH transcription factors. Such factors are the corticotroph-upstream transcription element-binding (CUTE) proteins, which, in synergy to Ptx1, activate POMC gene transcription *(20)*. (*See* Chapter 1 for in-depth review of pituitary development.)

Corticotroph-Cell Development

The corticotroph cells arise from an ectodermal progenitor cell *(18)*. In the ovine fetus they can be first identified in the pars distalis by the 40th d of gestation and in the pars intermedia by the 60th d. By midgestation, two distinct types of POMC-positive cells can be recognized: (a) the fetal -type cells, which are numerous, large, columnar and arranged in clusters; they are able to produce POMC but in low quantities, and (b) the adult-type cells, which are few and small but are able to produce large quantities of POMC and process it to ACTH and B-PLH. The population of fetal corticotrophs declines progressively during gestation, disappearing completely before term. In human fetuses, POMC-positive cells appear by the 8th wk of gestation. After the third month of gestation, the development of corticotroph cells depends heavily on hypothalamic neuropeptides and glucocorticoids. Anencephaly, fetal hypothalamo-pituitary disconnection, fetal paraventricular nucleus lesions or bilateral fetal adrenalectomy delay the maturation of anterior pituitary corticotrophs *(21,22)*.

Adrenocorticotropin (ACTH)

ACTH, a 39 amino acid peptide, is a post-translational product of POMC. ACTH is secreted into the systemic circulation in a pulsatile ultradian, diurnal, and stress-related manner. The biologic activity of ACTH resides in the N-terminal portion of its molecule with the first 24 amino acids being necessary for maximal biological activity. ACTH regulates glucocorticoid and adrenal androgen secretion by the zonae fasciculata and reticularis, respectively. It is also a secondary regulator of aldosterone synthesis by the zona glomerulosa. Specific ACTH receptors mediate all actions of ACTH. The receptor is activated upon binding to ACTH, resulting in the activation of the heterotrimeric G-protein complex, which subsequently activates adenylate cyclase. This enzyme catalyzes cyclic AMP generation, which results in stimulation of protein kinase A (PKA) and the release of the activated catalytic subunit. Subsequently, cholesterol ester hydrolase (the enzyme responsible for the conversion of cholesterol esters to cholesterol) is activated. Cholesterol is then transported inside the mitochondria for side-chain cleavage, the first step of steroidogenesis. ACTH also exerts important trophic effects on the adrenal cortex. There is no known transplacental passage of ACTH. It should be noted, however, that human placenta expresses the POMC gene and synthesizes ACTH and α-melanocyte-stimulating hormone (α-MSH) under the paracrine regulation of placental CRH *(23)*.

The ACTH Receptor

The ACTH receptor (melanocortin receptor type 2 or MC2-R) is a member of the G-protein-coupled membrane receptor superfamily, which consists of seven hydrophobic membrane-spanning domains connected by hydrophilic loops on either side of plasma membrane. The receptor consists of 297 amino acids with a molecular weight of 33 kDa in the unmodified form. However, it undergoes extensive glycosylation in the extracellular part of the N-terminal region, which increases its molecular weight to about 43 kDa. Each of the melanocortin receptors, including that for ACTH, couples to Gs and adenylate cyclase. The ACTH receptor exhibits an absolute specificity for ACTH, requiring two peptide domains for recognition and activation, the core H-F-R-W sequence, present in all melanocortin peptides, and a highly basic motif found only in the midportion of ACTH. The chromosomal localization of the intronless human ACTH receptor gene has been determined in the distal end of chromosome 18. The ACTH receptor transcript is detectable in all three adrenal zones. The other melanocortin receptors are MC1 in the skin, and MC3 and MC4 receptors in the brain. The fetal adrenal gland in the rat synthesizes and secretes corticosterone as early as d 13. Plasma corticosterone levels rise in parallel to ACTH from d 16 to d 19 and decrease thereafter. The number of adrenal ACTH receptors per µg of adrenal cell DNA reaches maximum values on d 19 and minimum at the 1st wk postnatally. In the perinatal period, there is correlation between the plasma immunoreactive ACTH levels, plasma corticosterone, and number of ACTH receptors/ µg DNA *(24)*. In the ovine fetus, there is an increase in cortisol levels in late gestation. A concomitant increase in plasma corticosteroid-binding capacity regulates free cortisol levels in the fetal circulation, thus attenuating negative glucocorticoid feedback prepartum *(25)*. The negative glucocorticoid feedback on the pituitary corticotrophs becomes functional late in gestation. Adrenalectomy during this period significantly stimulates the fetal HPA axis, whereas chronic dexamethasone administration in late-pregnancy drastically inhibits the fetal HPA axis at hypothalamic, pituitary, and adrenal levels. It is of major physiological significance that the negative glucocorticoid feedback to the hypothalamus is transiently blunted prepartum, allowing fetal plasma cortisol to rise.

Corticotroph Function and Glucocorticoids

The number of glucocorticoid receptors (GR) in the human pituitary peaks late in gestation and decreases during labor. The paradox of rising GR numbers in the fetal pituitary at term, namely at the time of rise of endogenous glucocorticoids, points to an altered efficacy of glucocorticoid feedback at term *(26)*. This alteration cannot be explained by a decrease in the density of pituitary GR. A 97kD (full-length receptor) and a 45kD (half-length receptor) immunoreactive GR protein have been detected in the ovine fetus. The proportion of the 45kD GR protein increases significantly with development, whereas the 97kD protein concentration is not altered during development *(27)*. Late-gestation dexamethasone treatment of the pregnant guinea pig modifies fetal hippocampal glucocorticoid receptors. Thus, in utero exposure to excess endogenous and synthetic corticosteroids may lead to a potentially permanent modification of HPA axis activity and of negative glucocorticoid feedback *(28)*.

6-8 week embryo

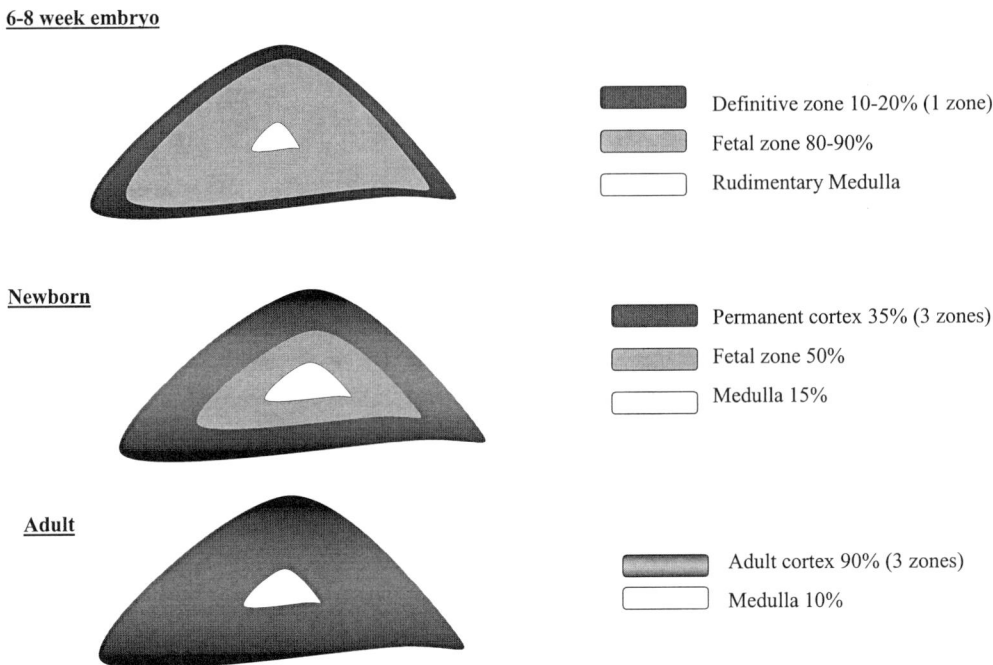

Definitive zone 10-20% (1 zone)

Fetal zone 80-90%

Rudimentary Medulla

Newborn

Permanent cortex 35% (3 zones)

Fetal zone 50%

Medulla 15%

Adult

Adult cortex 90% (3 zones)

Medulla 10%

Fig. 1. Human adrenal gland development.

DEVELOPMENT OF THE ADRENAL GLAND

The adrenal cortex and medulla have different embryologic origins. The adrenal cortex arises from mesodermal cells migrating from the dorsal celomic epithelium at the medial and cranial end of the developing mesonephros. In humans, the adrenal cortex is identifiable by the 4th wk of gestation. Between the 6th and 8th wk, the cortex develops two zones (Fig. 1). The inner fetal zone forms 80–90% of the adrenal cortex and is composed of cells with minimal mitotic activity. The definitive zone in the external part of the gland forms a very thin subcapsular rim of immature basophilic cells characterized by high mitotic activity. They proliferate rapidly and move centripetally into the enlarging inner fetal zone. An indistinct transitional area separates the two zones. The adrenal gland increases rapidly in size between the second and third month of fetal life reaching its maximum in proportion to total fetal weight at the end of this period. It continues to grow rapidly until term weighing 3–4 grams at birth. It rapidly regresses soon after birth, reaching half its fetal size by the end of the first month of life and its minimum by the first year. The postnatal reduction of adrenal-gland size is due to a gradual apoptosis of fetal-zone cells *(29)*. ACTH and a host of local neuropeptides, cytokines, and catecholamines regulate adrenocortical-cell differentiation and centripetal migration, affecting variably cellular proliferation, differentiation, and apoptosis *(30,31)*. In humans, complete maturation of the adrenal cortex is achieved later in life after adrenarche, by the 15th yr of age. When mature, the cortex makes up about 90% of the adrenal gland and surrounds the centrally located medulla. Adrenal cortical cells are layered in zones, the outermost being the zona glomerulosa, the medial zona fasciculate, and the innermost zona reticularis. A cortical cuff, resembling the zona glomerulosa centrally and the fasciculata peripherally, surrounds the central vein. The zona glomerulosa comprises about 5–10% of the cortex and is the location of mineralocorticoid aldosterone synthesis. The cells are small, with a dense nucleus, small mitochondria, scant smooth endoplasmic reticulum, and occasional lipid inclusions. The zona fasciculata comprises 75% of the cortex and is formed of large cells, with more abundant cytoplasm, endoplasmic reticulum, and lipid inclusions with prominent microvilli. Cells of the zona reticularis are more granular in appearance and contain smaller amounts of lipid inclusions, dense endoplasmic reticulum, and numerous microvilli. The zonae fasciculata and reticularis form a functional unit, having the capacity to secrete glucocorticoids, adrenal androgens, and adrenal estrogens. It is of interest that clusters and isolated cortical cells are widespread in the adrenal medulla. Similarly, clusters and isolated chromaffin cells are present in all zones of the adrenal cortex *(32)*.

Zonation Theories

Adrenal-gland development is complex and poorly understood at the molecular level. It is the result of a balance between cell proliferation, differentiation, and programmed cell death (apoptosis). Three hypothetical models attempt to describe the process of adrenal development and the formation of the adrenocortical zones. According to the transformation field theory, two fields of cortical-cell proliferation and apoptosis exist in the adrenal gland. The first one is located between the zona glomerulosa and the zona fasciculata, while a second between the fasciculata and reticularis. These two zones secrete the necessary substances controlling adrenal development. The migration theory proposes continuous cell-migration between the different adrenocortical zones, from areas of high mitotic activity to areas of higher differentiation or increased apoptosis. Cell-migration can follow a unidirectional pattern (from the glomerulosa to the reticularis), a bidirectional pattern (from the zona intermedia to the glomerulosa and the reticularis), or loop-type pattern (from the zona intermedia to the glomerularis and then to the adrenal medulla). Finally, according to the zonal theory, the three adrenocortical zones develop independently of each other and no zone-to-zone or transition zone-to-zone cell-migration exists *(33)*.

ACTH and Adrenal Development

ACTH, in addition to its effect on steroidogenesis, promotes adrenal development via regulation of adrenocortical proto-oncogene expression. Indeed, ACTH stimulates the expression of c-jun, c-fos, jun-B, and c-myc, which directly stimulate mitosis and cell differentiation. ACTH also increases the expression of several adrenal paracrine-growth factors in the zona glomerulosa including basic fibroblast growth factor (bFGF) and insulin-like growth factors 1 and 2 (IGF-1 and IGF-2) *(33)*. In addition to these effects, ACTH also exerts a potent anti-apoptotic action on the fetal adrenal cortex *(31)*.

The Intra-Adrenal Renin-Angiotensin System (RAS)

This system has emerged as a typical example of an intra-adrenal paracrine system, being functional by early gestation *(34)*. ACTH, changes in electrolyte balance, and the genetic background regulate the intra-adrenal renin production, which, in turn, modifies adrenal-zone characteristics. The intra-adrenal RAS paracrine loop regulates aldosterone synthesis by the zona glomerulosa cells, and controls cortical cell cycle via alterations in proto-oncogene expression, some steroidogenic enzyme activity, and apoptosis. It should be noted that angiotensin II exerts its biologic effect on the adrenal cortex via two types of angiotensin II receptors *(35)*. The Type 1 receptor mediates angiotensin II effects on aldosterone biosynthesis *(36)*, while the type 2 receptor mediates other effects including apoptosis *(37)*.

The Intra-Adrenal Immune System

Components of the immune system affect the HPA axis not only centrally, but also peripherally at the adrenal level. Thus, cytokines deriving from resident macrophages and medullary cells affect apoptosis, differentiation and steroidogenesis. Tumor necrosis factor alpha (TNF-α), for instance, induces apoptosis, interleukin-1 (IL-1) inhibits apoptosis, and interleukin-6 (IL-6) induces mitosis and steroidogenesis *(33,38)*. Major histocompatibility complex class II antigens first appear in the adrenal cortex around the fourth year of life. After that time, adrenal expression of MHC class II antigens parallels the functional maturation of the adrenal cortex. In the adult they are expressed in the zona reticularis *(39,40)* and there is evidence that they induce programmed adrenocortical cell death *(41)*. Apoptosis induction of adrenocortical cells by MHC class II molecules may be mediated by the CD95/Fas receptors. CD95/Fas are co-localized with MHC class II antigens in the inner cortical zones, along with adrenal macrophages. It is possible that resident macrophages play a significant role in apoptotic-body clearance from the adrenal cortex. As mentioned earlier, scattered clusters or isolated chromaffin cells are present in all zones of the adrenal cortex. Their role in regulation of adrenocortical organogenesis and function is not yet fully elucidated. It is suspected that they regulate adrenocortical functions in a paracrine manner *(42,43)*. The distribution of mitotic and apoptotic markers varies in each adrenocortical zone. For instance, the tumor-suppressor gene p53 and its downstream effector gene p21 promote cell-cycle arrest in G1-phase and are expressed in areas of DNA damage in the inner cortical zones. They seem to be related to both DNA repair and apoptosis *(44,45)*. Internucleosomal DNA fragmentation characterizes apoptotic cells and is found in the entire adrenal cortex. Proliferating cell nuclear antigen (PCNA), which is a marker of mitosis, is highly expressed in the inner cortical zones, whereas Ki-67 protein, a proliferation marker of cycling cells, predominates in the zona fasciculata *(46)*. The highest apoptotic index is detected in the outermost zones of the adrenal cortex, mainly in the zona glomerulosa *(41)*. In conclusion, it appears that there is a fine balance between apoptosis, proliferation, and differentiation in the adrenal gland, not only during development, but also throughout the adult life.

Development of Adrenal Steroidogenesis

Active adrenal steroidogenesis starts from the 6th wk of gestation in the fetal zone. Circulating LDL represents the most significant source of cholesterol for adrenal steroidogenesis in both fetal and adult adrenals. The steroidogenic activity of the fetal zone is routed towards DHEA production, since this zone lacks 3β-HSD activity. Production of DHEA starts early in gestation between the 6th and 12th wk of gestation. DHEA can be sulfated to DHEA-sulfate (DHEA-S) by fetal adrenal sulfokinase and along with DHEA is used by placenta as substrate for estrogen synthesis. Early in pregnancy, the transitional zone of the fetal adrenal has a similar function to the fetal zone. However, by the third trimester, it expresses enough of the necessary enzymes produce glucocorticoids. Most of the enzymes involved in cortisol and aldosterone synthesis are members of the cytochrome P450 family of oxidases. The first and rate-limiting step in steroid synthesis is cholesterol side-chain cleavage, a reaction catalyzed by ACTH. Cholesterol is converted in the inner mitochondrial membrane to the C21-steroid pregnenolone, by a six-carbon side-chain cleavage and addition of double-bonded oxygen at position 20. Pregnenolone is the common precursor for all other steroids. It is transferred into the smooth endoplasmic reticulum (SER), where it is converted to progesterone by 3β-hydroxy-steroid dehydrogenase/Δ5-isomerase (3β-HSD) or to 17OH-pregnenolone by 17-hydroxylase/17,20-lyase. Progesterone is the precursor for the 17-desoxysteroids and aldosterone, whereas 17OH-pregnenolone and 17OH-progesterone are the precursors for the 17-hydroxysteroids, cortisol and DHEA. In zona glomerulosa cells, steroidogenesis is routed towards 17-desoxysteroids and aldosterone production. In zona fasciculata, the major zone of the adrenal cortex, 17OH-progesterone undergoes two successive hydroxylations to produce cortisol. Finally, the zona reticularis produces adrenal androgens.

Factors Affecting Adrenal Development

Adrenal cortical organogenesis and steroidogenesis are closely related processes, regulated by endocrine, paracrine, and autocrine factors including chorionic gonadotropin, steroid hormones, ACTH, activin, inhibin, and other neuropeptides, as well as several growth factors including bFGF, epidermal growth factor (EGF), transforming growth factor-α and -β (TGF-α, TGF-β), IGF-1, IGF-2, and steroidogenic factor-1 (SF-1). The regulation of fetal adrenal steroidogenesis changes with advancing gestation. Human chorionic gonadotropin (hCG) plays a significant role in fetal adrenal growth and DHEA production during the first trimester of pregnancy. As pregnancy progresses, fetal adrenal steroids inhibit hCG production. Early in pregnancy there is a dual regulation of the fetal adrenal zone by hCG and ACTH, whereas after midgestation, ACTH-mediated regulation predominates. Studies in anencephalic fetuses show that growth of the adrenal gland is independent of fetal ACTH stimulation for the first 15 wk of gestation. After that time, however, the fetal and definitive cortical zones rapidly regress in weight, cellular size, and cellular organization in the absence of ACTH, suggesting that the development of adrenals during middle and late gestation is under hypothalamic-pituitary control (47). ACTH exerts its proliferative effect in fetal adrenocortical cells via a variety of growth factors, such as bFGF (48), activin/inhibin, and IGF-2. It upregulates P450SCC, P450C17, and 3β-HSD expression in fetal adrenal cells, having thus acute and long-term effects on adrenal growth and steroidogenesis. These effects are zone-specific and differentiation stage-specific. ACTH-stimulated induction of P450C17 at term, for instance, increases cor-tisol production and permits initiation of labor. EGF and TGF-α have been detected in adrenals of human fetuses and they are mitogenic to the fetal and definitive zone cells. EGF is a stimulator of the HPA axis. In the fetal adrenal, it increases 3β-HSD expression in the definitive and transitional zones (49), leading thus to increased cortisol secretion. bFGF is also a potent mitogen for human fetal adrenal cells of both the definitive and fetal zones. IGF-1 and 2, synergistically with EGF and bFGF, stimulate proliferation of fetal adrenal cortical cells in vitro. IGF-2 mRNA is found in abundance in all zones of the fetal adrenal gland, but is barely detectable in the adult adrenal. IGF-1 mRNA, in contrast, is found in low amounts in the fetal adrenal and in high concentrations in the adult

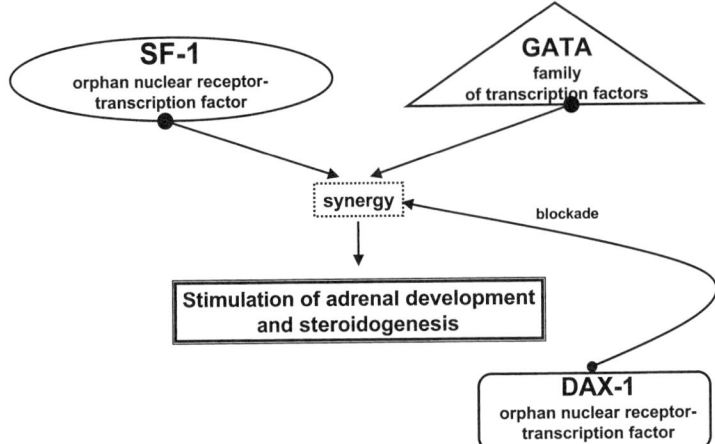

Fig. 2. The SF-1/GATA/DAX-1 system.

adrenal. Thus it is proposed that IGF-2 is the predominant of the two IGFs, mediating ACTH tropic actions in the fetal adrenal *(50)*. While ACTH and cAMP stimulate IGF-2 expression in the adrenal gland, IGF-2 increases the responsiveness of the adrenocortical cells to ACTH. IGF-2 also regulates P450SCC, P450C17, and 3β-HSD activity in fetal-zone cells, promoting DHEA-S and cortisol synthesis *(51)*. As in other tissues, TGF-β suppresses proliferation and increases apoptosis in human fetal adrenal cells in vitro *(52)*. In addition to its effect on proliferation and apoptosis, it decreases P450C17 mRNA expression and enhances ACTH stimulation of 3β-HSD mRNA expression in these cells *(53)*. Its overall effect is inhibitory for steroidogenesis *(54)* and stimulatory for the adrenal RAS system *(55)*. Activins and inhibins, which are structurally and functionally related to TGF-β, inhibit EGF-stimulated, but not bFGF-stimulated, growth of fetal-zone cells in vitro. Activin inhibits mitogenesis and induces apoptotic cell death of fetal-zone cells, but has no effect on growth and steroidogenesis of the adult adrenal cortex *(52)*. It also increases ACTH-stimulated production of cortisol by the fetal zone cells. Vascular endothelial growth (VEGF) factor is a potent angiogenic peptide that has been detected in adrenal cortical cells. It is expressed abundantly in the extensively vascularized fetal zone and in lesser amounts in the definitive zone. ACTH stimulates VEGF gene expression and protein secretion from fetal adrenocortical cells. VEGF may thus be a paracrine local regulator of adrenal cortical angiogenesis, coordinating cortical vascularization and ACTH-stimulated cortical growth *(56)*.

Steroidogenic Factor-1 (SF-1) and DAX-1 in Adrenal Development

A rapidly increasing number of recent publications suggest that the nuclear receptors/ transcription factors SF-1 and DAX-1 are major players in the development of the adrenal gland (Fig. 2). These are orphan receptors, as their ligands are still unknown. Human SF-1 is highly expressed throughout the developing adrenal cortex from very early in gestation *(57)* and in all zones of the adult adrenal cortex *(58)*. Studies in SF-1 knockout mice reveal that SF-1 is essential for adrenal organogenesis and development. It upregulates gene expression of P450C17 and other genes encoding cytochrome P450 steroid hydroxylases, by binding to their promoter regions. Additionally, it regulates the expression of the ACTH-receptor gene, the StAR protein gene controlling cholesterol uptake by adreno-cortical cells, and the scavenger receptor-class B-type I protein gene. Thus, SF-1 controls steroidogenesis at multiple levels *(59)*. Mice heterozygous for SF-1 gene mutations exhibit adrenal insufficiency resulting from profound defects in adrenal development and organi-zation *(60)*. Compensatory mechanisms, such as cellular hypertrophy and increased expres-sion of the rate-limiting steroidogenic protein StAR, help to maintain adrenal function at near-normal capacity under basal conditions. However, adrenal insufficiency becomes apparent following stress, suggesting that normal gene dosage of SF-1 is required for achieving an adequate stress response.

The DAX-1 nuclear receptor is highly expressed in fetal and adult adrenals. DAX-1 has similar tissue distribution as SF-1, but contrary to SF-1 it suppresses steroidogenesis. Indeed, DAX-1, SF-1, and the GATA family of factors are co-expressed in the pituitary, adrenals, and gonads. In these tissues, GATA family members synergize with SF-1. DAX-1 represses GATA/SF-1 synergism, an effect that may represent an important fine-tuning mechanism regulating SF-1-dependent genes in target tissues *(61)*. Indeed, DAX-1-induced effects on all SF-1-dependent transcription is mediated by disruption of transcriptional synergism between GATA-4 and SF-1 and does not involve direct repression of GATA-dependent transactivation. Mutations of the DAX-1 gene result in X-linked congenital adrenal hypo-plasia (AHC) and hypogonadotropic hypogonadism (HH). However, only a subset of patients with AHC carries mutations in DAX-1. Recently, it has been suggested that mid-kine (MDK, a member of the extracellular pleiotrophin/midkine heparin-binding protein family) is expressed early in rat fetal adrenal development and is involved in regulation of adrenal growth and differentiation. MDK may be a good candidate gene for AHC not due to DAX-1 mutations *(62)*. Recently, a novel mutation in the DAX-1 gene has been described that does not cause congenital adrenal hypoplasia but adrenal insufficiency of delayed-onset and an incomplete type of HH *(63)*.

Placental Estrogens and Adrenal Development

Placental estrogens derive from fetal adrenal DHEA-S. They stimulate placental ste-roidogenesis and progesterone production. In primates at midgestation, estradiol abol-ishes ACTH-induced increases in fetal adrenal DHEA production, whereas near term this effect is greatly diminished. It is thus possible that human placenta regulates maternal and fetal C19-steroid production, via estrogens *(64)*. Estrogens, in association with IGF-2, stimulate the fetal cortical zone into producing DHEA at the expense of cortisol. Inter-estingly, estrogens also stimulate the activity of 11β-hydroxysteroid dehydrogenase an enzyme catalyzing the inactivation of cortisol to cortisone.

HPA AXIS AND FETAL DEVELOPMENT

Products of the fetal HPA axis play important roles in the development of several fetal tissues including the lung *(65)*. Their effects are mediated by cortisol and DHEA. The latter regulates the production of estrogens from human placenta, which affect fetal and maternal adrenal steroidogenesis, maternal cardiovascular function, uteroplacental vascu-larization and blood flow, placental steroidogenesis, and the maintenance of pregnancy, via uterine quiescence *(66)*. The developing HPA axis has intense activity during the late fetal period and reduced basal and stress-induced ACTH and corticosterone secretion during the early postnatal period. Despite the uncertainty about the adaptive significance of glucocorticoid hypersecretion during the late fetal period, it is clear that elevated fetal cortisol levels near term are essential for the survival of the neonate. Low-circulating glucocorticoid levels in the first 2 wk of life are believed to be essential for normal brain and behavioral development. Excessive exposure of the developing brain to glucocorticoids may have life-long adverse effects.

HPA AXIS AND PARTURITION

Parturition is a well-orchestrated endocrine event that, once initiated, occurs to completion. The origin of the signals initiating parturition remains unknown. The fetus exerts a critical role in the process leading to birth by controlling activation of the fetal hypothalamic-pituitary-adrenal (HPA) axis. Fetal HPA axis activation leads to increased cortisol and estrogen-precursor secretion from the fetal adrenal gland in late gestation. The end result is an increase in placental estrogen production (67). Cortisol secreted by the fetal adrenal cortex late in gestation regulates the maturation of the fetus and initiates the cascade of events leading to parturition. In ovine fetuses at term activation of the fetal HPA axis increases fetal basal plasma cortisol and the cortisol secretory bursts, which lead to induction of placental estrogen biosynthesis relative to progesterone. The resulting increased estrogen to progesterone ratio induces myometrial contractility and initiation of labor, via induction of prostaglandin secretion and enhancement of myometrial response to oxytocin. The environment of the uterus on the other hand, remains rich in progesterone, which controls regionalization of the uterine activity, allowing fundal region contractility and concomitant lower uterine segment relaxation (67). Placental and fetal hypothalamic CRH rise greatly in pregnancy, especially near term. They drive fetal production of ACTH, by binding to type I CRH receptors, and are essential for the onset of parturition. Thus, type I CRH receptor blockade by antalarmin infusion in the ovine fetus can delay the onset of parturition (68). Placental CRH is secreted into the fetal circulation and is measurable in fetal plasma (69). It has paracrine effects within the placenta, the decidua, and the myometrium, regulating myometrial contractility, local prostaglandin release, and placental blood flow. It also has endocrine effects on the mother and the fetus, exerting a direct effect on the fetal adrenal cortex to preferentially increase the synthesis of DHEA-S, which is the principal substrate for placental estrogen synthesis (70). Glucocorticoids stimulate placental CRH secretion, in contrast to their inhibition of hypothalamic CRH secretion (71). Fetal ACTH is a key regulator of adrenal cortisol secretion in the ovine fetus and plays an essential role in maintaining the growth and responsiveness of the fetal adrenal. Its secretion, which increases near term, depends on the presence of an intact connection between the hypothalamus and the pituitary. Paraventricular nucleus (PVN) lesions in the fetus decrease CRH levels, as well as the responsiveness of the fetal pituitary to CRH. They also attenuate the normal preparturient ACTH and cortisol surge, thus delaying markedly the onset of parturition (72). The preparturient cortisol surge fails in hypothalamo-pituitary disconnected fetuses as well, but this defect can be reversed by low-dose ACTH infusion (73). As mentioned earlier, a decreased sensitivity of ACTH secretion to negative glucocorticoid feedback during the last days of fetal life seems to play an important role in initiation of parturition. Reduction in negative glucocorticoid feedback efficacy may have a permissive role for the preparturient increase of fetal ACTH and cortisol secretion. Prenatal maternal therapy with betamethasone suppresses endogenous fetal cortisol and DHEA-S production, but does not blunt the postnatal cortisol rise in response to stress.

THE NEONATAL WINDOW OF HPA AXIS HYPOFUNCTION

In the rat, the elevated fetal plasma ACTH and corticosterone at term decrease sharply during the first few days of life and remain low up to the 10th d, bouncing back by d 21 *(74)*. The physiological basis of this window of HPA axis hypofunction so early in life may be due to a combination of hypothalamic immaturity, decreased sensitivity of the adrenal gland to ACTH, low adrenal gland cholesterol stores, and low levels of adrenal steroidogenetic enzymes. It now appears that the most important etiological factor is an immaturity of the neonatal hypothalamus suggested by the decreased basal and stress-induced CRH gene transcription rate during the first postnatal week *(75,76)*. It is possible that because of several developmental alterations in the hypothalamic and limbic system, the density of glucocorticoid and mineralocorticoid receptors increases, leading to an enhanced negative glucocorticoid feedback on CRH synthesis in the immediate postnatal period *(76–78)*. Interestingly, exogenous steroid administration in the first week of life results in selective long-term glucocorticoid receptor downregulation *(79)*, while nurturing behavior results in glucocorticoid receptor upregulation in the neonate *(80)*. It is also possible that CRH receptor distribution in the limbic system affects the hippocampal input into the neonatal hypothalamus suppressing CRH synthesis *(76)*. In addition, it should be stressed here that the catecholaminergic innervation of the paraventricular hypothalamic nucleus matures after the 2nd wk of postnatal life, leaving the hypothalamus vulnerable to suppression from the limbic system *(81)*. Indeed, experimental β-adrenoceptor blockade reduces stress-induced ACTH release, whereas α2-adrenoceptor blockade increases basal and stress-induced ACTH response in neonatal rats *(82)*. One thing appears to be certain, though: contrary to the hypothalamus, the neonatal corticotrophs mature much earlier, being fully functional by the 1st d of birth. Indeed, they respond normally to the stimulatory effect of exogenous CRH and AVP *(74)*. However, the percentage of corticotrophs decline, from twice as many as in the adult pituitary on d 2 to below adult values between d 4 and 11. Recovery of corticotroph-cell population occurs on d 15. Corticotroph POMC mRNA parallels hypothalamic CRH mRNA levels, being low between d 4 and 7 and increasing steadily thereafter *(75)*. In humans, diurnal cortisol rhythmic secretion is established early in neonatal life *(83)*. In rodents, it begins on postnatal d 18. As for the adrenal gland per se, we know that its ACTH receptor density declines during the first week of life *(24)*. Increased adrenal cholesterol stores and basal and stimulated enzymatic activity in the adrenals may contribute to the gradual increase in corticosterone biosynthesis after postnatal d 10. After d 10, plasma corticosteroid-binding globulin (CBG) and corticosterone protein binding increase also, causing a decrease in the corticosterone volume of distribution. The resulting decline in corticosterone metabolic-clearance rate accounts for the subsequent increase of plasma corticosterone levels *(84)*. The developmental rise in CBG and corticosterone seems to be elicited by a normally occuring postnatal increase in serum thyroxine concentration. Thyroxine is required not only to initiate but also to sustain that CBG rise, by stimulation of CBG synthesis mainly in the liver. In fact, hepatic CBG mRNA rise precedes the increase of circulating CBG levels in early neonatal life.

STRESS AND HPA AXIS DEVELOPMENT

The nervous, endocrine, and immune systems are regarded as components of a complex functional unit, intercommunicating under normal and stress conditions by specific neurotransmitters, hormones, and immune mediators. During pregnancy, maternal, fetal, and placental mediators interact to preserve homeostasis, fetal well-being, and growth. Stress in general causes decreased negative feedback on CRH release and an increase in fetal or neonatal adrenal steroidogenesis. Stressed growth-retarded fetuses have elevated umbilical cord CRH, ACTH, and cortisol levels, as well as decreased DHEA-S levels, compared to normal fetuses (85). Maternal stress during pregnancy results in alterations of both maternal and fetal HPA axes. Activation of HPA axes during pregnancy may adversely affect length of gestation, timing of delivery, newborn neurobehavioral development, and infant birth weight (86,87). Indeed, pregnant monkeys exposed to stress, having excessive ACTH levels, deliver infants with altered neurobehavioral status, impaired motor coordination, and muscle tonicity, short attention span, irritability, and affected social skills (88). Chronic maternal stress may exert neurotoxic effects in fetal rat PVN neurons, whereas short-lasting stress facilitates differentiation and maturation of these cells (89). Intrauterine infection represents a major cause of HPA axis activation during pregnancy, resulting in a dramatic increase in fetal adrenal steroidogenesis. In the neonate too, endotoxemia stimulates adrenal steroidogenesis (90). Hypoxia represents a major stress for the fetus, causing increased CRH mRNA in the fetal PVN and increased ACTH production (91). Similarly, acute maternal hypoxia induces upregulation of fetal adrenal P450SCC, P450C21, and 3β-HSD mRNAs, but not P450C17mRNA, leading to increased fetal plasma cortisol and decreased plasma androstendione levels. Pregnancy-induced hypertension is also associated with activation of the fetal HPA axis (92), whereas gestational diabetes is associated with suppression of the fetal HPA axis. In the postnatal period, maternal deprivation, which represents a major stress for the neonate, causes age-dependent acute and persistent changes in basal and stress-induced ACTH and corticosterone secretion. Specifically, 4-d old neonatal rats subjected to 24 h of maternal deprivation have minimal acute changes in ACTH and corticosterone secretion, as well as exaggerated ACTH responses to stress at 20 d of life. In contrast, 12-d old rats subjected to 24 h of maternal deprivation show a marked acute elevation of ACTH and corticosterone, but a decreased ACTH response to stress at 20 d of life. Reinstitution of components of the maternal nurturing behavior, such as tactile stimulation and feeding, can reverse some of the neonatal endocrine effects evoked by maternal deprivation.

CONGENITAL ADRENAL HYPERPLASIA (CAH)

CAH is a group of autosomal recessive disorders of cortisol biosynthesis. Deficiency of 21-hydroxylase is responsible for over 90% of CAH, while 11-hydroxylase deficiency accounts for 5% of CAH. The remaining forms of CAH are relatively rare and involve other enzymes in the pathway of cortisol biosynthesis. The mechanism by which adrenocortical hyperplasia occurs is the following: an enzymatic block at any step in cortisol biosynthesis from cholesterol results in a decrease of glucocorticoid negative feedback upon the CNS leading to compensatory elevations of ACTH, which, in its attempt to increase cortisol secretion, causes oversecretion of intermediary steroid compounds and/or adrenal androgens. The cortisol (± aldosterone) deficiency and the excess of these substances cause the clinical manifestations of the CAH syndromes. Depending on the patient's gender, the affected enzyme, and the extent of enzymatic dysfunction, symptoms may include mild to severe female or male virilization, male undermasculinization of varying degrees, glucocorticoid and/or mineralocorticoid deficiency, and/or mineralocorticoid excess (*see* also Chapter 19).

21-Hydroxylase Deficiency

It is the most common cause of CAH inherited as an autosomal recessive trait and, in the US, it occurs in approx 1:10,000 live births. The clinical picture of the 21-hydroxylase deficiency depends on the time of its onset. The 21-hydroxylase deficiency of infancy has two distinct clinical presentations: salt-wasting (SW) and simple virilization (SV). In the SW type, most patients do not synthesize aldosterone effectively and have mild degrees of sodium wasting. Vomiting aggravates the clinical picture that leads to dehydration, occurring between d 7 and 14 of life. The condition is characterized by hyponatremia, hyperkalemia, dehydration, and acidosis. Serum aldosterone is low in spite of elevated plasma renin activity. The basal level of 17-hydroxyprogesterone, the intermediate substance just prior to the deficient enzyme, is high and diagnostic. The SV type of 21-hydroxylase deficiency represents the most common cause of intrauterine hyperandrogenism, which causes genital ambiguity in the female infant, presenting as clitoral hypertrophy and fusion of the labia. The masculinization of the female external genitalia may be such that it could lead to errors in sex assignment. Hyperandrogenism in the male fetus may cause increased size of penis, which is frequently missed at the nursery. The 21-hydroxylase of childhood usually presents as isosexual precocious puberty in boys and heterosexual precocious puberty in girls. Acceleration of bone maturation leads to early closure of the epiphyses and premature cessation of growth. Finally, late-onset 21-hydroxylase deficiency presents prior to or at puberty as premature adrenarche; hirsutism; acne; male pattern baldness; and menstrual irregularities (oligo-amenorrhea), causing later anovulation and infertility. The diagnosis is made by measurement of the serum 17-hydroxyprogesterone response to ACTH (1-24) stimulation. The gene encoding the 21-hydroxylase enzyme, CYP21, lies within the major histocompatibility complex on chromosome 6p. A highly homologous pseudogene, the CYP21P, is adjacent to CYP21. Thus, most gene mutations causing 21-hydroxylase deficiency result from recombinations between CYP21 and CYP21P. It should be stressed here that genotype does not always correlates with phenotype.

11-Hydroxylase Deficiency

Overproduction of 11-deoxycorticosterone and 11-deoxycortisol, the steroid intermediate substrates for 11-hydroxylase, characterize this syndrome. The elevated deoxycorticosterone, which has salt-retaining properties, causes salt retention, hypokalemia, alkalosis, and hypertension. If the 11-hydroxylase defect is severe enough to increase the levels of androgens during intrauterine life, the affected females are born with virilized external genitalia. If the defect is less severe, the increased androgen levels may cause isosexual precocious puberty in boys and heterosexual precocious puberty in girls. Attenuated forms of the disease have been described, with late-onset female hyperandrogenism and mild hypertension. High levels of plasma 11-deoxycortisol and its metabolic product tetrahydro-11-deoxycortisol in urine characterize the disease. Humans have two isoenzymes with 11-hydroxylase activity, each encoded by a different gene. The CYP11B1 gene encodes 11-beta-hydroxylase. This enzyme catalyzes the conversion of 11-deoxycortisol to cortisol. The CYP11B2 gene encodes a second 11-beta-hydroxylase, the aldosterone synthase, which is required for the conversion of deoxycorticosterone to aldosterone, a step regulated by angiotensin II and taking place in zona glomerulosa. Mutations of the CYP11B2 gene result in a syndrome characterized by aldosterone deficiency, i.e., salt loss, hyperkalemia, and hypovolemic shock in infancy, and frequently failure to thrive in childhood. Unequal cross-over of the CYP11B genes generates duplicated chimeric genes having the transcriptional regulatory region of CYP11B1 and the coding sequence of aldosterone synthase. The resulting disease is due to ACTH-regulated aldosterone biosynthesis the condition termed glucocorticoid-suppressible hyperaldosteronism.

17-Hydroxylase Deficiency

This involves adrenal cortices and gonads and results in decreased production of cortisol, androgens, and estrogens. To overcome the block in the production of cortisol, patients produce excessive amounts of 11-deoxycorticosterone, which causes hypertension and hypokalemia (i.e., a syndrome similar to that from 11-hydroxylase deficiency) and low levels of sex steroids responsible for ambiguous genitalia in the male infant or delayed puberty in both phenotypic XY and XX females. The biochemical profile consists of elevated serum or plasma progesterone, corticosterone and 11-deoxycorticosterone.

ADRENOLEUKODYSTROPHIES (ALD)

These are metabolic disorders characterized by malfunction of the adrenal cortex and progressive neuronal demyelination due to abnormalities of myelin metabolism. The underlying biochemical abnormality is the impairment of beta-oxidation of very-long-chain fatty acids (VLCFA) in peroxisomes resulting in an accumulation of saturated unbranched fatty acids. ALD are members of a larger family of peroxisomal disorders. These disorders are divided into three groups. The first group is characterized by defects in the biogenesis of peroxisomes; it is a group of lethal diseases, which include neonatal ALD, Zellweger syndrome, infantile Refsum disease, and hyperpipecolic acidemia. The patients have distinct peroxisomal protein import defects, i.e., their cells are unable to import proteins containing one or both peroxisomal targeting signals (PTS1 and/or PTS2). The second group includes peroxisomal disorders due to loss of a single peroxisomal function from isolated enzyme deficiencies. This group includes the X-linked ALD, the peroxisomal thiolase deficiency, bifunctional protein deficiency, the acyl-CoA oxidase deficiency, classic Refsum disease, hyperoxaluria type I, and acatalasaemia. Finally, the third group includes peroxisomal disorders arising from multiple enzyme deficiencies, one of the more recognized disorders being rhizomelic chondrodysplasia punctata.

Neonatal Form

This is a rare autosomal recessive disease, characterized by a decrease in the number and size of the peroxisomes, which exhibit generalized functional failure. Indeed, the function of at least six peroxisomal enzymes is impaired. Most patients have severe mental retardation. The onset of the neurological symptoms precedes that of the clinically evident adrenal insufficiency, although an abnormal response to ACTH stimulation test is present quite early.

X-Linked Form

This form of ALD affects mainly the white matter of the nervous system and adrenal cortex. It is one of the most common peroxisomal disorders, with an incidence of 1:20,000 males. The gene responsible for this disease is located in Xq28 and encodes an ATP-binding peroxisomal membrane transporter protein called ALDP. It belongs to a family of membrane transporters. The two most common forms of the X-linked ALD are the childhood cerebral form and the adult adrenomyeloneuropathy (AMN). Apart of the different age of onset, the two forms of the X-linked ALD also differ in their neurological presentations. Thus, the childhood form involves mainly the cerebral structures, while the adult form mainly the spinal cord and peripheral neurons. The childhood cerebral ALD is a severe disease, with neurological symptoms begining between 5 and 12 yr of age. The disease is characterized by progressive inflammatory cerebral demyelination, adrenal insufficiency, and sometimes hypogonadism. The typical case is a boy presenting with progressive visual and hearing loss, deterioration of speech and gait, and various behavioral abnormalities. Rarely, the onset of the disease may take the form of acute adrenal insufficiency (Addisonian crisis), with vomiting, fever, and metabolic coma, which resolves following the initiation of appropriate therapy. Within a few years, the disease progresses to dementia, blindness, and quadriplegia. Affected heterozygotic mothers may develop some neurologic deficit, usually spasticity, at mid-life, which is progressively deteriorating with time. The adult form of ALD, AMN is a milder disease with onset between 15 and 30 yr of age and a much slower progression. The disease primarily involves peripheral neurons and the spinal cord. However, early cognitive impairments are frequent in a large percentage of AMN patients since 60% of AMN patients demonstrate a significant neuropsychological impairment, most commonly a pattern of subcortical dementia. The illness may first present as an isolated Addison's disease without any apparent neurological involvement. Indeed, the adrenal insufficiency in AMN may long precede nervous-system dysfunction. In some cases adrenal insufficiency may remain the only clinical manifestation of the disease. It is prudent to consider the possibility of AMN in any boy with Addison's disease. AMN may also present as primary hypothyroidism and/or hypogonadism. Indeed, a certain degree of hypogonadism is present in all patients with AMN.

Adrenoleuko-Myeloneuropathy

ALMN is an ALD syndrome with characteristics of both childhood ALD and AMN. All forms of ALD are characterized by high levels of the VLCFA hexacosanoate (C26), and docosanoate (C22). Gas-chromatographic analysis of VLCFA from the demyelinated cerebral white matter shows increase of C26:0 fatty acid in cholesterol esters and C24:0 and C24: in gangliosides.

3 BETA-HYDROXYSTEROID DEHYDROGENASE (3β-HSD) DEFICIENCY

Deficiency of the 3β-HSD is an autosomal recessive disease, which may cause a severe form of CAH that impairs the steroidogenesis in both the adrenals and the testes. Affected newborns of either gender may exhibit symptoms and signs of adrenal insufficiency and ambiguous genitalia. The latter is a result of excessive adrenal androgens produced in females and defective testicular androgen production in males. The biochemical picture consists of elevated ratio of Δ5' to Δ4' steroids. The diagnostic steroid precursor is 17-hydroxypregnenolone. Humans have two highly homologous genes encoding the 3β-HSD, each encoding a 3β-HSD isoenzyme. Type I 3β-HSD gene is mainly expressed in the placenta and peripheral tissues, while type II 3β-HSD gene in the adrenals and gonads. The disease is the result of homozygous mutations of the type II 3β-HSD gene.

SYNDROMES OF GLYCEROL KINASE DEFICIENCY

Glycerol kinase deficiency occurs either as an isolated enzyme deficiency, presenting with hypotonia, apnea, developmental delay, and glyceroluria in neonates, without evidence of adrenal insufficiency or myopathy, or as part of a syndrome consisting of dystrophic myopathy (Duchenne's muscular dystrophy), AHC, primary adrenal insufficiency, and severe mental retardation. Hyperglycerolemia and glyceroluria characterize these syndromes. Prenatal diagnosis can be made by amniocentesis and measurement of high concentrations of glycerol in the amniotic fluid or low glycerol-kinase enzymatic activity in cultured amniotic fluid cells. Glycerol kinase deficiencies are inherited in an X-linked recessive fashion. A broad distribution of microdeletions in the p21 region of the short arm of chromosome-X have been described in several kindreds, with the dystrophic myopathy syndrome and the hypoplasia of the adrenal glands.

CONGENITAL ISOLATED GLUCOCORTICOID DEFICIENCY: ALLGROVE SYNDROME

Familial ACTH resistance is a rare form of primary adrenal insufficiency characterized by elevated plasma ACTH concentrations and low or undetectable plasma cortisol levels not responding to exogenous ACTH. Affected members from several kindreds were found to have inactivating mutations of the ACTH receptor. In addition to ACTH resistance, patients with the Allgrove syndrome also have alacrima and achalasia (triple A syndrome) as well as several neurological symptoms. No mutations of the ACTH receptor were identified in several kindreds with this syndrome.

REFERENCES

1. Baram TZ, Lerner SP. Ontogeny of corticotropin releasing hormone gene expression in rat hypothalamus-comparison with somatostatin. Int J Dev Neurosci 1991;9:473–478.
2. Matthews SG, Challis JR. Regulation of CRH and AVP mRNA in the developing ovine hypothalamus: effects of stress and glucocorticoids. Am J Physiol 1995;268:E1096–E1107.
3. Lugo DI, Pintar JE. Ontogeny of basal and regulated secretion from POMC cells of the developing anterior lobe of the rat pituitary gland. Dev Biol 1996;173:95–109.
4. Asa SL, Kovacs K, Singer W. Human fetal adenohypophysis: morphologic and functional analysis in vitro. Neuroendocrinology 1991;53:562–572.
5. Dupouy JP, Chatelain A. In-vitro effects of corticosterone, synthetic ovine corticotrophin releasing factor and arginine vasopressin on the release of adrenocorticotrophin by fetal rat pituitary glands. J Endocrinol 1984;101:339–344.
6. Saoud CJ, Wood CE. Ontogeny and molecular weight of immunoreactive arginine vasopressin and corticotropin-releasing factor in the ovine hypothalamus. Peptides 1996;17:55–61.
7. Sasaki A, Liotta AS, Luckey MM, Margioris AN, Suda T, Krieger DT. Immunoreactive corticotropin-releasing factor is present in human maternal plasma during the third trimester of pregnancy. J Clin Endocrinol Metab 1984;59:812–814.
8. Sasaki A, Shinkawa O, Margioris AN, Liotta AS, Soto S, Murakami O, et al. Immunoreactive corticotropin releasing factor in human plasma during pregnancy, labor and delivery. J Clin Endocrinol Metab 1987;64:224–229.
9. Sasaki A, Tempst P, Liotta AS, Margioris AN, Hood LE, Kent SBH, et al. Isolation and characterization of corticotropin-releasing hormone-like peptide from human placenta. J Clin Endocrinol Metab 1988; 67:768–773.

10. Grino M, Chrousos G, Margioris AN. The corticotropin releasing hormone gene is expressed in human placenta. Biochem Biophys Res Commun 1987;148:1208–1214.
11. Grammatopoulos DK, Hillhouse EW. Basal and interleukin-1beta-stimulated prostaglandin production from cultured human myometrial cells: differential regulation by corticotropin-releasing hormone. J Clin Endocrinol Metab 1999;84:2204–2211.
12. Simmons DM, Voss JW, Ingraham HA, Broide RS, Rosenfeld MG, Swanson LW. Pituitary cell phenotypes involve cell-specific Pit-1 mRNA translation and synergistic interactions with other classes of transcription factors. Genes Dev 1990;4:695–711.
13. Hermesz E, Mackem S, Mahon KA. Rpx: a novel anterior-restricted homeobox gene progressively activated in the prechordal plate, anterior neural plate and Rathke's pouch of the mouse embryo. Development 1996;122:41–52.
14. Takuma N, Sheng HZ, Furuta Y, Ward JM, Sharma K, Hogan BL, et al. Formation of Rathke's pouch requires dual induction from the diencephalon. Development 1998;125:4835–4840.
15. Treier M, Gleiberman AS, O'Connell SM, Szeto DP, McMahon JA, McMahon AP, Rosenfeld MG. Multistep signaling requirements for pituitary organogenesis in vivo. Genes Dev 1998;12:1691–1704.
16. Kioussi C, O'Connell S, St-Onge L, Treier M, Gleiberman AS, Gruss P, Rosenfeld MG. Pax6 is essential for establishing ventral-dorsal cell boundaries in pituitary gland development. Proc Natl Acad Sci USA 1999;96:14,378–14,382.
17. Tremblay JJ, Goodyer CG, Drouin J. Transcriptional properties of Ptx1 and Ptx2 isoforms. Neuroendocrinology 2000;71:277–286.
18. Rosenfeld MG, Briata P, Dasen J, Gleiberman AS, Kioussi C, Lin C, et al. Multistep signaling and transcriptional requirements for pituitary organogenesis in vivo. Recent Prog Horm Res 2000;55:1–13; discussion 13–14.
19. Parks JS, Brown MR, Hurley DL, Phelps CJ, Wajnrajch MP. Heritable disorders of pituitary development. J Clin Endocrinol Metab 1999;84:4362–4370.
20. Therrien M, Drouin J. Cell-specific helix-loop-helix factor required for pituitary expression of the proopiomelanocortin gene. Mol Cell Biol 1993;13:2342–2353.
21. Antolovich GC, McMillen IC, Robinson PM, Silver M, Young IR, Perry RA. Effect of cortisol infusion on the pituitary-adrenal axis of the hypothalamo-pituitary-disconnected fetal sheep. Neuroendocrinology 1992;56:312–319.
22. McDonald TJ, Hoffman GE, Nathanielsz PW. Hypothalamic paraventricular nuclear lesions delay corticotroph maturation in the fetal sheep anterior pituitary. Endocrinology 1992;131:1101–1106.
23. Margioris AN. Corticotropin releasing hormone and the placenta and fetal membranes. In: Brennecke S, Rice G, eds. Molecular Aspects of Placental and Fetal Membrane Autocoids, vol. 12. CRC Press, Boca Raton, FL, 1993, pp. 277–301.
24. Chatelain A, Durand P, Naaman E, Dupouy JP. Ontogeny of ACTH(1-24) receptors in rat adrenal glands during the perinatal period. J Endocrinol 1989;123:421–428.
25. Berdusco ET, Yang K, Hammond GL, Challis JR. Corticosteroid-binding globulin (CBG) production by hepatic and extrahepatic sites in the ovine fetus: effects of CBG on glucocorticoid negative feedback on pituitary cells in vitro. J Endocrinol 1995;146:121–130.
26. Yang K, Jones SA, Challis JR. Changes in glucocorticoid receptor number in the hypothalamus and pituitary of the sheep fetus with gestational age and after adrenocorticotropin treatment. Endocrinology 1990;126:11–17.
27. Saoud CJ, Wood CE. Developmental changes and molecular weight of immunoreactive glucocorticoid receptor protein in the ovine fetal hypothalamus and pituitary. Biochem Biophys Res Commun 1996;229:916–921.
28. Dean F, Matthews SG. Maternal dexamethasone treatment in late gestation alters glucocorticoid and mineralocorticoid receptor mRNA in the fetal guinea pig brain. Brain Res 1999;864:253–259.
29. Bocian-Sobkowska J, Wozniak W, Malendowicz LK. Postnatal evolution of the human adrenal fetal zone: stereologic description and apoptosis. Endocr Res 1998;24:969–973.
30. Feige JJ, Keramidas M, Chambaz EM. Hormonally regulated components of the adrenocortical cell environment and the control of adrenal cortex homeostasis. Horm Metab Res 1998;30:421–425.
31. Carsia RV, Nagele RG, Morita Y, Tilly KI, Tilly JL. Models to elucidate the regulation of adrenal cell death. Endocr Res 1998;24:899–908.
32. Bornstein SR, Ehrhart-Bornstein M, Usadel H, Bockmann M, Scherbaum WA. Morphological evidence for a close interaction of chromaffin cells with cortical cells within the adrenal gland. Cell Tissue Res 1991;265:1–9.

33. Wolkersdörfer GW, Bornstein SR. Reappraisal of adrenal zonation theories based on the differential regulation of apoptosis. In: Margioris AN, Chrousos GP, eds. Adrenal Disorders, vol. 3. Humana Press, Totowa, NJ, 2000, pp. 45–57.

34. Wintour EM, Moritz K, Butkus A, Baird R, Albiston A, Tenis N. Ontogeny and regulation of the AT1 and AT2 receptors in the ovine fetal adrenal gland. Mol Cell Endocrinol 1999;157:161–170.

35. Breault L, Lehoux JG, Gallo-Payet N. Angiotensin II receptors in the human adrenal gland. Endocr Res 1996;22:355–361.

36. Gupta P, Franco-Saenz R, Mulrow PJ. Locally generated angiotensin II in the adrenal gland regulates basal, corticotropin- and potassium-stimulated aldosterone secretion. Hypertension 1995;25:443–448.

37. Chamoux E, Breault L, Lehoux JG, Gallo-Payet N. Involvement of the angiotensin II type 2 receptor in apoptosis during human fetal adrenal gland development. J Clin Endocrinol Metab 1999;84:4722–4730.

38. Path G, Bornstein SR, Ehrhart-Bornstein M, Scherbaum WA. Interleukin-6 and the interleukin-6 receptor in the human adrenal gland: expression and effects on steroidogenesis. J Clin Endocrinol Metab 1997;82:2343–2349.

39. Marx C, Bornstein SR, Wolkersdörfer GW, Peter M, Sippell WG, Scherbaum WA. Relevance of major histocompatibility complex class II expression as a hallmark for the cellular differentiation in the human adrenal cortex. J Clin Endocrinol Metab 1997;82:3136–3140.

40. Khoury EL, Greenspan JS, Greenspan FS. Adrenocortical cells of the zona reticularis normally express HLA-DR antigenic determinants. Am J Pathol 1987;127:580–591.

41. Wolkersdörfer GW, Ehrhart-Bornstein M, Brauer S, Marx C, Scherbaum WA, Bornstein SR. Differential regulation of apoptosis in the normal human adrenal gland. J Clin Endocrinol Metab 1996;81:4129–4136.

42. Bornstein SR, Gonzalez-Hernandez JA, Ehrhart-Bornstein M, Adler G, Scherbaum WA. Intimate contact of chromaffin and cortical cells within the human adrenal gland forms the cellular basis for important intraadrenal interactions. J Clin Endocrinol Metab 1994;78:225–232.

43. Margioris AN, Venihaki M, Stournaras C, Gravanis A. PC12 cells as a model to study the effects of opioids on normal and tumoral adrenal chromaffin cells. Ann NY Acad Sci 1995;771:166–172.

44. Didenko VV, Wang X, Yang L, Hornsby PJ. DNA damage and p21(WAF1/CIP1/SDI1) in experimental injury of the rat adrenal cortex and trauma-associated damage of the human adrenal cortex. J Pathol 1999;189:119–126.

45. Didenko VV, Wang X, Yang L, Hornsby PJ. Expression of p21(WAF1/CIP1/SDI1) and p53 in apoptotic cells in the adrenal cortex and induction by ischemia/reperfusion injury. J Clin Invest 1996;97:1723–1731.

46. Sasano H, Imatani A, Shizawa S, Suzuki T, Nagura H. Cell proliferation and apoptosis in normal and pathologic human adrenal. Mod Pathol 1995;8:11–17.

47. Aberdeen GW, Leavitt MG, Pepe GJ, Albrecht ED. Effect of maternal betamethasone administration at midgestation on baboon fetal adrenal gland development and adrenocorticotropin receptor messenger ribonucleic acid expression. J Clin Endocrinol Metab 1998;83:976–982.

48. Mesiano S, Mellon SH, Gospodarowicz D, Di Blasio AM, Jaffe RB. Basic fibroblast growth factor expression is regulated by corticotropin in the human fetal adrenal: a model for adrenal growth regulation. Proc Natl Acad Sci USA 1991;88:5428–5432.

49. Coulter CL, Read LC, Carr BR, Tarantal AF, Barry S, Styne DM. A role of epidermal growth factor in the morphological and functional maturation of the adrenal gland in the fetal rhesus monkey in vivo. J Clin Endocrinol Metab 1996;81:1254–1260.

50. Mesiano S, Mellon SH, Jaffe RB. Mitogenic action, regulation and localization of insulin-like growth factors in the human fetal adrenal gland. J Clin Endocrinol Metab 1993;76:968–976.

51. Mesiano S, Jaffe RB. Interaction of insulin-like growth factor-II and estradiol directs steroidogenesis in the human fetal adrenal toward dehydroepiandrosterone sulfate production. J Clin Endocrinol Metab 1993;77:754–758.

52. Spencer SJ, Mesiano S, Lee JY, Jaffe RB. Proliferation and apoptosis in the human adrenal cortex during the fetal and perinatal periods: implications for growth and remodeling. J Clin Endocrinol Metab 1999;84:1110–1115.

53. Lebrethon MC, Jaillard C, Naville D, Begeot M, Saez JM. Regulation of corticotropin and steroidogenic enzyme mRNAs in human fetal adrenal cells by corticotropin, angiotensin-II and transforming growth factor beta 1. Mol Cell Endocrinol 1994;106:137–143.

54. Stankovic AK, Dion LD, Parker CR Jr. Effects of transforming growth factor-beta on human adrenal steroid production. Mol Cell Endocrinol 1994;99:145–151.

55. Gupta P, Franco-Saenz R, Gentry LE, Mulrow PJ. Transforming growth factor-beta 1 inhibits aldosterone and stimulates adrenal renin in cultured bovine zona glomerulosa cells. Endocrinology 1992;131:631–636.

56. Shifren JL, Mesiano S, Taylor RN, Ferrara N, Jaffe RB. Corticotropin regulates vascular endothelial growth factor expression in human fetal adrenal cortical cells. J Clin Endocrinol Metab 1998;83:1342–1347.

57. Hanley NA, Rainey WE, Wilson DI, Ball SG, Parker KL. Expression profiles of SF-1, DAX1 and CYP17 in the human fetal adrenal gland: potential interactions in gene regulation. Mol Endocrinol 2001;15: 57–68.

58. Ramayya MS, Zhou J, Kino T, Segars JH, Bondy CA, Chrousos GP. Steroidogenic factor 1 messenger ribonucleic acid expression in steroidogenic and nonsteroidogenic human tissues: northern blot and in situ hybridization studies. J Clin Endocrinol Metab 1997;82:1799–1806.

59. Ramayya MS. Adrenal organogenesis and steroidogenesis. In: Margioris AN, Chrousos GP, eds. Adrenal Disorders, vol. 2. Humana Press, Totowa, NJ, 2000, pp. 11–43.

60. Bland ML, Jamieson CA, Akana SF, Bornstein SR, Eisenhofer G, Dallman MF, Ingraham HA. Haploinsufficiency of steroidogenic factor-1 in mice disrupts adrenal development leading to an impaired stress response. Proc Natl Acad Sci USA 2000;97:14,488–14,493.

61. Tremblay JJ, Viger RS. Nuclear receptor Dax-1 represses the transcriptional cooperation between GATA-4 and SF-1 in sertoli cells. Biol Reprod 2001;64:1191–1199.

62. Dewing P, Ching ST, Zhang YH, Huang BL, Peirce RM, McCabe ERB, Vilain E. Midkine is expressed early in rat fetal adrenal development. Mol Genet Metab 2000;71:616–622.

63. Tabarin AC, Achermann JC, Recan D, Bex V, Bertagna X, Christin-Maitre S, et al. A novel mutation in DAX1 causes delayed-onset adrenal insufficiency and incomplete hypogonadotropic hypogonadism. J Clin Invest 2000;105:321–328.

64. Albrecht ED, Pepe GJ. Suppression of maternal adrenal dehydroepiandrosterone and dehydroepiandrosterone sulfate production by estrogen during baboon pregnancy. J Clin Endocrinol Metab 1995;80: 3201–3208.

65. Venihaki M, Carrigan A, Dikkes P, Majzoub JA. Circadian rise in maternal glucocorticoid prevents pulmonary dysplasia in fetal mice with adrenal insufficiency. Proc Natl Acad Sci USA 2000;97:7336–7341.

66. Albrecht ED, Aberdeen GW, Pepe GJ. The role of estrogen in the maintenance of primate pregnancy. Am J Obstet Gynecol 2000;182:432–438.

67. Challis JRG, Matthews SG, Gibb W, Lye SJ. Endocrine and paracrine regulation of birth at term and preterm. Endocr Rev 2000;21:514–550.

68. Chan EC, Falconer J, Madsen G, Rice KC, Webster EL, Chrousos GP, Smith R. A corticotropin-releasing hormone type I receptor antagonist delays parturition in sheep. Endocrinology 1998;139:3357–3360.

69. Nodwell A, Carmichael L, Fraser M, Challis J, Richardson B. Placental release of corticotrophin-releasing hormone across the umbilical circulation of the human newborn. Placenta 1999;20:197–202.

70. Smith R, Mesiano S, Chan EC, Brown S, Jaffe RB. Corticotropin-releasing hormone directly and preferentially stimulates dehydroepiandrosterone sulfate secretion by human fetal adrenal cortical cells. J Clin Endocrinol Metab 1998;83:2916–2920.

71. Majzoub JA, McGregor JA, Lockwood CJ, Smith R, Taggart MS, Schulkin J. A central theory of preterm and term labor: putative role for corticotropin-releasing hormone. Am J Obstet Gynecol 1999;180: S232–S241.

72. McDonald TJ, Nathanielsz PW. Bilateral destruction of the fetal paraventricular nuclei prolongs gestation in sheep. Am J Obstet Gynecol 1991;165:764–770.

73. Poore KR, Canny BJ, Young IR. Adrenal responsiveness and the timing of parturition in hypothalamo-pituitary disconnected ovine foetuses with and without constant adrenocorticotrophin infusion. J Neuroendocrinol 1999;11:343–349.

74. Grino M, Dakine N, Paulmayer-Lacroix O, Oliver C. Ontogeny of the hypothalamo-pituitary-adrenal axis. In: Margioris AN, Chrousos GP, eds. Adrenal Disorders, vol. 1. Humana Press, Totowa, NJ, 2000, pp. 1–9.

75. Grino M, Young WS III, Burgunder JM. Ontogeny of the corticotropin-releasing factor gene in the hypothalamic paraventricular nucleus and of the proopiomelanocortin gene in rat pituitary. Endocrinology 1989;124:60–68.

76. Baram TZ, Yi S, Avishai-Eliner S, Schultz L. Development neurobiology of the stress response: multilevel regulation of corticotropin-releasing hormone function. Ann NY Acad Sci 1997;814:252–265.

77. Rosenfeld P, van Eekelen JA, Levine S, de Kloet ER. Ontogeny of corticosteroid receptors in the brain. Cell Mol Neurobiol 1993;13:295–319.

78. Yi SJ, Masters JN, Baram TZ. Glucocorticoid receptor mRNA ontogeny in the fetal and postnatal rat forebrain. Mol Cell Neurosci 1994;5:385–393.

79. Felszeghy K, Gaspar E, Nyakas C. Long-term selective down-regulation of brain glucocorticoid receptors after neonatal dexamethasone treatment in rats. J Neuroendocrinol 1996;8:493–499.

80. Sarrieau A, Sharma S, Meaney MJ. Postnatal development and environmental regulation of hippocampal glucocorticoid and mineralocorticoid receptors. Brain Res 1988;471:158–162.

81. Borisova NA, Sapronova AY, Proshlyakova EV, Ugrumov MV. Ontogenesis of the hypothalamic catecholaminergic system in rats: synthesis, uptake and release of catecholamines. Neuroscience 1991;43: 223–229.

82. Grino M, Paulmyer-Lacroix O, Faudon M, Renard M, Anglade G. Blockade of alpha 2–adrenoceptors stimulates basal and stress-induced adrenocorticotropin secretion in the developing rat through a central mechanism independent from corticotropin-releasing factor and arginine vasopressin. Endocrinology 1994;135:2549–2557.

83. Hindmarsh KW, Tan L, Sankaran K, Laxdal VA. Diurnal rhythms of cortisol, ACTH and beta-endorphin levels in neonates and adults. West J Med 1989;151:153–156.

84. Schroeder RJ, Henning SJ. Roles of plasma clearance and corticosteroid-binding globulin in the developmental increase in circulating corticosterone in infant rats. Endocrinology 1989;124:2612–2618.

85. Goland RS, Jozak S, Warren WB, Conwell IM, Stark RI, Tropper PJ. Elevated levels of umbilical cord plasma corticotropin-releasing hormone in growth-retarded fetuses. J Clin Endocrinol Metab 1993;77: 1174–1179.

86. Drago F, Di Leo F, Giardina L. Prenatal stress induces body weight deficit and behavioural alterations in rats: the effect of diazepam. Eur Neuropsychopharmacol 1999;9:239–245.

87. Schneider ML, Roughton EC, Koehler AJ, Lubach GR. Growth and development following prenatal stress exposure in primates: an examination of ontogenetic vulnerability. Child Dev 1999;70:263–274.

88. Schneider ML, Coe CL, Lubach GR. Endocrine activation mimics the adverse effects of prenatal stress on the neuromotor development of the infant primate. Dev Psychobiol 1992;25:427–439.

89. Fujioka T, Sakata Y, Yamaguchi K, Shibasaki T, Kato H, Nakamura S. The effects of prenatal stress on the development of hypothalamic paraventricular neurons in fetal rats. Neuroscience 1999;92:1079–1088.

90. Dent GW, Smith MA, Levine S. The ontogeny of the neuroendocrine response to endotoxin. Brain Res Dev Brain Res 1999;117:21–29.

91. Matthews SG, Challis JR. Regulation of CRH and AVP mRNA in the developing ovine hypothalamus: effects of stress and glucocorticoids. Am J Physiol 1995;268:E1096–E1107.

92. Emanuel RL, Robinson BG, Seely EW, Graves SW, Kohane I, Saltzman D, et al. Corticotrophin releasing hormone levels in human plasma and amniotic fluid during gestation. Clin Endocrinol (Oxf) 1994;40: 257–262.

17 Molecular Genetics of Adrenal Disease

Perrin C. White, MD

CONTENTS

INTRODUCTION
CONGENITAL ADRENAL HYPERPLASIA AND RELATED CONDITIONS
ADRENOLEUKODYSTROPHY
DEVELOPMENTAL DEFECTS
REFERENCES

INTRODUCTION

This chapter provides an overview of inherited disorders of adrenal function. Taken together, the most common of these are a series of inborn errors of steroid-hormone biosynthesis, often collectively termed congenital adrenal hyperplasia (CAH). However, other inherited disorders can affect adrenal function. Adrenoleukodystrophy is a disorder of oxidation of very long chain fatty acids which therefore accumulate in various tissues, particularly the adrenal gland and the brain. There are also rare syndromes such as adrenal hypoplasia congenita (AHC), which are caused by mutations in transcription factors that control adrenal development.

CONGENITAL ADRENAL HYPERPLASIA AND RELATED CONDITIONS

Normal Physiology

BIOCHEMISTRY OF NORMAL STEROID SYNTHESIS

Congenital adrenal hyperplasia (CAH) is a general term for the inability to synthesize cortisol and other glucocorticoids due to any of several enzymatic deficiencies, each of which is inherited in an autosomal recessive manner. The synthesis of various other steroids may be impaired depending on the enzyme involved, and thus these enzymatic deficiencies disrupt normal physiology in different ways. To understand why this is so, it is necessary to review the normal pathways of steroid biosynthesis in the adrenal cortex (Fig. 1) *(1)*.

The human adrenal cortex consists of three concentric zones: the outermost is the zona glomerulosa, followed by the zona fasciculata and zona reticularis. These three zones are

From: *Contemporary Endocrinology: Developmental Endocrinology: From Research to Clinical Practice*
Edited by: E. A. Eugster and O. H. Pescovitz © Humana Press Inc., Totowa, NJ

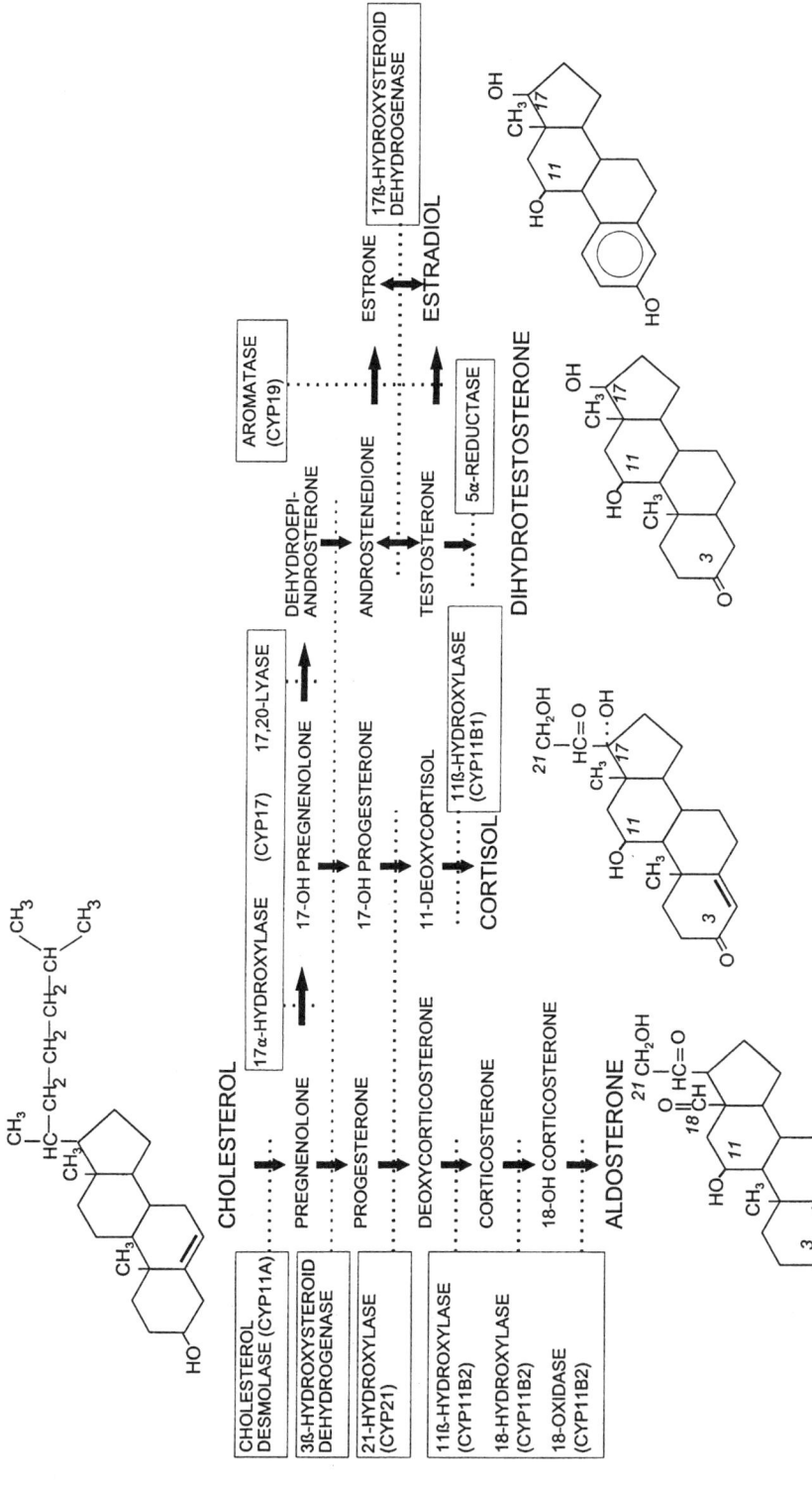

Fig. 1. Pathways of steroid biosynthesis. The pathways for synthesis of progesterone and mineralocorticoids (aldosterone), glucocorticoids (cortisol), androgens (testosterone and dihydrotestosterone), and estrogens (estradiol) are arranged from left to right. The enzymatic activities catalyzing each bioconversion are written in boxes. For those activities mediated by specific cytochromes P450, the systematic name of the enzyme ("CYP" followed by a number) is listed in parentheses. CYP11B2 and CYP17 have multiple activities. The planar structures of cholesterol, aldosterone, cortisol, dihydrotestosterone, and estradiol are placed near the corresponding labels.

responsible for the synthesis of mineralocorticoids (salt-retaining hormones), glucocorticoids ("stress" steroids), and androgen precursors, respectively.

In all zones, the first and rate-limiting step in steroid biosynthesis is importation of cholesterol from cellular stores to the matrix side of the mitochondria inner membrane, where the cholesterol side-chain cleavage system is located. This system consists of cholesterol desmolase (CYP11A, P450scc) and two accessory proteins, adrenodoxin and adrenodoxin reductase. Importation into mitochondria is controlled by the steroidogenic acute regulatory (StAR) protein (2,3), the synthesis of which is increased within minutes by trophic stimuli such as ACTH or, in the zona glomerulosa, increased intracellular calcium. StAR is a synthesized as a 37 kD phosphoprotein that contains a mitochondrial importation signal peptide. However, importation into mitochrondria is not necessary for StAR to stimulate steroidogenesis, and it now seems likely that, on the contrary, mitochondrial importation rapidly inactivates StAR. The mechanism by which StAR mediates cholesterol transport across the mitochondrial membrane is not yet known. Perhaps it interacts with the so-called peripheral benzodiazepine receptor, an 18 kD protein that is also required for cholesterol transport (4).

Once inside mitochondria, cholesterol is cleaved to pregnenolone by cholesterol desmolase. Pregnenolone is the common precursor for all other steroids, and as such this hormone may undergo metabolism by several other enzymes.

To synthesize mineralocorticoids in the zona glomerulosa, 3β-hydroxysteroid dehydrogenase (3β-HSD) in the endoplasmic reticulum converts pregnenolone to progesterone (5). This is 21-hydroxylated in the endoplasmic reticulum by 21-hydroxylase (CYP21, P450c21) to produce deoxycorticosterone (DOC). Aldosterone, the most potent mineralocorticoid, is produced by the 11β-hydroxylation of DOC to corticosterone (compound B), followed by 18-hydroxylation and 18-oxidation of corticosterone. The final three steps in aldosterone synthesis are accomplished by a single mitochondrial P450 enzyme, aldosterone synthase (CYP11B2, P450aldo) (6).

To produce cortisol, the major glucocorticoid in man, 17α-hydroxylase/17,20 lyase (CYP17, P450c17) in the endoplasmic reticulum of the zona fasciculata and zona reticularis converts pregnenolone to 17α-hydroxypregnenolone (7). 3β-HSD in the zona fasciculata utilizes 17α-hydroxypregnenolone as a substrate, producing 17α-hydroxyprogesterone. The latter is 21-hydroxylated by CYP21 to form 11-deoxycortisol, which is converted to cortisol by 11β-hydroxylase (CYP11B1, P450c11) in mitochondria.

In the zona reticularis of the adrenal cortex and in the gonads, the 17,20-lyase activity of CYP17 converts 17α-hydroxypregnenolone to dehydroepiandrosterone (DHEA), a sex-hormone precursor. DHEA is further converted by 3β-HSD to androstenedione. In the gonads, this is reduced by an isozyme of 17β-hydroxysteroid dehydrogenase to testosterone. In pubertal ovaries, aromatase (CYP19, P450c19) can convert androstenedione and testosterone to estrone and estradiol, respectively (8). Testosterone may be further metabolized to dihydrotestosterone by steroid 5α-reductase in androgen target tissues (9).

REGULATION OF ADRENAL STEROID SECRETION

Cortisol Secretion. Cortisol secretion is regulated mainly by adrenocorticotropic hormone (corticotropin, ACTH). ACTH is a 39-amino acid peptide that is synthesized in the anterior pituitary as part of a larger molecular weight precursor peptide, pro-opiomelanocortin (POMC). ACTH acts through a specific G protein-coupled receptor to increase intracellular levels of cyclic AMP (cAMP, 3',5'-adenosine monophosphate) *(10)*. Cyclic AMP has short-term (minutes to hours) effects on cholesterol transport into mitochondria by StAR protein but longer term (hours to days) effects on transcription of genes encoding the enzymes required to synthesize cortisol *(11)*.

ACTH also influences the remainder of the steps in steroidogenesis as well as the uptake of cholesterol from plasma lipoproteins and maintenance of the size of the adrenal glands.

Cortisol is the primary regulator of resting activity of the hypothalamic-pituitary-adrenal (HPA) axis through negative feedback effects on ACTH and CRH. These are exerted at the level of both the hypothalamus and the pituitary and are mediated by type II corticosteroid receptors (i.e., classic glucocorticoid receptors) *(12)*.

Aldosterone Secretion. The rate of aldosterone synthesis, which is normally 100- to 1000-fold less than that of cortisol synthesis, is regulated mainly by angiotensin II and potassium levels, with ACTH having only a short-term effect *(13)*. Angiotensin II occupies a G protein-coupled receptor *(14)* activating phospholipase C. The latter protein hydrolyzes phosphatidylinositol bisphosphate to produce inositol triphosphate and diacylglycerol, which raise intracellular calcium levels and activate protein kinase C (PKC) and calmodulin-regulated (CaM) kinases. Similarly, increased levels of extracellular potassium depolarize the cell membrane and increase calcium influx through voltage-gated L-type calcium channels. Phosphorylation of as-yet-unidentified factors by CaM kinases increases transcription of the aldosterone synthase (CYP11B2) enzyme required for aldosterone synthesis.

21-Hydroxylase Deficiency

CLINICAL PRESENTATION

Different biosynthetic pathways are affected by the various forms of CAH, which thus have distinct sets of adverse effects (Table 1). Approximately 90–95% of CAH cases are caused by 21-hydroxylase deficiency, which occurs in 1:10,000–1:15,000 births in most populations *(15,16)*.

Patients with 21-hydroxylase deficiency cannot adequately synthesize cortisol because they cannot convert 17-hydroxyprogesterone to 11-deoxycortisol. Inefficient cortisol synthesis signals the hypothalamus and pituitary to increase CRH and ACTH, respectively. Consequently, the adrenal glands become hyperplastic. But rather than cortisol, the adrenals produce excess sex-hormone precursors that do not require 21-hydroxylation for their synthesis. Once secreted, these hormones are further metabolized to active androgens (testosterone and dihydrotestosterone) and to a lesser extent estrogens (estrone and estradiol). The net effect is prenatal virilization of girls, and rapid somatic growth with early epiphyseal fusion in both sexes. Approximately three-quarters of patients cannot synthesize sufficient aldosterone to maintain sodium balance because they cannot convert progesterone to deoxycorticosterone. They are termed "salt wasters" and are predisposed to episodically develop potentially life-threatening hyponatremic dehydration.

Patients with adequate aldosterone production and no salt-wasting who nevertheless have signs of prenatal virilization and/or markedly increased production of hormonal precursors of 21-hydroxylase (e.g., 17-hydroxyprogesterone), are termed "simple virilizers." In addition, a mild "nonclassic" form of the disorder is recognized in which affected females have little or no virilization at birth, but children develop signs of androgen excess during childhood or (for girls) at puberty. Many patients detected by family studies

Table 1

Clinical, Biochemical, and Genetic Characteristics of Congenital Adrenal Hyperplasia and Related Conditions

Deficiency	21-hydroxylase	11β-hydroxylase	Aldosterone synthase	Glucocorticoid suppressible aldosteronism	17α-hydroxylase	3β-hydroxysteroid dehydrogenase	Lipoid adrenal hyperplasia
Enzyme/ gene	CYP21	CYP11B1	CYP11B2	CYP11B1/ CYP11B2	CYP17	HSD3B2	STAR
Alias	P450c21	P450c11	P450aldo		P450c17	3β-HSD	
Incidence	1:14,000	1:100,000	Rare	Rare	Rare	Rare	Rare
Hormones							
Glucocorticoids	↓	↓			↓	↓	↓
Mineralocorticoids	↓ in SW	↑	↓	↑	↑	↓ often	↓
Androgens	↑↑	↑		↑	↓	↓ in ♂ ; ↑ weak androgens in ♀	↓
Estrogens							
↑ Metabolites	++ 17-OHP	DOC, S	B, 18-OHB	aldo, 18-oxoF	DOC, B	DHEA, 17Δ5Preg	None
Clinical signs							
Ambiguous genitalia	♀	♀			♂	severe in ♂ mild in ♀	♂
Salt-wasting crisis	+ in SW		+			+	+
Hypertension		+		+	+		
Na balance	↓ in SW	↑	↓	↑	↑	↓	↓
K balance	↑ in SW	↓	↑	↓	↓	↑	↑

+, present; ↓, diminished quantity; ↑, increased quantity; ♂, male; ♀, female; nl, normal; SW, salt-waster; P450, cytochrome P450; 17-OHP, 17-hydroxyprogesterone; DOC, deoxycorticosterone; S, 11-deoxycortisol; B, corticosterone; 18-OHB, 18-hydroxycorticosterone; aldo, aldosterone; 18-oxoF, 18-oxocortisol; DHEA, dehydroepiandrosterone; 17Δ5Preg, 17-Δ5-pregnenolone.

or neonatal screening are asymptomatic. Nonclassic 21-hydroxylase deficiency occurs more frequently than the classic disease; a frequency of 1:500 has been suggested for the general population, and up to 2% of Ashkenazi (Eastern European origin) Jews.

GENETICS

Steroid 21-hydroxylase (P450c21, CYP21) is a microsomal cytochrome P450 enzyme that converts 17-hydroxyprogesterone to 11-deoxycortisol and progesterone to deoxycorticosterone. As with other microsomal P450s, the enzyme accepts electrons from an NADPH-dependent cytochrome P450 reductase, thus reducing molecular oxygen and hydroxylating the substrate.

The structural gene encoding human CYP21 (CYP21, CYP21A2, or CYP21B) and a pseudogene (CYP21P, CYP21A1P, or CYP21A) are located in the HLA major histocompatibility complex (MHC) on chromosome 6p21.3 about 30 kb apart, adjacent to and alternating with the C4B and C4A genes encoding the fourth component of serum complement (Fig. 2) *(17,18)*. Nonfunctional fragments of adjacent genes are included in the duplicated segment. CYP21 and CYP21P each contain 10 exons spaced over 3.1 kb. Their nucleotide sequences are 98% identical in exons and about 96% identical in introns. However, CYP21P contains several mutations that prevent synthesis of an active enzyme. These include an A→G substitution 13 nucleotides (nt) before the end of intron 2 that results in aberrant splicing of pre-mRNA, an 8 nt deletion in exon 3, and a 1 nt insertion in exon 7, each of which shifts the reading frame of translation, and a nonsense mutation in codon 318 of exon 8. There are also 8 missense mutations *(19,20)*.

MUTATIONS CAUSING 21-HYDROXYLASE DEFICIENCY

Most mutations causing 21-hydroxylase deficiency that have been described thus far are apparently the result of either of two types of recombinations between CYP21, the normally active gene, and the CYP21P pseudogene: unequal crossing-over during meiosis resulting in a complete deletion of C4B and a net deletion of CYP21 *(21)*, and apparent gene-conversion events resulting in the transfer to CYP21 of deleterious mutations normally present in CYP21P. Because particular mutations occur in many unrelated kindreds, each mutation, and the degree of enzymatic compromise it causes, may be correlated with the different clinical forms of 21-hydroxylase deficiency (i.e., salt wasting, simple virilizing, and nonclassic disease).

The classification of 21-hydroxylase deficiency into salt-wasting, simple-virilizing, and nonclassic types is a useful way roughly to grade the severity of the disease and to predict the therapeutic interventions that will likely be required. If molecular diagnosis could predict this classification, it would increase the utility of prenatal diagnosis and neonatal screening and it might serve as a useful diagnostic adjunct to ACTH-stimulation tests.

The simplest way to correlate genotype and phenotype is to see which mutations are characteristically found in each type of 21-hydroxylase deficiency. This is most informative for frequently occurring mutations. Deletions and large conversions are most often found in salt-wasting patients, the intron 2 nt656g mutation is found in both salt-wasting and simple-virilizing patients, I172N (Ile-172→Asn) is characteristically seen in simple-virilizing patients, and V281L (Val-281→Leu) and P30L (Pro-30→Leu) are found in nonclassic patients. This distribution is consistent with the compromise in enzymatic activity conferred by each mutation *(22,23)*.

However, patients are usually compound heterozygotes for different mutations, and so this approach has little predictive value in itself. A useful analytic strategy is to consider

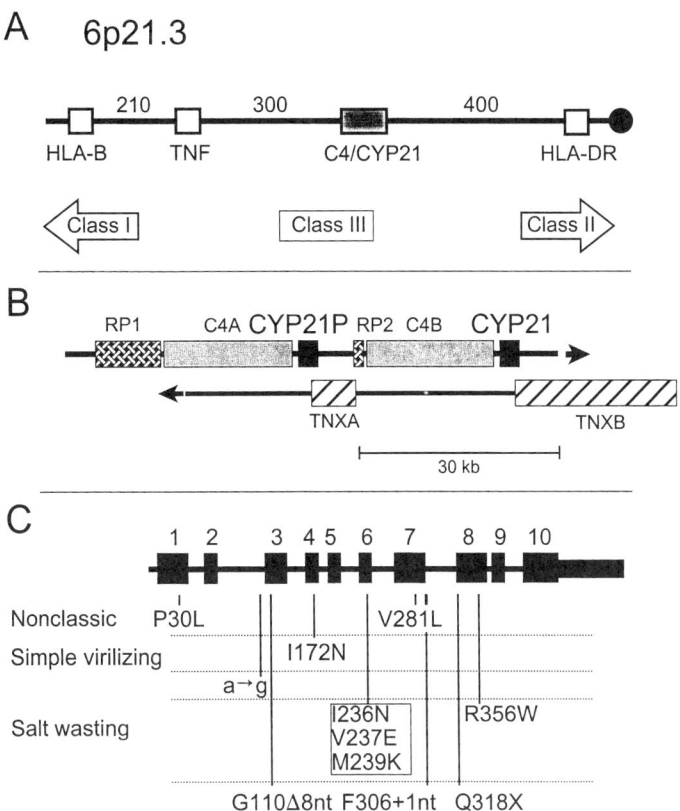

Fig. 2. (A) Location of the *CYP21* genes within the *HLA* major histocompatibility complex on chromosome 6p21.3. There are many more genes in this region than are indicated. The direction of the centromere is indicated by the circle at the right end of the line. Numbers denote distances between genes in kilobasepairs (kb). *HLA-B* is the nearest "Class I" transplantation antigen gene to *CYP21*, and *HLA-DR* the nearest Class II gene. The region between these classes of genes is termed "Class III." *TNF*, tumor necrosis factor (actually two genes). The *C4/CYP21* region is diagrammed in B. **(B)** Map of the genetic region around the 21-hydroxylase (*CYP21*) gene. Arrows denote direction of transcription. *CYP21P*, 21-hydroxylase pseudogene; *C4A* and *C4B*, genes encoding the fourth component of serum complement; *RP1*, gene encoding a putative nuclear protein of unknown function; *RP2*, truncated copy of this gene. *TNXB*, tenascin-X gene and *TNXA*, a truncated copy of this gene, are on the opposite chromosomal strand. The 30 kb scale bar is positioned to show the region involved in the tandem duplication. **(C)** Mutations causing steroid 21-hydroxylase deficiency. Exons are numbered. *CYP21P* has nine deleterious mutations that may be transferred into *CYP21* by gene conversion, causing 21-hydroxylase deficiency. The three mutations in the box are invariably inherited together. These mutations are characteristically associated with different forms of 21-hydroxylase deficiency; the mutations at the bottom of the panel cause the most severe enzymatic deficiency. There are several dozen additional rare mutations that collectively account for 5% of all 21-hydroxylase deficiency alleles; these are not shown. As an example of mutation terminology, P30L is Proline-30 to Leucine. Δ, deletion, +, insertion. Other single letter amino acid codes: A, alanine; C, cysteine; D, aspartic acid; E, glutamic acid; F, phenylalanine; G, glycine; H, histidine; I, isoleucine; K, lysine; L, leucine; M, methionine; N, asparagine; P, proline; Q, glutamine; R, arginine; S, serine; T, threonine; V, valine; W, tryptophan; Y, tyrosine.

that 21-hydroxylase deficiency is a recessive disease, and thus the phenotype of each patient is likely to reflect his or her less severely impaired allele. If mutations are provisionally classified by the degree of enzymatic compromise—severe, moderate, or mild—then one might hypothesize that salt-wasting patients would have severe/severe genotypes; simple-virilizing patients would have severe/moderate or moderate/moderate genotypes; and nonclassic patients would have severe/mild, moderate/mild, or mild/mild genotypes. This approach predicts the severity of the disease approx 80% of the time *(22)*.

Several explanations for the less than complete correspondence between genotype and phenotype are possible. The most obvious is that the severity of the disease falls on a continuum and patients with disease severity near the "borders" of the various classifications may easily fall on either side of these borders. The intron 2 nt656g mutation is particularly associated with this problem; it is classified as severe but is clearly "leaky" and may yield enough normally spliced mRNA to ameliorate the enyzmatic deficiency in some patients *(24)*. Genetic or environmental factors other than 21-hydroxylase activity may influence also phenotype. The degree of salt wasting tends to improve with time, even in subjects who are genetically predicted to have no 21-hydroxylase activity *(25)*, and genetically identical siblings are occasionally discordant for severity of salt wasting. Thus this clinical parameter must be influenced by other factors. Similarly, genetically based variations in androgen biosynthesis or sensitivity to androgens would be expected to influence the phenotype.

Disorders of 11β-Hydroxylase Isozymes

STEROID 11β-HYDROXYLASE ISOZYMES

Humans have two 11β-hydroxylase isozymes that are responsible for cortisol and aldosterone biosynthesis, CYP11B1 (P450c11, 11β-hydroxylase) and CYP11B2 (P450aldo, aldosterone synthase, respectively). These isozymes are mitochondrial cytochromes P450 located in the inner membrane on the matrix side.

CYP11B1 11β-hydroxylates 11-deoxycorticosterone to corticosterone and 11-deoxycortisol to cortisol. It can also convert 11-deoxycorticosterone to 18-hydroxy,11-deoxycorticosterone, but it 18-hydroxylates corticosterone poorly. It cannot convert corticosterone into aldosterone. In contrast, CYP11B2 has strong 11β-hydroxylase activity but also 18-hydroxylates and then 18-oxidizes corticosterone and cortisol to aldosterone and 18-oxocortisol, respectively *(26–28)*. When deoxycorticosterone is converted to aldosterone, the same steroid molecule probably remains bound to the enzyme for all three conversions without release of the intermediate products.

In humans, CYP11B1 and CYP11B2 are encoded by two genes *(29)* approx 40 kb apart *(30,31)* on chromosome 8q24; CYP11B2 is on the left (if the genes are pictured as being transcribed left to right) (Fig. 3). The nucleotide sequences of these genes are 95% identical in coding sequences, and the predicted proteins are 93% identical in amino acid sequence *(29)*.

Mutations or rearrangements involving these genes cause three different diseases: 11β-hydroxylase deficiency, aldosterone synthase deficiency, and glucocorticoid-suppressible hyperaldosteronism.

CLINICAL PRESENTATION OF 11β-HYDROXYLASE DEFICIENCY

Steroid 11β-hydroxylase deficiency comprises 5–8% of cases of CAH, occurring in about 1:100,000 births in the general Caucasian population *(6)*. Patients with this disorder are

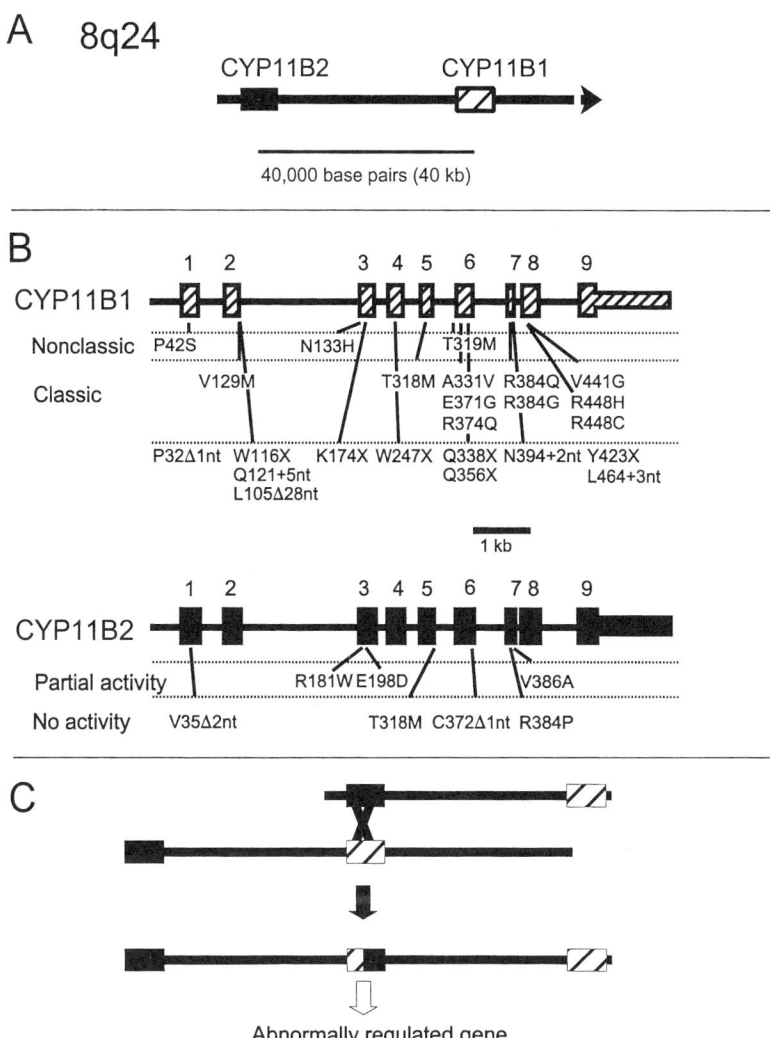

Fig. 3. Mutations involving the 11β-hydroxylase (CYP11B1) and aldosterone synthase (CYP11B2) genes. (**A**) The arrangement of genes is diagrammed. (**B**) Mutations in CYP11B1 causing nonclassic or classic 11β-hydroxylase deficiency, and mutations in CYP11B2 causing aldosterone synthase deficiency. These are arranged in the diagram so that those causing increasing enzymatic compromise are arrayed from top to bottom. Dotted lines divide mutants into groups with similar activities. Although there are two types of aldosterone synthase deficiency, they do not correspond exactly to in vitro levels of enzymatic activity. R181W and V386A do not cause disease separately, but double homozygosity causes CMO II type aldosterone synthase deficiency. Other combinations with this phenotype include T318M+V386A and R181W+C372Δ1nt. Homozygosity for either V352nt and R384P, or double homozygosity for E198D+V386A, has been associated with CMO I type deficiency. (**C**) Unequal crossing-over generating a chimeric *CYP11B1/2* gene that has aldosterone synthase activity but is expressed in the zona fasciculata. This causes glucocorticoid suppressible hyperaldosteronism.

unable to convert 11-deoxycortisol to cortisol. As occurs in 21-hydroxylase deficiency, elevated levels of ACTH cause steroid precursors of cortisol to accumulate. These are shunted into the pathway for androgen biosynthesis, leading to signs of androgen excess.

A parallel defect usually exists in the synthesis of 17-deoxy steroids in the zona fasciculata, so that deoxycorticosterone is not converted to corticosterone and instead accumulates. Because deoxycorticosterone and some of its metabolites have mineralo-corticoid activity, elevated levels may cause hypertension and hypokalemia. About two-thirds of untreated patients become hypertensive, sometimes early in life. This clinical feature distinguishes 11β-hydroxylase deficiency from 21-hydroxylase deficiency, in which poor aldosterone synthesis causes renal salt wasting in the majority of patients. Although the conversion of deoxycorticosterone to corticosterone is also required for aldo-sterone biosynthesis in the zona glomerulosa, this step is mediated by a distinct enzyme, aldosterone synthase, that is not affected in 11β-hydroxylase deficiency.

Nonclassic 11β-hydroxylase deficiency has the same presentation as nonclassic 21-hydroxylase deficiency and is not associated with hypertension, but it occurs much less frequently than that disorder.

As with 21-hydroxylase deficiency, the cortisol deficiency and elevated levels of cor-tisol precursors in 11β-hydroxylase deficiency are treated with glucocorticoids. This will usually treat associated hypertension, although supplemental antihypertensive therapy, often with calcium-channel blockers, may be required, especially in long-standing cases. Mineralocorticoid supplementation is rarely necessary, although transient suppression of the zona glomerulosa is occasionally seen when glucocorticoid therapy is instituted in a hypertensive patient.

CLINICAL PRESENTATION OF ALDOSTERONE SYNTHASE DEFICIENCY

Aldosterone synthase (corticosterone methyloxidase) deficiency is an autosomal reces-sive inherited defect of aldosterone biosynthesis. Patients with this disorder are subject to potentially fatal electrolyte abnormalities as neonates and a variable degree of hypo-natremia and hyperkalemia combined with poor growth in childhood, but they may have no symptoms as adults. Cortisol and sex-steroid synthesis are entirely unaffected. Two types of this disorder have been described; patients with type I deficiency have low serum levels of 18-hydroxycorticosterone, whereas patients with type II deficiency have high levels of this aldosterone precursor and thus an elevated ratio of 18-hydroxycorticoster-one to aldosterone. Both are caused by mutations in the gene encoding the aldosterone syn-thase enzyme (see *Genetics of Aldosterone Synthase Deficiency and Genetics of Gluco-corticoid-Suppressible Hyperaldosteronism*) *(6)*.

This disorder is treated with salt supplementation and mineralocorticoid replacement, usually with fludrocortisone.

CLINICAL PRESENTATION OF GLUCOCORTICOID-SUPPRESSIBLE HYPERALDOSTERONISM

Glucocorticoid suppressible hyperaldosteronism (also called dexamethasone-suppres-sible hyperaldosteronism or glucocorticoid-remediable aldosteronism) is a form of hyper-tension inherited in an autosomal dominant manner with high penetrance. It is characterized by moderate hypersecretion of aldosterone, suppressed plasma renin activity, and rapid reversal of these abnormalities after administration of glucocorticoids. It is clearly a rare disorder but until several years ago the absence of reliable biochemical or genetic markers made it difficult to ascertain.

Hypokalemia is usually mild and may be absent. Absolute levels of aldosterone secretion are usually moderately elevated in the untreated state but may be within normal limits. Plasma renin activity is strongly suppressed, so that the ratio of aldosterone secretion to renin activity is always abnormally high. Levels of 18-hydroxycortisol and 18-oxocortisol are elevated to 20–30 times normal. The ratio of urinary excretion of tetrahydro metabolites of 18-oxocortisol to those of aldosterone exceeds 2.0, whereas this ratio averages 0.2 in normal individuals *(32)*. Elevation of 18-oxocortisol is the most consistent and reliable biochemical marker of the disease, although it may also be elevated in cases of primary aldosteronism. This steroid may be of pathophysiologic significance; it is an agonist for the mineralocorticoid receptor and has been shown to raise blood pressure in animal studies *(33)*.

Once an affected individual has been identified in a kindred, additional cases may be ascertained within that kindred using biochemical (18-oxocortisol levels) *(32)* or genetic (*see* below) markers. It is apparent from these studies that affected individuals have blood pressures that are markedly elevated as compared to unaffected individuals in the same kindred, although some patients may in fact have normal blood pressures. Even young children typically have blood pressures greater than the 95th percentile for age, and most are frankly hypertensive before the age of 20. The hypertension is often of only moderate severity and blood pressures exceeding 180/120 are unusual. Associated signs of hypertension are frequent including left ventricular hypertrophy on the electrocardiogram and retinopathy. Some affected kindreds have remarkable histories of early (before age 45) death from strokes in many family members *(32)*.

Steroid biosynthesis is otherwise normal so that affected individuals have normal growth and sexual development.

Most laboratory and clinical abnormalities are suppressed by treatment with glucocorticoids, whereas infusion of ACTH exacerbates these problems *(34)*. This suggests that aldosterone is being inappropriately synthesized in the zona fasciculata and is being regulated by ACTH. Moreover, 18-hydroxycortisol and 18-oxocortisol, the steroids that are characteristically elevated in this disorder, are 17α-hydroxylated analogs of 18-hydroxycorticosterone and aldosterone, respectively. Because 17α-hydroxylase is not expressed in the zona glomerulosa, the presence of large amounts of a 17α-hydroxy, 18-oxo-steroid suggests that an enzyme with 18-oxidase activity (i.e., aldosterone synthase, CYP11B2) is abnormally expressed in the zona fasciculata *(35)*.

The initial treatment of choice in adults is dexamethasone (1–2 mg/d). Children with this condition should be treated cautiously because of potential adverse effects of glucocorticoid therapy on growth. If therapy is indicated, children should be treated with the lowest effective dose of hydrocortisone. If hypertension is of long standing, it may not completely respond to glucocorticoids. This problem is similar to that observed in patients with 11β-hydroxylase deficiency and the choice of adjunctive therapy is governed by the same considerations. Patients with this disorder usually respond poorly to conventional antihypertensive medications unless they are also treated with glucocorticoids.

GENETICS OF 11β-HYDROXYLASE DEFICIENCY

Deficiency of 11β-Hydroxylase Results from Mutations in CYP11B1. In Moroccan Jews, a group that has a high prevalence of 11β-hydroxylase deficiency (1:5000–7000) *(36)*, almost all affected alleles carry the same mutation, R448H (Arg-448→His) *(37)*, which probably affects interactions with the heme group of the enzyme. Many additional mutations have been identified including missense, nonsense, and frameshift mutations *(38–41)*. In contrast to 21-hydroxylase deficiency, deletions and gene conversions have not been identified in patients with 11β-hydroxylase deficiency. Although CYP11B1 and CYP11B2, like CYP21 and CYP21P, are closely linked homologs, CYP11B1 and CYP11B2 both encode active enzymes. Thus, gene conversions that transfer polymorphic sequences between CYP11B1 and CYP11B2 should not produce 11β-hydroxylase deficiency alleles. This may explain why 11β-hydroxylase deficiency is less frequent than 21-hydroxylase deficiency.

Unequal crossovers between CYP11B1 and CYP11B2 should yield a chromosome carrying a single CYP11B gene with a 5' end corresponding to CYP11B2 and a 3' end corresponding to CYP11B1. Like CYP11B2, such a gene should be expressed at low levels and only in the zona glomerulosa and thus might function as an 11β-hydroxylase deficiency allele. As yet, such chromosomes have not been detected. On the other hand, the reciprocal product of an unequal crossover, a chromosome carrying three CYP11B genes, has been observed in glucocorticoid suppressible hyperaldosteronism (*see Genetics of Glucocorticoid Suppressive Hyperaldosteronism*).

GENETICS OF ALDOSTERONE SYNTHASE DEFICIENCY

Aldosterone synthase deficiency results from mutations in CYP11B2 that reduce enzymatic activity to less than 1% of normal *(42,43)*. Individuals who are homozygous for mutations that severely compromise but do not destroy enzymatic activity have entirely normal aldosterone biosynthesis with normal ratios of plasma renin activity to aldosterone *(42)*. Similarly, patients with 21-hydroxylase deficiency carrying CYP21 mutants that retain 1–2% of normal activity are able to synthesize aldosterone normally *(44)*. The finding that such reductions in enzymatic activity are not rate-limiting may reflect the very low levels at which aldosterone is normally secreted. This suggests that the apparent rarity of aldosterone synthase deficiency may reflect problems of ascertainment, because any but the most severe defects will in fact have no obvious phenotypic effects.

Patients with type I and type II deficiencies differ in having low or high levels of the immediate precursor of aldosterone, 18-hydroxycorticosterone. It might be supposed that type I deficiency would result from more severe enzymatic defects *(45,46)*, but patients with similar genotypes have been identified with both types of the disorder *(43,47)*. The difference between these disorders may be due to associated polymorphisms in the adjacent CYP11B1 gene *(48)*.

GENETICS OF GLUCOCORTICOID-SUPPRESSIBLE HYPERALDOSTERONISM

All patients with glucocorticoid suppressible hyperaldosteronism have the same type of mutation, a chromosome that carries three *CYP11B* genes instead of the normal two (Fig. 3) *(30,31,49)*. The middle gene on this chromosome is a chimera with 5' and 3' ends corresponding to *CYP11B1* and *CYP11B2*, respectively. The chimeric gene is flanked by presumably normal *CYP11B2* and *CYP11B1* genes. In all kindreds analyzed thus far, the breakpoints (the points of transition between *CYP11B1* and *CYP11B2* sequences) are located between intron 2 and exon 4. As the breakpoints are not identical in different kindreds, these must represent independent mutations.

The chromosomes carrying chimeric genes are presumably generated by unequal crossing-over. The high homology and proximity of the *CYP11B1* and *CYP11B2* genes makes it possible for them to become misaligned during meiosis. If this occurs, crossing-over between the misaligned genes creates two chromosomes; one carries one *CYP11B* gene (i.e., a deletion), the other carries three *CYP11B* genes.

The invariable presence of a chimeric gene in patients with this disorder suggests that this gene is regulated like *CYP11B1* (expressed at high levels in the zona fasciculata and regulated primarily by ACTH) because it has transcriptional regulatory sequences identical to those of *CYP11B1*. If the chimeric gene has enzymatic activity similar to that of *CYP11B2*, a single copy of such an abnormally regulated gene should be sufficient to cause the disorder, consistent with the known autosomal dominant mode of inheritance of this syndrome. Abnormal expression of the chimeric gene in the zona fasciculata was directly demonstrated by *in situ* hybridization studies of an adrenal gland from a patient with this disorder *(50)*.

The chimeric genes causing glucocorticoid suppressible hyperaldosteronism may be readily detected by hybridization to Southern blots of genomic DNA, or they may be specifically amplified using the polymerase chain reaction (PCR) *(51)*. As these techniques are widely used in molecular genetics laboratories, direct molecular genetic diagnosis may be more practical in many cases than assays of 18-oxocortisol levels, which are not routinely available *(52)*.

The limited region in which crossover breakpoints have been observed in glucocorticoid-suppressible hyperaldosteronism alleles suggests that there are functional constraints on the structures of chimeric genes able to cause this disorder. One obvious constraint is that sufficient *CYP11B2* coding sequences must be present in the chimeric gene so that the encoded enzyme actually has aldosterone synthase (i.e., 18-hydroxylase and 18-oxidase) activity. As determined by expressing chimeric cDNAs in cultured cells, chimeric enzymes with amino termini from *CYP11B1* and carboxyl termini from *CYP11B2* have 18-oxidase activity only if at least the region encoded by exons 5–9 corresponds to *CYP11B2*. If the sequence of exon 5 instead corresponds to *CYP11B1*, the enzyme has 11β-hydroxylase but no 18-oxidase activity *(30)*. This is entirely consistent with the observation that no breakpoints in glucocorticoid suppressible hyperaldosteronism alleles occur 5' to exon 4. The chimeric enzymes either have strong 18-oxidase activity or none detectable and there does not appear to be any location of crossover that yields an enzyme with an intermediate level of 18-oxidase activity. Thus, there is no evidence for allelic variation in this disorder (i.e., variations in clinical severity are unlikely to be the result of different cross-over locations).

Other factors such as kallikrein levels may affect the development of hypertension in this disorder *(52)*. One study found that blood pressure in persons with glucocorticoid-suppressible hyperaldosteronism is higher when the disease is inherited from the mother than when it is paternally inherited *(53)*. It is theoretically possible that the gene is imprinted (i.e., the maternal and paternal copies are expressed differently), but it seems more likely that exposure of the fetus to elevated levels of maternal aldosterone subsequently exacerbates the hypertension.

17α-Hydroxylase/17,20 Lyase Deficiency

CLINICAL PRESENTATION

Steroid 17α-hydroxylase deficiency is a relatively rare cause of CAH, accounting for about 1% of cases. It is characterized biochemically by poor synthesis of 17-hydroxylated steroids such as cortisol and elevated levels of 17-deoxy steroids *(7)*. Deoxycorticosterone is one such steroid. Thus, patients with 17α-hydroxylase deficiency often have hyperten-sion and other signs of mineralocorticoid excess similar to those seen in 11β-hydroxylase deficiency. However, whereas patients with 11β-hydroxylase deficiency have signs of androgen excess, patients with severe 17α-hydroxylase deficiency are unable to synthe-size sex steroids. Males are born with female-appearing external genitalia indistinguish-able in appearance from those seen in lipoid adrenal hyperplasia (*see Lipoid Adrenal Hyperplasia*) or androgen insensitivity, although the latter condition is readily distin-guished by elevated levels of androgens. Testes are often palpable in the inguinal canals or the labio-scrotal folds. Females appear normal at birth but remain sexually infantile. The ovaries have poor follicular development and in rare cases appear as streak gonads.

Some patients with mild 17α-hydroxylase deficiency are able to synthesize at least some sex steroids so that males have partially masculinized ambiguous genitalia and females develop some signs of puberty. Some (mostly female) patients have been reported to have isolated 17α-hydroxylase deficiency with normal 17,20-lyase activity. Conversely, a few patients have isolated 17,20-lyase deficiency *(54)*.

BIOCHEMISTRY

Steroid 17α-hydroxylase/17,20 lyase (CYP17, P450c17) is a microsomal cytochrome P450 with 508 amino acids; it bears 35% amino acid identity with CYP21. It catalyzes conversion of pregnenolone to 17α-hydroxypregnenolone. It also catalyzes an oxidative cleavage of the 17,20 carbon-carbon bond, converting 17α-hydroxypregnenolone and 17α-hydroxyprogesterone to dehydroepiandrosterone and androstenedione, respectively. A pair of electrons and a molecule of O_2 are required for each hydroxylation or lyase reac-tion. CYP17 is a microsomal cytochrome P450 and accepts these electrons from NADPH-dependent cytochrome P450 reductase.

Activity of 17α-hydroxylase is required for the synthesis of cortisol, whereas both 17α-hydroxylase and 17,20-lyase activities are required for androgen and estrogen bio-synthesis. As significant amounts of 17α-hydroxylated steroids are secreted by the human adrenal cortex but not by the gonads, it is apparent that the 17,20-lyase activity of CYP17 is stronger in the gonads than in the adrenals, relative to 17α-hydroxylase activity. Tissue specific variations in lyase activity may reflect the activity of the electron transport pro-tein, cytochrome b5, or perhaps phosphorylation of the enzyme *(55)*.

GENETIC ANALYSIS

In humans, a single copy of the CYP17 gene is located on chromosome 10q24.3 *(56–58)*. It consists of 8 exons spread over 6.7 kb. At this time, at least 18 different mutations have been identified in 27 individuals *(7,59)*. All known mutations are in coding regions. A 4 bp duplication in the last exon causing a shift in the reading frame has been found in 10 patients in the Netherlands or of Dutch Mennonite ancestry; this presumably repre-sents a founder effect *(60)*. Complete deficiency is associated with frameshifts or non-sense mutations. In one kindred, two exons were replaced by a segment of the *Escherichia coli* lac operon; the mechanism by which this rearrangement occurred is not known but it may have involved viral integration into the genome *(61)*.

Partial deficiency is associated with missense mutations in *CYP17* or, in one case, dele-tion of a single codon (ΔF53 or 54) maintaining the reading frame of translation *(62,63)*. These mutations have been introduced into cDNA and expressed in cultured cells. These studies suggest that greater than 20% of normal activity is required to synthesize sufficient androgens to permit normal male sexual development; 50% of normal activity must be sufficient for normal development because obligate heterozygous males are asymptomatic. Patients with isolated 17,20 lyase deficiency have mutations in CYP17 that interfere with electron transfer from cytochrome P450 reductase *(64)*.

3β-Hydroxysteroid Dehydrogenase Deficiency

CLINICAL PRESENTATION

Deficiency of 3β-hydroxysteroid dehydrogenase interferes with synthesis of mineralocorticoids, glucocorticoids, and sex steroids. Thus, severely affected patients may succumb in the neonatal period to shock from glucocorticoid and mineralocorticoid deficiency similar to that seen in 21-hydroxylase deficiency. However, because testosterone cannot be synthesized, affected males are born with ambiguous genitalia, as seen in 17α-hydroxylase/17,20 lyase deficiency. Unlike the latter disorder, affected individuals secrete large amounts of dehydroepiandrosterone, which is a weak androgen. Thus, affected females also are sometimes born with ambiguous genitalia. As is the case with other forms of CAH, the internal genital structures correspond to the chromosomal sex.

Although classic 3β-hydroxysteroid dehydrogenase deficiency is rare, comprising less than 1% of cases of CAH, a mild or nonclassic form of the disease has been postulated to be a frequent cause of hirsutism and/or menstrual irregularities (particularly polycystic ovary syndrome [PCOS]) in women. However, reliable clinical diagnostic criteria for the nonclassic disorder are difficult to establish, consisting mainly of altered ratios of dehydroepiandrosterone to androstenedione.

BIOCHEMISTRY

Conversion of Δ5-3β-hydroxysteroids (pregnenolone, 17-hydroxypregnenolone, dehydroepiandrosterone) to Δ4-3-ketosteroids (progesterone, 17-hydroxyprogesterone, androstenedione) is mediated by 3β-hydroxysteroid dehydrogenase. These conversions are mediated by several isozymes in the endoplasmic reticulum, all of which are of the short-chain alcohol dehydrogenase type. They utilize NAD+ as an electron acceptor. In addition to 3β-hydroxysteroid dehydrogenase activity, these enzymes mediate a Δ5-Δ4-ene isomerase reaction that transfers a double bond from the B ring to the A ring of the steroid so that it is in conjugation with the 3-keto group.

Thus far, two isozymes have been identified in humans. The human type I enzyme is expressed in the placenta, skin, and adipose tissue, whereas the type II enzyme is expressed in the adrenal gland and the gonads. There are as many as six *HSDB3* genes in humans, all of which are located on chromosome 1p11-13, but only two, HSD3B1 and HSD3B2, encode active enzymes *(65–67)*.

GENETICS

Patients with the classic form of the disease have mutations in the HSD3B2 gene that abolish activity *(68,69)*. As this gene is expressed in the adrenals and gonads, these mutations account fully for the pathogenesis of the disease. Because the HSD3B1 gene is intact, steroid biosynthesis in the placenta should be normal during gestation. Moreover, 3β-hydroxysteroid dehydrogenase activity in the skin and adipose tissue should remain intact postnatally, suggesting that complete 3β-hydroxysteroid dehydrogenase deficiency should occur rarely if at all.

Although nonclassic 3β-hydroxysteroid dehydrogenase deficiency has been reported to occur frequently, mutations in HSD3B2 have rarely been identified in such patients, and this disorder is apparently not usually due to a specific enzymatic deficiency *(70)*.

Lipoid Adrenal Hyperplasia

Clinical Presentation

Lipoid adrenal hyperplasia is a defect in importation of cholesterol into mitochondria in steroid-synthesizing cells of the adrenals and gonads. This decreases but does not completely abolish steroid synthesis. However, it leads to accumulation of cytoplasmic lipid droplets containing cholesteryl esters and consequent death of the cells. Thus, this defect ultimately abolishes synthesis of all steroids in the adrenals and gonads, although transient synthesis of estrogens can occasionally occur in the ovaries of affected girls at puberty, because primary ovarian follicles are endocrinologically dormant before puberty and are thus not destroyed by lipid accumulation.

Because affected individuals are unable to synthesize cortisol or aldosterone, they develop salt wasting and shock as seen in 21-hydroxylase deficiency. Because sex steroids cannot be synthesized, males are born with female-appearing external genitalia. Females usually remain sexually infantile although transient secretion of estrogens at puberty occurs rarely *(3)*.

Biochemistry/Genetics

By analogy with other forms of CAH, it was originally hypothesized that patients with lipoid adrenal hyperplasia had mutations in the cholesterol desmolase (CYP11A, P450scc) enzyme, but no such mutations have been detected *(71)*. Because the maintenance of human pregnancy is critically dependent on placental progesterone synthesis, such mutations may be embryonically lethal. Instead, mutations have been detected in all affected individuals in the gene encoding the StAR protein *(72,73)*. The affected gene is located on chromosome 8p11.2; a processed pseudogene is located on chromosome 13 and is not involved in this disease.

ADRENOLEUKODYSTROPHY

Clinical Presentation

Adrenoleukodystrophy is an X-linked disorder of oxidation of very long-chain (>24 carbon) fatty acids (VLCFA) *(74)*. It is characterized by progressive nervous-system demyelination and adrenal insufficiency. It occurs in approx 1:20,000 males and may account for as much as 25% of cases of adrenal insufficiency in boys. There are several phenotypes, of which the most severe is the childhood cerebral form. Patients suffering from this form have onset of brain demyelination before age 10, with severe progressive neurologic compromise leading to death within 5–10 yr. These problems can also have their onset in adolescence or adulthood, in which case neurologic deterioration is correspondingly slower. Other patients present in adult life with adrenomyeloneuropathy, which is paraparesis due to spinal-cord disease; this subsequently progresses to cerebral involvement in 45% of cases. Adrenal insufficiency may precede or follow the onset of neurologic signs; it typically affects the zona fasciculata before the zona glomerulosa.

Although the disease is X-linked, approx half of female carriers (typically mothers of affected males) have some degree of neurologic involvement, which, in 20%, is similar to adrenomyeloneuropathy in males. However, only 1% of females develop adrenal insufficiency. The severity of disease within a single kindred can vary considerably; factors influencing disease progression have not been firmly identified. The disease is diagnosed biochemically by demonstrating elevated blood levels of VLCFA; female carriers usually have mild elevations that can often overlap the normal range.

As described in the film *Lorenzo's Oil*, dietary therapy with glycerol trioleate and glycerol trierucate reduces blood levels of VLCFA, but its efficacy in reducing brain levels of these compounds is limited, and it has little effect on the disease once neurologic deterioration is evident. It is not yet known if this therapy might be effective if administered before signs of neurologic disease develop (e.g., in prospectively ascertained members of an affected kindred). Bone-marrow transplantation may arrest progression in patients with mild nervous-system involvement.

Genetics

The affected *ALD* gene is located on chromosome Xq28. The gene has been positionally cloned; it encodes a peroxisomal membrane protein of the "ABC" transporter family and is structurally related to the protein affected in cystic fibrosis *(75)*. The ALD protein contains 745 amino acids and includes 6 transmembrane domains and an ATP binding domain. The functional protein is probably a dimer. The gene contains 10 exons spaced over 20 kb *(76)*.

The mutations causing ALD have been characterized in more than 80 kindreds *(74,77)*. Most mutations are unique to a single kindred, but a frameshift in exon 5 has been observed in one-sixth of unrelated families. Deletions, frameshifts, nonsense, and missense mutations have all been reported; approx 70% prevent synthesis of immunoreactive protein. There is apparently no correlation between genotype and phenotype.

DEVELOPMENTAL DEFECTS

Mutations in Steroidogenic Factor-1

Steroidogenic factor-1 (SF-1, also called Ad4BP) is a transcription factor that structurally resembles nuclear hormone receptors, but its physiologic ligand, if any, is unknown (i.e., it is an "orphan" receptor). It is required for normal expression of most steroidogenic enzymes in the adrenal cortex and the gonads *(78)*. "Knockout" mice lacking SF-1 fail to develop adrenal glands or gonads and also have hypothalamic abnormalities *(79)*. One mutation of the human SF-1 gene has been reported in an XY phenotypic female who presented shortly after birth with adrenal failure *(80)*. This patient had streak gonads with normal Mullerian structures including a uterus. She carried a heterozygous missense mutation (G35E), which involves part of the putative DNA binding domain just after the first of two zinc fingers.

Considering that heterozygous knockout mice are phenotypically normal, it is not clear why a heterozygous missense mutation caused such significant abnormalities in this patient. When expressed in cells, the mutant SF-1 fails to transactivate a known SF-1 response reporter gene (CYP11A), but it does not act as a dominant negative when co-expressed with wild-type SF-1. Perhaps it has dominant negative activity on other promoters, or normal adrenal and gonadal levels of SF-1 may be sufficiently limiting in humans that haploinsufficiency accounts for the observed phenotypic effects.

Adrenal Hypoplasia Congenita

CLINICAL PRESENTATION

Adrenal hypoplasia congenita (AHC) is a rare disorder characterized by failure of development of the adrenal gland along with hypogonadotropic hypogonadism (HH). It is inherited as an X-linked disease. The typical presentation is a male infant with undescended testes who develops severe adrenal insufficiency a few weeks after birth, but adrenal insufficiency develops later in childhood in some boys. Patients occasionally have micropenis.

Puberty does not occur spontaneously. Although gonadotropin levels are very low in the baseline state, there is often some response to a single pulse of exogenous gonadotropin releasing hormone (GnRH). However, gonadotropin secretion in response to a week of pulsatile GnRH (which is normally an effective stimulus of gonadotropin release) is quite low. Thus, there are probably both hypothalamic and pituitary defects in gonadotropin secretion. Moreover, patients with AHC may have oligospermia that is unresponsive to gonadotropins, suggesting that DAX-1 (*see* genetics section) has effects on the testes independent from its effects on gonadotropins. Females may exhibit delayed puberty but are fertile *(81)*.

Adrenal insufficiency is treated with glucocorticoid and mineralocorticoid replacement. Hypogonadism is treated with testosterone replacement.

GENETICS

Some patients have a deletion of part of the short arm of the X-chromosome (Xp21). Some patients with such deletions also have glycerol kinase deficiency and Duchenne muscular dystrophy, a "contiguous gene syndrome" due to a deletion affecting closely linked genes. Of note, duplication of an overlapping genetic region causes 46 XY male-to-female sex reversal. These findings permitted positional cloning of the *DAX-1* (dosage-sensitive sex reversal, AHC, X-linked) gene *(82)*.

The C-terminal half of the putative DAX-1 protein resembles the ligand-binding domain of other nuclear hormonereceptors. The N-terminal half of the protein bears no amino acid homology to other nuclear receptors, which typically contain a DNA-binding domain with two "zinc fingers." Instead, it contains 3½ repeats of a 65–67 amino acid motif which contain two putative zinc fingers *(83)*.

Thus, DAX-1 protein might affect gene expression by binding to DNA or binding to other transcription factors. SF-1 is an obvious candidate for an interaction partner, considering that its tissue distribution of expression is very similar to that of DAX-1, and mutations in the two genes have similar phenotypic effects. Indeed, DAX-1 and SF-1 physically interact through their C-terminal domains, and DAX-1 inhibits SF-1's ability to transactivate other genes *(84)*. One mechanism by which this repression occurs is via recruitment of the corepressor N-CoR by DAX-1 *(85)*. All mutations causing AHC affect the presence or structure of the C-terminal domain of DAX-1 and destroy the ability of DAX-1 to repress the transcriptional effects of SF-1.

In addition, DAX-1 may bind directly to hairpin loops in the 5' flanking regions of SF-1 responsive genes such as STAR *(86)*. On the other hand, SF-1 stimulates DAX-1 expression through specific DNA elements in the 5' flanking region of the *DAX-1* gene *(87)*.

It is puzzling that mutations in *SF-1* and *DAX-1* have similar phenotypes, yet SF-1 and DAX-1 behave antagonistically in functional assays. SF-1 and DAX-1 might actually act cooperatively to regulate certain genes in particular tissues, but further studies are required to address this question.

REFERENCES

1. White PC. Genetic diseases of steroid metabolism. Vitam Horm 1994;49:131–195.
2. Stocco DM, Clark BJ. Regulation of the acute production of steroids in steroidogenic cells. [Review] [268 refs]. Endocr Rev 1996;17:221–244.
3. Stocco DM. A review of the characteristics of the protein required for the acute regulation of steroid hormone biosynthesis: the case for the steroidogenic acute regulatory (StAR) protein. [Review] [95 refs]. Proc Soc Exp Biol Med 1998;217:123–129.
4. Papadopoulos V. Structure and function of the peripheral-type benzodiazepine receptor in steroidogenic cells. [Review] [113 refs]. Proc Soc Exp Biol Med 1998;217:130–142.
5. Rheaume E, Lachance Y, Zhao HF, Breton N, de Launoit Y, Trudel C, et al. Structure and expression of a new cDNA encoding the almost exclusive 3 beta-hydroxysteroid dehydrogenase/delta5-delta4 isomerase in human adrenals and gonads. Mol Endocrinol 1991;5:1147–1157.
6. White PC, Curnow KM, Pascoe L. Disorders of steroid 11 beta hydroxylase isozymes. Endocr Rev 1994; 15:421–438.
7. Yanase T, Simpson ER, Waterman MR. 17 alpha-hydroxylase/17,20-lyase deficiency: from clinical investigation to molecular definition. Endocr Rev 1991;12:91–108.
8. Simpson ER, Mahendroo MS, Means GD, Kilgore MW, Hinshelwood MM, Graham-Lorence S, et al. Aromatase cytochrome P450, the enzyme responsible for estrogen biosynthesis. Endocr Rev 1994;15: 342–355.
9. Wilson JD, Griffin JE, Russell DW. Steroid 5 alpha-reductase 2 deficiency. [Review]. Endocr Rev 1993; 14:577–593.
10. Mountjoy KG, Robbins LS, Mortrud MT, Cone RD. The cloning of a family of genes that encode the melanocortin receptors. Science 1992;257:1248–1251.
11. Waterman MR, Bischof LJ. Cytochromes P450 12: diversity of ACTH (cAMP)-dependent transcription of bovine steroid hydroxylase genes. [Review] [42 refs]. FASEB J 1997;11:419–427.
12. Evans RM, Arriza JL. A molecular framework for the actions of glucocorticoid hormones in the nervous system. [Review] [72 refs]. Neuron 1989;2:1105–1112.
13. Rainey WE, White PC. Functional adrenal zonation and regulation of aldosterone biosynthesis. Curr Opin Endocrinol Diab 1998;5:175–182.
14. Matsusaka T, Ichikawa I. Biological functions of angiotensin and its receptors. [Review] [99 refs]. Annu Rev Physiol 1997;59:395–412.
15. White PC, Speiser PW. Congenital adrenal hyperplasia due to 21-hydroxylase deficiency. Endocr Rev 2000;21:245–291.
16. Wedell A. Molecular genetics of congenital adrenal hyperplasia (21-hydroxylase deficiency): implications for diagnosis, prognosis and treatment. [Review] [30 refs]. Acta Paediatr 1998;87:159–164.
17. Carroll MC, Campbell RD, Porter RR. Mapping of steroid 21-hydroxylase genes adjacent to complement component C4 genes in HLA, the major histocompatibility complex in man. Proc Natl Acad Sci USA 1985;82:521–525.
18. White PC, Grossberger D, Onufer BJ, Chaplin DD, New MI, Dupont B, et al. Two genes encoding steroid 21-hydroxylase are located near the genes encoding the fourth component of complement in man. Proc Natl Acad Sci USA 1985;82:1089–1093.
19. Higashi Y, Yoshioka H, Yamane M, Gotoh O, Fujii-Kuriyama Y. Complete nucleotide sequence of two steroid 21-hydroxylase genes tandemly arranged in human chromosome: a pseudogene and a genuine gene. Proc Natl Acad Sci USA 1986;83:2841–2845.
20. White PC, New MI, Dupont B. Structure of human steroid 21-hydroxylase genes. Proc Natl Acad Sci USA 1986;83:5111–5115.
21. White PC, Vitek A, Dupont B, New MI. Characterization of frequent deletions causing steroid 21-hydroxylase deficiency. Proc Natl Acad Sci USA 1988;85:4436–4440.
22. Speiser PW, Dupont J, Zhu D, Serrat J, Buegeleisen M, Tusie-Luna MT, et al. Disease expression and molecular genotype in congenital adrenal hyperplasia due to 21- hydroxylase deficiency. J Clin Invest 1992;90:584–595.
23. Wilson RC, Mercado AB, Cheng KC, New MI. Steroid 21-hydroxylase deficiency: genotype may not predict phenotype. J Clin Endocrinol Metab 1995;80:2322–2329.
24. Higashi Y, Hiromasa T, Tanae A, Miki T, Nakura J, Kondo T, et al. Effects of individual mutations in the P-450 (C21) pseudogene on the P-450 (C21) activity and their distribution in the patient genomes of congenital steroid 21-hydroxylase deficiency. J Biochem (Tokyo) 1991;109:638–644.

25. Speiser PW, Agdere L, Ueshiba H, White PC, New MI. Aldosterone synthesis in salt-wasting congenital adrenal hyperplasia with complete absence of adrenal 21-hydroxylase. N Engl J Med 1991;324:145–149.

26. Curnow KM, Tusie-Luna MT, Pascoe L, Natarajan R, Gu JL, Nadler JL, et al. The product of the CYP11B2 gene is required for aldosterone biosynthesis in the human adrenal cortex. Mol Endocrinol 1991;5:1513–1522.

27. Kawamoto T, Mitsuuchi Y, Toda K, Yokoyama Y, Miyahara K, Miura S, et al. Role of steroid 11 beta-hydroxylase and steroid 18-hydroxylase in the biosynthesis of glucocorticoids and mineralocorticoids in humans. Proc Natl Acad Sci USA 1992;89:1458–1462.

28. Ogishima T, Shibata H, Shimada H, Mitani F, Suzuki H, Saruta T, et al. Aldosterone synthase cytochrome P-450 expressed in the adrenals of patients with primary aldosteronism. J Biol Chem 1991;266: 10,731–10,734.

29. Mornet E, Dupont J, Vitek A, White PC. Characterization of two genes encoding human steroid 11 beta-hydroxylase (P-450 (11) beta). J Biol Chem 1989;264:20,961–20,967.

30. Pascoe L, Curnow KM, Slutsker L, Connell JM, Speiser PW, New MI, et al. Glucocorticoid-suppressible hyperaldosteronism results from hybrid genes created by unequal crossovers between CYP11B1 and CYP11B2. Proc Natl Acad Sci USA 1992;89:8327–8331.

31. Lifton RP, Dluhy RG, Powers M, Rich GM, Gutkin M, Fallo F, et al. Hereditary hypertension caused by chimaeric gene duplications and ectopic expression of aldosterone synthase. Nat Genet 1992;2:66–74.

32. Rich GM, Ulick S, Cook S, Wang JZ, Lifton RP, Dluhy RG. Glucocorticoid-remediable aldosteronism in a large kindred: clinical spectrum and diagnosis using a characteristic biochemical phenotype. Ann Intern Med 1992;116:813–820.

33. Hall CE, Gomez-Sanchez CE. Hypertensive potency of 18-oxocortisol in the rat. Hypertension 1986;8: 317–322.

34. Oberfield SE, Levine LS, Stoner E, Chow D, Rauh W, Greig F, et al. Adrenal glomerulosa function in patients with dexamethasone-suppressible hyperaldosteronism. J Clin Endocrinol Metab 1981;53:158–164.

35. White PC. Defects in cortisol metabolism causing low-renin hypertension. Endocr Res 1991;17:85–107.

36. Rosler A, Leiberman E, Cohen T. High frequency of congenital adrenal hyperplasia (classic 11 beta-hydroxylase deficiency) among Jews from Morocco. Am J Med Genet 1992;42:827–834.

37. White PC, Dupont J, New MI, Leiberman E, Hochberg Z, Rosler A. A mutation in CYP11B1 (Arg-448-His) associated with steroid 11 beta-hydroxylase deficiency in Jews of Moroccan origin. J Clin Invest 1991;87:1664–1667.

38. Curnow KM, Slutsker L, Vitek J, Cole T, Speiser PW, New MI, et al. Mutations in the CYP11B1 gene causing congenital adrenal hyperplasia and hypertension cluster in exons 6, 7, and 8. Proc Natl Acad Sci USA 1993;90:4552–4556.

39. Helmberg A, Ausserer B, Kofler R. Frame shift by insertion of 2 basepairs in codon 394 of CYP11B1 causes congenital adrenal hyperplasia due to steroid 11 beta- hydroxylase deficiency. J Clin Endocrinol Metab 1992;75:1278–1281.

40. Naiki Y, Kawamoto T, Mitsuuchi Y, Miyahara K, Toda K, Orii T, et al. A nonsense mutation (TGG [Trp116]—TAG [Stop] in CYP11B1 causes steroid 11beta-hydroxylase deficiency. J Clin Endocrinol Metab 1993;77:1677–1682.

41. Geley S, Kapelari K, Johrer K, Peter M, Glatzl J, Vierhapper H, et al. CYP11B1 mutations causing congenital adrenal hyperplasia due to 11β-hydroxylase deficiency. J Clin Endocrinol Metab 1996;81: 2896–2901.

42. Pascoe L, Curnow KM, Slutsker L, Rosler A, White PC. Mutations in the human CYP11B2 (aldosterone synthase) gene causing corticosterone methyloxidase II deficiency. Proc Natl Acad Sci USA 1992;89: 4996–5000.

43. Zhang G, Rodriguez H, Fardella CE, Harris DA, Miller WL. Mutation T318M in the CYP11B2 gene encoding P450c11AS (aldosterone synthase) causes corticosterone methyl oxidase II deficiency. Am J Hum Genet 1995;57:1037–1043.

44. Tusie-Luna MT, Traktman P, White PC. Determination of functional effects of mutations in the steroid 21-hydroxylase gene (CYP21) using recombinant vaccinia virus. J Biol Chem 1990;265:20,916–20,922.

45. Mitsuuchi Y, Kawamoto T, Miyahara K, Ulick S, Morton DH, Naiki Y, et al. Congenitally defective aldosterone biosynthesis in humans: inactivation of the P450C18 gene (CYP11B2) due to nucleotide deletion in CMO I deficient patients. Biochem Biophys Res Commun 1993;190:864–869.

46. Geley S, Johrer K, Peter M, Denner K, Bernhardt R, Sippell WG, et al. Amino acid substitution R384P in aldosterone synthase causes corticosterone methyloxidase type I deficiency. J Clin Endocrinol Metab 1995;80:424–429.

47. Portrat-Doyen S, Tourniaire J, Richard O, Mulatero P, Aupetit-Faisant B, Curnow KM, et al. Isolated aldosterone synthase deficiency caused by simultaneous E198D and V386A mutations in the CYP11B2 gene. J Clin Endocrinol Metab 1998;83:4156–4161.
48. Russell DW, White PC. Four is not more than two [comment]. Am J Hum Genet 1995;57:1002–1005.
49. Lifton RP, Dluhy RG, Powers M, Rich GM, Cook S, Ulick S, et al. A chimaeric 11 beta-hydroxylase/ aldosterone synthase gene causes glucocorticoid-remediable aldosteronism and human hypertension. Nature 1992;355:262–265.
50. Pascoe L, Jeunemaitre X, Lebrethon MC, Curnow KM, Gomez-Sanchez CE, Gasc JM, et al. Glucocorticoid-suppressible hyperaldosteronism and adrenal tumors occurring in a single French pedigree. J Clin Invest 1995;96:2236–2246.
51. Jonsson JR, Klemm SA, Tunny TJ, Stowasser M, Gordon RD. A new genetic test for familial hyperaldosteronism type I aids in the detection of curable hypertension. Biochem Biophys Res Commun 1995;207: 565–571.
52. Dluhy RG, Lifton RP. Glucocorticoid-remediable aldosteronism (GRA): diagnosis, variability of phenotype and regulation of potassium homeostasis. Steroids 1995;60:48–51.
53. Jamieson A, Slutsker L, Inglis GC, Fraser R, White PC, Connell JM. Glucocorticoid-suppressible hyperaldosteronism: effects of crossover site and parental origin of chimaeric gene on phenotypic expression. Clin Sci 1995;88:563–570.
54. Yanase T, Waterman MR, Zachmann M, Winter JS, Simpson ER, Kagimoto M. Molecular basis of apparent isolated 17,20-lyase deficiency: compound heterozygous mutations in the C-terminal region (Arg (496)-Cys, Gln (461)-Stop) actually cause combined 17 alpha-hydroxylase/17,20-lyase deficiency. Biochim Biophys Acta 1992;1139:275–279.
55. Miller WL, Auchus RJ, Geller DH. The regulation of 17,20 lyase activity. [Review] [77 refs]. Steroids 1997;62:133–142.
56. Kagimoto M, Winter JS, Kagimoto K, Simpson ER, Waterman MR. Structural characterization of normal and mutant human steroid 17 alpha-hydroxylase genes: molecular basis of one example of combined 17 alpha-hydroxylase/17,20 lyase deficiency. Mol Endocrinol 1988;2:564–570.
57. Picado-Leonard J, Miller WL. Cloning and sequence of the human gene for P450c17 (steroid 17 alpha-hydroxylase/17,20 lyase): similarity with the gene for P450c21. DNA 1987;6:439–448.
58. Sparkes RS, Klisak I, Miller WL. Regional mapping of genes encoding human steroidogenic enzymes: P450scc to 15q23-q24, adrenodoxin to 11q22; adrenodoxin reductase to 17q24-q25; and P450c17 to 10q24-q25. DNA Cell Biol 1991;10:359–365.
59. Yanase T. 17 alpha-Hydroxylase/17,20-lyase defects. [Review]. J Steroid Biochem Mol Biol 1995;53: 153–157.
60. Imai T, Yanase T, Waterman MR, Simpson ER, Pratt JJ. Canadian Mennonites and individuals residing in the Friesland region of The Netherlands share the same molecular basis of 17 alpha-hydroxylase deficiency. Hum Genet 1992;89:95–96.
61. Biason A, Mantero F, Scaroni C, Simpson ER, Waterman MR. Deletion within the CYP17 gene together with insertion of foreign DNA is the cause of combined complete 17 alpha- hydroxylase/17,20-lyase deficiency in an Italian patient. Mol Endocrinol 1991;5:2037–2045.
62. Ahlgren R, Yanase T, Simpson ER, Winter JS, Waterman MR. Compound heterozygous mutations (Arg 239-stop, Pro 342-Thr) in the CYP17 (P45017 alpha) gene lead to ambiguous external genitalia in a male patient with partial combined 17 alpha-hydroxylase/17,20-lyase deficiency. J Clin Endocrinol Metab 1992;74:667–672.
63. Yanase T, Kagimoto M, Suzuki S, Hashiba K, Simpson ER, Waterman MR. Deletion of a phenylalanine in the N-terminal region of human cytochrome P-450 (17 alpha) results in partial combined 17 alpha-hydroxylase/17,20-lyase deficiency [published erratum appears in J Biol Chem 1989 Dec 15;264(35): 21,433]. J Biol Chem 1989;264:18,076–18,082.
64. Geller DH, Auchus RJ, Mendonca BB, Miller WL. The genetic and functional basis of isolated 17,20-lyase deficiency. Nat Genet 1997;17:201–205.
65. Lachance Y, Luu-The V, Labrie C, Simard J, Dumont M, de Launoit Y, et al. Characterization of human 3 beta-hydroxysteroid dehydrogenase/delta 5-delta 4-isomerase gene and its expression in mammalian cells [published erratum appears in J Biol Chem 1992 Feb 15;267(5):3551]. J Biol Chem 1990;265: 20,469–20,475.
66. Lachance Y, Luu-The V, Verreault H, Dumont M, Rheaume E, Leblanc G, et al. Structure of the human type II 3 beta-hydroxysteroid dehydrogenase/delta 5-delta 4 isomerase (3 beta-HSD) gene: adrenal and gonadal specificity. DNA Cell Biol 1991;10:701–711.

67. Morissette J, Rheaume E, Leblanc JF, Luu-The V, Labrie F, Simard J. Genetic linkage mapping of HSD3B1 and HSD3B2 encoding human types I and II 3 beta-hydroxysteroid dehydrogenase/delta 5-delta 4-isomerase close to D1S514 and the centromeric D1Z5 locus. Cytogenet Cell Genet 1995;69: 59–62.

68. Rheaume E, Simard J, Morel Y, Mebarki F, Zachmann M, Forest MG, et al. Congenital adrenal hyperplasia due to point mutations in the type II 3 beta-hydroxysteroid dehydrogenase gene. Nat Genet 1992; 1:239–245.

69. Simard J, Rheaume E, Mebarki F, Sanchez R, New MI, Morel Y, et al. Molecular basis of human 3 beta-hydroxysteroid dehydrogenase deficiency. [Review]. J Steroid Biochem Mol Biol 1995;53:127–138.

70. Zerah M, Rheaume E, Mani P, Schram P, Simard J, Labrie F, et al. No evidence of mutations in the genes for type I and type II 3 beta-hydroxysteroid dehydrogenase (3 beta HSD) in nonclassical 3 beta HSD deficiency. J Clin Endocrinol Metab 1994;79:1811–1817.

71. Lin D, Gitelman SE, Saenger P, Miller WL. Normal genes for the cholesterol side chain cleavage enzyme, P450scc, in congenital lipoid adrenal hyperplasia. J Clin Invest 1991;88:1955–1962.

72. Lin D, Sugawara T, Strauss JF, Clark BJ, Stocco DM, Saenger P, et al. Role of steroidogenic acute regulatory protein in adrenal and gonadal steroidogenesis. Science 1995;267:1828–1831.

73. Bose HS, Sugawara T, Strauss JF3, Miller WL. The pathophysiology and genetics of congenital lipoid adrenal hyperplasia. International Congenital Lipoid Adrenal Hyperplasia Consortium. N Engl J Med 1996;335:1870–1878.

74. Moser HW. Adrenoleukodystrophy: phenotype, genetics, pathogenesis and therapy. [Review] [173 refs]. Brain 1997;120:1485–1508.

75. Mosser J, Douar AM, Sarde CO, Kioschis P, Feil R, Moser H, et al. Putative X-linked adrenoleukodystrophy gene shares unexpected homology with ABC transporters. Nature 1993;361:726–730.

76. Sarde CO, Mosser J, Kioschis P, Kretz C, Vicaire S, Aubourg P, et al. Genomic organization of the adrenoleukodystrophy gene. Genomics 1994;22:13–20.

77. Kok F, Neumann S, Sarde CO, Zheng S, Wu KH, Wei HM, et al. Mutational analysis of patients with X-linked adrenoleukodystrophy. Hum Mutat 1995;6:104–115.

78. Parker KL, Schimmer BP. Steroidogenic factor 1: a key determinant of endocrine development and function. Endocr Rev 1997;18:361–377.

79. Ikeda Y, Luo X, Abbud R, Nilson JH, Parker KL. The nuclear receptor steroidogenic factor 1 is essential for the formation of the ventromedial hypothalamic nucleus. Mol Endocrinol 1995;9:478–486.

80. Achermann JC, Ito M, Hindmarsh PC, Jameson JL. A mutation in the gene encoding steroidogenic factor-1 causes XY sex reversal and adrenal failure in humans. Nat Genet 1999;22:125–126.

81. Seminara SB, Achermann JC, Genel M, Jameson JL, Crowley WFJ. X-linked adrenal hypoplasia congenita: a mutation in DAX1 expands the phenotypic spectrum in males and females. J Clin Endocrinol Metab 1999;84:4501–4509.

82. Muscatelli F, Strom TM, Walker AP, Zanaria E, Recan D, Meindl A, et al. Mutations in the DAX-1 gene give rise to both X-linked adrenal hypoplasia congenita and hypogonadotropic hypogonadism. [Review]. Nature 1994;372:672–676.

83. Burris TP, Guo W, McCabe ER. The gene responsible for adrenal hypoplasia congenita, DAX-1, encodes a nuclear hormone receptor that defines a new class within the superfamily. [Review] [94 refs]. Recent Prog Horm Res 1996;51:241–259.

84. Ito M, Yu R, Jameson JL. DAX-1 inhibits SF-1-mediated transactivation via a carboxy-terminal domain that is deleted in adrenal hypoplasia congenita. Mol Cell Biol 1997;17:1476–1483.

85. Crawford PA, Dorn C, Sadovsky Y, Milbrandt J. Nuclear receptor DAX-1 recruits nuclear receptor corepressor N-CoR to steroidogenic factor 1. Mol Cell Biol 1998;18:2949–2956.

86. Zazopoulos E, Lalli E, Stocco DM, Sassone-Corsi P. DNA binding and transcriptional repression by DAX-1 blocks steroidogenesis. Nature 1997;390:311–315.

87. Yu RN, Ito M, Jameson JL. The murine Dax-1 promoter is stimulated by SF-1 (steroidogenic factor-1) and inhibited by COUP-TF (chicken ovalbumin upstream promoter-transcription factor) via a composite nuclear receptor-regulatory element. Mol Endocrinol 1998;12:1010–1022.

INDEX